# Health Promotion

## *Effectiveness, efficiency and equity*

### THIRD EDITION

**Keith Tones and Sylvia Tilford**

Faculty of Health and Environment, Leeds Metropolitan University, Leeds, UK

First published in 1990 by:
Chapman & Hall
Second edition published in 1994 by:
Stanley Thornes (Publishers) Ltd

Third edition published in 2001 by:
Nelson Thornes Ltd
Delta Place
27 Bath Road
CHELTENHAM
GL53 7TH
United Kingdom

03 04 05 / 10 9 8 7 6 5 4 3

A catalogue record for this book is available from the British Library

ISBN 0 7487 4527 0


Page make-up by Northern Phototypesetting Co. Ltd
Printed in Great Britain by Ashford Colour Press

# CONTENTS

# Introduction

At first glance, the most obvious change to this third edition of *Effectiveness, Efficiency and Equity* has been the title. '*Health Education*' has been replaced by '*Health Promotion*'. This does not mean that we have abandoned Health Education – quite the reverse in fact. Rather, it reflects a change in nomenclature, which, arguably, started with the Ottawa Charter and associated developments. As a result, the emergence of health promotion has been paralleled by the marginalisation of health education. This has not just been due to mere fashion but has been indicative of an underlying dissatisfaction with aspects of the theory and practice of public health. As we note in Chapter 1, the demise of the conventional approach to health education centres on its 'victim-blaming' philosophy – real or imagined. Unfortunately, the health education baby was thrown out with the proverbial bath water! We therefore assert with some assurance in this book that a 'new' (or rather resurrected) and radical form of health education is essential for the promotion of the public health.

Although health promotion has replaced health education in the title, this new edition still centres on the pursuit of effectiveness and efficiency – a pursuit that has become increasingly important since the last edition. In the context of our discussions of the fundamental determinants of health, the question of equity has also assumed greater prominence.

As mentioned above, one of the major reasons for the change in nomenclature has been a certain dissatisfaction with the failure of health and medical services to seriously address the problems of health and illness at the national and international levels. This has been accompanied by an increasing acknowledgement of the importance of socio-economic, cultural and material factors in determining health status. At the same time, the complexity of the inter-relationships between these manifold influences has also been recognised. It seems that even politicians, who routinely seek simple solutions, are beginning to accept the existence of a multi-level web of diverse social, environmental and individual determinants of health. It is, therefore, clear to those who have seriously studied the situation that such a convoluted complex of causal mechanisms requires an equally complex and sophisticated set of solutions. Two related phenomena have accompanied this situation. First, it would seem that the 'medical model' is becoming less tenable and acceptable as a paradigm for explaining health and its promotion and is being replaced by a broader-based social empowerment model. Secondly, the very complexity of the analysis has resulted in a degree of confusion and uncertainty about how to proceed. This, in turn, is doubtless reflected in the definitional doubts that resulted in changes in terminology – including the adoption of health promotion as a replacement for health education.

Definitional difficulties, however, did not end with the Ottawa Charter and World Health Organization's (WHO) espousal of health promotion. At the present time in the UK there is considerable debate about the relationship between health promotion, public health and public health medicine. It is possible to argue that public health incorporates both health promotion and public health medicine. It is also possible to argue that health promotion should be the envelope that incorporates both public health and public health medicine. Logically, of course, both public health medicine and health promotion should enhance the public health but there is, unsurprisingly, a degree of controversy over the question of power and seniority! Webster and French (2001) nicely illustrate the current ferment of debate and action in the UK. They argue that:

*The phrase 'public health' as currently used embodies many of the confusions, vested interests and singular interpretations that have resulted from a simplistic interpretation of its historical development. It could even be argued that the term public health is often used in a spirit of what might be described as conspiratorial confusion.*

Webster and French cite a recent speech by the UK secretary of state for health that presents a decidedly forceful government view:

*'Public health' understood as the epidemiological analysis of the patterns and causes of population health and ill health gets confused with 'public health' understood as population-level health promotion, which in turn gets confused with 'public health' understood as public health professionals trained in medicine. So by series of definitional sleights of hand, the argument runs that the health of the population should be mainly improved by population-level health promotion and prevention, which in turn is best delivered, or at least overseen and managed, by medical consultants in public health. The time has come to abandon this lazy thinking and occupational protectionism.*

Interestingly, the English national 'Health Education Authority' (which was, arguably, a health promotion authority) has been replaced by a 'Health Development Agency'. 'Health Development', a term adopted by WHO, may thus be replacing 'Health Promotion' as the most appropriate vocabulary to describe what this present text is all about. However, for the present, we retain the title 'Health Promotion'!

Taking account of the various observations above, it would not be surprising if theoreticians and practitioners who believe they are involved in promoting public health were to become confused and disaffected. Those who subscribe to post-modernism would, of course, feel quite at home with the uncertainty. Kelly *et al.* (1993), writing about research into Healthy Cities, observe that 'To be paradoxical: the core idea of post-modernity is that there are no core ideas!' They are,

nonetheless, prepared to posit the following 'core idea':

*The core idea of post-modernity is that the social and moral conditions pertaining in the world at the present time mark a fundamental break with the past ... in philosophy, interpretation displaces system; in politics, pragmatism displaces principle; and in science chaos displaces order.*

(p159)

In the present text the purpose (to use Antonovsky's terminology) is quite determinedly negentropic. We argue, quite forcibly, that it is both possible and desirable to theorise: a sound theoretical framework is essential to the development of effective health promotion programmes and evaluating them. Indeed, the more complex and potentially confusing the situation, the more important theory becomes. Accordingly, *pace* post-modernism, theory figures prominently again in this 3rd edition. As will be apparent from Chapter 2, theory derived from psychological models still provides the more detailed and, perhaps, coherent basis for practice. While we are convinced that a judicious choice from these several theories will not only assist explanation and understanding but also enhance programme development and evaluation, we believe there is a need to develop and operationalise theory from the social as well as the behavioural sciences. By way of example we have discussed the concept of social capital, which offers a good prospect for explaining the effect of some of the broader social influences; we do, however, comment on the need for more precise clarification of the ways in which social capital apparently achieves its effect on health – directly and indirectly – and, above all, the ways in which social capital can be created. We also feel there is a need for integration of theories and models; apart from seeking to wed behavioural and social science perspectives, there is some evidence that important work is being achieved in making connections between the social, psychological and the biological. We make some mention in Chapter 1, for example, of what has been called 'socio-biological transition'. Such work offers the prospect of explaining how, for instance, inequity, individual empowerment beliefs and capabilities might impact on the biological and physiological factors that contribute to coronary heart disease. At a different level of model, such work can help bring together the apparently conflicting ideologies of preventive medicine and social empowerment models of health promotion.

The present book presents a number of different kinds of model. It argues for adopting a kind of continuum that charts a logical progression from models that seek to explain the factors inherent in different ideological approaches to health promotion through models that explain the social and individual actions pertaining to given ideological approaches and then on to models governing programme design before finally discussing models that describe approaches to evaluation. Following an operational principle that health promotion consists of a synergistic relationship between health education and 'healthy public policy', the ideological model of choice is described as an *Empowerment Model*. It acknowledges that there is still a need for individually focused health education but that this should be based on well-documented empowerment strategies. It asserts quite forcefully that individual empowering strategies are not a new (or old) version of victim blaming, provided that they do not ignore the power of environmental and social circumstances. Furthermore, while acknowledging the importance of lobbying and advocacy in order to 'build healthy public policy', the primacy of health education in achieving such policy change is emphasised. This is achieved through the well-recognised and documented processes of critical consciousness raising and advocacy. Indeed, the importance of media advocacy is reiterated and reinforced in this 3rd edition's chapter describing the nature and effectiveness of mass media in health promotion. Further, in the interest of integration (and reconciliation?) it is argued that the empowerment approach mentioned above is the most effective way of achieving the goals of preventive medicine. However, we note that the major difference between the *Medical*

*Model* and the *Empowerment Model* has to do with commitment to public and client participation – which, in turn, doubtless reflects personal and professional philosophies about the nature of humanity!

Despite our reluctance to lose the rubric 'health education' from the title of this edition of the book, we are sanguine about its replacement with 'health promotion'. In short, the ideological basis of the version of health promotion to which we subscribe is quite congruent with our views about the values base of health education. It matches the underpinning principles adopted by WHO and, as we note in Chapter 1, the Ottawa Principles have been re-affirmed in the Jakarta Declaration and embodied in a new WHO resolution. Underpinning all of these principles is the notion of social justice and equity. The empowerment of individuals and communities and the removal of barriers to the attainment of health, through the judicious application of 'healthy public policy', are the means whereby equity is to be achieved.

Again, within the UK it is interesting to note the major political shift, in a relatively short period of time, in the emphasis of government policy documents. As we note in the book *The Health of the Nation* (Department of Health, 1992) was essentially based on a *Preventive Medical Model* with an emphasis on individual behaviour. In contrast, recent government policy, expressed in *Our Healthier Nation: Saving Lives* (Department of Health, 1999) focuses on broader social issues and the overriding requirement of tackling inequality. A number of major initiatives have been launched in pursuit of this policy. These centre on multi-sector working involving community participation and establishing coalitions. The complexity of developing and evaluating such potentially unwieldy alliances is accordingly addressed in this edition of the text.

We have noted a particularly important development since the last edition of this book. In short, the pressure that we described in the last edition for health education to 'prove that it works' has increased. However, this increase has largely occurred within the broader context of an evidence-based medicine (EBM) imperative. The result has been a demand that health- and illness-related initiatives of all kinds must demonstrate that, in the interests of client welfare and economics, genuine health gain has been achieved. Accordingly, we have witnessed the emergence of an increasing number of publications that not only relate to public health and health promotion but also to medicine generally. Certainly, several books have examined research and questions of effectiveness in health promotion (see for example Davies and Kelly, 1993; EC/IUHPE, 2000; Popay and Williams, 1994; Perkins *et al.*, 1999; Rootman *et al.*, 2001; Thorogood and Coombs, 2000). The International Union of Health Education and Health Promotion has also produced a collection of texts containing exemplar reviews of a number of health promotion initiatives (IUHPE, 1995). Above all we have seen the flowering of meta-analysis in the form of a number of 'effectiveness reviews' – including reviews of health promotion. This phenomenon will receive further attention in Chapter 3.

The pursuit of evidence of success has certainly not been accepted with rejoicing! Apart from anticipated threats to occupational and individual self-interest, serious concern has been expressed about the nature of evidence and the appropriateness with which it has been used. Indeed, rather dramatically, the term 'paradigm wars' has been used to describe these concerns. The 'gold standard' that is embodied in the randomised controlled trial (RCT) has even been challenged! These issues will be discussed in some detail in Chapter 3, but Sir Douglas Black, with whom the classic and seminal review of health inequalities is associated, can preface these here with some observations. Black, in a discussion of the limitations of evidence, comments on EBM in general and the relative value of evidence from RCTs (Black, 1998). He acknowledges Bradford Hill and Doll's major contribution to medical history in their development of the RCT. As he puts it,

*It was a brilliant response to the increasing problems set by the proliferation of agents that are highly effective but also potentially hazardous from their side effects; ...*

however,

*... the extent that Cochrane and Sackett imply a primacy over other sources of therapeutic evidence, I think they take a step too far, and one that would perhaps take them beyond Doll and Hill themselves. ... The quality of evidence should be assessed not by the method by which it is obtained but by its strength or weakness. RCTs can produce evidence of great strength ... when a clinical situation is: common, so that the trial can be carried out in one centre; easily defined, so that inclusion and exclusion are simple; and has little variation between patients.*

Black argues that in many complex situations – such as coronary thrombosis and nephrotic syndrome – clinical decision making must be derived from many sources:

*...the basic medical sciences; the social sciences; the science of the 'seats and causes' of disease; the natural history of disease; epidemiology; the skills of diagnosis, of which speaking with the patient is paramount; and the range of possible therapies, graded for practicability and efficacy.*

It will be apparent from the description above that Black is discussing clinical decisions. As we hope to show convincingly in this book, contemporary health promotion programmes are inherently of considerably greater complexity. We will, therefore, be pressing the case for a careful and thoughtful consideration of the kinds of evidence needed to demonstrate success and the evaluation strategies needed to assemble such evidence. Reference will be made to the value of adopting, in some circumstances at least, a 'judicial principle'. In Black's words,

*I suggest that we are more commonly persuaded by a balance of likelihoods than we are driven forward by the iron laws of evidence.*

Since the last edition there has been increased recognition in most settings of the importance of evaluation and full consideration has been given to identifying appropriate methodologies and techniques for evaluating the complex interventions associated with health promotion. The debates between advocates of positivist and interpretivist styles have been ongoing but there is a growing consensus that the triangulation of evidence – often derived from methods crossing the so-called methodological divide – most satisfactorily provides answers to questions about success. In tune with the values of health promotion, we have also seen growing attention to facilitating the participation of communities in evaluation activities. Most recently there has been growing adoption in health promotion of what are described as 'theory of change' or 'realist' models of evaluation. The national and local evaluations of Health Action Zones in the UK are key examples where such methods have been used.

The format of this new edition is fundamentally similar to the 2nd edition. There are two parts – which have been more clearly signalled in the present book. The first part considers the nature of health promotion, effectiveness and associated theory. Part 2 concentrates on a number of settings. Since the last edition the 'settings approach' has received greater prominence and been actively promoted by WHO. The approach is particularly significant in the context of our theoretical discussion in that it emphasises the importance of a 'whole systems approach' to achieving the goals of health promotion. In other words, unlike a good deal of previous practice, settings should be much more than locations for delivering health education. The whole ethos should contribute to effectiveness – and, typically, a given setting should interact productively with its local community and different settings should collaborate as part of a 'community coalition'.

As with the 2nd edition, this version of the book lays no claim to providing a comprehensive review of health promotion programmes – successful or ineffective. We do, however, provide a wide variety of examples of both kinds of intervention to illustrate key themes that have emerged during our general discussion.

## REFERENCES

Black, D. (1998) *The limitations of evidence. Journal of the Royal College of Physicians of London*, 32 (1), 23–26.

Davies, J. K. and Kelly, P. (Eds) (1993) *Healthy Cities: Research and Practice*. Routledge, London.

Department of Health (1992) *Health of the Nation*. HMSO, London.

Department of Health (1999) *Our Healthier Nation: Saving Lives*. TSO, London.

EC/IUHPE (2000) *The Evidence of Health Promotion Effectiveness: Shaping Public Health in a New Europe*. EC, Brussels.

International Union for Health Promotion and Education, Regional Office for Europe (1995) *Improvement of the Effectiveness of Health Education and Health Promotion: A Series of Publications and a Database*. NIGZ, Woerden.

Kelly, M. P., Davies, J. K. and Charlton, B. G. (1993) *Healthy cities: a modern problem or a post-modern solution?* In J. K. Davies and M. P. Kelly (Eds), *Healthy Cities: Research and Practice*. Routledge, London.

Perkins, E. R., Simnett, I. and Wright, L. (Eds) (1999) *Evidence-Based Health Promotion*.

Popay, J. and Williams, G. (Eds) (1994) *Researching the People's Health*. Routledge, London.

Rootman, I., Goodstadt, M., Hyndman, B., McQueen, D.V., Potvin, L., Springett, J. and Ziglio, E. (2001) *Evaluation in Health Promotion: Principles and Perspectives*. WHO, Copenhagen.

Thorogood, M. and Coombes, Y. (eds.) (2000) *Evaluating Health Promotion, Practice and Methods*. Oxford University Press, Oxford.

Webster, C. and French, J. (2001) *The cycle of conflict: the historic development of the public health and health promotion movements*. In *Working For Health – Politics and Practice*. Sage, London.

# INTRODUCTION TO SECOND EDITION

*Editor: Then you would regard education as an essential part of a progressive health policy?*

*Minister: There is no doubt about that ... one of the most noticeable characteristics of the dark ages was fatalism; men were overwhelmed by circumstances; they existed under a sense of impending disasters that they could neither see nor prevent. Men who feel as they did – that external circumstances control their fate – despair of reform or progress; but let men once recognise that in large and increasing measure they are masters of their own destiny, and their life takes on a new, more hopeful, more purposeful aspect. Thus education is the instrument of reform, the giver of hope, the guide which directs the conscious individual effort without which health cannot be attained.*

The above extract is part of a dialogue between the UK Minister of Health, the Rt Hon Ernest Brown, and the editor of the *Health Education Journal*. The date was 1943 and it featured in the very first issue of that journal.

Apart from being a kind of panegyric for an empowerment model of health education, it is notable for the high hopes for progress which characterized those heady days leading up to the launch of the welfare state. We still have high hopes for health education but since those immediate post-Beveridge days, we have been increasingly expected to actually prove that those expectations and aspirations are justifiable.

It could be said with some justification that the task of education is to safeguard people's right to learn about important aspects of human culture and experience. Since health and illness occupy a prominent place in our everyday experience, it might reasonably be argued that everyone is entitled to share whatever insights we possess into the state of being healthy and to benefit from what might be done to prevent and treat disease and discomfort. Health education's role in such an endeavour would be to create the necessary understanding. No other justification would be needed.

In recent years, however, questions have been posed with increasing insistence and urgency about efficiency – both about education in general and health education in particular. We can be certain that such enquiries about effectiveness do not reflect a greater concern to know whether or not the population is better educated: they stem from more utilitarian motives.

It is apparent, even to the casual observer, that economic growth and productivity have become a central preoccupation in modern Britain. Economic success is seen as depending on the competitive urge which, among other things, should generate efficiency. It is, therefore, not surprising that health education should be required to prove itself – especially since both the education and health sectors have been subjected to critical scrutiny. In the first place, educational institutions are alleged to have failed to generate an entrepreneurial spirit; reforms have been urged which include setting attainment targets by which efficiency may be measured. Again, in the health service, alarm has been expressed at the seemingly insatiable demands for health care and ensuing galloping inflation. Economies have been required – again in the interest of efficiency; performance indicators have been developed to assess progress.

Moreover, since publication of the first edition of this book, we have witnessed the appearance of the first genuine attempt in England to develop a health policy for the nation (DoH, 1992). Not surprisingly, it sets specific targets and the justification it provides for selecting those particular targets and the associated five key diseases is that they should not only be epidemiologically important but they should also be feasible and measurable.

Unlike many traditional educational disciplines, health education has consistently sought not merely to provide understanding about its substantive subject matter but has concerned itself also with such goals as attitude change and lifestyles modification. Indicators of successful health education have, for this reason, defined much more than gains in knowledge and understanding. Moreover, since health education is regarded as an arm of preventive medicine (at any rate by health professionals), it has been subjected to the same economic imperative as other branches of the health service. Furthermore, since health education occasionally, and usually unwisely, claims that prevention can save money by reducing the need for expenditure on curative medicine, it is not at all surprising that the question 'Does health education work?' really means 'Is it successful in preventing unhealthy behaviours and reducing health service costs?'. Such a perspective is, of course, as limited as the narrowly conceived view that economic growth and productivity is the most important recipe for human happiness. It is nonetheless important to recognize the impetus which economic philosophy provides in creating a demand that health education should prove itself.

We discussed the relationship between health education and health promotion in the first edition of this book. Since then the star of health promotion has continued in the ascendant – though its continuing popularity has not necessarily been accompanied by a reduction in the ambiguities and conflicting notions associated with the term. Paradoxically perhaps, the main philosophical and practical thrust of *The Health of the Nation* is much more consistent with a 'traditional' model of preventive health education than with the more radical ideology of the World Health Organization (WHO) and Health for the All by the Year 2000 (HFA 2000).

As we will see, arguably the most significant impact of the doctrine of health promotion has been its emphasis on the environmental determinants of health and illness and the consequent need for the development of 'healthy public policy' together with a continuing concern to foster empowered participating communities. It could indeed be asserted that after the Alma Ata Conference (see Chapter 1), which confidently asserted the centrality of health education in achieving health for all, health education has been somewhat marginalized in later developments, such as the Ottawa Charter, in the headlong drive to tackle health issues through the medium of policy and politics. As we will endeavour to show in Chapter 1, health education is viewed as making a major contribution to health promotion while not being synonymous with it. Indeed, an admittedly somewhat simplistic formula is used to capture the essence of the synergistic relationship between policy and education. It asserts that Health Promotion = Health Education × Healthy Public Policy.

This book then maintains its focus on health education and is concerned with its effectiveness and efficiency. Clearly we need to know whether our efforts are effective. We need to know whether, for example, programmes designed to reduce barriers to the utilization of mammography services actually increase service uptake while minimizing women's concerns and anxieties. We need to know whether an empowerment stratagem centring on local concerns over damp housing in an urban ghetto has had a positive effect on people's feelings of helplessness and influenced local politicians and decision makers. We need to know whether anticipatory guidance in the clinical setting has, for instance, helped diabetics cope with and manage their disease in the context of an empowering partnership with their health care providers.

At a simple level we can unequivocally answer the question, 'Does health education work?' with a simple affirmative: yes, it does! The reason for such a confident assertion derives from the fact that there have been major changes in health-related behaviours over the past decade and, in many instances, an associated decline in premature death and the incidence of disease. In the USA, Britain and many other developed nations, there has been a substantial reduction in smoking and other risk factors implicated in coronary heart disease (CHD). In many countries there has been a significant improvement in cardiovascular health. Since the factors influencing these changes – cultural, behavioural and, arguably, epidemiological – must have been mediated by various forms of information, communication, persuasion and other educational activities, it would be churlish not to credit health education with the achievement.

For instance, Warner (1989) provides an update on the effects of the US antismoking campaign. He argues convincingly that:

> *In the absence of the antismoking campaign, adult per capita cigarette consumption in 1987 would have been an estimated 79–89 per cent higher than the level actually experienced. The smoking prevalence of all birth cohorts of men and women born during this century is well below that which would have been expected in the absence of the campaign. As a consequence, in 1985 an estimated 56 million Americans were smokers; without the campaign, an estimated 91 million would have been smokers. As a result of campaign-induced decisions not to smoke, between 1964 and 1985 an estimated 789 200 Americans avoided or postponed smoking-related deaths and gained an average of 21 additional years of life expectancy each; collectively that represents more than 16 million person-years of additional life each.*
>
> (p.144)

Since the first edition of this book went to press, a new review of the effectiveness of health education was published by Liedekerken *et al.* (1990) at the request of the Dutch Health Education Centre. Its avowed purpose was to '... clarify the conceptual and methodological issues about the question of effectiveness and provide a state of the art review of effectiveness research'. It also sought to make recommendations for health education practice and policy. The book includes a useful

brief review of 19 'subsectors' which provides a categorization of research by diseases and topics, settings and target groups. Interestingly, in seeking to respond to the question, 'Is health education effective?', the authors reach a similar conclusion to the one we reached in the introduction to the first edition. The conclusion: it depends!

Certainly, many people directly involved in programme development and evaluation are convinced that health education can be effective. Admittedly the cynic might contend that health educators must of necessity reach such a conclusion since they have an emotional (and political) investment in being seen to be successful. A recent WHO press release issued on 22 June 1992 is quite adamant.

> *Mass media campaigns, creative condom marketing programmes and the right messages from friends and co-workers have succeeded in slowing the spread of HIV, the AIDS virus, in projects around the world, a new analysis by the WHO reports.*

In a review of 15 HIV prevention projects carried out in 13 countries, doctors and scientists from the WHO Global Programme on AIDS have confirmed the effectiveness of a handful of approaches in producing significant changes in people's sexual behaviour.

In Zaire, the most outstanding achievement is the dramatic year-by-year increase in condom use. In 1987 fewer than half a million condoms were distributed – mainly by government clinics – for a population of more than 30 million people. Sales of condoms totalled less than 100 000. But by 1991 condom sales had soared to over 18 million.

Condoms are also being promoted extensively in Thailand, where almost all new HIV infections are a result of heterosexual transmission. Many such infections occur among Thailand's estimated 100 000 sex workers and the men who buy their services. Thai health workers set themselves an ambitious goal – to back up sex workers' demands that clients use condoms by imposing a policy of '100% condom use' in the sex entertainment industry. The project worked with both the brothel owners and women, assuring each group that their income would not be affected if condom use became mandatory. They were also informed that non-compliance with the policy would be met with penalties for the brothel owner.*

The strategy is working. In Samut Sakhon in Thailand, client use of condoms is now nearing 100%. The number of condoms used by men who have sex with prostitutes in the province has gone up from less than 15000 a month to over 50000, and in Chiang Mai condom use has increased from 30% to 80-90% of sexual contacts. Encouragingly, the project has now been extended nationwide to 66 of Thailand's 73 provinces.

In the introduction to the first edition of the book we reminded readers of existing general reviews of published studies of the success of health education and noted that they all provided evidence of effectiveness. For in stance, Gatherer et al. (1979) asked, 'Is Health Education Effective?'. He and his fellow authors then provided abstracts of research and an overview of evaluated studies. Bell et al. (1985) provide an annotated bibliography of health education research in the UK which includes many studies of effectiveness. Green and Lewis (1986) have been assiduous over the years in producing comprehensive and detailed lists of evaluated work together with critiques of research design which make it possible to judge the reliability and validity of the studies. It is, however, difficult to draw conclusions of a general nature from this kind of work – except that many of the interventions they describe have been effective in the sense in which the term has been used above. Gatherer's review, for example, reported that 85% of 62 reported studies demonstrated an improvement in knowledge while 65% of 39 studies indicated that there had been a change of attitudes 'in the desired direction'. Of 123 studies which sought to produce behavioural change, 75% actually succeeded in doing so. However, apart from elementary questions about research design such as whether the claimed changes could really be attributed to the health education intervention, there are more funda-

mental issues to be addressed. Foremost among these is the question of practical as opposed to statistical significance. For instance, how big were the changes in knowledge, attitude and practice? Were they big enough to justify claims of success? How big should they have been before we could argue a programme had been effective? Do the studies which apparently showed no change demonstrate the inefficiency of health education – or was it merely the case that the methods used and the available resources were inappropriate to the task? Or was the task intrinsically unsuitable for treatment by health education? Certainly, the observations of Gatherer et al. support the notion of ineffective delivery of the programme: 'The overall impression from much of the literature on health education is that too much of the health education practised is inappropriate for many, perhaps the majority, of the people for whom it is supposedly intended'.

It is, then, not possible to use reported research on effectiveness and efficiency – even when the research design has been impeccable – to reach conclusions about the success of health education. Before this is possible, we must be clear about the criteria by which a programme may be assessed and we must know a good deal about the circumstances associated with the design and delivery of the education. Two examples will serve to underline this assertion. The first of these describes a dietary intervention mounted in Spring, 1981, in a rural community in Finland (Koskela, personal communication).

Thirty Finnish couples were matched with 30 couples in southern Italy and an attempt was made to bring the Finns' dietary status more in line with the healthier status of the Italian group. They received intensive counselling and were provided with several '... strategic food items free of charge'. One dietitian visited six families frequently and also met them when they made a twice weekly visit to clinics for blood pressure measurement. The intervention was manifestly effective: by the end of the counselling the Finnish families' diets approximated to the healthier Mediterranean type of diet. The proportion of energy derived from fats declined from 39% to

---

*An interesting example of healthy public policy!

24%; the ratio of polyunsaturated to saturated fats increased from less than 0.2 to more than 1.0 (as compared with a shift in the P/S ratio from 0.24 to 0.32 recommended by NACNE (1983). The total serum cholesterol level also declined and there was a reduction in blood pressure in every subject. The intervention lasted six weeks and afterwards, subjects reverted to their normal (and presumably preferred) diets. The various physiological indicators followed suit along with their risk status.

The study appears to have been methodologically sound and the results genuine. Criteria of success were certainly consistent with a medical model – behaviour change associated with clinical improvement. Educational methods were appropriate and the choice of face-to-face counselling and behaviour modification techniques was consistent with learning theory. It was in most ways an efficient as well as an effective programme since it is hard to imagine how alternative educational strategies might have been used to achieve a better result. However, it is unlikely that such an approach would be widely used since the use of one dietitian per six families would almost certainly be considered too expensive. We cannot ignore the values underlying evaluation and the political factors which determine the priorities to be accorded to these. For instance it might well be the case that the alternative to the intervention described above would be to undertake the much more substantial costs involved in treating the disease which the intervention might well have prevented – probably because the necessary shift in resources from acute to preventive sectors would be politically unacceptable. The net result of the process of prioritization might well be a token mass media campaign which would be neither effective nor efficient.

The second example concerns the teaching of breast self-examination (BSE). This is a relatively inexpensive screening strategy designed to achieve early detection of potentially lethal abnormalities on the assumption that early intervention will result in a better chance of cure. A more expensive alternative device for detecting breast lumps in post menopausal women is the technique of mammography. The study described here sought to compare the efficiency of BSE with mammography. Its starting point was that BSE is often ineffectively performed due to the use of inappropriate teaching techniques. Indeed, common sense, let alone learning theory, would suggest that the acquisition of the psychomotor skill involved in BSE will not be efficiently acquired by the use of, for instance, pamphlets or even filmed models. Pennypacker *et al.* (1982) utilized learning theory to create the proper conditions for the acquisition of the skill: they provided an opportunity for skills practice and provided immediate knowledge of results of successful examination of breast tissues. They employed not only silicon models of the breast to provide practice but also supplied television and computer-assisted display of information when women transferred their learning from the silicon models to their own breasts. As a result women not only acquired efficient scanning techniques but also learned to exert the right degree of pressure and discriminate normal from abnormal tissue. According to the researchers, the sample studied was more efficient than a mammography unit at detecting small lumps (a 5.8% hit rate compared with 5.3%). However, rather like the first study cited above, although the relative effectiveness (i.e. the efficiency) of the method, was superior to competing techniques, the costs involved in the high technology, staffing and training would render it inappropriate for general use.

Apart from illustrating the complexity of determining efficiency and the political problems associated with basing decisions purely on the evidence of the relative effectiveness of competing strategies, the two studies allow us to make an important generalization. Provided that a given teaching method is based on sound educational theory, it is usually possible to achieve desired objectives. A good understanding of the psychosocial factors underpinning decision making and behaviour will help us design specific interventions which will be successful. However, the application of this understanding will often be severely curtailed by practical and political considerations. For instance there may be insufficient skilled personnel and resources to supply the condition for efficient learning; the theoretically appropriate methods may be too time consuming or even unethical.

It seems clear, then that health education can be effective but the important issue is about efficiency. In other words we need to know not merely whether health education has been successful but rather how successful it has been. Efficiency is thus concerned with the extent to which health education has achieved a given outcome by comparison with some alternative intervention. In the economic context outlined above, the criterion might be one of relative cost. In another context the yardstick might be the extent to which dietary behaviour has changed and the explicit or implicit comparison might be between individually directed health education or the introduction of labelling or other controls on food production and distribution. It is much more difficult to respond to the question of how efficient a given programme has been in achieving some desirable goal than it is to examine the issue of effectiveness. The answer to such a question will almost inevitably be 'it depends'. It depends, for instance, on the nature of goals, the criteria of success, the way in which the education is provided, the resources available? This is one of the issues which the book will seek to illuminate.

It might have been noted that the title of this edition of the book has acquired an appendage in the form of the word 'equity'. While we do not purport to provide a comprehensive discussion of this key issue for health education, we feel it provides a useful indicator of our own value position.

First of all, as we suggest in Chapter 1, it could be argued that the pursuit of equity and tackling inequalities in health are the major tasks facing health promotion. Although we have just presented in some detail two case studies of health education interventions which are concerned with conventional preventive medical outcomes, it will become clear that this book emphasizes the importance of broader empowering strategies which acknowledge the significance of those social, structural and environmental factors which ultimately determine our health status. Accord-

ingly, we will argue that our evaluation goals must move beyond a narrow individualistic, preventive orientation. Above all, this book is concerned with the **meaning** of success. It is concerned to examine and explore the values and ideological issues which underpin different models of an approach to health promotion and health education – and the practices which result from such 'philosophical' concerns.

A natural consequence of this stance is what one might call a need for 'methodological equity'. Although the randomized controlled trial and the various experimental designs associated with more traditional research approaches have an important part to play, they are not the only relevant evaluation method. Indeed, we will comment that their use in some instances may be ethically, epistemologically and technically inappropriate for many of the purposes of health education research.

This book is concerned, then, with general questions of success. It will not provide a detailed compendium of exemplars of effectiveness, nor is it intended to be an evaluation primer – although in Chapter 2 it does seek to remind readers of major research issues and approaches to evaluation. The first issue it addresses has to do with the meaning of success. Chapter 1 shows how the measurement of effectiveness and efficiency must ultimately depend on how success is defined. The definition of success will, in turn, be based on ideology and philosophy. Since there are wide divergences of view about the purpose of health education, indicators of performance should logically be derived from a statement of the values underpinning programme goals.

The second issue is more technical and concerns the design of evaluations. Research design, despite its image, is not a mechanically scientific process involving the choice of an off-the-peg formula. It requires careful thought about the nature of the successful outcome, the use to which results will be put and the degree of insight which these results will provide into programme efficiency. It will remind us that there are different kinds of evaluation all having different capabilities for application to practice; it will also remind us that, like health education itself, there are important ethical issues to be considered in the research process.

The third issue concerns the role of theory. Reference has already been made to the importance of learning theory in determining the choice of teaching method. The whole book, in fact, is based on the premise that sound theory is essential to the design of effective, efficient and practical programmes. This contention is illustrated by the particular case of the choice of indicators. There are a wide variety of markers which might be used as measures of performance and selecting those which most readily reflect the nature and degree of success achieved by any given health education enterprise is no easy matter. Chapter 3 attempts to show how theoretical considerations should influence choice of indicator. It illustrates the point by describing how the Health Action Model and Communication of Innovations Theory provide a basis for reasoned choice of measures of outcome and both indirect and intermediate indicators of programme efficiency.

The remainder of the book seeks to illuminate the various issues discussed above within the general framework of five settings: schools, health service, mass media, workplace and community. Although some reference will be made, both directly and obliquely, to more specific methods, these will not figure prominently in our analysis.

Since terms such as 'setting', 'sector', 'context', 'strategy' and 'method' often feature in discussions about designing and implementing health education programmes – and sometimes may be used interchangeably – it may be useful to engage in some definition and clarification at this juncture. Moreover, given the observations made above about the centrality of values in any discourse about evaluation, it is important to recognize that such expressions as 'programme delivery' or 'strategic intervention' are themselves value laden and carry particular connotations. The following observations are more fully explored elsewhere (Tones, 1993).

First of all, the terms 'setting' or 'context' are relatively unambiguous: both refer to location and indicate **where** health education might take place. Some of the more popular settings include,

for example, workplace, school, health care system and voluntary organization. Although 'setting' is currently favoured, we might just as well talk about 'context'. Indeed, the connotation of an interweaving of elements is particularly appealing since the peculiar mixture of organizational and interpersonal factors inherent in a given setting will influence the 'texture' of any health education programme provided in that setting.

Rather rarely the term 'sector' might be used – implying some kind of subdivision. Those who have been imbued with the spirit of the Ottawa Charter (Chapter 1), with its emphasis on 'intersectoral collaboration', might well prefer to use that particular word.

This discussion of terminological niceties is not as pedantic as it might first appear: choice of a particular term may – as mentioned above – signal some underlying ideological principle. For example, the word 'strategy' might be thought of as synonymous with setting or context. It might be said to be 'strategically sound' to use mass media to achieve the *Health of the Nation* objective of reducing the prevalence of cigarette smoking to no more than 20% by the year 2000. An alternative strategy might emphasize the importance of using the workplace as a locus for the efficient 'delivery' of health education.

Etymologically, though, the word strategy (or, more precisely, 'stratagem') does not only imply a military campaign but also incorporates the notion of 'trick'. Therefore for those whose ideological commitment is to build health education programmes on people's 'felt needs' and who seek to facilitate the achievement of self-empowered choice, these 'top-down' connotations of the term would strike a discordant note.

There would be much less disagreement about the meaning of methodology (i.e. a system of methods) when employed in health education. Methods are relatively specific (by comparison with strategies); they operate at the micro rather than the macro level. Very similar methods may be used in a wide variety of settings or contexts and may form part of or adjuncts to such strategies as mass media or community development. For instance, one or more different varieties of group discussion may form an integral part of strategies designed to stimulate community participation or be used as a follow-up to televised smoking cessation groups.

Whatever the terminology employed, it is clear that we are discussing initiatives which operate at different levels ranging from macro to micro – as may be seen in Figure A.

At the macro level we must include national policy and mass media. At the organizational or setting level we would identify key contexts for providing health education such as school, workplace, medical service, voluntary bodies and settings which are somewhat less easy to classify such as youth clubs. Clearly policy may be 'built in' to each of these intermediate levels.

Finally, at the micro level, a substantial array of specific methods together with ancillary audiovisual aids and learning resources may be deployed.

Two generalizations may be made at this point about settings. Firstly, any particular programme goals will be more effectively attained when different settings have congruent aims and operate synergistically. This principle will apply both to programmes which have a preventive orientation, such as the various CHD prevention programmes described in Chapter 8, and also to programmes

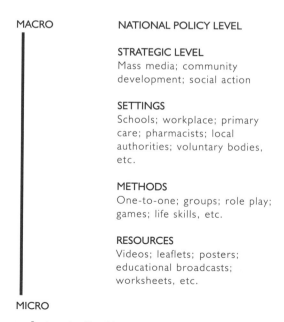

**Figure A** Levels of health education operation.

having such goals as the achievement of empowerment or community participation. Secondly, there is a synergistic effect when health education is supported by policy: maximal efficiency will therefore occur when a coherent health education programme is supported by appropriate legal, fiscal, economic and environmental measures – and vice versa. Although this book does not directly address the effectiveness of social policy changes in enhancing health, the postulated synergism between education and social policy should always be borne in mind when considering the efficiency of either kind of intervention.

The education system has been widely seen as a major institution for the delivery of health education. Chapter 4 will assess the contribution it makes at a number of levels – from individual outcomes within the classroom to national policies and activities which support school activities. Both hospital and primary care services have been urged to develop the educational component of their activities – not least because, as we have seen above, educational inputs have been viewed as means of contributing to cutting health care costs. Chapter 5 will examine the philosophical approach adopted to education in a health care context, the success of education as exemplified by a small number of outcomes and will conclude with a general discussion of factors which enhance educational activity in primary care and in hospitals.

Chapter 6 seeks to provide a theoretical analysis of the use of mass media as a delivery strategy and identifies the features which distinguish this from all other strategies and settings discussed here. In general it supports the view that the proper application of social marketing principles will increase the chances of success while at the same time noting the fallacy of assuming that the process of marketing health is basically the same as that which is involved in selling commercial products. The chapter also reinforces the book's general contention about synergy and asserts that mass media are most effectively employed in the context of an integrated community programme. A larger and wider variety of specific evaluations have been included in this chapter compared with those chapters considering alternative delivery systems. This decision has been made because of the typically inflated aspirations entertained for mass media use. Attempts are therefore made to indicate the limitations of this particular strategy and also to show how different features of programme construction – the content of the messages, the target population and the intrinsic variations in the type of media used – can influence the chances of achieving success. It is hoped in this way to generate more realistic expectations of what mass media can achieve.

Chapter 7 examines health promotion in the workplace – a strategy which offers several interesting insights into the meaning of effectiveness and efficiency. The workplace provides excellent examples of the way in which different philosophies and models of health education give rise to widely divergent criteria of success. Moreover, the worksite illustrates the potential synergy between health policy and education in the form of, for instance, alcohol policy development and employee assistance programmes. In addition, evaluation of health education in the workplace provides us with some of the hardest evidence of effectiveness and efficiency.

The final chapter in this book focuses on the community. In doing so, it recapitulates themes explored in Chapter 1. More particularly, it compares and contrasts the essentially democratic, 'bottom-up' approach associated with community development with the 'top-down' approach exemplified by the strategic delivery of a number of well known international heart disease prevention projects. In making this comparison, we will also note that the notion of a simple dichotomy between top-down and bottom-up is not tenable in practice. However, we will be able to provide suggestions for a wide range of indicators of success which might be used in these different programmes and projects. We will also, in doing so, provide some evidence of effectiveness – and even efficiency.

No attempt is made in this book to relate the contents specifically to the UK scene – nor to review the international literature systematically.

Rather it selects eclectically whatever examples suit the purposes of any given chapter. We choose from whatever source seems most appropriate to provide evidence in support of our arguments and assertions. However, because our experience is primarily of UK situations and the available evidence of effectiveness and efficiency tends to have been generated in North America, most examples will be derived from Britain and the USA.

## REFERENCES

Bell, J. *et al.* (1985) *Annotated Bibliography of Health Education Research completed in Britain from 1948-1978 and 1979–1983*, Scottish Health Education Group, Edinburgh.

Department of Health (1992) *Health of the Nation*, HMSO, London.

Editorial. (1943) *Health Education Journal*, 1,1.

Gatherer, A., Parfit, J., Porter, E. and Vessey, M. (1979) *Is Health Education Effective?*, Health Education Council, London.

Green, L.W. and Lewis, F.M. (1986) *Measurement and Evaluation in Health Education and Health Promotion*, Mayfield, Palo Alto, California.

Liedekerken, P.C. *et al.* (1990) *The Effectiveness of Health Education*, Van Gorcum, Assen, Netherlands.

NACNE (1983) *A Discussion Paper on Proposals for Nutritional Guidelines for Health Education in Britain*, Health Education Council, London.

Pennypacker, H.S., Goldstein, M.K. and Stein, G.H. (1982) Efficient technology of training breast self-examination, in *Public Education About Cancer*, (ed. P. Hobbs), UICC Technical Report Series, UICC, Geneva.

Tones, B.K. (1993) Methods and strategies in health education. *Health Education Journal* 52 (3)125-39.

Warner, K.E (1989) Effects of the antismoking campaign: an update. *American Journal of Public Health*, 79 (2)144 51.

WHO (1992) Aids prevention does work, says the World Health Organization. Press release WHO/44, 22 June.

# PART ONE

# 1 SUCCESSFUL HEALTH PROMOTION: THE CHALLENGE

## THE PROBLEMATIC NOTION OF HEALTH AND ITS DETERMINANTS

*Health Education* is an essential and major component of *Health Promotion*. Health promotion, as a quasi-political movement and professional activity, might with justification be described as the militant wing of *Public Health*. As we will note later at some length, health promotion is an essentially contested concept: it means different things to different people. Since health itself is a nebulous, multi-dimensional notion – open to multiple interpretations – it is unsurprising that the definition of health promotion is itself problematic. Accordingly, if we are to provide a coherent, critical and useful account of health education and its evaluation, it would be sensible to provide a reminder of some of the more important interpretations of this phantasmagoric construct that is health.

In relatively recent times, the classic definition of health incorporated into the constitution of the World Health Organization (WHO, 1946) has served both as an inspiration to those subscribing to a holistic philosophy of life and an irritant to those faced with the practical and pressing demands of managing and preventing disease on a day-to-day basis!

**Box 1**

> Health is a state of complete physical, mental and social well-being and not merely the absence of disease or infirmity.
>
> (WHO, 1946)

The etymology of the word health, i.e. *hal* or whole, provides an indication that WHO's holistic definition has a long philosophical history. Operationalising most definitions of health that emphasise its multi-dimensional nature and its positive aspects is, however, notoriously difficult.

## Health as mirage

Dubos (1959), having observed the evanescent and ephemeral nature of health, notably likened it to a mirage: unattainable but, arguably, worth pursuing!

> *The concept of perfect and positive health is a utopian creation of the human mind. It cannot become reality because man will never be so perfectly adapted to his environment that his life will not involve struggles, failures, and sufferings.*
>
> *… we are more exacting than our ancestors in matters of health, and especially are we less willing to accept the infirmities, pains, and blemishes, the catarrhs, coughs, and nauseas that used to be regarded as inevitable accompaniments of life … it is also true that the modern ways of life are creating problems of disease that either did not exist a few decades ago or are now more common than in the past.*
>
> *Nevertheless, the utopia of positive health constitutes a creative force because, like other ideals, it sets goals and helps medical science to chart its course toward them.*
>
> Dubos (1965 pp346–7)

Tarlov (1996) referred to what he considered to be three key characteristics of a non-medical approach to defining health:

- *…capacity to perform…*;
- the capacity to *…effectively negotiate the demands of the social environment*;
- a process of achieving *…individual fulfilment such as the pursuit of values, tasks, needs, aspirations and potential.*

Clearly holistic definitions of health are susceptible to accusations of omni-pretentiousness. Indeed, there is a danger that the 'individual fulfilment' mentioned above by Tarlov – together with its associated values and aspirations – will become synonymous with what individuals, society as a whole and their religious systems deem to be the 'good life'. For health promoters to seriously aspire to such goals is not merely impracticable, it represents delusions of grandeur! There are, however, holistic and positive aspects of health that can be rather more readily translated into measurable operations. One of these is the concept of self-actualisation.

## Health as self-actualisation

The third of these criteria for healthful living was, of course, more completely developed by Maslow (1967, 1970) and encapsulated in his concept of *self-actualisation*. Self-actualisation is the apex of his pyramid of human needs and only achieved after other more mundane and basic needs – such as food and safety – have been met. It may be defined as:

> *The inherent tendency towards self fulfilment, self expression and the attainment of autonomy from external forces. A self actualising individual is deemed to be realistic, spontaneous and demonstrative, able both to engage and transcend problems, being particularly resistant to social pressures.*
>
> (Harre and Lamb, 1983 p559)

Readers may find this concept surprisingly relevant to current health promotion concerns with empowerment and such notions as 'coherence'. Interestingly, it was used some years ago to underpin an approach by a national organisation to its health education campaigns using the catchphrase Be all You Can Be! In practice, however, some not inconsiderable ingenuity was needed to match a self-actualising approach to what was an essentially preventive medicine agenda, e.g. *'Don't Use Drugs – Be All You Can Be!*, *Walk About a Bit – Be All You Can Be!'*

## Health as empowerment

As will be readily apparent later in this book, empowerment is considered to be highly important for the achievement of health promotion goals. It could also legitimately be seen as a worthwhile health goal in its own right. Antonovsky's (1979, 1984) popular ideal of salutogenesis provides a good illustration of such a goal. One important outcome has been described as a sense of coherence. It is interesting as an example of what many would consider to be a worthwhile mental health target which, at the same time, contains a significant empowerment dimension together with a (potentially contradictory) component that is related to the creation of a sense of community – a broader social health goal which is of current interest.

***Box 2*** Health as a Sense of Coherence

> - *Comprehensibility*: life is predictable and makes sense.
> - *Manageability:* possession of empowering resources to meet life's demands.
> - *Meaningfulness*: life makes sense emotionally.

## Health and medicine

Apart from reiterating an earlier observation that the pursuit of holistic, 'wellness' goals has been known to cause extreme irritation in medical practitioners, we should recall that there has been a long history of conflict between those concerned with the cure of disease and those having a more wide ranging interest. McKeown (1979), in his seminal work, comments on the ... *dual nature of medicine which resulted from ideas which have been promoted with varying emphasis in all periods down to the present day: health preserved by way of life and health restored by treatment of disease.*

He cites approvingly Dubos (1959, 1965) as follows:

*The myths of Hygieia and Asclepius symbolise the never-ending oscillation between two different points of view in medicine. For the worshippers of Hygieia, health is the natural order of things, a positive attribute to which men are entitled if they govern their lives wisely. According to them, the most important function of medicine is to discover and teach the natural laws which will ensure a man a healthy mind in a healthy body. More sceptical, or wiser in the ways of the world, the followers of Asclepius believe that the chief role of the physician is to treat disease, to restore health by correcting any imperfections caused by the accidents of birth or life.*

(McKeown, 1979 p3).

We will return later to a discussion of the 'medical model' in health promotion, but the existence of this tension should be noted now. We should also observe that the quotation from Dubos implies that the tension is due to conflict between curative medicine and *individual* behaviour – although much of Dubos' work, and certainly McKeown's focus on social conditions, does not support the 'individualistic' hypothesis – a point that will be reiterated later. Indeed, Peter Draper would frequently refer to those committed to prevention via lifestyle change as *false prophets of Hygieia!*

Before moving on to look critically at the determinants of health and illness, two points should be made rather forcefully: few doctors can nowadays fail to acknowledge that there are 'positive' dimensions to health – often expressed in terms of 'quality of life'. Secondly, a large body of research clearly demonstrates that the laity – the general public – not only recognise the existence of broad wellness criteria for health but are apt to ascribe greater importance to these than to narrower medical goals in 'needs assessment' exercises. See Box 3 below for an observation from one patient which provides a telling illustration (Tones and Green, 1999).

**Box 3**   A Lay View of Health

*… if there isn't enough money to pay for the rent or food or clothes, then you can't begin to think of other things. You have to have these things, like a roof over your head, a job, for self-respect, a coat on your back and food in the stomach. I've got 'good health'. I've not been in hospital, I don't take tablets, but that's not health to me. I'm sick because I have trouble paying my bills, I have trouble feeding the kids at times, so bodily I'm all right, but here (indicates head) I'm terrible, 'cos I worry and that's not health is it?*

Durrant (1993, p98).

A nice interpretation of the holistic dimension of health is provided by Sweeney in the 1997 James Mackenzie lecture (Sweeney, 1998). He cites approvingly Cassell's (1991) concept of '*personhood*'. This includes:

*… personality and character; a past with life experiences that provide a context for illness; a family with ties that may be positive or negative; a cultural background; a variety of roles and relationships; a body and a self-image of that body; a secret life of fears, desires, hopes, and fantasies; a perceived future and … a transcendental dimension (that is some sort of life of the spirit, however that is expressed).*

*… each aspect of personhood is susceptible to injury and damage, and … this injury is what causes suffering…. Suffering can occur in relation to any aspect of a person and it occurs when the person perceives his or her impending destruction or disintegration. The sort of injuries that cause suffering are the death and suffering of loved ones, powerlessness, helplessness, hopelessness, the loss of a life's work, deep betrayal, isolation, homelessness, memory failure, unremitting fear, and physical agony.*

Most of these concepts are entirely congruent with more technical (and less poetic) constructs that are discussed more completely in this and following chapters and which relate both to health and to the determinants of health.

## Holistic health and bio-medicine: essential conflict?

It might, with some justification, be argued that it is counter-productive to overemphasise the differences between a broad, 'salutogenic' approach to the promotion of health and a medically oriented concentration on disease and symptoms (especially given the relatively high status and power of the institution of medicine!). The nature of any such dichotomy will receive further discussion later in the chapter when we consider the so-called 'medical model' of health promotion. We might, however, as an adjunct to the present discussion about the nature of health make the following observations about the possibilities of harmonious working.

- Doctors increasingly recognise the significance of 'quality of life'. Indeed in the context of the 'managerial revolution' in the UK national health service, 'Quality Adjusted Life Years' (QUALYs) are receiving attention as a device to reduce the limitations of focusing solely on such measures as life expectancy as indicators of health gain. Admittedly, since QUALYs are the invention of health economists, doctors are unlikely to find them especially endearing.
- It is inappropriate, not to say churlish, to fail to acknowledge that the cure of disease and relief of symptoms actually contributes to health and quality of life. As Blane *et al.* (1996) rightly observe:

   *Surgery for things such as hernias, cataracts, prostate, varicose veins and hip joints may not be glamorous or do very much to improve life expectancy, but they are important to the quality of life of old people.*

   (p. 11)

- Since it is unreasonable to expect even health promoters to do everything, the ordinary dictates of efficiency require appropriate role differentiation. It is, therefore, reasonable to expect doctors and those health professionals employed by medical services to focus on disease, its treatment and prevention.
- Nonetheless, a bio-medical focus inevitably provides a blinkered outlook on the public health and can be dramatically misleading – not just in connection with holistic and 'positive' health goals but also in connection with the prevention of such major health concerns as cardiovascular disease. Health and medical practitioners ignore the psychosocial dimensions of health and health care at their peril. Effective, efficient – and equitable – health care in its broadest aspect requires an understanding of what might be called the social ecology of health and the psychological determinants of individual actions.

## THE SOCIAL ECOLOGY OF HEALTH

Whatever its preferred definition of health, productive action to promote health is not possible without a sound understanding of its determinants. The position adopted here is that, on the basis of a considerable body of evidence, the major determinant of health and illness is a complex web of social, psychological and structural interactions. One of the earlier and, from the perspective of health promotion, most important analyses of these interactions featured in the Lalonde Report (Lalonde, 1974). It became known as the '*Health Field Concept*'.

### The Health Field Concept

The Lalonde Report (thus named after the Minister of Health) was a working document that reviewed the health of Canadians (and was far from satisfied with the results). The Health Field Concept was in fact derived from a conceptual schema outlined by LaFramboise (1973) which provided a simple, so-called map of 'health territory'. Health and illness were considered to result from the interplay of four key influences: genetic factors, the environment, lifestyle and medical services. Although this formulation was hardly novel, it acquired a special status when endorsed by a government agency!

Moreover, since the 'simple map' claimed to identify the major influences on health and since health promotion might be described as any deliberate or planned attempt to foster health and/or prevent and manage disease, it would seem logical that the goals of health promotion might be achieved by the creation of some judicious mix of the four 'inputs' that are described in Figure 1.1 below. Some further reflection on these four inputs would, therefore, seem appropriate at this juncture.

## The genetic dimension

Despite the somewhat jocular assertion that the best way to ensure living to a ripe old age is to be very careful in the selection of one's parents, the current evidence would seem to be that the genetic contribution to variations in health and disease is relatively small. As Tarlov (1996) notes, the influence of single gene inheritance is likely to be of the order of between 1 and 5%. He acknowledges that evidence is building for the influence of *polygenic* inheritance but is unwilling

to estimate its contribution to health – particularly since ... *the expression of the polygenes in a specific disease requires association with non-biological antecedents that are social* (p73).

## The health and medical services

Apart from the exhortation to 're-orient medical services' as part of a more general trend to demedicalisation, curative medicine has often been excluded from the health promotion field, leaving lifestyle and environment as the main areas of interest. This is perhaps rather churlish, given our earlier comment about the beneficial impact of many curative procedures on quality of life. However, research evidence would seem to support this relegation of the medical services. Tarlov (1996) cites a World Bank Report (World Bank, 1993) which stated that *at any level of income and education, higher health spending should yield better health, all else being equal. But there is no evidence of such a relation* (p53).

Bunker *et al.* (1994) are more specific. They recall that life expectancy in the USA increased from 45 to 75 years during the 20th century. Using a variety of evidence and a raft of measures, they calculate that 5 years of the 30 year gain (17%) was due to medical services. They also

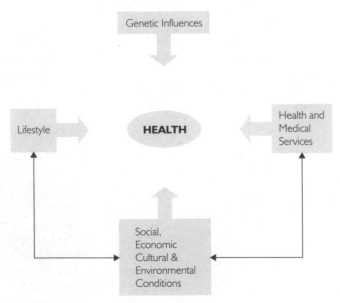

**Figure 1.1**  The Health Field Concept

extrapolated that if the services were more equitably distributed an additional gain of 1.5 years might have been expected.

Wilkinson (1996) makes a similar point.

*Both within and between developed countries, there is no clear relationship between medical provision – such as doctors per head or medical expenditure – and mortality rates.*

(p114)

Wilkinson notes that deaths from diseases regarded as 'amenable to medical treatment' are, admittedly, falling faster than deaths from other causes. However, 'amenable' diseases account for only a small proportion of all deaths.

Furthermore, Wilkinson refers to Mackenbach *et al.*'s (1990) study of avoidable mortality and the health services. This demonstrated convincingly that the (real) benefits of medical interventions are substantially dwarfed by social and environmental factors.

Again Wilkinson reminds us that even if medicine doubled the survival time of those suffering from major, life-threatening diseases, the gain would be relatively insignificant compared with halving of the incidence of the diseases (through effective preventive measures).

Bearing in mind this latter point, we should be careful to distinguish the impact of those medical services concerned with treatment and cure from those whose major purpose is prevention. As we will note later, this would involve a re-definition and 're-framing' of what legitimately comprises a health service.

## Social and behavioural determinants

If genetic inheritance and medical services contribute some 22% to health gain, it requires little mathematical skill to conclude that the remaining two inputs in the Health Field Concept must be of particular concern to health promotion. Determining the *relative* contribution of individual behaviours (or lifestyles), on the one hand, and the broader social, economic and physical environment, on the other, has led to some extensive debate and considerable acrimony. The underly-

ing reasons for the debate are by no means merely scientific or technical but, as we will demonstrate later, reflect certain key ideological issues, which are significantly reflected in discussion of the main purposes of health promotion. For now, we will merely note that Tarlov (1996) completed his analysis of the relative contributions to health gain by ascribing between 25 and 60% to 'health-related behavioural risk factors'. The 35 percentage point difference between the upper and lower estimate is, of course, due to the inseparability of the relative influences of individual behaviour and the broader social and environmental circumstances in which the individual behaviours are manifested.

## Limitations of lifestyle explanations

There is doubtless no need to provide further explication here of the contribution of lifestyle to the aetiology of disease – especially since a focus on individual sins of omission and commission characterised the approach of preventive medicine and health education for the better part of the 20th century! Increasingly, however, explanation of the determinants of health and disease is shifting away from this narrow concentration on individual behaviours and beginning to emphasise the importance of environmental influences.

Syme (1996) provides a lively discussion of the limitations of an individualistic strategy for health promotion. He chooses coronary heart disease to illustrate his contention that a new approach is needed – largely because this disease has been extensively researched and there is virtually universal agreement about the contribution of three cardinal risk factors: smoking, high blood pressure and elevated serum cholesterol. He also acknowledges the (debatable) claims of several other risk factors but makes the dramatic point that when risk factors of all kinds are added together, they account for about 40% of coronary heart disease. As he puts it, *How is it possible that, after fifty years of massive effort, all of the risk factors we know about, combined, account for less than half of the disease that occurs?* Of course some individual risk factors might still be awaiting discovery. Not only is this highly unlikely, but their contribution would have to be extremely substantial to account for the 'missing' 60% of the variance. The strategic importance for health promotion practice and evaluation of the limitations of behavioural risk factors is of great significance. Box 4 below reiterates the evidence.

**Box 4**  Limited Contribution of Individual Risk Factors to Explanation of CHD

---

- *Mortality rates from CHD have declined by over 40% in the U.S. since 1968. This cannot be accounted for by changes in behaviours.*
- *With the exception of smoking related cancers, there has been a decline in all causes of death in the U.S. since 1968.*

(Syme, 1996)

- *In the British 'Whitehall Study', the social gradient in mortality from CHD was similar among smokers and non-smokers.*
- *A combination of all risk factors measured in the Whitehall Study accounted for only a quarter of the mortality gradient.*
- *At least half the social gradient must have been due to factors other than: smoking, plasma total cholesterol, blood pressure, body mass index, physical inactivity and height.*

(Marmot *et al.*, 1984; Marmot, 1986)

---

Syme notes two other problems associated with the emphasis on individual behaviours:

- It is very difficult to achieve change in those behaviours that have been identified. As Syme observes in relation to the 'flagship' MRFIT (Multiple Risk Factor Intervention Trial),

    *... highly motivated men in the top 10 per cent risk category for coronary heart disease were able to make only minimal changes in their eating and smoking behaviours in spite of*

*intensive intervention over a six-year period (MRFIT, 1982).*

- Even where people succeed in changing their behaviour and thus reducing their risk, new recruits take their place. Indeed, the major strategy adopted by the tobacco industry is to attract new smokers to replace those who have quit the habit or who have died.

The second of these two observations is indisputable. The first, however, needs to be treated with some caution, since we must be convinced that the intervention is sufficiently intensive and sophisticated. One of the points made later in this book is the importance of the often ignored '*Type 3 Error*', i.e. concluding that a health promotion initiative has been unsuccessful despite the fact that the intervention was so badly designed that it could not possibly have achieved its stated goals.

Having provided this caveat, we must admit that it is exceedingly difficult to change deeply entrenched behaviours that are profoundly satisfying to the individual in question! We should also note that addressing the environmental determinants of health is by no means an easy option. It is at least as difficult to change these social and environmental factors that influence health and behaviour as it is to change personal lifestyle.

## The importance of environment

The environmental contributions to the health field can be quite simply categorised at this juncture. They include: the physical environment – such as natural disasters, pollution, unsafe work places and other material circumstances; socioeconomic circumstances – including social group and forms of deprivation; the social environment – including the nature of communities and social networks; the cultural environment – the complex of values, beliefs and norms that exert a socialising influence on individuals. Clearly, none of the determinants of health discussed above act alone and multiple interactions may operate between two or more of the various inputs. Indeed, we should note that not only do the social and environmental determinants make a major direct contribution, they also indirectly influence the individual characteristics that constitute the risk factors for various diseases. It is also worth noting that the various inputs operate at different levels. The *macro level* refers, for example, to national or international influences; at the *meso level* regional institutions and local organisations – such as workplace and school – may exert their effects; on the other hand, at the *micro level* we can identify the more intimate and direct effects of immediate and extended family, peer group and local community. This concentric circle of influences will be re-visited in a later chapter when we consider the factors contributing to individual health and illness-related decisions and behaviour.

Given the mounting evidence that social and environmental factors play a more significant part in the aetiology and management of disease – and in the promotion of health generally – it may, at first glance, appear surprising that public health, medicine and health promotion (albeit reluctantly) continue to emphasise the individualistic behaviour change approach. We should not be surprised! The clinical/medical tradition has been concerned with individual patients; clinical medicine has relatively greater professional power than those involved in public health (and certainly those working in health promotion and health education) and its pronouncements still have considerable influence with the public; it is easier to focus on specific disease entities and gain funding for '*vertical*' programmes designed to tackle these diseases.

Again, whereas traditionally the public at large has been relatively amenable to legislation and other forms of 'social engineering' and associated coercive measures to deal with epidemics and major threats to the social fabric not under individual control, people are notoriously resistant to efforts by the 'nanny state' to harangue them about their self-inflicted health problems and to control their individual behaviours. More important still, it is politically problematic to seek to achieve changes in the social and economic structure of societies – as we will note later.

## THE INEQUALITIES ISSUE

Undoubtedly the most important single phenomenon relating to health is the undisputed fact that the incidence, prevalence and experience of health, disease and sickness – and their determinants – are unequally distributed. There are blatant and systematic inequalities in individuals' genetic potential, their life chances and their exposure to pathogens of all kinds; there are inequalities in the extent to which they adopt lifestyles that contribute to or militate against disease experience; there are inequalities in their child-rearing experience; there are inequalities in their psycho-social attributes – such as emotional stability, self-esteem, self-confidence and the values, attitudes, beliefs and skills that contribute indirectly to their health status. Since most of these inequalities are not inevitable, certain individuals and social groups are the beneficiaries of health advantages: others are relatively disadvantaged and deprived. The unequal and hierarchical distribution of health and its determinants is consistently associated with various measures of social status – most commonly defined in terms of social class or socio-economic status. Assuming that unavoidable and damaging inequalities are not desirable – and since a majority of nations at least pay lip-service to the principle of equity, health inequalities are a matter of major philosophical and political concern. Accordingly, once the existence of inequities has been acknowledged, debate and speculation about the most appropriate strategies and policies for remedying the situation tend to be urgent and heated. As we will assert later in this chapter, attempts to remedy inequities are certainly central to the ideology of health promotion. However, it is clear that the effectiveness and efficiency of strategies for action must depend on understanding both the nature and distribution of these ubiquitous inequalities and the various ways in which they contribute to health status. Accordingly, we will now briefly review some of the current issues.

**Box 5**   The Reality of Inequality

*UK Inequity – late 1960s*

Children aged seven who were born into the lowest socio-economic category (social group V, unskilled manual) were more likely than average children to:

- be premature or overdue
- weigh less
- be shorter
- be clumsy
- stammer or squint
- have convulsions
- have suppurating ears
- be neither immunised nor vaccinated
- have never attended clinic or dentist
- to die or suffer damage at birth
- be bed-wetters and nail-biters
- be aggressive and destructive
- be maladjusted
- come from overcrowded homes
- come from broken homes and homes lacking normal amenities
- have less well-educated parents
- speak unintelligibly
- be less creative
- have poorer general knowledge
- be poor readers
- be poor at arithmetic.

From Davie *et al.* (1972): the National Child Development Study of 17,000 babies born 3–9 March, 1958.

Given that measures to tackle inequalities are ideologically problematic (at least for those of certain political persuasions) and (for those of any political persuasion) bound to be extremely expensive, it is not surprising that attempts have been made to challenge the reality and/or inevitability of inequalities in health. It is not possible to overestimate the dramatic impact of the *Black Report* on inequalities in health in Britain (Townsend and Davidson, 1992). Its contents and conclusions are well known. However, in the light of the above observations about the political pre-

cariousness of tackling inequality, it is worth reminding readers of the reaction of government to the report. Patrick Jenkin, the then Secretary of State for Social Services, commented in his Foreword:

> *I must make it clear that additional expenditure on the scale which could result from the report's recommendations – the amount involved could be upwards of £2 billion a year (1980 prices) – is quite unrealistic in present or any foreseeable economic circumstances, quite apart from any judgement that may be formed of the effectiveness of such expenditure in dealing with the problems identified.*

The minister then noted he was making the report available for discussion but *without any commitment by the government to its proposals.* The way in which the report was made available has entered the folklore. Only 260 duplicated copies were released. No press release or press conference was arranged and a few copies were sent to selected journalists on the Friday before the August Bank Holiday (thus guaranteeing the lowest possible level of publicity). Of course, such manoeuvrings also virtually guarantee that a publication becomes a *cause celebre* and the demand was such that the report is now safely enshrined in the publication to which reference was made above! The *British Medical Journal* commented that the official discarding of the report demonstrated 'shallow indifference'. A subsequent leader in the same journal compared the *Black Report* to the Bible: *... much quoted, occasionally read and largely ignored when it comes to action* (*British Medical Journal*, 1986).

Writing in the introduction to *Inequalities in Health*, Townsend *et al.* (1992) comment on the tendency of history to repeat itself and comment on a sense of *deja vecu* in connection with the next key UK publication on health inequalities – *The Health Divide* (Whitehead, 1992). This report was commissioned by the Director General of the Health Education Council (HEC) and not only reiterated the findings of the earlier *Black Report* but demonstrated that the gap between rich and poor had continued to increase. As the chair of the HEC noted at the time, the report was *political dynamite in an election year!* Accordingly, a previously arranged press briefing was cancelled. An alternative press launch was, however, held in the offices of the Disability Alliance; entirely predictably, this rather clumsy attempt at censorship resulted in *The Health Divide* also developing into a fully fledged *cause celebre*! It subsequently – with revisions – joined the *Black Report* in the publication co-authored by Townsend *et al.* (1992). Devotees of conspiracy theory were not surprised to note the departure of the Director General of the HEC prior to the abolition of that body and its re-emergence as the Health Education Authority.

Bearing in mind observations to be made later in this chapter, it is worth reiterating at this point the intrinsic difficulties facing those seeking to pursue a radical, political agenda in health promotion – even when government is apparently ideologically committed to action!

At all events, in addition to providing a comprehensive catalogue of inequalities, the authors of the *Black Report* and *The Health Divide* felt it necessary to deal with challenges to the reality of the existence of the inequalities in health (and indeed in society generally) that they had so thoroughly explored and explicated. They identified four classes of possible explanation for the phenomena they reported. These were as follows.

- *The artefact explanation*: e.g. the data on inequality were artificial variables. For instance, the findings might be explained by a 'shrinkage' in the proportion of the population in the poorest occupational classes.
- *Natural and social selection*: in short the gaps were due to the gravitation of the weak and ill to the lower social groups.
- *Cultural/behavioural explanations*: the explanation centres on individual lifestyle and associated cultural factors. It is a useful way of constructing reality for those who wish to demonstrate that the health gap is due to 'irresponsible' behaviour, i.e. it is essentially 'victim blaming'. Clearly, it should be noted that it is

also possible to accept the validity of cultural/lifestyle explanations without blaming the individual.
- *Materialist/structuralist explanations*: accounts for inequality in terms of social and economic factors – for instance in respect of the direct or indirect effects of poverty.

As a result of extensive research, it is now generally accepted that the first two explanations make only a minor contribution to the overall experience of inequality. They should, therefore, be discounted in formulating strategies for action. Accordingly, the interaction of lifestyle and socio-environmental factors, as noted in Figure 1.1, must be the focus for health promotion.

## Social class, occupation and education

The relationship between social class or, more accurately, socio-economic status and health is by now so well established that its existence may be viewed as a truism. However, it is more important to understand just what aspects of this social gradient account for its influence on health so that realistic action may be taken. The *Black Report* (Townsend and Davidson, 1992) defined 'social class' as *... segments of the population sharing broadly similar types and levels of resources, with broadly similar styles of living and (for some sociologists) some shared perception of their collective condition* (p39). It also discusses the problems of selecting appropriate and useful indicators. Occupational status, education, income and economic development are all considered to be associated with social status and their correlates and can serve as proxy measures. Occupation has been used most frequently as an indicator of social class and its relationship with both education and income is doubtless obvious.

For instance, the second 'Whitehall Study' of 10,308 civil servants in London demonstrates, among other things, both a finely detailed hierarchy between the employment grades of the civil servants in question and an almost equally precise relationship between grade and salary level. This gradient is also mirrored by the civil servants' experience of disease (Brunner, 1996) – a point reiterated by Syme (1996), who also gives a flavour of the reality of social class differentials in Britain:

> ... *those one step down from the top of the hierarchy, civil servants who are professionals and executives (such as doctors and lawyers), have heart disease rates that are twice as high as those at the very top: upper-class directors of agencies, almost all of whom have been educated at Oxford and Cambridge, and whose career usually ends with a knighthood.*
>
> (pp26–7)

## Using indices of deprivation

In order to sharpen and clarify those components of social status that contribute most to the variance in inequalities in health, a number of indices have been developed. British indices include, for example, the Jarman Underprivileged Area Scores (Jarman, 1984); the Townsend Index (Townsend *et al.*, 1988) and the Carstairs Index (Carstairs and Morris, 1989). These indices incorporate such specific indicators as: percentage of private households containing economically active members who are unemployed; the proportion of private households with more than one person per room; households which do not possess a car; households that are not owner occupiers. Combinations of these measures serve as efficient proxy measures of health. It is, however, more difficult to identify the precise mechanisms whereby the deprivation measured by the indices actually contributes to health status.

Blane *et al.* (1996) provide an interesting example of research that, on the one hand, demonstrates the indirect effect of education on health and illness and, on the other, demonstrates the difficulty mentioned above of discovering causal mechanisms. It also illustrates the way in which deprivation indices can predict health status and shows how different indices seem to 'plug into' different socio-economic influences. The authors used the Townsend and Carstairs Indices and also assessed the levels of educational attainment in 107 local education authorities (e.g. the

relative success rates in GCSE examinations). Both the deprivation indices and the measures of educational attainment were significantly associated with mortality in the study areas. Educational attainment accounted for some 30–40% of the variance in mortality However, since the measures of mortality clearly could not refer to the students whose examination results had been (recently) recorded but rather were derived from infant deaths and deaths occurring in parents' or grandparents' generations, it seemed that the education measure was reflecting some more general community characteristic. To compound the complexity of the inter-relationships between the various measures used by the researchers, when assessments of deprivation assessed by the Carstairs Index were controlled, the association between education and mortality was virtually demolished. On the other hand, when the Townsend Index was used, the association between mortality and education largely survived!

## Health, wealth and poverty

Common sense would predict that poverty is the active ingredient in deprivation and would account for health inequalities. In fact, it seems clear that the relationship between wealth and health is by no means simple. For instance, Preston (1976) concluded that no more than 10% of an increase in life expectancy is due to increased gross national product. In the light of this observation, it is interesting to consider Marmot's (1996) remarks on what can only be described as the grotesque fact that the life expectancy at birth in Guinea-Bissau and Afghanistan in 1992 was 43 years, compared with a life expectancy in Japan of 78.6 years. Equally grotesque is his observation that the real gross domestic product per capita in the former countries is $700–750, while that in Japan is $19,400. It is, however, unwise to jump to causal conclusions: for instance, the United Nations Human Development Report (1994) demonstrated a number of situations where there is no direct relationship. By way of example, Guinea and Sri Lanka had similar levels of per capita income but life expectancy in Guinea is 43.9 years, compared with 71.2 in Sri Lanka.

Marmot cites Caldwell, who suggested that countries which achieve good life expectancies despite low income have the following features in common:

> ... a substantial degree of female autonomy, dedication to education, an open political system, a largely civilian society without a rigid class structure, a history of egalitarianism and radicalism, and of national consensus.
>
> (Caldwell, 1986)

Clearly, a *high* degree of poverty must be detrimental to health and Wilkinson's (1996) observation seems very reasonable: up to about $5000 per capita income there is a high correlation between income and life expectancy. Above that level other factors come into play and explanation involves what Wilkinson refers to as an *'income gearing factor'*, i.e. *If 10 per cent of the improvement in mortality is directly associated with income, then 90 per cent is associated with something which improves the gearing between income and health* (p112). It is likely that the important factor is *relative* income (Wilkinson, 1992, 1994) and, therefore, relative inequality. However, although this is an important piece of evidence and does have implications for social policy in relation to the re-distribution of income, it does not provide detailed insights into the relationship between the socio-economic phenomenon and individual or community health. Some attempts will be made to remedy this deficiency later. For now we might usefully consider a controversial notion related to the phenomenon of deprivation: the concept of *underclass*.

## In pursuit of the 'underclass'

The notion of 'underclass' is highly contentious. It gives rise to heated debate and angry exchanges – rooted in conflicting political ideologies. Although, at first glance, its demonstration of major inequalities would appear to be consistent with concerns about inequalities, the explanation it offers for those inequalities attracts considerable opprobrium. In fact, Townsend *et al.* (1992) caution against the pitfall of concentrating on the 'dangerous notion of an "underclass"'. They cite an editorial in the *Lancet* (1990):

> *The emotion of the well-heeled towards underclasses is fear, often voiced as blame and articulated in exhortation to uphold the family, obey the law, be industrious, and make use of the opportunities of the market. More appropriate emotions might be shame and indignation. One cannot walk about London – an exercise eschewed by Prime Ministers – without a strong measure of both.*

The invention of the term 'underclass' has been attributed to Ken Auletta, an American journalist writing in the 1980s. However, the most notorious advocate of the concept is Charles Murray, who made a messianic visit to Britain in 1989 at the invitation of the *Sunday Times* and made a second visit in 1994 to ascertain whether his apocalyptic forecast that Britain would shortly be in the same unfortunate predicament as the USA was becoming reality. His *Sunday Times* articles were subsequently published by the Institute of Economic Affairs (Lister, 1996).

In short, Murray distinguished between the deserving and undeserving poor. As Green noted in his foreword to the conclusions Murray drew from his first visit and published under the title of *The Emerging British Underclass* (Lister, 1996), the term 'underclass' was applied only to those poor who were ... *distinguished by their undesirable behaviour, including drug-taking, crime, illegitimacy, failure to hold down a job, truancy from school and casual violence* (p19).

In the publication resulting from his second visit – and tellingly entitled *Underclass: the Crisis Deepens* (Lister, 1996) – Murray indicated his intention to focus on three 'symptoms': crime, illegitimacy and economic inactivity among working-aged men. In reality his major concern was with illegitimacy. Within this latter context, he compared unfavourably the *'New Rabble'* of the 'underclass' with the *'New Victorians'*. His solution to the problem was to substantially abandon welfare funding and emphasise 'authentic self government'. He was, incidentally, reticent about the meaning of 'authentic' and the means for achieving this.

## The underclass: explanations and definitions

Inevitably, Murray's analysis created a furore. Some opponents challenged the very existence of an 'underclass' and the associated notion of a 'culture of dependency'. For example, Lister cites Kempson's (1996) conclusions from a review of 31 research studies supported by the Joseph Rowntree Foundation:

> ... people who live on low incomes are not an underclass. They have aspirations just like others in society: they want a job; a decent home; and an income that is enough to pay the bills with a little to spare. But social and economic changes that have benefited the majority of the population, increasing their incomes and their standard of living, have made life more difficult for a growing minority, whose fairly modest aspirations are often beyond their reach.
>
> (p163)

Others, however, accept the existence of an 'underclass' – or something like it. Willetts (1992, cited by Lister, 1996), for example, identifies three problematic groups: the long-term unemployed, unskilled workers in erratic employment and younger single mothers. Of greater importance, however, is the nature of the disagreements about explanations and causes between those who accept the existence of a problematic socio-economic group or sub-culture but cannot accept Murray's diagnosis nor his proposed remedies.

The crux of the debate about explanations centres on the distinction between those who view the problem as 'structural' oppression and those who consider that it arises from individual ineptitude. Wilson (1987) seemed to subscribe to both in his definition of 'underclass' as:

> ... that heterogeneous grouping of families and individuals who are outside the mainstream of the American occupational system. Included ... are individuals who lack training and skills

and either experience long-term unemployment or are not members of the labor force, individuals who are engaged in street crime and other forms of aberrant behaviour, and families that experience long-term spells of poverty and/or welfare dependency.

> (p8)

Field (1996), too, is prepared to use the term 'underclass' for the current situation in Britain.

> ... I accept that Britain does now have a group of poor people who are so distinguished from others on low income that it is appropriate to use the term 'underclass' to describe their position in the social hierarchy.
>
> (p57)

Field, however, distinguishes the British from the American context by asserting that, unlike the US experience, there is no racial basis to Britain's underclass. He also emphasises its structural causes and identifies three major constituent groups:

> the very frail, elderly pensioner, the single parent with no chance of escaping welfare under the existing rules and with prevailing attitudes, and the long-term unemployed.

Again, it is possible to agree with some of the problems identified by Murray without subscribing to an individualistic explanation. Phillips (1996) (while likening Murray to *a bit of chewing gum that gets stuck to the sole of your shoe!*), nonetheless believes that ... *the progressive collapse of the intact family is bringing about a set of social changes which is taking us into uncharted and terrifying waters.* Additionally, she recognises that

> ... there are now whole communities, framed by structural unemployment, in which fatherlessness has become the norm. These communities are truly alarming because children are being brought up with dysfunctional and often antisocial attitudes as a direct result of the fragmentation and emotional chaos of households in which sexual libertarianism provides a stream of transient and unattached men servicing their mothers.
>
> (pp156–7)

## The individual dimension

Despite the popularity of the structural explanation among social scientists and many health care workers, it would be unwise to completely exclude the possibilities of individual capacities and responsibilities. Buckingham (1996) provides a 'statistical update' and, not without a degree of courage, directly addresses the question 'Are the underclass workshy?'. While he emphasises the primacy of structure he does provide some evidence that there may well be – for some people – alternative explanations. He utilised the invaluable 1958 cohort originally recruited for the National Child Development Survey (Davie *et al.*, 1972) and compared the responses of a sample of working class men with 'underclass' men to the following two statements:

- I would pack in a job I didn't like even if there was no job to go to.
- Almost any job is better than none.

There was a statistically significant difference between the two samples. Some 39% of the underclass group agreed with the former statement, compared with 16% of the working class group. And 47% of the underclass considered that 'any job was better than none', compared with 59% of the working class sample.

Buckingham also chose to challenge the dictates of political correctness by addressing the question of cognitive ability and even asserted that *Even when compared with the below average scoring working class, the underclass are significantly less intelligent* (a full standard deviation below the mean male score). 'Underclass women', for instance, whose child was illegitimate scored 30.6 (out of 80) on a standardised score of general ability, whereas the mothers of children born within marriage scored 41.2.

Lister's (1996) thoughtful review of the 'underclass' issue also observes that an emphasis on structural explanations needs to be balanced by an acknowledgement that individuals can, *in certain circumstances*, make a difference. As Lister puts it

*... there is ample evidence of the ways in which, both individually and collectively,*

*people in poverty (and especially women) struggle to gain greater control over their own lives and to improve their situation and that of the communities in which they live.*

(p12)

This observation will find a strong echo in our later discussion of health promotion's empowerment imperative. In the meantime, it will be useful to conclude this discussion of inequalities and the social determinants of health by referring to Galbraith's valuable contribution to the critique of the concept of 'underclass'.

## Challenging the 'culture of contentment'

Galbraith (1992a) noted what he termed the *present and devastated position of the socially assisted underclass* but vigorously attacked Murray's formulation and the associated 'trickle down' theory of the beneficial effects of enriching what might be called the 'overclass'. He quoted one of the Reagan administration's metaphors that ... *if one feeds the horse enough oats, some will pass through to the road for the sparrows.* Galbraith's wholehearted espousal of structural economic solutions is made explicit:

*Life in the great cities in general could be improved, and only will be improved, by public action – by better schools with better-paid teachers, by strong, well-financed welfare services, by counseling on drug addiction, by employment training, by public investment in the housing that in no industrial country is provided for the poor by private enterprise, by adequately supported health care, recreational facilities, libraries and police.*

In the light of contemporary attempts to deal with 'underclass' problems within existing fiscal and economic strategies, his final observation is especially relevant:

*The question once again, much accommodating rhetoric to the contrary, is not what can be done but what will be paid.*

**Box 6**  Inequity in the Late 1990s

- The income gap between the high-paid and the low-paid widened rapidly and only that in New Zealand has surpassed the rate of divergence in Britain. Between 1977 and 1992 top wages in Britain grew by 50% and median wages by 35%. Low wages ended the period in real terms less than in 1975 (Blane *et al.*, 1996).

- 

|  | Springburn, Glasgow | Wokingham Berks |
|---|---|---|
| Chronic illness (per 1000) | 155 | 36 |
| Infant mortality (deaths per 10,000 live births) | 67.9 | 53.2 |
| GCSE failures (%) | 77 | 46 |
| Poverty (% households) | 41 | 10 |

(Townsend Centre for International Poverty Research, 1999)

- The death rate from CHD in people under 65 is almost three times higher in Manchester than in Oxfordshire.

- In the 45–64 age group, 25% of professional women and 17% of professional men report a limiting long-standing illness, compared with 45% of unskilled women and 48% of unskilled men.

- In 1996/7 4.5 million children were brought up in families with below half average income – three times the number 20 years ago.

- Long-standing illness in unskilled men over 65 was 72%; in professional groups this was 53%.

- A middle-aged man who loses his job doubles his chances of dying in the next five years.

- In 1996 there were at least 4.3 million 'fuel poor' householders who needed to spend 10% of their income to keep their homes warm.

- Pedestrian fatality rates for children of unskilled parents are five times higher than those of professional parents.

- In 1996 12% of men in professional jobs smoked compared with 40% in unskilled manual occupations; proportions among women were 11% and 36%.

- Teenage girls from poor neighbourhoods are more likely to become pregnant and teenagers account for more than one in 10 births in some inner city areas.

- The median age at which people first have sex is two years lower among both males and females from manual households than those from professional ones.

- People in lower socio-economic groups eat less fruit and vegetables and less food rich in dietary fibre than other groups.

- People in lower income groups tend to pay more for their food because of the physical inaccessibility of large retail outlets and higher prices in small local shops (Department of Health, 1999a).

Reference has been made above to inequalities in society and their impact on health. The importance of *relative* inequality has also been emphasised. The most important macro policy would thus seem to be one of reversing the trend and achieving the relatively narrow differential between social groups that appears to characterise healthier nations and which characterised Britain in the early 1950s. The difficulties of achieving change of this order cannot be overestimated and Galbraith's concept of the culture of contentment also has major implications for health promotion strategies seeking to achieve such policy change of this order. He argues that the problems of the underclass will only be addressed by challenging the self-satisfaction experienced by the vast majority of the populations in the USA and UK: there may be a small proportion of the population owning most of the wealth but, he argues, the rest of the population – other than the underclass – are quite satisfied with their lot (in the oft-quoted words of a former British Prime Minister, *They have never had it so good!*). They are unwilling to rock the boat and jeopardise their current circumstances and bank balances by taking up cudgels on behalf of the disadvantaged.

## Pathways from socio-economic influence to individual health experience

We noted earlier the interaction between the various social and environmental determinants of health and other influences, such as lifestyle and health service provision. Given that social factors such as poverty and personal lifestyle do not have a one-to-one relationship with health, one of the more challenging tasks facing researchers is to disentangle the pathways whereby macro influences are translated into individual behaviours – and the psycho-social factors determining those behaviours. For example, just how does relative poverty increase the likelihood of premature death in individuals? The efficiency of health promotion strategies should be considerably enhanced if such mechanisms could be firmly established.

Wilkinson (1996) discusses the impact of economic development and refers to a need to explore the qualitative aspects of material change and to identify the 'gearing' between income and health. We need, for example, to look for factors such as psycho-social pathways between, say, GNPpc (gross national per capita product) and life expectancy. He comments on two main sources of change that might provide such gearing:

> *The first is the continuous stream of technical innovations which yield qualitative improvements in material life, and the second is an amorphous series of changes in the nature of psychological and social life. Though invisible to indices of economic growth, both may be inextricably bound up with the process of qualitative change, which we know as economic development.*

More particularly, he speculates on the importance of 'social capital', a commodity that we will examine later in this chapter.

## The psychology of control and biological transition

Of particular relevance to the model of health promotion adopted in this book are the observations of those researchers who consider aspects of control to be the important mediating factor between socio-economic influence and individuals' health-related responses. Syme (1989) makes reference to such well-known constructs as self-efficacy, perceived locus of control and learned helplessness. Karasek and Theorell (1990) also emphasise the importance of control together with discretion over tasks in a work context. Brunner (1996) uses results from the second Whitehall study of English civil servants to explore the basis of cardiovascular disease. Not only does he reiterate the importance of control, he also argues for a quite direct link between these psychological variables and specific physiological effects. As he puts it:

> *Lower grade office staff tend to experience their work as monotonous and lacking in opportunities to control how and what they do. A relatively low income will often accompany these characteristics of work. The long-term psychological demands imposed by such life circumstances, compared with those of higher status workers, may produce an excess of psychiatric illness such as depression … but is it plausible that an adverse psychosocial environment could produce an excess of coronary disease?*

> *If the biologically important gradients shown in Whitehall II and other data are put together, i.e. those relating to impaired glucose tolerance, insulin resistance, fibrinogen, HDL cholesterol, triglycerides, and central obesity, a coherent explanation can be proposed to account for these specific effects. This pathway links the chronic stress response of the hypothalamic pituitary adrenal system with resulting elevated levels of corticosteroids, to central obesity, insulin resistance, poor lipid profile and increased tendency for the blood to clot.*

(p290)

Tarlov (1996) also speculates about the probability of what he calls a 'sociobiological translation' process. His perspective centres on the process whereby people's environmental, social and personal circumstances exert an effect *that may take decades before becoming clinically apparent*. He addresses directly the issue of inequality and considers it possible that later in young people's development,

> ... *perhaps when youths start to make specific plans for their own future, but also throughout the life course the stark reality of inequality becomes appreciated. Observations and experiences of inequity, limitations in opportunities for jobs, housing, and income, employment instability, and social segregation intersect with expectations derived from identity. When expectations and reality clash, we speculate, the chronic, persistent, inescapable dissonance between what a person would like to do or become and what seems accomplishable triggers biological signals that are antecedents of chronic disease development ... the biological signals are probably subtle, but steady and long-term.*

(pp85–6)

The proposed mechanism involves a 'lipid–vascular endothelial interaction' resulting in the formation of atherosclerotic plaque.

It might, of course, legitimately be argued that the reduction of inequalities, achieving an improvement in working conditions and helping people gain control over their lives are entirely justifiable reasons in their own right for the development of health promotion programmes. Given the importance of salutogenic goals, this is entirely true. However, taking account of political realities, it remains a fact that 'salutogenic programmes' are more likely to be financed if there is a likelihood of reducing the incidence of major diseases – especially if there is some bio-medical substantiation!

Before moving on to discuss the nature and philosophy underpinning health promotion programmes in general, it is worth summarising the multiple factors that influence health – taking account of the preceding discussions. Figure 1.2 provides such a summary.

## THE MEANING OF HEALTH PROMOTION

It would be entirely logical to identify health promotion as *any* measure which promotes health. It is, however, reasonable to assume that health promotion should refer only to *planned* activities. Of course, serendipitous events may result in a health gain, just as health learning may occur without any deliberate attempt to persuade or educate. However, the perhaps optimistic assumption is made in this book that the intentional planning of policy initiatives and the organisation of learning experiences are more likely to result in a positive outcome than reliance on happenstance. Clearly, it is assumed that the superiority of planned interventions will depend on the skills of the health promotion practitioner – although we must, however, regrettably accept that not all intentional attempts at health promotion will be in competent hands!

The simple definition outlined above would be consistent with WHO's approach that considered health promotion as a

> ... *unifying concept for those who recognize the need for change in the ways and conditions of living, in order to promote health.*

(WHO, 1984)

Elaborating slightly on this simple notion, we might, logically, define health promotion as any planned intervention that seeks to improve health and/or prevent disease by engaging with the four main domains comprising the Health Field Concept: individual behaviour and lifestyle, social and environmental determinants, health services and, assuming that real intervention possibilities exist, the genetic pre-disposition. To do so, however, would not only provide a superficial account but would ignore the complex web of values and ideologies that underpin research programme planning and professional practice. We will, therefore, give some thought to the emergence of the health promotion 'movement' and, particularly, consider the seminal and continuing influence of WHO on philosophy and practice.

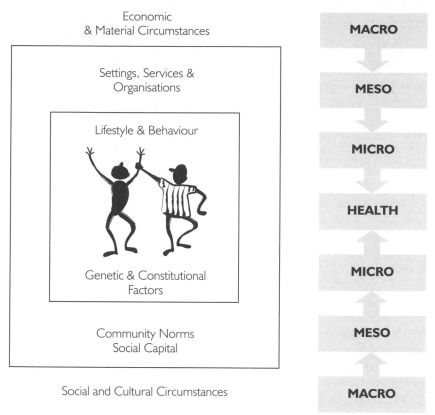

**Figure 1.2**  Macro, Meso and Micro Influences on Health

## Different ideologies: different perspectives

A complete and comprehensive account of health promotion and its historical roots is beyond the scope of this book. However, for the reasons stated above, some further discussion is needed. This will involve separately analysing health promotion as ideology, on the one hand, and as structure, on the other. In other words, the values underpinning dominant notions of health promotion will be considered; subsequently a model operationalising the concept will be presented. This model will highlight its main component parts and *inter alia* demonstrate the relationship between health education and other major processes contributing to the promotion of health.

Before doing this, it might be illuminating to consider some of the different meanings ascribed to health promotion.

Many publications have provided definitions of and perspectives on health promotion during the last few years (Anderson, 1984; Tones, 1985; Green and Raeburn, 1988; Minkler, 1989). For example, the term has been used to refer to the approaches listed below.

- The attainment of positive health or well-being – or even 'high level' well-being.
- A high visibility media-centred approach derived from an over-optimistic view of what marketing methods can achieve and confusing the sale of commercial products with the 'sale' of health. In its more reflective and respectable form it utilises

principles of social marketing; on the other hand, what might be called a 'hullabaloo model' is somewhat similar but merely involves much superficial publicity signifying very little.

- A preventive approach emphasising the importance of objectives and performance indicators. It is best exemplified by an influential series of publications, including *Objectives for the Nation* and those produced by the US Department of Health, Education and Welfare (1978, 1979) and the Department of Health and Human Services (1980). This initiative contrasted '*health protection*' and '*preventive health services*' with health promotion. While the two former strategies involved the development of legislative, environmental and other policy measures to achieve health gain, the latter, 'health promotion', was distinguished by a focus on individual behaviours and involved the adoption of early primary preventive practices.

In short, the concept of health promotion is rather like virtue: it means all things to all people – who are united only in their agreement that it is rather desirable! Green and Raeburn (1988) describe rather nicely how a wide variety of different interest groups have laid claim to this essentially contested concept.

*Ideologues, professionals, interest groups, and representatives of numerous disciplines have attempted to appropriate the field for themselves. Health and education professionals, behavioral and social scientists, public administrators, town planners, futurists, holistic health and self-care advocates, liberals, conservatives, voluntary associations, funding agencies, governments, community groups, and many others all want something from health promotion, all want to contribute something, and all bring their own orientation to bear on it.*

(p30)

## The contribution of the World Health Organization

The stance adopted in this book is essentially consistent with the ideological canons of WHO. For

this reason, and again acknowledging the significance of WHO's contribution, we should perhaps remind ourselves of the various 'milestones' in WHO's progress towards its current formulation of health promotion.

The seeds of health promotion may be found in WHO's original and classic definition of health (WHO, 1946), with its holistic emphasis and its accentuation of the positive. In more recent time a major impetus was provided with the clarion call to achieve 'Health for All by the Year 2000' (HFA 2000). Interestingly, in the context of developing indicators of performance, the HFA initiative included a more realistic definition of health than the classic 1946 version. As the then Director General of WHO pointed out:

*The challenging constitutional objective of the Word Health Organization: the attainment by all peoples of the highest possible level of physical, mental and social wellbeing, is now being transformed into the dynamic notion of a Health for All movement. With this change in emphasis, public health is reinstating itself as a collective effort, drawing together a wide range of actors, institutions and sectors within society toward a goal of a '<u>socially and economically productive life</u>' (authors' emphasis). This social goal ... moves health from being the outcome measure of social development to being one of its major resources.*

(Mahler, 1986 p1)

More recently WHO reiterated the more tangible definition of health and asserted its commitment to equity (WHO, 1998):

*The concept and vision of Health for All were defined in 1977, when the Thirtieth World Health Assembly decided that the main social target of governments and WHO in the coming decades should be 'the attainment by all the citizens of the world by the year 2000 of a level of health that will permit them to lead a socially and economically productive life'. The Declaration of Alma-Ata, adopted in 1978 by the International Conference on Primary Health Care, ... jointly sponsored* *and organized by WHO and UNICEF, stated that primary health care was the key to attaining Health for All ... This call for HFA was, and remains fundamentally, <u>a call for social justice</u> (authors' emphasis).*

(p2).

The above definition signals the importance of the Declaration of Alma Ata – a major event in the progress towards health promotion (WHO, 1978). It made several important assertions, which were later to be incorporated into health promotion. Above all, it declared that the existence of gross inequalities between advantaged and disadvantaged peoples was 'politically, socially and economically' unacceptable. In pursuit of equity, economic and social development was, therefore, essential to the achievement of health. On the other hand, people themselves have not only a right but also a duty to participate individually and collectively in the planning and implementation of their health care. *Primary Health Care* (PHC) was considered to be the key to achieving HFA 2000, and PHC was seen as not only more than primary *medical* care but ideologically different. Alma Ata broadened considerably the definition of health services by redefining agriculture, animal husbandry, food, industry, education, housing, public works, communications and other sectors as services essential for the promotion of health.

The original primary health care elements are listed in Appendix 1.1.

As mentioned above, Alma Ata might with justification be viewed as a prototype for *Health Promotion* (WHO, 1984). A flavour of its ideological dynamic is provided by the following quotation from Kickbusch (1986) – a major figure in the proselytisation of health promotion – which she describes as ... *a new forcefield for health* (which) *integrates social action, health advocacy and public policy*. It incorporates:

*... diverse, but complementary, methods or approaches, including communication, education, legislation, fiscal measures, organizational change, community development and spontaneous local activities against health*

*hazards. It offers new challenges to existing professional groups, commercial and corporate bodies, cultural norms and the inertia of health institutions ... it reiterates the Health for All components of intersectoral action and advocacy for health, stressing the need to go beyond health care and equity in access to a healthy life.*

(pp437–8)

The Ottawa Charter (WHO, 1986; *Health Promotion*, 1986) provided a powerful drive for international action towards the creation of a new public health. It embodied the principles of health promotion; its major thrust was for social change and political activity. Although it urged the development of personal skills, its paramount recommendation was the need to 'build healthy public policy'. In so doing it could be argued that it marginalised health education – dislodging it from the centre stage position which Alma Ata bestowed on it. This point will be revisited later in the chapter.

**Box 7** The Ottawa Charter: Key Principles

- Build healthy public policy
- Create supportive environments
- Strengthen community action
- Develop personal skills
- Reorient health services

It would be interesting to know just how many of the signatories of the Ottawa Charter understood the policy implications of what they were signing or, if they did, whether they were fully committed to the ideological principles embodied in the Charter. According to Green and Raeburn (1988), Canada's policy framework did in fact adopt an empowering approach congruent with Charter principles. On the other hand, the publications of the US Department of Health and Human Services, to which reference was made earlier, do have a rather narrower concern with individual behaviours. Green and Raeburn, however, invite us to note that the reputation of this US conceptualisation for focusing only on rugged individualism is somewhat undeserved. They point out that of the 15 prioritised areas for disease prevention and health promotion in *Objectives for the Nation*, two thirds are addressed to environmental measures or health care systems.

Bearing in mind the importance of operationalising the notion of health in the context of developing performance indicators and measurable objectives, we should at this point note that the Ottawa Charter was preceded by the development of 38 targets for achieving HFA 2000 in the European Region (WHO, 1985).

Following the Ottawa Charter, WHO was active in the development of the '*Settings Approach*'. The precursor of this initiative was the influential Healthy Cities Project, which established a number of 'test beds' for health promotion – initially in 11 European cities; this subsequently acted as a catalyst for similar developments in another 300 or more cities (Fryer, 1988; Kickbusch, 1989).

> *The city with its own political mandate and often highly developed sense of civic pride is ... uniquely placed to develop the kind of citizen-responsive health promotion initiatives which are necessary to tackle the new health problems of the 21st century. As the most decentralized level which can marshal the necessary resources and which has wide-ranging responsibilities and networks it is in an ideal position to support the kind of intersectoral process which leads to creative, effective and efficient action.*
>
> (Morris, 1987)

As we will note later in this book, 'settings' for health promotion are more than convenient locations for the delivery of health: health promoting settings are required to ensure that all aspects of the ethos and environment of the setting in question are designed to foster health development. A number of key settings and networks were subsequently established, of which the most significant are the school, the hospital, the workplace and health promoting villages and islands. As we will state later, it is not unreasonably assumed that greater progress will be made towards achieving 'health for all' when the majority of settings operate in a coherent and co-

ordinated fashion. Accordingly, the importance of 'intersectoral working' receives consistent emphasis in WHO publications.

Continuing the description of the development of health promotion, we should note two conferences designed to further the application of the Ottawa Charter principles. The first of these, the Second International Conference on Health Promotion in Adelaide (*Health Promotion*, 1988) generated a number of recommendations in the further pursuit of healthy public policy and included four key points:

- improving the health of women – the world's primary health promoters;
- food and nutrition – ensuring adequate amounts of healthy food for all;
- tobacco and alcohol – major health hazards that deserve immediate action;
- creating supportive environments – so that health is nurtured and protected.

The second and, perhaps, more influential conference took place in Sundsvall in 1991. This highlighted the contribution that the 'spiritual, social, cultural, economic, political and ideological dimensions' of the environment could make to health. It focused on six areas:

- education;
- food and nutrition;
- home and neighbourhood;
- work;
- transport;
- social support and care.

Strategies for environmental change were separately identified as:

- policy development;
- regulation;
- reorientation of organisations;
- advocacy;
- building alliances/creating awareness;
- enabling;
- mobilizing/empowering.

(WHO, 1991; Haglund *et al.*, 1993)

The most recent and fourth of the landmark conferences on health promotion was held in

Jakarta in 1997 and gave rise to the Jakarta Declaration (WHO, 1997). The main purpose of the conference was three-fold:

- to review and evaluate the impact of health promotion;
- to identify innovative strategies to achieve success in health promotion;
- to facilitate the development of partnerships in health promotion to meet global health challenges.

It is interesting to note that the conference reaffirmed the five basic Ottawa strategies. In relation to this present book's concern with effectiveness and efficiency, it is also interesting to note the confident assertion that

> There is now clear evidence that comprehensive approaches to health development are the most effective. Those that use combinations of the five strategies are more effective than single-track approaches. (The term 'health development' is now frequently used interchangeably with 'health promotion'.)

It reiterates the importance of a settings approach:

> ... particular settings offer practical opportunities for the implementation of comprehensive strategies. These include mega-cities, islands, cities, municipalities, local communities, markets, schools, the workplace, and health care facilities.

Participation and community involvement, major health promotion mantras, are endorsed:

> ... participation is essential to sustain efforts. People have to be at the centre of health promotion action and decision-making processes for them to be effective.

and

> Health learning fosters participation. Access to education and information is essential to achieving effective participation and the empowerment of people and communities.

At approximately the same time as the Jakarta Conference, WHO reiterated the importance of addressing the *social* determinants of health (WHO, 1998).

## Health For All revisited

Three evaluations of the global HFA strategy concluded that progress had been made but a number of significant barriers to progress were identified (Box 8 below). Nonetheless, Resolution WHA48.16 requested the Director-General

> ... to take the necessary steps for renewing the health-for-all strategy together with its indicators, by developing a new holistic global health policy based on the concepts of equity and solidarity, emphasising the individual's, the family's and the community's responsibility for health, and placing health within the overall development.

**Box 8**  Evaluation of HFA, 1979–1996

In many countries progress towards HFA is hampered by:

- insufficient political commitment to the implementation of HFA;
- failure to achieve equity in access to all PHC elements;
- the continuing low status of women;
- slow socio-economic development;
- difficulty in achieving inter-sectoral action for health;
- unbalanced distribution of, and weak support for, human resources;
- widespread inadequacy of health promotion activities;
- weak health information systems and no baseline data;
- pollution, poor food safety and lack of safe water supply and sanitation;
- rapid demographic and epidemiological changes;
- inappropriate use of, and allocation of resources for, high cost technology;
- natural and man-made disasters.

*Reproduced from Health for All in the 21st Century (WHO, 1998 p6)*

A final step in WHO's progress in the development of Health for All, Primary Health Care and Health Promotion was achieved and celebrated in 1998. In short, the Executive Board of the WHO adopted a resolution formally signalling the importance of health promotion. The full text is given in Appendix 2 and a résumé of some of WHO's 'milestones' listed in Box 9.

**Box 9**  World Health Organization: Milestones in the Development of Health Promotion

- WHO Constitution. Health not merely the absence of disease but also mental, physical and social well-being.
- 1978: *Health for All by the Year 2000* launched (HFA 2000).
- 1978: Conference of Alma Ata. Importance of *Primary Health Care* emphasised.
- 1984: Statement of principles of *Health Promotion*. Discussion document on concepts and principles.
- 1986: *Ottawa Charter*. Health promotion as the process of enabling people to increase control over their lives and health. Emphasises:
  - building healthy public policy;
  - creating supportive environments;
  - strengthening community action;
  - developing personal skills;
  - reorienting health services.
- 1988: *Adelaide Conference*. Health as a fundamental human right and a sound social investment. Importance of linked economic, social and health policies. Stresses importance of equity in health. Emphasis on inter-sectoral working.
- 1988: Development of *Healthy Cities* initiative – followed by *settings approach*.
- 1991: *Sundsvall Conference*. Focus on environments and their spiritual, social, cultural, economic, political and ideological dimensions.
- 1997: *Jakarta Conference*. Reviews and evaluates impact of health promotion; re-asserts the primacy of the Ottawa Charter principles. Re-asserts importance of settings approach and health promoting schools, workplaces, communities and islands. Sets out priorities for health promotion in the 21st century.
- 1998: World Health Assembly *Resolution on Health Promotion* (WHA51.12).
- *Health for All in the 21st Century*. Continues thrust of HFA 2000. Sets out global priorities and targets for the first two decades of the 21st century for helping people worldwide to reach and maintain the highest attainable level of health throughout their lives.
- July, 2000: The *Verona Initiative*. Development of the 'Investment Triangle' – health, social development and economic development in pursuit of 'empowerment, equity, communication and commitment'.

## Ideology and health promotion

As we have noted, evaluation is concerned to assess the extent to which certain valued outcomes have been achieved. It is therefore important for us at this stage to give some further consideration to the values which permeate different approaches to health promotion. In short, we must consider the ideology of health promotion and, subsequently, the ideological basis of those different manifestations, which are sufficiently distinct to have been categorised as 'models'. First, though, some brief clarification of how the term ideology is being used here.

Although not as ambivalent and ambiguous a concept as health promotion, the term ideology is open to many interpretations. Indeed, one influential work on the subject (Eagleton, 1991) lists 'more or less at random' some 16 definitions in common use. These include: the process of production of meanings, signs and values in social life; the medium in which conscious social actors make sense of their world; the confusion of linguistic and phenomenal reality; a body of ideas characteristic of a particular social group or class; false ideas which help to legitimate a dominant political power. The term will be used here simply to describe the complex of values and associated beliefs which provide people with meaning in their personal and professional lives and which, by way of example, would influence their preference for one or other 'model' of health education and their preferred way of working. Ideology would thus be used not only to justify adoption of a given model but might also serve as a basis for vigorously attacking competing models and associated practice!

The ideological basis of the WHO formulation of health promotion will have been evident in the principles of the Ottawa Charter and associated publications and pronouncements. The ethical and moral view of humanity enshrined in this perspective on health promotion and the general pronouncements of WHO are summarised below.

## Pursuit of holistic goals

Following the guiding principle enshrined in the 1946 Constitutional definition, health should be viewed holistically as a positive state and as an essential commodity which people need in order to lead socially and economically productive lives. Health promotion should, therefore, not only be concerned with the management and prevention of disease but actively pursue mental, physical and social well-being.

## The pursuit of equity

Health will not be achieved nor illness prevented and controlled unless existing health inequalities between and within nations and social groups have been eradicated. The paramount concern of health promotion should, therefore, be with the attainment of equity. Indeed, equity is viewed by WHO not just as a goal for health promotion but as the linchpin for the achievement of *Health for All in the 21st Century* (WHO, 1998). Box 10 illustrates this observation by identifying some of the more important challenges to equity.

**Box 10**  Equity: Foundation of *HFA in the 21st Century* (WHO, 1998)

---

Equity underpins the concept of Health for All

- The call for HFA was – and remains, fundamentally – a call for social justice.
- Equity requires the removal of unfair and unjustified differences between individuals and groups.

New Challenges to equity since the Alma-Ata Conference:

- more people living in absolute poverty;
- widening gaps between rich and poor within and between many countries, communities and groups;
- strong evidence linking absolute and relative poverty to ill-health;
- environmental risks threatening equity across generations;
- uneven benefits of globalization;
- uneven access to health systems.

(p22)

---

As Whitehead (1990) argues, equity is not the same as equality and, therefore, inequity is different from inequality.

*The term 'inequity' has a moral and ethical dimension. It refers to differences, which are unnecessary and avoidable but, in addition, are also considered unfair and unjust. So, in order to describe a certain situation as inequitable, the cause has to be examined and judged to be unfair in the context of what is going on in the rest of society.*

(p5)

Seven examples of situations which, according to the criteria mentioned above, should be judged equitable or inequitable are provided by Whitehead (1992) and are produced in Table 1.1.

We might also remind ourselves that the UK Beveridge Report stated that the prevention and treatment of disease by any future National

**Table 1.1**  Which health differentials are inequitable?

| Determinant of health differentials | Potentially avoidable | Commonly viewed as unacceptable |
|---|---|---|
| 1. Natural, biological variation | No | No |
| 2. Health damaging behaviour if freely chosen | Yes | No |
| 3  Transient health advantage of groups who take up health promoting behaviour first (if other groups can easily catch up) | Yes | No |
| 4. Health damaging behaviour where choice of lifestyle is restricted by socio-economic factors | Yes | Yes |
| 5. Exposure to excessive health hazards in physical and social environment | Yes | Yes |
| 6. Restricted access to essential health care | Yes | Yes |
| 7. Health-related downward social mobility (sick people move down social scale) | Low income Yes | Low income Yes |

Health Service was just one part of a more comprehensive plan of general social welfare designed to combat the now almost legendary 'five sources of misery' – the 'giants' of 'want, disease, ignorance, squalor and idleness'. It is interesting to note increasing contemporary recognition that the giant of disease is most likely to be slain by tackling the remaining four !

## Voluntarism and the empowerment imperative

A healthy nation is not only one which has an equitable distribution of resources but one which also has an active empowered community which is vigorously involved in creating the conditions necessary for a healthy people. Accordingly, one of the key principles and a major driving force in health promotion is the notion of voluntarism – that people should, other things being equal, be encouraged to make free choices and should be trusted to act independently and in a responsible manner. As we will note later, other things are rarely equal. Therefore, health promotion, in accordance with democratic principles, has a responsibility not just to value and trust individuals and communities but to ensure that they have the power to freely choose and efforts are made to create a sense of responsibility for their fellow human beings.

A further underlying assumption of health promotion is that health, like warfare, is too important to be left to the professionals – in this case, medical practitioners. Moreover, following the precepts of Illich and empirical observations of iatrogenesis, it is clear that medical services may not only fail to meet the needs of the public but

actually create harm. The problem, in the context of the goals of health promotion, is not so much that clinical iatrogenesis may occur but rather that the traditional *modus operandi* of medicine is depowering. People are frequently passive recipients of care and good advice. On the other hand, the pre-eminent concern of health promotion should be to enable rather than coerce. The goal should be cooperation rather than compliance.

Accordingly, following the exhortation of the Ottawa Charter, there must be a 'reorientation of health services'. The changes in direction and emphasis are not just to ensure that services are accessible, equitable and empowering but, even more important, to recognise that a wide and varied range of public and private services and institutions influence health for good or ill. They should, therefore, be incorporated in health promotion planning and their energies and expertise harnessed, within a 'healthy alliance', for the promotion of health. We will have more to say on this point when we later discuss the 'settings approach' and the important issue of *inter-sectoral collaboration*.

## UPSTREAM OR DOWNSTREAM? THE CHALLENGE OF VICTIM BLAMING

People's health is not just an individual responsibility; our health is, to a large extent, governed by the physical, social, cultural and economic environments in which we live and work. To cajole individuals into taking responsibility for their health, while at the same time ignoring the social and environmental circumstances which conspire to make them ill, is a fundamentally defective strategy – and unethical. It is, in short, *victim blaming*. For these reasons, 'building healthy public policy' is considered to be at the very heart of health promotion.

## Zola's river analogy

Zola's celebrated 'river analogy' of medical care (Zola, 1970, cited by McKinlay, 1979) has frequently been used to explicate objections to the narrow individualistic 'victim blaming' focus of many health education tactics. This parable describes a doctor's increasingly frenzied rescue efforts as (s)he struggles to drag drowning people from the flood. The doctor remarks *You know, I am so busy jumping in, pulling them to shore, applying artificial respiration, that I have no time to see who the hell is upstream pushing them all in.* McKinlay considered the individually directed approach of health education as a 'downstream' endeavour. He pointed out the ultimate futility of this kind of strategy and argued that we should ... *cease our preoccupation with this short-term problem-specific tinkering and begin focusing our attention upstream.* Pursuing the nautical metaphor, and using a currently popular image, the preventive model of health education may be likened to the rearranging of the deck chairs on the Titanic.

**Box 11** A Case for Refocusing Upstream

> *'You know', he said, 'sometimes it feels like this. There I am standing by the shore of a swiftly flowing river and I hear the cry of a drowning man. So I jump into the river, put my arms around him, pull him to shore and apply artificial respiration. Just when he begins to breathe, there is another cry for help. So I apply artificial respiration, and then just as he begins to breathe, another cry for help. So back in the river again, reaching, pulling, applying, breathing and then another yell. Again and again, goes the sequence. You know, I am so busy jumping in, pulling them to shore, applying artificial respiration, that I have no time to see who the hell is upstream pushing them all in'.*
>
> McKinlay (1979)

We might note a related metaphor, in which paramedics are shown loading various injured people into an ambulance strategically placed at the foot of a steep cliff. Rather pointedly, a lone advocate of preventive medicine is shown busily building a fence at the cliff edge and observers are expected to draw the conclusion that prevention is better than cure. Clearly, it is possible to elaborate on the aquatic metaphor: presumably the hospital and mortuaries are located somewhere near the river mouth with the first-aider working somewhat further upstream. The fence builders will be working further upstream still. However, Zola's observation about the importance of the 'political economy' of illness makes it clear that he is arguing for work at the very fountainhead or source of the river – addressing the social and economic determinants of health and illness.

## Blaming the victim

Some years ago in Britain a former Junior Minister of Health committed an interesting gaffe during a visit to the North of England that illustrates nicely the victim blaming tendency. It is of course a matter of epidemiological record that the diet in Northern Britain leaves a lot to be desired! The minister's advice to northerners was that they should act responsibly and eat prudently. The scarcely disguised implication of the exhortation was that failure to eat sensibly was due to ignorance at best and, at worst, to fecklessness.

The reality is that the problem is rarely if ever due to ignorance; if poor diet is related to any personal characteristic, that personality trait is not fecklessness. As we will see later, it would be more legitimate to ascribe unhealthy behaviours to general apathy and 'learned helplessness' resulting from chronic exposure to debilitating social conditions – and lack of money.

The importance of social and structural factors in determining whether or not individuals select and eat a prudent diet is certainly well documented. Charles and Kerr's (1986) research demonstrates categorically that women – the dietary 'gatekeepers' in most cultures – were well aware of the difference between healthy and unhealthy food. Although they might not possess detailed technical knowledge, they not only knew enough to produce nutritionally sound meals for their families, they were positively motivated to do so. They were, however, prevented from doing this by a series of barriers, of which one was quite simply the financial cost of healthy meals.

It is, of course, naive to argue that cost is the only barrier to the adoption of healthy behaviour in general and sensible eating in particular. It is nonetheless of paramount importance. Lang *et al.* (1984), for instance, demonstrated convincingly that in Britain healthy food was both more expensive and less accessible for people living in disadvantaged circumstances. More recently the National Consumer Council (1992) commented that the cost of food in local corner shops was at least 20% more expensive than in (frequently less accessible) supermarkets. It noted too that 47% of families seeking help from the Family Welfare Association did not have enough money for food after paying for rent, fuel and other necessities. More than half were £10 per week short. The Council also argued that, contrary to popular belief, poor people often adopt a very rational course of action in managing their limited resources: they acquire more nutrients per penny than those who are better off. Unfortunately, in doing so, they exist on a diet high in sugar and saturated fats and low in fruit and vegetables. The minister, it would appear, was indeed guilty of blaming the victim.

Although 'victim blaming' is readily used as a condemnatory term of narrow preventive programmes, it is worth clarifying its origin and the peculiar slant given to it by its inventor – William Ryan (1976).

Victim blaming, according to Ryan, is a tendency which relates not only to health and illness, but is at the heart of many contemporary social phenomena such as crime, poverty and racism. In common with Navarro (1976), Ryan views victim blaming as an ideological process, which serves to justify inequalities in society, including inequalities in health. Inequality is not merely a regrettable by-product of the pursuit of wealth but is an essential and enduring feature of capitalism. He describes John D. Rockefeller celebrating the virtues of inequality in Sunday school:

*The growth of a large business is merely a survival of the fittest ... . The American Beauty rose can be produced in the splendor and fragrance which bring cheer to its beholder only by sacrificing the early buds which grow up around it. This is not an evil tendency in business. It is merely the working out of a law of nature and a law of God.*

(p21)

Galbraith (1992a) makes a similar point in his observations about the victim blaming tendency of economists:

*Such was the service of economics to early capitalism. And such service has continued. Toward the end of the last century, in what has now come down to us as the Gilded Age, Herbert Spencer avowed the economic and social doctrine of the survival of the fittest – it is to him and not to Darwin that we owe those words. Though British, Spencer was a figure of heroic proportions in the United States, as were his disciples. His most distinguished acolyte, William Graham Sumner of Yale, (Sumner, 1914, p.90) served the gilded constituency in remarkably explicit language: 'The millionaires are a product of natural selection ... . They may fairly be regarded as the naturally selected agents of society for certain work. They get high wages and live in luxury, but the bargain is a good one for society.'*

(pp80–1)

We should note that the crude social darwinism expressed by Rockefeller and Spencer is not, according to Ryan, victim blaming proper. Liberal socially concerned professionals who are genuinely committed to deal with the effects of inequality and help its victims espouse victim blaming. Their victim blaming lies in the fact that they concentrate on the victims and seek to help them through various individually focused enterprises. Their failure results from their not tackling the social origins of the problem.

For Ryan the solution is dramatically simple: he encapsulates it in a subsection of his book entitled *'In Praise of Loot and Clout'*. Power and money, in effect, provide the solution to the problem of inequality and its by-products. In support of this contention he quotes the vaudeville star Fanny Brice's celebrated aphorism: *I've been rich*, she said, *and I've been poor; and, believe me, rich is better.*

Ryan elaborates on the effects of poverty:

> *Being poor is stressful. Being poor is worrisome; one is anxious about the next meal, the next dollar, the next day. Being poor is nerve-wracking, upsetting. When you're poor, it's easy to despair and it's easy to lose your temper. And all of this is because you're poor. Not because your mother let you go around with your diapers full of bowel movement until you were four; or shackled you to the potty-chair before you could walk. Not because she broke your bottle on your first birthday or breast-fed you until you could cut your own steak. But because you don't have any money.*

(p157)

Ryan's scathing attack on essentially psychological (or rather psychoanalytical) remedies to social problems is undoubtedly timely. As we have emphasised previously, it is not possible to deny the central importance of poverty in general, and relative poverty in particular, in the aetiology of health and social problems. However, to argue only for a shift in the distribution of wealth as a solution to these problems is both politically problematic and technically naive, as we will later indicate.

Before considering the relevance of our discussion of ideological matters for the adoption of one or other 'model' of health promotion, we should, for the sake of completeness, make a passing reference to the culpable concept of 'healthism'. We observed earlier that health promotion was welcomed by some people as a salutary alternative to what they saw as the negative messages of preventive medicine and its handmaiden, health education. In short, they espoused a definition that urged the pursuit of well-being. Crawford (1980) described this commitment to *individual* well-being as 'healthism'. It was still victim blaming –

possibly with a more cosmetically attractive patina!

## HEALTH PROMOTION MODELS AND THEIR IDEOLOGICAL BASIS

Luck and Luckman (1974) provide a useful general definition of a model (see Box 12).

**Box 12** The Meaning of Model

> *A model is a representation of the significant features of the problem under study. It can be a simple verbal description or a three-dimensional design such as is produced by architects or engineers, or it can be an abstract logical or mathematical representation. Since it is usually too expensive and risky to experiment blindly with the problem in the real world we need a model to allow us to examine the effect of a range of possible changes, either initiated by the decision makers or coming spontaneously from the environment. The model builder always has to satisfy two conflicting needs: (s)he wants (the) model to be a faithful representation of the problem; (s)he also wants (the) model to be a powerful tool for examining a wide range of alternative courses of action, which implies that it must be simple to apply.*
>
> Luck and Luckman (1974)

In short, then, a model should provide a simplified representation of some aspect of reality that, nonetheless, incorporates all of the key elements needed to provide a meaningful account of the subject under review. Health promotion or health education models are of two sorts: ideological and technical. The former seek to provide a simplified but reasonably accurate explanation of how sets of values can give rise to different constructions of the major strategic purpose of health- and illness-related action. In other words, they assert what the purpose of health promotion and health education *ought* to be about. If seriously and systematically adopted they should, within the limits of political realities, govern professional and lay practice. Good 'technical' models, on the other hand, should provide a comprehensive account, which helps practitioners to translate their ideological commitments into practice. Further and detailed discussion of technical health promotion models will be examined in Chapter 2.

A comprehensive account of contemporary models of health education and health promotion is beyond the scope of this book – although several interesting analyses have been provided (for example, Draper *et al.*, 1980; Draper, 1983; French and Adams, 1986; Beattie, 1991, Downie *et al.*, 1992). We will content ourselves here with a tripartite conceptual analysis, which is considered to incorporate major distinctions in approach to philosophy and practice. This comprises:

- an Educational Model;
- a Preventive Model;
- an Empowerment Model.

## Education and the promotion of health

It is worth recalling that, in this present chapter, we are discussing *ideological* models. Accordingly, we might note the existence of two assumptions which are often made about education for health and which certainly cannot be said to be consciously ideological, nor dignified by the appellation 'model'. These assumptions do not only apply to health education but rather to any educational initiative. They can be characterised as:

- education as *communication*;
- education as *teaching*.

The first of these two assumptions has only a very limited ideological dimension, centring on the beliefs that people have a right to knowledge and that knowledge is power. Those subscribing to the list of values associated with WHO's formulation of health promotion would doubtless agree people do indeed have a right to knowledge. Hopefully, however, they would also recognise that the assertion that knowledge is power is a half-truth. Associated with this half-truth is the ingenuous

view that if knowledge is shared with a client, client group or any other kind of audience, the recipient of that knowledge will be capable of making health choices and making decisions (typically in accordance with the particular prejudices of the communicator!). In short, then, education has been confused with communication.

Communication is certainly one indispensable component in the educational process, but it includes much more, as the 'technical' definition of health education demonstrates (Box 13).

**Box 13** Health Education: A 'Technical' Definition

> Health education is any intentional activity that is designed to achieve health- or illness-related learning, i.e. some relatively permanent change in an individual's capability or disposition. Effective health education may, thus, produce changes in knowledge and understanding or ways of thinking; it may influence or clarify values; it may bring about some shift in belief or attitude; it may facilitate the acquisition of skills; it may even effect changes in behaviour or lifestyle.

The technical perspective provided by the above definition derives from viewing education as synonymous with '*teaching*' – since teaching is any planned or deliberate activity designed to achieve intended learning outcomes. To some extent this is a reasonable stance to adopt since any educational endeavour, *whatever its ideological orientation*, will be concerned to achieve learning outcomes. The ideological underpinning, however, will determine what learning outcomes are or are not acceptable.

## Education and ethics

Long before those involved in health education became immersed in ideological and philosophical debate, educationalists had explored and expatiated on such matters. Education was critically compared with and distinguished from a number of other activities, deliberate or unintentional, that resulted in learning. The main factor characterising education and distinguishing it from many of these other activities is that it must be *morally acceptable*. (Clearly, we must acknowledge that moral acceptability is culturally determined but we will ignore this for the moment – apart from noting that most cultures would at least pay lip service to WHO's ideological canons.)

Figure 1.3 depicts a spectrum of ethical activities – all concerned with promoting learning of one kind or another. Education is firmly located at the virtuous end of the continuum while '*brainwashing*' is relegated to the negative pole. Teaching, training and instruction occupy a neutral position, as their ethicality will depend on the learning goals for each specific instance. For example, training people to acquire the social interaction skills necessary for empathic relating to clients is clearly an ethical activity. On the other hand, instructing delinquents in the skills needed to become fully fledged criminals would not normally be considered an ethical activity – however efficient and effective it might be! '*Primary socialisation*' is located some way towards the 'brainwashing' end of the spectrum since the way many, if not most, parents shape their children's values and behaviours has more in common with that particular technique than with other forms of training and instruction (although admittedly the techniques of primary socialisation may well be more enduring than those in the armamentarium of brainwashing!).

## Voluntarism and the limits to choice

One of the most significant values central to edu-cation's ethical position on the moral high ground – and distinguishing it from the other activities in Figure 1.3 – is the principle of voluntarism (Tones, 1987). This derives in part from the views of philosophers of education, such as Hirst (1969), who considered that the cardinal characteristic of education was rationality and freedom of choice. As we mentioned earlier, the definitional criteria of education typically incorporate notions of an ethically acceptable goal; according to Hirst and other philosophers of similar persuasion, it also must use morally justifiable methods. In essence, the learner must fully comprehend what is happening to him or her during the educational process – and why. Accordingly, any kind of coercion or techniques that conceal the purpose of the communication – including persuasion – is by definition unacceptable.

Several 'official' health education pronouncements have, in the past, acknowledged this voluntaristic principle. For instance, the North American Society of Public Health Educators' Code of Ethics talked about informed consent and *change by choice, not by coercion* (SOPHE, 1976). Again, Green and Kreuter's (1991) oft-quoted definition of health education incorporated the principle of voluntarism:

> *In short, health education is aimed primarily at the voluntary actions people can take on their own, individually or collectively, as citizens looking after their own health or as decision makers looking after the health of others and the common good of the community.*

(p14)

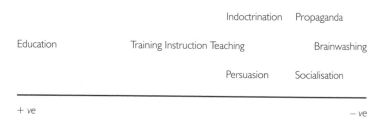

**Figure 1.3**   An Ethical Continuum of Influences on Learning

To reiterate then, voluntarism remains a cardinal principle of Health Promotion.

Not surprisingly, the methods recommended for a voluntaristic educational approach are much more sophisticated than those involved in mere communication. Clearly *understanding* is emphasised in relation to the acquisition of information, but this would be supplemented by an insistence that learners go through a process of values and belief clarification before they are in a position to make a voluntaristic choice. The values clarification exercise would in turn require specific techniques such as the use of group discussion. If this educational process goes according to plan, students will have acquired necessary information, have gained a thorough understanding of all the relevant issues and clarified their beliefs and values and thus, apparently, be in a state of readiness to make their decisions, either now or at some future time. The word 'apparently' is used advisedly since their state of readiness would also require the acquisition of decision making skills (a rather vague notion but probably involving the acquisition of some sort of '*minimax*' strategy for scanning alternative courses of action, calculating likely outcomes and comparing these with the values which have been previously clarified and then making an anticipatory decision designed to maximise benefits and minimise costs). Again, this latter would require the use of 'informal' teaching techniques such as simulation, gaming or role play. A more refined version of the approach would go one stage further and build into the curriculum the possibility for practising decision making – typically in a simulated setting. Certainly, health education curriculum projects in the early 1970s were at least paying lip-service to a need not only to provide information but to help students make informed decisions (admittedly there was a strong, not very well hidden agenda, that informed decisions should be the 'right' decisions – decisions which would lead to an approved preventive outcome). Again, various drug education programmes were at the forefront in recognising that knowledge and understanding must be supplemented by belief and values clarification and the practice of skills in simulated situations when the learner would be subjected to offers of legal or illegal substances.

## Challenges to an educational model

Now although the educational model, in its more sophisticated guise, is morally rather satisfying, it has its detractors. The first criticism is levelled against an apparent assumption that education will have been successful provided only that the learners are in full possession of the facts, have an in-depth understanding of the situation, have clarified their beliefs and values and acquired some practice in making decisions. In other words, an implicit suggestion that it does not matter what choice learners ultimately make as long as it is rationally based. Some of the exponents of the North American values clarification 'movement' were in fact taken to task over their apparent lack of interest in having a moral or ethical basis to their pedagogic concerns, apart from that of the process of values clarification itself. For example, Forcinelli (1974) took exception to the apparent amorality of the approach, noting that:

> ... *an educational system can produce a dishonest and potentially dysfunctional product and then merely say these are legitimate expressions of individual values. It is possible to conceive of one going through (a process of values clarification) and deciding that (s)he values intolerance or thieving.*

Some particular issues, of course, should be treated in a morally neutral way and many democratic societies consider it right that its citizens should disagree about important social matters and even encourage a degree of dissent. In other words, the 'values clarification' approach is entirely appropriate for encouraging decision making about controversial issues, i.e. significant social issues on which different groups and individuals in society urge different and conflicting courses of action. One prime example of such an approach in Britain has been the Humanities Curriculum Project (Stenhouse, 1969). Nonetheless, most educational programmes are not values neutral: they are firmly rooted, explicitly or implicitly, in quite conventional values. Many curriculum projects, for example, while emphasising the importance of personal growth and fulfilment, actively promote respect and concern for other people's right to self-fulfilment. McPhail (1977) encapsulated this principle in the phrase 'considerate way of life'. We have, by now, shown how health promotion should be rooted in concerns about equity and other key values – including McPhail's 'considerate way of life'. It must therefore be acknowledged that the notion of freely choosing which seems to be at the heart of the educational model is, in fact, curtailed by moral imperatives.

In the last analysis, it is doubtless self-evident that the voluntaristic principle that is at first glance sacrosanct to the educational model must be tempered by an equally powerful imperative to actively promote, rather than clarify, a number of fundamental values. However, the major weakness of a classic educational model is its failure to acknowledge the extent to which freedom to choose is curtailed by a number of internal, psychological factors and external constraints – including cultural norms and pressures. Genuine freedom of choice is a very rare commodity indeed.

Clearly ignorance is a barrier to informed choice but ignorance is relatively easily rectified; certainly this particular obstacle poses no threat to the educational model. On the other hand, a 'pure' educational approach would be unable to assist health educators to cope with two much more significant barriers to rational decision making: the first of these centres on individual limitations, while the second reminds us again of the potentially unhealthy influence of environmental factors.

First, it is apparent that in many cases individuals are not free to choose: their freedom of choice may, for example, be constrained by the presence of 'addictions' or other compulsive behaviours. As McKeown (1979) pointed out:

> ... it is said that the individual must be free to choose (whether he wishes to smoke). But he is not free; with a drug of addiction the option is open only at the beginning.

(p125)

**Box 14**  Charlie Brown and the Limitations to Choice

The dilemma of freedom of choice was nicely illustrated a few years ago by one of Schultz's *Peanuts* cartoons.

Charlie Brown is shown on a snowy day balancing a large snowball in his hand and looking quizzically at Lucy.

Lucy sternly returns his gaze and makes the following considered observation:

> *Life is full of choices. You may choose, if you wish, to throw the snowball at me ... You may choose if you wish, not to throw the snowball at me. Now if you wish to throw the snowball at me, I'll pound you right into the ground!*
>
> *If you choose not to throw the snowball at me, your head will be spared.*

Charlie Brown is shown on his own – without snowball and looking contemplative. He concludes that

> *Life is full of choices; but you never get any.*

More important, however, are negative socio-economic and material circumstances and the effect of these on individual attributes. For these reasons, two major challenges have been directed at the educational model. The first of these quite simply asserts that even the more sophisticated version (perhaps especially the more sophisticated version) will not lead to the abandonment of unhealthy behaviours and the adoption of a healthy lifestyle. One group of critics therefore advocates a much tougher and allegedly more realistic stance associated with a *Preventive Model* of health promotion. A second group of critics note that the *Educational Model*'s occupancy of the moral high ground is based on false pretences. In short, it might well stand accused of fostering a new and more subtle, albeit less harsh, form of victim blaming. The position adopted here is that neither the *Educational Model* nor a model centring solely on prevention are adequate to satisfy the ideological requirements of health promotion nor ensure that these are translated into effective practice. Before examining and justifying this assertion and providing a detailed explanation of a competing *Empowerment Model*, it is important to subject the previously dominant ideology and practice of prevention to some quite close scrutiny.

## HEALTH PROMOTION AND THE PREVENTION OF DISEASE

The second health promotion model to be discussed here derives from that well-established construct the *Medical Model*. The characteristics of this model are sufficiently well known not to need elaboration here. It may be summarised as having a mechanistic focus on microcausality; the body is viewed as a machine whose component parts are subject to attack from microbes or other pathogens. The prime function of medicine is to repair the machine when it malfunctions and to keep it in good running order. Health tends to be defined in terms of absence of disordered functioning – or, at any rate, in relation to the machine functioning as well as might be expected for its age and any possible inherent design flaws.

Apart from its focus on object rather than person – its enthusiasm for investigating the component part at the most reductionist level – the *Medical Model* has also been associated with another significant ideological imperative – the tendency for Western medicine to lay claim to ever larger areas of human experience. As we have seen, the health promotion movement, with its emphasis on reorientation of health services and lay competence, has provided a substantial and sustained challenge to this process of *medicalisation* – a process which, according to Kelleher *et al.* (1994)

> ... led to doctors being cast more and more in the role of secular priests whose expertise encompassed not only the treatment of bodily ills but also advice on how to live the good life, and judgements on right and wrong behaviour.

This challenge can also be viewed at its most vitriolic in the writings of Illich (1976) and his notion of '*cultural iatrogenesis*', i.e. the way in which medicine depowers whole cultures by sapping their self reliance.

In case the ideological basis of what lay people in Western society would regard as a perfectly normal way of thinking about health is not absolutely clear, it is worth recalling Doyal's (1981) lucid review of the ways in which health and illness are socially constructed. In common with writers such as Navarro (1979) she reflects a common critique that, apart from its reductionist tendencies, medicine reflects a capitalist value system. Since many commentators have subscribed to the view that capitalism is intrinsically 'unhealthy' ('wealth nor health'), it is unsurprising that a medical model should attract a degree of opprobrium. As Doyal points out, the functional definition of health by medicine reflects a capitalist value system which ... *defines people primarily as producers...* and is ... *concerned with their 'fitness' in an instrumental sense, rather than with their own hopes, fears, anxieties, pain or suffering.* Doyal cites Stark (1977) as follows:

> *Disease is understood as a failure in and of the individual, an isolatable 'thing' that attacks the physical machine more or less arbitrarily from 'outside' preventing it from fulfilling its essential 'responsibilities'. Both bourgeois epidemiology and 'medical ecology' ... consider 'society' only as a relatively passive medium through which 'germs' pass en route to the individual.*

The preventive model of health education, by definition, is concerned to contribute to the goals of preventive medicine and would thus be subject to the same ideological objections as the *Medical Model* proper. It would, however, be wrong to assume that the goals of health education and prevention were *necessarily* congruent with the dominant ideology of medicine (for which read curative *medicine*). Rather, it represented a revisionist tendency, a point which merits a little further consideration.

The history of preventive medicine in the late 19th and the 20th centuries may be rather simply described as revealing a decline in the public health movement paralleled by the ascendancy of curative medicine. With the rising incidence of chronic degenerative disease, preventive medicine enjoyed something of a revival at the same time as the hegemony of curative medicine was increasingly being challenged – primarily by public health doctors. McKeown's (1979) critique is now well known and generally accepted. Professor Knox succinctly described medicine's contribution to the public health in a tribute to McKeown shortly after the latter's death:

> Before 1900, doctors probably did more harm than good; between 1900 and 1930, they broke even; only since 1930, by which time the major health improvements of the present era were established, was it clear that doctors were beginning to win.

Doctors such as Cochrane (1972) also began to ask rather awkward questions about the effectiveness of many routinely accepted medical procedures and writers such as McKeown also suggested that curative medicine was not only experiencing some difficulty with chronic degenerative diseases, it was also neglecting its traditional caring functions. He detected ... *a new note of severity in contemporary criticism* of medicine and, rather mischievously, quoted Nancy Mitford's comparison of medical practice in the time of Louis XIV with the contemporary activities of curative medicine:

> In those days, terrifying in black robes and bonnets, they bled the patient; now terrifying in white robes and masks, they pump blood into him. The result is the same: the strong live; the weak, after much suffering and expense, both of spirit and money, die.
>
> (Mitford, 1969)

As we will see later, we argue that the apparently yawning ideological chasm between medicine and health promotion may be (and should be) narrower than the above critical comments might lead us to believe. For now, however, it is useful to provide a reminder of the classic rationale for health education's contribution to preventive medicine. It may be summarised as follows:

- Curative medicine has a limited capability for managing the major (western) burden of chronic degenerative disease and key infectious diseases such as AIDS. Moreover, its practice is characterised by accelerating costs and it incorporates not insubstantial iatrogenic 'side effects'.
- Prevention is, therefore, better (and cheaper) than cure.
- Since human behaviour plays a significant part in the aetiology of many diseases and in the management of all of them, education is needed to persuade people to behave appropriately.

The functions of health education in relation to the goals of preventive medicine are listed in Table 1.2.

It should be noted that the term 'health education' rather than 'health promotion' is deliberately employed in Table 1.2. The reasons will doubtless be clear after earlier observations about the importance of taking environmental circumstances into account and the need to avoid 'victim blaming'.

At any rate, after many years of neglect, the belated recognition of the importance of health education was greeted with a certain degree of satisfaction by health educators – even though the proportion of resources devoted by the UK, and most other health services, to health education was still diminutive. Moreover, preventive medicine itself still occupied a relatively lowly position in the medical pecking order and its subsequent metamorphosis into community medicine (and, more recently, public health medicine) did not necessarily improve matters. Again, it is a matter of conjecture whether the most recent change of name to public health medicine has signified any real rise in the status of public health. However, as we will note later, the most recent of all developments in the UK, i.e. since the change of government in 1997, has resulted in a remarkable emphasis on broad-based *health promotion* initiatives.

**Table 1.2** The Preventive Model and levels of prevention.

| Level of prevention | Function of health promotion |
|---|---|
| *Primary prevention* | *Health Education.* Concerned with health behaviour, i.e. those activities undertaken by individuals believing themselves to be healthy in order to prevent future health problems or detect them asymptomatically |
| Aim: to prevent onset of disease/reduce its incidence | *Aims:* to persuade individuals to adopt behaviour believed to reduce the risk of disease by adopting 'healthy' lifestyle; to persuade individuals to utilise preventive health services appropriately<br>*Policy aims:* to engineer environmental circumstances in order to prevent disease (typically involving legislation, economic and fiscal measures and actual structural changes to the environment); to ensure availability of and access to relevant services and provide staff training |
| *Secondary prevention* | *Health Education:* Concerned with illness behaviour, i.e. those activities undertaken by individuals experiencing symptoms in order to determine their state of health; subsequent adoption of measures designed to meet perceived need |
| Aim: to prevent development of existing disease, minimise its severity, reverse its progress, reduce prevalence | *Aims:* to persuade individuals to utilise screening services appropriately, learn appropriate self-care and seek early diagnosis and treatment for amenable conditions; to persuade individuals to comply with medical recommendations<br>*Policy aim:* to ensure availability and access to relevant services and provide staff training |
| *Tertiary prevention* | *Health Education.* Concerned with adoption and relinquishing of sick role |
| Aim: to prevent deterioration, relapse and complications, promote rehabilitation and help adjustment to terminal conditions | *Aims:* to persuade individuals to comply with medical treatment, including palliative measures, and to adjust to limitations resulting from effects of disease; to persuade patients to resume normal behaviours consistent with impairment; to provide terminal care counselling where relevant<br>*Policy aim:* to provide appropriate services and training for staff |

Certainly, the 1970s version of the preventive model of *health education* received a good deal of official support – though still with a relatively small proportion of the health and education budgetary provision. Ironically, this happened at a time when the model espoused by government was being subjected to increasingly vigorous criticism for its victim blaming tendency. The reasons for this apparent paradox was quite clear and entirely consonant with Doyal *et al.*'s critique of the enterprise culture. First there was the economic imperative: it was assumed that money could be saved for the hard pressed medical services if people could be persuaded to adopt healthy lifestyles; second there was the ideological imperative: it was right that individuals should take responsibility for their own health and, additionally, should become good consumers (and, thus, it was acceptable and even desirable to challenge the status and alleged restrictive practices of medicine). In short, the pre-ventive model was ideologically and practically consonant with an individualistic, enterprise-oriented culture.

In the context of our earlier discussion of the ideological principles of health promotion it is not surprising that the preventive model of health education has come under attack in recent years. In part, the critique has derived from a view that medicine has somehow 'hijacked' education as part of a process of 'professional medicalisation' (Vuori, 1980). The *Preventive Model* of health promotion is summarised in Figure 1.4.

## The radical challenge

Various '*radical*' approaches to health promotion have been proposed as more acceptable alternatives to the *Preventive Model* discussed. Bearing in mind Zola's exhortation to 'refocus upstream', they might reasonably have been called 'upstream models' or, again, acknowledging the primacy of

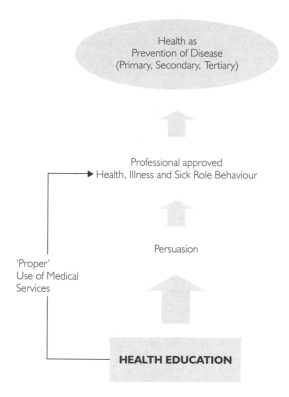

**Figure 1.4**   A Preventive Model of Health Education

centred on the preventive model's inherent victim blaming (Brown and Margo, 1978; Labonte and Penfold, 1981; Coreil and Levin, 1985; Rodmell and Watts, 1986), which, in turn, derives substantially from the dominant ideology of health associated with the *Medical Model*.

We have, of course, already observed how the *Preventive Model* of health education relates to its bed-fellow the *Medical Model* (though not always very comfortably). We also noted its relationship to the process of medicalisation while commenting on the alleged congruence between the *Medical Model* and the ideology of capitalism. It is, therefore, worthwhile at this juncture reiterating the close ties between the values and beliefs underlying the individually focused preventive imperative and the key Western ideology of capitalism. In short, capitalism and the pursuit of profit are viewed as intrinsically unhealthy. For instance, concern for the environment is of secondary importance to profit; the workplace is frequently a source of illness (Watterson, 1986); the enterprise culture gives virtually free rein to the marketing of products irrespective of their effects on health. Indeed, it can be argued that health and wealth are in some fundamental way incompatible (Draper *et al.*, 1977). This point of view is, of course, central to Marxist tradition. As de Kadt (1982) succinctly points out:

> ... *they see ideologies as weapons in the class struggle whereby, for example, hegemonic groups portray reality in such a way as to make those dominated conform to their fate, which may then give rise to 'false consciousness' on the part of the latter.*

He goes on to cite the *Communist Party Manifesto*:

> ... *the ruling ideas of each age have ever been the ideas of its ruling class.*

Navarro's often quoted attack on 'conventional' health education is consonant with this interpretation. As he notes,

> ... *rather than weakening, [health education] ... strengthens the basic tenets of bourgeois*

social and environmental influences on health, they might alternatively have been designated as 'social-structural' models of health promotion – or, in recognition of a need for collective action to influence health and social policy, the term 'collectivist' might have been employed. As it is, and after etymological consideration, we have employed the word 'radical' above to indicate a need to scrutinise the *roots* of health problems and develop programmes accordingly. It might be argued that this is rather a weak justification, since advocates of the preventive model would probably consider the roots of ill health were to be found in an individual's errors of omission or commission. However, the notion of radicalism can also serve to indicate a challenge to a dominant ideology (in this case, the *Preventive Medical Model*). The major source of dissatisfaction has *individualism ... far from being a threat to the power structure, this lifestyle politics complements and is easily cooptable by the controllers of the system.*

(Navarro, 1976)

While the traditionally individualistic focus of medicine and the preventive model's – perhaps unthinking – concentration on individual lifestyle and behaviours fit readily with capitalism's concern with individual enterprise and effort, many medical practitioners would be horrified to find themselves accused of collusion with capitalism's oppression of the masses. This may, of course, represent false consciousness, but we should comment that there is one other reason for doctors' apparently unreasonable victim blaming ideology. Before developing this observation, let us first of all emphasise that the essence of victim blaming is not just working with individuals. If this were the case the only really ethical health promotion activity would be the use of mass media (and, as we will note in a later chapter, mass media are frequently used in a highly unethical fashion!). Again, teaching children in the classroom would automatically involve victim blaming! Clearly, victim blaming consists of ignoring the broader social, material, economic and cultural factors determining individual behaviour and placing the entire burden of responsibility for action on individuals (victims) themselves while, at the same time, not recognising the limits to the individual's power to act and, on occasions, denying the individual the opportunity to take responsibility when he or she actually has some scope for making choices. Therefore, any victim blaming associated with health promotion in the medical setting has nothing to do with medical personnel working with individual patients (if it were true, then individual counselling of an asthmatic would be victim blaming while providing patient education in a group would be ideologically acceptable); rather, it has to do with the locus of responsibility and the extent to which opportunities are provided for empowerment.

## De-powering effects of the sick role

We mentioned above that there was a second possible reason for medicine to espouse a victim blaming

approach to health promotion – other than a commitment to right-wing entrepreneurial policies. In short, this derives from the way in which the perceived need for patients to adopt a *'sick role'* has led to the imperative for patients to *comply* with medical advice. As noted elsewhere (Tones, 1998), the very term 'compliance' is incompatible with the values of health promotion (even in its more recent sanitised translation as 'adherence').

An extensive discussion of the sick role (Talcott Parsons, 1951, 1979) is not appropriate here. However, the process can be summarised as follows.

- Sick persons are unable both to fulfil their social roles and lack the power to overcome their incapacity; they cannot thus be *held responsible* (authors' emphasis) for their incapacity and some therapeutic intervention is needed to aid recovery.
- They thus enter the sick role and are, consequently, exempt from their normal social obligations.
- Although this sick role has been medically legitimated, being ill is to occupy a deviant status and is undesirable.
- Accordingly, people in general have an obligation to seek medical help and patients have an obligation to *comply with* medical advice (authors' emphasis).

The complementary practitioner role involves the provision of non-judgemental support while, at the same time, clearly approving appropriate behaviour and disapproving inappropriate behaviour. Of particular interest in the context of the centrality of empowerment for health promotion, the therapist should maintain a degree of detachment related to the *'competence gap'* existing between professional and client. As DiMatteo and DiNicola (1982) observe, *The disparity in power and control carves an emotional chasm between physician and patient – a chasm that is bridged only by the physician's altruism and orientation to serving people* (p51). Doctors must 'deny reciprocity' in order to avoid the kinds of interpersonal relationships associated with other normal social interactions.

It has of course been acknowledged quite widely that the sick role 'prescription' is problematic. It becomes immediately untenable once the treatment involves more than taking prescribed medication. Moreover, if patients are expected to comply unswervingly with medical advice on the one hand but, on the other, are expected to take decisions, change their unhealthy lifestyles and generally 'look after themselves', both they and the doctor are placed in an ambivalent and unenviable position. Doctors too can face a difficult dilemma: suppose they consciously try to cast off their traditional authoritarian role and work in a patient-centred way, then those patients who have been socialised into expecting to be told by the doctor what to think and what to do may doubt the doctors' competence and express dissatisfaction if they are consulted about the nature of their symptoms and treatment!

In Chapter 2 we will offer a model of an empowering and ethically 'correct' encounter between medical practitioner and client which should go some way to achieving both a satisfactory preventive outcome and at the same time reduce the regularly lamented but typically observed 40–50% rate of non-cooperation between practitioner and client. However, such an encounter could not possibly work within the strictures of the traditional doctor–patient interaction described above.

A further manifestation of the imbalance of power associated with the Parsonian view of patient and practitioner has to do with effect of hospitalisation on patients. In short, following Goffman's (1961) classic analysis of the hospital as a total institution, observers such as Taylor (1979) have commented on how hospitals are one of the few places in which individuals forfeit control over virtually every task they customarily perform. This has particular relevance for our later discussion of the *Health Promoting Hospital*.

At this juncture it is probably useful to note the emergence of a rather broader challenge to medicine than the political and sociological critiques to which reference has been made so far. Gabe *et al.* (1994), for instance, having reminded their readers of the power and authority of medicine in the following somewhat colourful manner,

*… the occupation of healing changed from being frequently seen as a rattlebag of quacks and rogues to a profession with considerable power, authority and status.*

then proceeded to list a number of diverse influences that currently challenged medicine. They included the challenge from an increasingly powerful management culture in the UK health services (Hunter, 1994); the effect of professionalisation of occupations allied to medicine and, in particular, nursing (Witz, 1994) and the increasing threat of litigation (Dingwall, 1994); the important influence of the feminist movement (Doyal, 1994); the anti-vivisectionist movement (Elston, 1994); *some* self-help groups (Kelleher, 1994); the phenomenon of 'trial by television' (Bury and Gabe, 1994).

## HEALTH PROMOTION AND EMPOWERMENT

Having explored the nature of so-called educational and preventive models of health promotion – and their limitations – we turn now to an analysis of an approach which is favoured in this book and which is consistent with the ideological commitment to equity and the values inherent in WHO's formulation of health promotion. Its central concern is with the empowerment of communities and individuals. It is not, however, merely an extension of an educational model – and thus subject to accusations of a more genteel and sanitised form of victim blaming. Rather, it incorporates the main elements of what we earlier described in terms of a radical challenge to the narrow preventive approach. Central to the 'anatomy' and functioning of this model is the reciprocal relationship between the environment and the individual; between individual and community empowerment; between empowerment, 'healthy public policy' and engineering those aspects of the environment that will make the healthy choice the easy choice. These relationships are shown diagrammatically in Figure 1.5.

Following our earlier emphasis on inequalities and equity, Figure 1.5 reiterates the view that the underlying goal of health promotion and health education is the achievement of equity, i.e. a fair

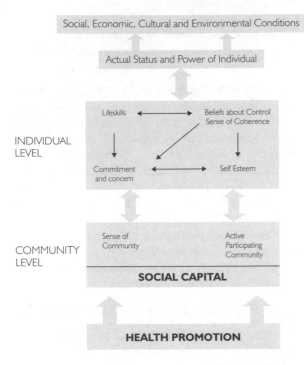

**Figure 1.5**   Reciprocal Determinism: Health Promotion
and the Environment

distribution of power and resources. Figure 1.5 focuses on the contribution of health education. As we have seen, whether or not equity is achieved depends on the material, social, economic and cultural circumstances obtaining in a given country, city or neighbourhood. These environmental factors and associated political systems will either facilitate or militate against the achievement of health.

As regards empowerment, it can reasonably be argued that the state of empowerment is fundamentally healthy and therefore worth pursuing in its own right. In Figure 1.5 its *instrumental* function is portrayed: an *active, participating community* (i.e. an empowered community) is shown as a prerequisite for the development of healthy public policy which, in turn, will act as moderating influence on the environment.

A reciprocal relationship is deemed to exist between community empowerment and self-empowerment. An empowered community facili-

tates the development of self-empowerment in its members. On the other hand, although there is strength in numbers, an empowered community is no more than the sum total of its empowered members.

The relationship between people and their environment is also reciprocal. Clearly, the environment may exert a powerful controlling influence on people, but people can also influence their environments – provided only that the environment is not so completely oppressive as to stifle all individual activity. Two directions of popular influence are shown in Figure 1.5. Individuals and communities may interact directly with their environment and/or may exert pressure on government or other authorities at national, regional, organisational and local levels in order to achieve the implementation of healthy public policy.

## The notion of empowerment

Many references have been made in this chapter to empowerment – in particular the ideological dimension. The detailed dynamics of empowerment and its operationalisation will be the subject of further discussion in Chapter 2. For the present we will merely define individual or self-empowerment as a set of competences and capabilities which, together with certain related personality characteristics, contribute to a relatively high degree of actual control over a given individual's life and health.

**Box 15**

Self-empowerment is a state in which an individual possesses a relatively high degree of actual power – that is, a *genuine* potential for making choices.

Self-empowerment is associated with a number of beliefs about causality and the nature of control that are health promoting. It is also associated with a relatively high level of realistically based self-esteem together with a repertoire of *life skills* that contribute to the exercise of power over the individual's life and health.

As we will see in Chapter 2, aspects of a *Sense of Coherence* (Antonovsky, 1979), to which reference was made at the beginning of this chapter, are associated with self-empowerment. Community empowerment will also receive further consideration in Chapter 2. For the present, we will provide a little additional elaboration on the earlier statement that an active participating community is the sum of the empowered individuals it contains. At one level, the importance of such a dynamic community is self-evident – a community that has confidence, a range of skills and a commitment to act will be in a better position to influence its material and social circumstances than a community that is apathetic and alienated.

Furthermore, there have been suggestions that in some way an empowered community consists of more than the sum of its parts. Indeed, the very definition 'community' implies a sense of shared goals and circumstances together with a more or less extended network of relationships and interactions. The term *'sense of community'* is used to describe this kind of 'gestalt' and, according to McMillan and Chavis (1986), has four main characteristics:

- membership: a feeling of belonging;
- influence: a sense of mattering;
- integration and fulfilment of needs;
- shared emotional connection.

One of the most comprehensive analyses of the concept was provided by Maton and Rappaport (1984) who looked for the *... correlates and contexts of empowerment among members of a Christian, non-denominational religious setting.* The researchers defined a sense of community in terms of *... a sense of closeness with a loving God who actively transforms* (i.e. empowers) *members' lives .... (i.e. increased compassion and humility and a desire to serve and help others).* The researchers' summary of church members' verbalisations of their religious ideals illustrates the centrality of *'meaningfulness'* to this particular definition of empowerment. This is revealed by

> *... a desire for increased closeness with God and for God to meet personal needs together*

> *with a desire to become more compassionate and self-sacrificing as people; the goal of developing deep trust and childlike dependence on God together with the need to retain intellectual honesty in dealing with doubts and personal responsibility for one's decisions; and a desire for the fellowship to be a 'family' which provides both interpersonal and material support for members together with a desire to involve everyone in decision making and to be able to change structures and traditions whenever they begin to rigidify and interfere with members' spiritual and personal growth.*

(p42)

## Social support and social capital

As we will see in a later chapter, one of the most thoroughly replicated research findings is that access to and therefore the provision of social support is almost inevitably beneficial for the promotion of health and being a member of a 'genuine community', having a shared sense of purpose and a network of mutually supportive relationships, must surely be fundamentally healthy. However, although it might seem churlish to question the apparent sanctity of a 'sense of community', it is possible to envisage such a community being prey to 'false consciousness' and living cosily contented within a generally unhealthy and unjust system (a similar challenge will be made in the next chapter to the apparent beneficence of an individual 'sense of coherence'). We must, therefore, keep in mind health promotion's firm commitment to the creation of 'active participating communities' rather than a contented community. Indeed, membership of a 'virtual' community, i.e. connection with other people but *across* geographical boundaries, may be more beneficial in terms of provision of support for community members. The currently popular notion of *'social capital'* may very well contribute to a sense of community but encapsulates and emphasises the importance of engagement and action (Mustard, 1996).

At the time of writing – certainly in the UK – the development of social capital is viewed as a kind of antidote to 'social exclusion' and the kinds of social and health problems associated with descriptions of disadvantaged neighbourhoods and the characteristic disorders associated with the 'underclass'. The work of Putnam (1993a, b, 1995) has been most influential in the formulation of the concept and has been formally defined as those ... *features of social organisation, such as networks, norms, and trust, that facilitate co-ordination and co-operation for mutual benefit* (Putnam *et al.*, 1993, pp35–6.)

According to Putnam, '*Civic Societies*' possess *stocks of social capital* such as *trust, norms and networks* that tend to be self-reinforcing, cumulative and generate *virtuous circles* that result in *co-operation, civic engagement and collective wellbeing*. Of particular interest from the perspective of this book is the fact that most of the desirable features can in principle be specifically defined and measured and thus serve as indicators of effective programmes. Equally important, however, is the prior process of accurately operationalising the feature of community participation. Again, a similar concern for the promotion of community participation and action may be seen in the idea of 'active citizenship' as promoted by the European Foundation for the Improvement of Living and Working Conditions (Chanan, 1997). A former president of the EU is approvingly quoted:

> *There is a need to mobilize people. Dialogue is essential and nothing can be done without grassroots involvement. We must set out on the road towards a more active participatory society.*
>
> (p1)

Campbell *et al.*'s (1999) critical appraisal of social capital and its influence on health provides an important cautionary note about not being too readily seduced by the attractions of this popular notion's putative solutions to the problems of alienation and helplessness. For instance, they reiterate our earlier observation that sources of social capital often cross geographical boundaries and 'diverse and geographically dispersed network types' might be more health enhancing than

other types of traditional community. Moreover, contrary to Putnam's references to involvement in voluntary association and organisations, Campbell *et al.*'s research in the UK found that *informal* networks of friends and neighbours constituted the bulk of any existing social capital. Furthermore,

> *Putnam's essentialist conceptualisation of a cohesive civic community bore a greater resemblance to people's romanticised reconstruction of an idealised past than to people's accounts of the complex, fragmented and rapidly changing face of contemporary community life – characterised by relatively high levels of mobility, instability and plurality.*
>
> (p156)

In general, though, the time would seem to be ripe for collaboration between national and international bodies in pursuit of policies designed to achieve the virtuous circle of factors that promote health and social regeneration through an active, committed citizenry. The kinds of substantial policy change involved in such an ambitious venture is not easy to achieve. Education must figure prominently in this venture.

## Education and policy: a symbiotic relationship

The relative contributions of social, economic, cultural and material environmental and individual action have been central to our discussion so far. We have noted how the 'primitive' form of the *Preventive Model* has rightly been accused of victim blaming because of the way it has emphasised the individual at the expense of the social and environmental. We have also observed how the Ottawa Charter and related pronunciamentos have repeatedly underlined the importance of 'building healthy public policy' in order to create a supportive environment. At the same time, health education has, arguably, been sidelined – having been contaminated by its victim blaming history. The position adopted here is that both education and policy are essential to the achievement of health promotion goals. Accordingly, we would suggest that a basic 'anatomy' of health promotion can be incorporated in the following simple 'formula':

**Box 16**  The Anatomy of Health Promotion

> health promotion = health education × healthy public policy

The rationale for this assertion is doubtless obvious: on the one hand health education can expect to achieve limited success unless it operates within a supportive environment. For instance, a general sense of dissatisfaction with what they perceived as the relatively ineffectual efforts of health education in reducing the incidence of smoking in young people inspired the '*BUGA UP*' crusaders in Australia to launch a high profile – and generally illegal – campaign to achieve a shift in public policy relating to smoking. In other words, education to persuade people to quit smoking was severely hampered by the advertising tactics and the calculated misinformation produced by the tobacco industry. Accordingly, it was argued that political action and the implementation of policy measures to ban advertising and sponsorship was essential to promote the public health. As we will note in our later discussion of mass media, the strategy seems to have been largely successful.

It can, of course, be argued that health education alone may achieve satisfactory results – as has been demonstrated on a number of occasions in the field of patient education. However, even when people are quite well motivated to learn and to change their behaviours, it would be unusual if better results could not be achieved by providing a supportive environment – such as enhanced material circumstances and access to social support.

On the other hand, those who, often obsessively, promoted the policy route have frequently had to acknowledge that the implementation of healthy public policy is exceedingly difficult to achieve when powerful individuals, organisations and vested interests are firmly opposed to change. Governments and others who hold the reins of power will often make mere token gestures to

healthy policy without the radical and empowering contribution of education – as we hope to demonstrate later. At this juncture, however, some elaboration of the importance of healthy public policy is justified

## The primacy of policy in health promotion

Following our earlier discussion of equity and inequality, it is not surprising to find that those concerned with placing policy at the centre of health promotion's activities frequently focus on this key issue. For instance, Milio (1986), in an influential book on the subject, reminds us that

> *Most, if not all, of the variations in the modern illness profiles of men and women ... can be understood as responses to the differing environments which they ... typically experience.*

She suggests two ways in which health promoting policy might be developed. First, a principle of equity might guide policy formation such that all groups of people might be exposed to the

> *... same excesses and deficits of both health-promoting and health-damaging circumstances.*

Alternatively

> *Policy ... might be developed with a view of some attainable optimum in health, for instance, the level achieved by some groups (within the USA) or by certain other nations. Not only would all people be equally exposed to the pluses and minuses of environment, but the policy objectives would center on minimizing health-damaging circumstances and on minimizing or eliminating both excesses and deficits of health-promoting resources, such as selected food and energy supplies.*

(p71)

As we previously observed, healthy public policy is at the heart of an ecological approach to health promotion such as that embodied in the Ottawa Charter and in its list of prerequisites for health the Charter included: *food and education;*

*shelter; a stable ecosystem and sustainable resources, peace; equity and justice.* Central to the attainment of all these policy goals is the imperative of redistributing economic resources. If a reminder of the significance of the Charter's assertions should be needed, a particularly timely jog to the memory was recently provided by Doll (1992) in his Stallones Memorial Lecture. In this he concluded that

> ... *the principal environmental hazards worldwide are those associated with poverty of individuals within the market economy and of communities in the developing countries ... . In future ... they will be the effects of overpopulation and the production of greenhouse gases.*

In a very real sense, then, economic policy is health policy. It is, therefore, especially appropriate that the World Health Organization has emphasised the importance of taking account of the health dimensions of economic reform (WHO, 1992) – especially in relation to developing countries. The notion of '*health conditionality*' should be applied to all economic developments. In other words, the implications for health of any economic measure should be considered at the very start of the planning process and should be taken into account at the development and implementation stages of planning;

> ... *the objective of economic decision making should from the beginning include the objective of protecting and promoting the quality of life.*

(WHO, 1992, pix)

Anderson and Draper (1991) adopted an even more radical stance in their call for a fundamental review of economic policy. They have *inter alia* called for a re-think in the way we define economic benefits. Of particular interest for our present discussion, they argued for the replacement of inappropriate indicators, such as Gross National Product (GNP), with new measures of economic success which are congruent with the goals of health promotion.

Dahlgren and Whitehead (1991) gave a num-

ber of examples of healthy public policy related to the pursuit of equity (see Box 17).

**Box 17** Examples of Healthy Public Policies

---

*A French policy resulted in 'foyers' – a scheme that combined housing for young people with opportunities to obtain training and employment skills and the provision of preventive services, health education and leisure facilities.*

(p25)

*The 'Newpin' Project in London was devised to deal with high rates of maternal depression, isolation, poor child health and child abuse in a severely disadvantaged area. It comprised a voluntary befriending service at home with a neighbourhood drop-in centre.*

(p25)

*The Swedish government created a 'Swedish Working Life Fund' by imposing a tax on business that raised 2000 million ECUs. This was paid back over a five year period to companies that produced sound proposals for improving conditions in their workplaces.*

(p28)

*In Liverpool, the health authority devised schemes, using government grant aid, to employ 250 long-termed unemployed people in socially useful work such as dental health education and hospital security.*

(p32)

*Norway's food and nutrition policy, initiated in 1975, addresses equity issues by means of pricing policies, farming subsidies and improvements in transport and distribution of food to ensure that cheap, nutritious food is more readily available in local shops. Supportive educational services are also made available.*

Dahlgren and Whitehead (1992)

---

More recently, the Acheson Report (Department of Health, 1998) on inequalities in health directed attention to eight areas for future policy development:

- income;
- tax and benefits;
- education;
- employment;
- housing and environment;
- mobility;
- transport and pollution;
- nutrition.

It made

*three crucial recommendations ... all policies likely to have an impact on health should be evaluated in terms of their impact on health inequalities; a high priority should be given to the health of families and children; further steps should be taken to reduce income inequalities and improve the living standards of poor households.*

A further 36 more specific policy recommendations were made – and these should ... *demand the commitment of the government as a whole.*

The recommendations are listed in Appendix 3.

In July 1999 the UK government did in fact provide an indication of its commitment: it listed several examples of inequality and inequity together with the actions that it was taking to reduce these (Department of Health, 1999b). As the report put it,

*We are ensuring that the needs of people who have suffered the effects of inequality for too long are placed at the centre, rather than the margins, of plans for health and social improvement.*

(p39).

Bearing in mind Galbraith's observation, cited earlier, it remains to be seen whether the resources needed for quite fundamental changes will be forthcoming.

## Meso and micro level policy

Of course, policy does not only operate at the macro level and involve political manoeuvring on the national and international stage. It also oper-

ates at a meso level – for instance in relation to the development of smoking policy in the workplace or the achievement of supportive policy measures in the health promoting school. Box 18 provides a nice example of 10 key points associated with the development of a policy designed to facilitate the adoption of breastfeeding in hospital and increase its incidence and prevalence. The policy itself involves not only organisational and environmental changes but also includes a requirement for staff training and education of the new mothers. It reminds us that not only is education required to bring about policy change, policy is required to facilitate the provision of education and educational services in a range of settings. We can also imagine the kinds of organisational and attitudinal barriers that might have to be overcome before the policy is accepted and fully implemented.

Again, at the micro level policy measures would be necessary to facilitate the provision of health education (e.g. by providing financial incentives for doctors) and they would also be required to provide a supportive environment to facilitate clients' or patients' adoption of new behaviours. For instance, as we will note in Chapter 2 when we consider the 'anatomy' of a face-to-face encounter between health practitioner and client, a doctor might seek to influence policy measures relating to the provision of benefits or social services support for a depressed patient who is fearful that she might physically abuse her children.

**Box 18**  Ten Steps to Successful Breastfeeding

Every facility providing maternity services and care for newborn infants should:

1 Have a written breastfeeding policy that is routinely communicated to all healthcare staff.

2 Train all healthcare staff in skills necessary to implement the breastfeeding policy.

3 Inform all pregnant women about the benefits and management of breastfeeding.

4 Help mothers initiate breastfeeding within half an hour of birth.

5 Show mothers how to breastfeed and how to maintain lactation even if they are separated from their infants.

6 Give newborn infants no food or drink other than breast milk, unless *medically* indicated.

7 Practise rooming-in, allowing mothers and infants to remain together 24 hours a day.

8 Encourage breastfeeding on demand.

9 Give no artificial teats or pacifiers (also called dummies or soothers) to breastfeeding infants.

10 Foster the establishment of breastfeeding support groups and refer mothers to them on discharge from the hospital or clinic.

*UNICEF Baby Friendly Initiative*

(Note also the seven point plan involved in the *community* Baby Friendly Initiative.)

## Healthy public policy: the coercion trap

The role of health and social policy in addressing the fundamental determinants of health has already received some detailed consideration. Indeed, as we have noted above, the development of policy has been regarded by some 'radicals' as the only serious way of avoiding victim blaming and implementing sound public health measures. It is easy to see why. The use of legislation, taxation and measures designed to change the physical environment and material circumstances can in principle have a rapid and often proven effect on the determinants of health, health services and health-related behaviours. However, a determined pursuit of such social engineering strategies can be – somewhat paradoxically – more appropriate to a narrow, authoritarian preventive model of health promotion. Not unreasonably it can also leave health promotion open to those pseudo-libertarians who are always ready to label health promoters as 'health fascists'! Certainly, those who espouse an empowerment approach to health promotion can be faced with a challenging dilemma since many, if not most, policy measures

militate against the principle of voluntarism. And voluntarism is perhaps the main plank in the platform of those who follow the path of 'true' education. It is also an underlying principle in an empowerment approach to the promotion of health.

Garrison Keillor provides an entertaining and ironic cameo of the application of swingeing policy measures (and in certain US states, not too far from the truth!).

*Box 19*  End of the Trail

> *The last cigarette smokers in America were located in a box canyon south of Donner Pass in the High Sierra by two federal tobacco agents in a helicopter who spotted the little smoke puffs just before noon. One of them, Ames, the district chief, called in the ground team by air-to-ground radio. Six men in camouflage outfits, members of a crack anti-smoking joggers unit, moved quickly across the rugged terrain surrounding the bunch in their hideout, subdued them with tear gas, and made them lie face down in the hot August sun. There were three females and two males, all in their mid-forties. They had been on the run since the adoption of the Twenty-eighth Amendment.*
>
> Keillor (1990 p3)

The implementation of healthy public policy typically limits freedom of choice. In an extreme case, legislation designed to raise the wages of the poorly paid and reduce the earnings of the rich (probably one of the most fundamentally effective health policy measures) would actually restrict wealthy people's capacity to make money!

Even when the focus is on facilitation, removing barriers that limit some individuals' capacity to make healthy choices can limit other individuals' freedom to do as they want. The process of achieving equity and a socially and economically productive life is to some extent a zero sum strategy.

Of course, those who exist in relative poverty would doubtless accept that imposing limitations on the excesses of the wealthy classes would be an entirely laudable policy measure. On the other hand, measures to restrict their own unhealthy behaviours would be greeted with a chorus of disapproval: banning smoking in workplace or bar; draconian increases in the price of alcohol and tobacco; ensuring that only healthy food was served in the works canteen – all such policies would doubtless be considered an inappropriate intrusion into private life and an infringement of liberty.

The degree of coercion involved in the implementation of policy clearly varies from case to case. Figure 1.6 depicts this 'Spectrum of Coercion'. One pole is the location for various legislative measures, such as banning tobacco advertising and smoking in public places, that involve prohibition.

At the other pole are located those measures that, in general, facilitate choice. For instance, the coercive fiscal policy of regular increases in taxation on cigarettes will undoubtedly impose a disproportionate burden on the impoverished smoker; on the other hand, the provision of free nicotine substitutes for those affected is essentially facilitative and will reduce the negative effects of the coercive measure and increase the likelihood of smokers quitting their habit. The provision of cycle tracks and good, accessible exercise facilities will reduce barriers to making healthy choices (admittedly it may well antagonise those who resent state 'interference' and the related tax burden).

We also re-visit earlier observations about the *Educational Model*'s commitment to voluntarism and indicate how the 'educational spectrum' in Figure 1.3 relates to the symbiotic relationship of education and policy. Figure 1.6 reminds us that coercion is not only due to policies that provide environmental restrictions but also to strategies that range from ethically acceptable, voluntaristic approaches to manipulative tactics that involve different degrees of psychological coercion. Not surprisingly, empowerment is at the facilitative end of the continuum. Again, in accordance with Figure 1.3, 'brainwashing' features at the coercive end. Those who have a somewhat idealised image of parent–child interaction might be somewhat offended at the placing of primary socialisation at the extreme pole of psychological coercion! Since primary socialisation can involve a range of often latent activities, such as modelling, emotional blackmail and other techniques akin to brainwashing, this categorisation should be unremarkable. In the somewhat sanitised words of Philip Larkin, *They screw you up, your mum and dad.*

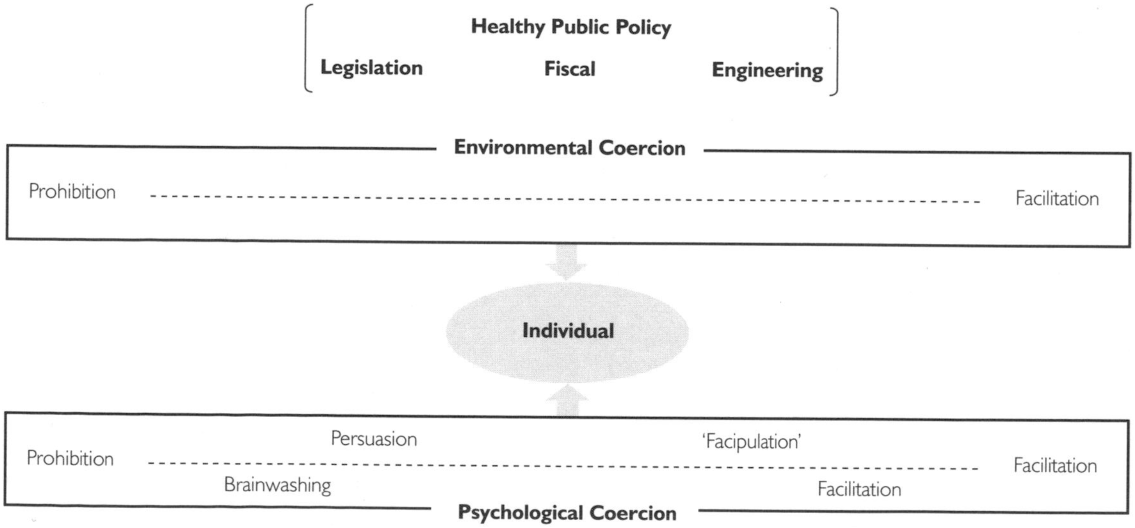

**Figure 1.6** A Spectrum of Coercion

Of course, it is both possible and desirable that primary socialisation should emphasise such child rearing devices as independence training and the enhancement of self-esteem. To the extent that these are effective, primary socialisation might appear at the empowerment end of the continuum.

In the context of future discussion of community development, the term *'facipulation'* merits some brief explanation. Community development would seem to epitomise an ethical, voluntaristic, empowering and generally ideologically sound approach to health promotion. However, Constantino David (1982) noted the temptation for community workers to subtly influence community members – under the guise of participation. Perhaps with the praiseworthy intention of demolishing 'false consciousness', they seek to indoctrinate the client group with the political ideology that motivates the community workers themselves. This is the process of *'facipulation'*; it may also appear in an equally subtle form in face-to-face counselling – again an educational and therapeutic proceedure that should be both empowering and voluntaristic.

It is, hopefully, clear then that there is quite considerable ambivalence involved in the adoption of the view that health promotion should comprise the synergistic mix of education and policy – especially since the notion of education itself can be paradoxical. It would, however, be foolish to naively accept the principle of voluntarism. As we have seen, there are clearly stated values underpinning the health promotion enterprise and these should be quite transparent and openly stated. Although the empowerment model adopted here is least likely to damage the principle of voluntarism, commitment to that principle must be limited by the pursuit of these 'higher' values. Following this argument, it is possible to justify the use of coercion in certain cases. Briefly, the adoption of coercive measures is justified (and has been justified for many centuries) in terms of the twin concepts of *utilitarianism* and *paternalism*.

The principle of utilitarianism states that people's freedom of action should be respected as long as it does not interfere with the general good.

As John Stuart Mill (1961) put it,

> *The only purpose for which power can be rightfully exercised over any member of a civilised community, against his will, is to prevent harm to others. His own good, either physical or moral is not sufficient warrant.*

There are, of course, a surprisingly large number of instances where power is exercised in order to prevent harm to others – or at any rate to the public purse. Health promotion is not at all unique in seeking to use healthy public policy to avoid damage to individuals, communities and the national good.

Although Mill argued that power should not be exercised over other people for their *own* good, on utilitarian grounds, the principle of paternalism legitimises such interference in certain cases. In short, we may coerce others who are deemed to be incapable for whatever reason of making 'rational' decisions themselves. Whereas ignorance may not justify paternalistic intervention (since ignorance is relatively easily rectified), being young has frequently been considered to be sufficient grounds for adults making decisions for children! The educational system itself not only places a legal requirement on attendance (at least in developed countries) but determines what students will be taught. Lefanu (1994), in a publication whose main purpose was to challenge the 'health fascist' tendency of health promoters, complained that health education in schools seemed to be ... *qualitatively different from most other forms of education whose aim is to impart knowledge or intellectual skills.* It was, of course, naïve or ingenuous of him to make an assumption that schools operated in a values-free way – merely providing knowledge and intellectual skills. As we noted earlier, educational philosophers such as Hirst (1969) considered rationality to be the true purpose of education but the application of such a principle in practice has been rare indeed.

Certainly in UK in the 1960s and early 1970s schools at least paid lip-service to notions of encouraging children's growth and development and creativity – and considered it important to foster social education and debate about controversial issues. However during the heydays of the Thatcher years, indoctrination was barely concealed in the eager ideological thrust to 'get back to basics' (which seemed to involve support for often out-dated methodologies such as rote learning and a keen desire to convert the curriculum into a device to engender a narrow notion of 'enterprise' for economic growth together with a concern to promote certain equally narrow and dogmatic 'family values'). What the curriculum signally failed to do was to foster voluntaristic decision making.

We must, therefore, reiterate the point that health promotion's value position must be quite transparent. It centres on the pursuit of social justice and employs democratic principles. It must, therefore, accept the principle of utilitarianism and take account of the common good; in the interests of individuals' welfare it must on occasions subscribe to the principle of paternalism since it is clear that some individuals are not capable of looking after themselves or, alternatively, have given their informed consent to health promotion 'treatment'. We could reasonably assume that since some 60–70% of smokers regularly declare that they would prefer not to smoke, various measures which might be viewed as coercive may be used for the good of the 'de-powered' client group. Such coercion should, clearly, not be used merely because the health promoter happens to disagree with the preferences and passions of this client group!

A further paradox might be suggested at this point. If voluntarism and empowerment should be central ethical concerns for health promotion, should empowerment not only be a central concern in dealing with clients and the public but also govern relationships with politicians and others in power who will be the subject of lobbying and advocacy? Or is it legitimate to use various manipulative, coercive and persuasive tactics associated with a top-down preventive approach with this latter group ? Is there to be one law for the public and clients and another for those whom health promoters are concerned to influence? For instance, are health service managers to be treated as clients whereas 'opponents', such as the tobacco industry and others promoting unhealthy products, should be subjected to whatever cunning weapons experts in media advocacy have in their armamentarium ?

## AN *EMPOWERMENT MODEL* OF HEALTH PROMOTION

Having considered an *Educational Model* and a *Preventive Model* of health promotion – and having found these lacking both ideologically and practically, a model is now proposed that seeks to remedy the deficiencies of these two alternative models. As the name suggests, particular emphasis is placed on the primacy of empowerment – and the synergism between education and policy. The model is shown in Figure 1.7.

Two major categories of 'input' are shown in Figure 1.7 as promoting health; the first of these is concerned with creating health public policy, the second with influencing individual choices. The policy dimension figures prominently and, in a manner that has been earlier explored in some detail, is viewed as one of the major devices for managing the social, economic and material circumstances that have such an important influence on health. In short, there is a major 'upstream' focus in this particular model of health promotion.

As with the *Educational Model* and *Preventive Model*, the empowerment approach depicted in Figure 1.7 is also concerned to acknowledge the importance of influencing individual choices. After all, the most common health promotion work involves some kind of face to face encounter with individuals or small groups of individuals. However, whereas the *Preventive Model* seeks to persuade and coerce and the *Educational Model* merely aims to provide information, the model favoured here seeks to empower choice by building individual capacity – as defined in an earlier reference to self-empowerment. Additionally, of course, the measures defined in the model are designed to remove the broader environmental barriers militating against genuine freedom to choose.

Furthermore, whereas the opponents of the victim blaming inherent in the narrow educational

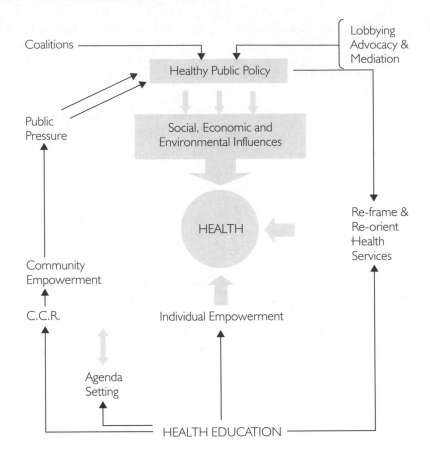

**Figure 1.7**   An Empowerment Model

and preventive approaches to health promotion have emphasised the importance of achieving radical political action (principally through the processes of lobbying and advocacy) the present model argues forcefully for the inclusion of a '*radical-political*' educational process having as its raison d'être a challenge to social rather than individual pathogens and the creation of public policy designed to counter these.

In short, the proposed characteristics for effective and ethical health education include the following principles.

• It makes a direct contribution to *individual* health by influencing health- and illness-related behaviours. It does not, however, operate in a discredited 'top-down' fashion; it does not seek to persuade, coerce and cajole, but rather contributes to self-empowerment: if successful it enhances individuals' control over their lives and their health.

• It follows the *Preventive Model*'s precedent in its concern to influence health services. Its function is, however, considerably different: it does not aim to promote the 'development and proper use of services' by, for example, persuading clients to use services in a medically approved fashion but aims to re-orient those services by reducing barriers to access and making the services more 'user friendly'. More importantly it contributes to 're-framing' perceptions of what health services should be: for instance, it demonstrates how such diverse organisations as housing, transport and economic development corporations can make a significant contribution to health – or illness.

- Finally and, arguably most important, it seeks to mobilise community opinion and concentrate public pressure on government and other powerful agencies such that they are impelled to create policies designed to address the broad determinants of health. It does this by a process of *'critical consciousness raising'* (CCR) and community empowerment.

The synergy of policy and education can be seen, particularly, in relation to the re-orientation and re-framing of services. On the one hand, health education can provide empowering education for patients relating to service utilisation and, on the other, can provide education and training for service personnel – for example, training of occupational health nurses or first aid personnel in the workplace. The three lobbying processes can seek to change policy relating to the health services, for instance, in tackling inequity of provision encapsulated in the 'Inverse Care Law' (i.e. those most in need of health promotion services are least likely to benefit from them).

We will examine this educational process in greater detail below but, first of all, we should give some consideration to the varieties of lobbying activities that have been viewed as the methods of choice for combating unhealthy circumstances.

## Lobbying, advocacy, mediation and community coalitions

This 'triad' that occupied a prominent place in the Ottawa Charter is shown in Figure 1.7 and comprises powerful tools for influencing the material and social determinants of health. The meaning of lobbying is well enough defined in everyday parlance and is a traditional avenue for those seeking to influence governments and other powerful individuals and organisations. It is used here as any attempt by individuals or organised interest

groups to exert pressure on those having the power to introduce new policies or change existing policies. Advocacy is a particular variety of lobbying and, although the term is open to more than one interpretation, advocates have one trait in common: they actively seek to represent the interest of relatively under-privileged groups and thus redress, at least in part, imbalances in power.

Advocates have, by definition, greater power and influence than their clients and particular skills, which they put at their clients' disposal. The reality is, however, that even highly competent advocates may make little impact on dominant power structures. Indeed, in a recent critique of the notion of advocacy, Baric (1988) commented on the Acheson Report (Department of Health, 1998) on public health in the UK. This report proposed the establishment of directors of public health who might reasonably have been expected to have an advocacy function. However, these new public health specialists, unlike their forebears – the medical officers of health – were effectively forbidden from challenging authority, even though to do so might well have been in the public interest. Important instances of powerful bodies interceding on behalf of the disadvantaged and unhealthy have been recorded – for example, the British Medical Association and the Church of England (Canterbury, 1985) have taken up the cudgels on behalf of a socio-economic underclass – such efforts tend to merely dent the dominant ideology of prevailing power structures. It would, indeed, be a brave government – some might say suicidal – which would be prepared to court electoral resentment at the kinds of fiscal policy needed, for example, to redistribute wealth. Governments of all political persuasions might feel it wiser to have recourse to pious hopes of achieving some future economic growth which would allow them to improve the status of the impoverished by the dubious mechanism of 'trickle down', to which reference was made earlier in this chapter.

It is, of course, much more convenient when ideology can be used as a basis for inaction. The relevant ideological arguments have been well rehearsed by many right-wing politicians. They usually centre on commitment to the values of robust individualism and enterprise. It is considered to be not only possible but actually a worthwhile and edifying experience to rise above poverty and achieve success. Such points of view are typically buttressed by assertions that it is in fact possible (by employing appropriate management skills) to live on state benefits. An equally popular rationalisation is that there is, anyway, no genuine poverty in today's Western democracies (compared, say, with previous eras or with the current situation in developing countries). Our earlier discussion of inequity will hopefully have given the lie to such assertions.

Given the problems in achieving change in the face of powerful opposition, the notion of mediation is useful since it reminds us that health promoters are but one of a number of stakeholders in a *policy community*. These stakeholders typically indulge in a process of negotiation and bargaining within an arena of conflicting demands for policy implementation. Moreover, since health promoters may well be relatively low in the political pecking order, compromise may be the only viable outcome. Examples of a particularly unsatisfactory compromise have been demonstrated over many years in the negotiation between the 'health lobby' and the tobacco manufacturers and resulted in, for example, the various 'voluntary agreements' – although due credit should be accorded to the UK government which, at the time of writing, has promised implementation of a complete advertising ban on tobacco products. '*Consultative collaboration*' between media producers and health promoters has often been more productive and resulted in a 'win-win' situation in which changes have been made to potentially health damaging images, presentations or programmes without insult to the entertainment value of the media productions in question.

Reference is also made in Figure 1.7 to the term 'coalition', in recognition of the potentially powerful effect on policy of the creation of health promoting alliances. Further reference will be made later in this book to this concept but for now we need only note that there is quite convincing evidence that coalitions can make an effective contribution to building healthy public policy. The alliance between health promoters and the great, the good and the powerful – with an added ingredient of community participation – might achieve more than lobbying, advocacy and mediation. Reference to community participation leads us to consideration of what we argue here is potentially the most powerful of all determinants of policy change – radical, consciousness-raising education.

## Education for radical action: critical consciousness raising

The so-called 'new' public health has been associated with radical challenge. However, it is worth reminding ourselves of the role health education played in the 'old' public health and there are indeed many interesting parallels between the first public health movement and the doctrine of health promotion. For instance, the sanitary reforms of the 19th century were associated with a general reforming zeal directed at the overall squalor, poverty and poor working conditions of the populace. Moreover, the reformers met with vigorous opposition and, as is the case today, their demand for state intervention was seen as ideologically unsound. We have already noted Rockefeller's recourse to social Darwinism to support his Panglossian assertion that all is for the best in the best of possible worlds – and how, in the 19th century, the writings of Herbert Spencer were used to show how poverty was part of the natural order of things (a role played today by economists judiciously selected by politicians!). Again, the perceived threat to profit stimulated angry reactions from commercial interests.

Health education was not recognised as such but health 'propagandism' and pamphleteering were in evidence – and greatly resented! Sutherland (1979) quotes a petulant article in *The Times* newspaper which declared that the people would *... prefer to take the chance of cholera and the rest than to be bullied into health* (p7). Incidentally, Sutherland also described a rather nice example of early 19th century victim blaming when he referred to the Manchester and Salford Sanitary Association's employment of working class women as indigenous health education aides to teach the 'laws of health' to the poor! We might also note the suggestion that one of the most significant influences on public health reforms was the perception by the wealthy that they themselves were at risk from the unrest and diseases of the underclass – a matter of some significance for contemporary predictions that the 'overclass' might well have to take refuge in fortified ghettos to keep the militant underclass at bay. Hopefully, appropriate consciousness raising will convince members of the 'overclass' to shrug off the 'culture of contentment' and recognise that the most comfortable solution all round is to tackle disadvantage and relative poverty. At all events, the pamphleteering of the 19th century would appear to have points in common with the radical health education process of modern times and the most appropriate formulation for this is Freire's invention of '*critical consciousness raising*'. The term critical consciousness raising is derived from the Brazilian-Portuguese term *conscientização* – translated as ... *the development of the awakening of critical awareness* (Freire, 1974 p19).

Freire contrasts critical consciousness with '*magical consciousness*', which apprehends facts and fatalistically attributes them to some superior power (the relationship with external locus of control will no doubt be self-evident). '*Naive consciousness*', on the other hand, involves a more realistic perception of causality but accepts it uncritically. In other words, it represents the 'false consciousness' of those who have accepted the rightful reality of a dominant ideology. The purpose of CCR is to help people break free of false consciousness and it does so by using the following four-step process.

• Fostering reflection on aspects of personal reality.
• Encouraging a search for, and collective identification of, the root causes of that reality.
• Examination of implications.
• Development of a plan of action to alter reality.

This integral process of planning and action rooted in critical reflection was referred to as '*praxis*' by Freire. The techniques and methods employed centred on group work ('*culture circles*') and used a '*dialectical*' problem solving approach to discussion. A more comprehensive discussion of Freire's radical strategy is beyond the scope of this book. However, Minkler and Cox (1980) provide a succinct analysis of the approach with case studies of work in Honduras and San Francisco. Macdonald and Warren (1991) also offer a useful application of Freirean theory to primary health care.

The *quality* of the knowledge resulting from CCR is distinctly different from other educational approaches. Those who have participated in the group dialogue will have not only a deeper understanding of their circumstances (as opposed to their personal risk) but also some important beliefs about self, i.e. their capacity to influence their circumstances. Again, the implications of praxis are not at first glance dissimilar to the action planning built into the process of attitude change central to a preventive model. However, the commitment is to social rather than personal change and incorporates a powerful affective element: if CCR is effective, people will not only be aware of social issues, understand them and believe that it is possible to change their circumstances, they will also feel indignant and want to translate understanding into action.

The implication of what has been said so far about the Freirean approach might lead to the conclusion that in challenging the dominant ideology and presenting an alternative meaning system the radical model is in some way educating rather than persuading; is providing a 'true' picture of reality. This is not necessarily the case and de Kadt (1982) strikes a cautionary note:

> *In post-revolutionary situations, in countries with Marxist governments, conscientisacion may be bound up with wider political activities and mobilization behind the party line ... Freire insists that people must be allowed to discover things for themselves, that meanings must not be imposed for them on their world. Yet, of course, the discussion leader cannot but make available certain facts, give certain leads, encourage certain interpretations, which effectively turn the perception of the 'learners' in certain directions. This is*

*above all true for the party militant, mobilizing the people for a particular social transformation. One type of consciousness is thereby replaced by another ... the new consciousness will also be a partial interpretation of reality. It may show little realism about the obstacles that stand in the way of changing present structures, or may provide little more than ringing generalizations and abstractions about the social arrangements to replace those at present stigmatized.*

(p743)

There are parallels here with our earlier recording of Constantino-David's caveat about community development approaches.

There is a further limitation to Freire's philosophy and methods: an empowered community – as depicted in Figure 1.7 – has not only been elevated to a state of critical consciousness, it has a sense of community and a high level of social capital together with a range of skills and competences that can be used to convert consciousness into action. Hopefully it will also have powerful allies!

Again, although on occasions Freire would aim to provide some actual skills to those whose consciousness had been raised (after all, his original programme was concerned with adult literacy), there is no guarantee that the learners will have been equipped to change social circumstances. Apart from any possible misrepresentations of reality created by the teacher-activist, merely to raise consciousness in a general oppressive environment is considerably more unethical than victim blaming. In short, CCR can be dangerous! A cartoon – ascribed to Morley – illustrates the tightrope that political activists have to tread if they are to be effective and remain alive. The health worker is depicted as an ostrich confronting an authoritarian regime. (S)he is exhorted not to stick her head over the parapet – else it might be blown off – but, on the other hand, not to stick her head in the sand!

### Agenda setting

Reference to Figure 1.7 will reveal an educational process paralleling the 'mainstream' radical CCR/community empowerment function. It has been labelled 'agenda setting'; it is superficially similar to CCR in its concern to raise health issues for public consumption and in its potential effect on health policy. We can identify two main operations. The first of these might merely consist of raising issues in order to facilitate decision making about policy matters. This function might be illustrated by the use of a television documentary to inform the public about any currently controversial issue. More typical, though, is the political use of agenda setting. In this latter mode government may test the temperature of public opinion with a view to ascertaining the acceptability of new legislation. As we observed earlier, public policy measures are highly likely to result in some restriction of people's liberty or involve them in financial cost; psychological reactance (or, less technically, bloody mindedness!) is a predictable outcome.

Government is, of course, reluctant to court electoral unpopularity and can therefore use agenda-setting tactics via mass media as a kind of 'softening up' process – an elaborated and extended version of policy 'leaks' to journalists. Agenda setting may well happen incidentally. For instance, a series of mass media campaigns in Britain set the scene for the introduction of legislation making the wearing of seat belts in cars compulsory. While the campaigns achieved only moderate success in persuading individual drivers and front seat passengers to voluntarily use seat belts, raising public consciousness about the problem of traffic accidents and the benefits of seat belts doubtless laid the foundations for legislation – despite the fact that it restricted individual liberty – without generating any serious electoral costs for the government of the day.

It could, of course, be argued that agenda setting and CCR are not qualitatively different processes. It could indeed be postulated that policy measures could be located on a spectrum of political acceptability. On the assumption that government can afford to be only one small step ahead of public opinion, this spectrum would reflect the public's latitude of acceptance. For example, government might be favourably disposed to measures designed to alleviate inequalities in health but consider that the increased cost in taxation would be met with furious opposition by tax payers and therefore deemed to be electoral suicide. In short, the 'culture of contentment', to repeat Galbraith's important notion, might prove too strong.

It is, in fact, possible to conceive of such a spectrum of acceptability however, it is more useful to consider the agenda setting and CCR functions as qualitatively rather than quantitatively distinct. As we have noted, CCR involves a *radical* challenge to dominant ideology and should be reserved for situations where such a challenge can be demonstrated. Consider for instance the above-mentioned challenge to health inequalities. A left-wing government might be ideologically committed to remedying inequalities but be persuaded that the cost of the radical measures would be electorally unacceptable; realpolitik might therefore dictate inaction plus some degree of agenda setting designed to produce a climate of public opinion conducive to some limited policy implementation. On the other hand, a right-wing government might be totally opposed ideologically to state intervention irrespective of cost. Firm commitment to enterprise, the pursuit of profit and rampant individualism would be incompatible with radical healthy public policy. In this latter scenario more dramatic public pressure would be needed – perhaps in extreme cases leading to refusal to re-elect a recalcitrant government.

Consider the following less politically challenging – but nonetheless problematic – case of fluoridation of public water supplies. Now it is firmly established that the fluoridation of public water supplies is the most effective public health strategy for reducing the incidence of dental caries – particularly in lower social groups. Clearly, any such policy constrains individuals' freedom to drink non-fluoridated water. The scene is therefore set for an ideological confrontation between, on the one hand, the values of dental and public health practitioners and, on the other, proponents of voluntaristic choice – possibly represented by members of the Pure Water League or similar pressure groups. Despite some qualms about

accusations of fostering the 'nanny state', the ideological concerns of right-wing politicians – together with the conviction that money might be saved for the health service – may well be congruent with the wishes of the medical lobby. However, in the last analysis perceptions of electoral gain may be the sole determinant of action. For instance, if agenda setting were to result in opinion surveys and focus groups revealing an increased level of acceptability for fluoridation, legislation would be enacted without further delay.

## IDEOLOGICAL DIVIDES, FALSE DICHOTOMIES AND THE MEASUREMENT OF SUCCESS

So far we have explored the ideological basis of health education and examined a number of models. We identified a *Preventive Medical Model* and contrasted that with an *Educational Model* and an *Empowerment Model* – incorporating a radical dimension in the latter. We also enshrined the principle of voluntarism in this empowerment model and could thus be accused of annexing the educational model! This is not merely some meaningless sleight of hand; rather it reflects the fact that *any* model is just an attempt to impose meaning on complex realities. This particular attempt to simplify and make sense of the reality of debates about the 'true' purposes of health education and health promotion has apparently resulted in the construction of two separate models: a *Preventive Model* with an authoritarian disease-oriented focus and a radical, person-centred *Empowerment Model*. However, even this distinction is far from cut and dried. For instance, as we observed earlier, it is probably the case that empowering people is more likely to achieve successful preventive medical outcomes than an authoritarian approach employing coercive tactics. On the other hand, there is no logical reason why medical workers should not pursue preventive goals in a non-authoritarian client-centred way.

We are not, of course, denying the existence of ideological divides in health education: from earlier discussions it is quite apparent that there are often substantial variations in people's values and philosophies. It is, however, important to avoid reification; we must beware of false dichotomies and be sensitive to the fact that there may be several complex overlapping purposes in the practice of health education and health promotion. It is therefore our intention now to look for genuine conflicts in value and ideology and comment on false distinctions. A useful way of doing this is to briefly revisit Figure 1.7 and note how aspects of the different models of health promotion discussed so far are nested in this particular analysis of the empowerment imperative. For instance, although not explicitly labelled in Figure 1.7, the central goal of 'health' is considered to include both the results of the successful prevention and management of disease as well as more holistic and 'positive' formulations; accordingly, the importance of primary, secondary and tertiary prevention is acknowledged. However, given the ideological principles of health promotion adopted in this chapter, it is not surprising that two features of the classic medical model are not represented. First, health education's traditional emphasis on persuasion has been replaced by an emphasis on the empowerment and support of voluntaristic choice. Second, the territorial claims of a *Medical Model* have succumbed to the challenge of demedicalisation and 'reoriented' medical services are shown as just one part of a wider range of health promoting services. Thirdly, and most importantly, a 'bottom-up', non-authoritarian stance is adopted together with the radical, political challenge to a health damaging status quo and associated with critical consciousness raising and social mobilisation. In other words, a determined challenge to the power base of society.

## Ideological divides and personal prejudices

This would seem to be a useful point at which to consider the compatibility of the various health education and health promotion functions examined so far. We might, for instance, ask about the possibility of compromise in the radical challenge to dominant values. This in turn raises two further questions: to what extent are radicals prepared to compromise and is compromise logically impossible?

Essentially the issue centres on whether or not meaningful change is possible without radical confrontation with a value system. It is an issue too complex to be addressed here in any depth but it is interesting to note that de Kadt (1982), in his discussion of ideological aspects of critical consciousness raising, clearly believes that useful change has occurred without any fundamental change in capitalism, i.e. through a process of reform rather than by a 'radical transformation of the social system'. In support of his argument he cites the emergence of legislation to curtail the unbridled pursuit of profit: safety at work legislation, legislation about health standards of products and, 'more timidly', environmental pollution.

Interestingly, de Kadt refers to the influence of moderate left-wing writers such as J. K. Galbraith in achieving reforms. Whether or not these reforms are viewed as significant or minor and counter-productive, Galbraith has recently argued (1992b) that compromise is the only way of changing the 'unacceptable face of capitalism'. In a lecture to the Institute of Public Policy he commented on the success of previous left-wing challenges to capitalism but advocated abandoning polarised attitudes.

*Ours is an age of constructive pragmatism ... There can be no escape from thought into theology.*

*Inter alia* we must recognise that revolutionary challenge to capitalism is unlikely to be acceptable to the public; whether this be on account of self-interest or false consciousness is a matter of only academic importance.

In the context of this discussion about the efficacy and feasibility of espousing a radical ideology we might usefully revisit the notion of victim blaming. It will be recalled that victim blaming refers to the prescription of individual solutions to socially determined problems. A single-minded radical ideology would assert that for this reason only social/environmental solutions are acceptable – for instance by implementing appropriate health and social policy change. However, irrespective of any debate about compromise and the art of the possible, the radical solution in this instance is logically flawed. To reiterate an earlier observation, the assertion is naive in that individual learning will always be a necessary part of health education. First, there are instances where social or environmental measures are to a greater or lesser extent irrelevant. For example, patients need information and they need to acquire certain beliefs and attitudes together with actual skills if they are to manage their diabetes or their ostomies. Social/structural factors are important only to the extent that patients cannot afford to pay for the treatment or facilities are not available – or, more subtly, to the extent that their will and self-esteem has been sapped by negative social circumstances. Second, as we indicated in our comments on empowerment, individuals need a number of competencies before they can engage in radical challenge: these cannot be magically supplied through some sort of community action.

Therefore, one of the important false ideological dichotomies in health education derives from a misinterpretation of the true nature of victim blaming. It centres on an ill thought out tendency to deride the empowering and supportive function adopted by health educators working with individuals or groups of individuals. The use of life skills, for instance, to facilitate and support personal choice may be condemned as a new form of victim blaming. As we noted earlier, the reality is that the only form of education which is not concerned with individual clients is the use of unsupported mass media – which in the history of health education have, wittingly or unwittingly, adopted a victim blaming stance! If we consider more politically correct activities, such as the development of community coalitions or community development, we will find individually focused educational activities at their core. The formation of coalitions of community groups in order to create a power base from which to mount a radical challenge is an important strategy for remedying inequalities. However, the actual component educational activities involve work with groups and influential individuals such as community leaders.

Again, a classic element of community development consists of educational activities designed to empower small groups of individuals – quite commonly women – in a neighbourhood context. In fact, as we also noted earlier, consciousness raising without providing appropriate educational skills and competencies may be self-indulgent posturing and as unethical as true victim blaming! Therefore, to reiterate, it is more meaningful to reserve the term victim blaming for those circumstances in which any kind of health promotion activity fails to take account of relevant social, structural or environmental factors.

We have so far discussed a number of health education models and their ideological peculiarities and, as we observed earlier, these models are social constructions: they differentially represent people's beliefs about significant aspects of their world and the values they attach to them. If, therefore, we ask why people subscribe to one model or another we are enquiring into the beliefs and values they have acquired through the process of socialisation. General experience and socialisation will, for example, have created beliefs and prejudices about human nature and the purpose of life; professional socialisation will have generated notions and feelings about the proper courses of action to adopt in any given occupational practice.

The results of both kinds of socialisation may be observed in the ideological commitments espoused by health educators. Three dimensions of belief and value would seem to be especially significant in defining the purpose of health promotion and health education and, therefore, in defining the meaning of success. One of these might be described in terms of radicalism and conservatism; a second could usefully be described in relation to either a democratic view of people or, at the opposite pole, an authoritarian perspective. The third dimension, which we will now consider, concerns the beliefs and values associated with the *Medical Model*, which is contrasted with an alternative, holistic view of health.

The nature of the *Medical Model* has already been quite fully discussed and its major features identified as:

- a mechanistic, reductionist disease-oriented conception of health;

- the territorial imperative derived from this notion and described by the term medicalisation;
- a tendency towards paternalistic authoritarianism.

As indicated earlier, ideological dimensions are not necessarily 'factorially' unique. Insofar as medical practitioners still tend to be located at the authoritarian rather than the democratic end of the spectrum, then we might ascribe this phenomenon to the process of professional socialisation which, rightly or wrongly, was derived from a belief that the effectiveness and status of doctors depended on patients adopting a passive role! Alternatively or additionally, those of an authoritarian disposition might have been attracted to this particular profession.

It is not uncommon, of course, to associate the *Medical Model* also with the first of the three dimensions mentioned above: that of radicalism versus conservatism. We have already noted Navarro's (1976) identification of medicine with capitalism and this is by no means an uncommon view. Clearly, in many cultures – of which the USA would provide the archetypal example – medicine is virtually synonymous with the pursuit of profit. On the other hand, it would be unfair to tarnish socialist medicine with such an appellation. The essential nature of the *Medical Model* is more reasonably related to its narrow, mechanistic disease orientation. As such, any challenge derives from those who question its over-emphasis on physical aspects of health and the scant attention its pays to holistic approaches to well-being, 'positive health' and 'quality of life'.

We have discussed in various contexts the nature of radical challenge to dominant ideologies, of which the critique of capitalism and the victim blaming tendency is a prime example. Again, insofar as the *Medical Model* represents the status quo, critics may legitimately be defined as radicals. On the other hand, acceptance of the status quo *in toto* characterises extreme conservatism.

Just as people may well be normally distributed (statistically speaking) on a scale of radicalism versus conservatism, they may equally be located at some point on the third dimension – authoritarianism versus democracy. Those whose convictions result in their location at the authoritarian end of the scale would presumably believe that, since most people are more or less inadequate and not to be trusted, it is legitimate to make decisions on their behalf. In other words, in the context of the continuum shown in Figure 1.6, they will adopt a paternalist solution to most health issues. On the other hand, democratically inclined health educators would be convinced of the moral rightness of voluntarism and be committed to 'bottom-up' programmes based on the felt needs of the population – even when it might be naïve to do so!

This analysis is, of course, not new. It has been debated in general psychology for some time. For instance, McGregor's (1966) analysis of two extreme styles of management centred on the notion that there were two extreme and opposing views of human motivation. He described these as 'theory X' and 'theory Y'. Theory X was based on an essentially authoritarian and 'top-down' perspective characterised by such beliefs as people are by nature indolent, lacking in ambition, self-centred, resistant to change and gullible.

Cattell (1965) reminded us of the ways in which personality attributes can generate prejudices which frequently underpin what are superficially rational arguments. He cited William James, stating that

> ... *differences in intellectual conclusions among philosophers could be traced more to their differences in temperament than to any differences in facts available to them.*
>
> (p358)

According to this viewpoint, ideological inclinations and the choice of health education model may be determined, at least in part, by temperamental factors. Interestingly, two of the personality traits which Cattell incorporated into his factorially determined system have parallels with the two dimensions under discussion here. They are 'radicalism' versus 'conservatism' and a factor most conveniently described as 'toughminded' versus 'tenderminded'. Again, one of the better known personality typologies developed by Eysenck (1960) incorporates a two-dimensional model which seeks to explain various social attitudes, including political orientation. These two dimensions are radicalism versus conservatism and toughmindedness versus tendermindedness. Thus communist tendencies would be consistent with toughminded radicalism while fascism would be characterised by toughminded conservatism.

It would undoubtedly be rash to apply these insights from personality theory to health educators' predilections for different models and ideologies, at any rate without support from substantial factor analytic studies. Nonetheless, it is tempting to speculate that toughminded conservatives would more likely be enthusiastic advocates of the *Medical Model* whereas toughminded radicals would subscribe to movements seeking to challenge capitalist-inspired victim blaming. Presumably tenderminded radicals would be well represented in advocates of holistic health and, perhaps, the gentler versions of community development.

At all events, whether it be personality traits or clusters of beliefs and values which influence theoretical preferences, we should recognise that values and subjective interpretation rather than rational and technical analyses actually determine choice of model.

Suffice it to say at this juncture that the position advocated by the *Empowerment Model* depicted in Figure 1.7 makes it possible to reconcile some of these diverse personal philosophical positions. However, since it is fully consistent with the principles of health promotion outlined at the beginning of this chapter, it is predicated on a relatively optimistic view of humanity and is intrinsically opposed to a *narrow Medical Model*. Indeed, subject to the limitations defined in our earlier discussion of utilitarianism and paternalism, any approach which adopts an authoritarian stance is unacceptable – including those radical-political strategies that also seek to make the healthy choice the only choice. This assertion is, of course, itself a value statement and clearly readers

are free to pursue their own personal ideological goals – insofar as their professional circumstances allow this to happen! This chapter will now conclude with a quite brief discussion of the meaning of success from the standpoint of devotees of different models and ideologies.

## EVALUATION AND THE MEANING OF SUCCESS

Evaluation research seeks to provide answers to questions about the effectiveness of health promotion and health education. Its purpose is to measure success. Statements about success depend on the aims and goals of the health promotion or health education initiative. These aims and goals – as we have been at some pains to suggest – depend on ideological models. The *efficiency* of any given initiative is concerned with the degree of success achieved, i.e. with *relative* effectiveness, and involves explicit or implicit comparison with some alternative, competing initiative. The question of efficiency will be considered in Chapter 2. Our present interest is to discuss what success would look like when viewed from the standpoint of different models.

If WHO's litany of principles is followed then, in general, success must be judged in relation to these key ideological principles. For instance, in the last analysis we would look for evidence that people's lives were more socially and economically productive than they were prior to health promotion interventions. We might look for evidence of greater equity – that progress had been made in the campaign to slay the 'five giants of disease, idleness, ignorance, squalor and wa advocated by Sir William Beveridge over 50 ago. We would look for indications that public policy had been implemented, s tal was more widely distributed and were actively participating in improve their health. It would alistic to use such broad out success: we would need cators, a point discusse ter 2. For now w exemplify the c assess success for health promotion ventures operating in accordance with the different models discussed above. Firstly, the *Educational Model*.

## Effectiveness and the *Educational Model*

As we have seen, in its simplest form this model consists of merely providing knowledge. Success is not only easy to define but easy to achieve. For example, evaluation of a programme of education designed to reduce unwanted pregnancies in teenage mothers would need only to demonstrate that the client group had understood and remembered the various negative aspects of teenage pregnancy and the nature of contraception and contraceptive practice necessary to avoid pregnancy. A more thorough approach that was based on insights from educational psychology would provide more detailed and comprehensive insights into the various facts, concepts and principles – together with related and subordinated notions such as the physiology of reproduction. A more sophisticated model would require evidence that additional capabilities had been acquired and an evaluator would expect to find evidence that individuals had clarified their beliefs and values relating to sexuality and, for example, acquired certain cognitive strategies to help them make decisions consistent with their values. The learners might also be assessed on their capacity to show their competence in making decisions in a simulated real life setting.

success for this particular model it will, hopefully, be enlightening to refer to the two most recent health policy documents produced by the UK government, *Health of the Nation* (Department of Health, 1992) *and Saving Lives: Our Healthier Nation* (Department of Health, 1999a). This will also provide an opportunity to note the way in which a change of government has resulted in a change of stance which represents a shift from one ideological model in the direction of an approach that is much more consistent with the *Empowerment Model* advocated in this book.

Although the ministerial preamble to the *Health of the Nation* claimed a commitment to *... the pursuit of 'health' in its widest sense...* the *Preventive Model* best defines its dominant ideology. In the light of our earlier observations about compromise between radical and conservative ideology, it is noteworthy that *Health of the Nation* itself demonstrated some movement from an earlier more conservative and authoritarian position in that, unlike previous major official pronouncements, it accepted the importance of public policy and the need for inter-sectoral collaboration and inter-agency working. Moreover, some reference was also made to 'quality of life' in accepting that improvement to the public health would be made not only by 'adding years to life' (i.e. increase in life expectancy and reduction in premature death) but also by 'adding life to years' (minimising effects of illness and disability, promoting healthy lifestyles, physical and social environments and improving quality of life).

Again, in a section discussing the health needs of people in specific population groups, socio-economic variations in health status were acknowledged – albeit fleetingly and with a sense of some trepidation! However, in respect of this latter acknowledgement of the possibility of broader social determinants of ill health, a passing reference was made to a complex interplay of genetic, biological, social, environmental, cultural and behavioural factors. It was noted that the variations in public health produced by this complex interplay *... are by no means fully understood*, but more specific reference was made to *individual* risk behaviours: higher rate of smoking, poorer diets, heavier drinking and lower take-up of preventive health services *in groups whose health is worst*.

Five key areas for action were listed in *Health of the Nation*: CHD and stroke; cancers; mental illness; HIV/AIDS and sexual health; accidents. These are, of course, classic epidemiological targets, but even in the two action areas where 'health' was mentioned, the focus was on disease. For instance, in the section appropriately headed 'mental illness', the only reference to mental health was about making an (unspecified) improvement to the mental health of mentally ill people. The objectives and targets of the chapter on sexual health (and HIV/AIDS) were concerned solely with the prevention of sexually transmitted disease and drug misuse.

We noted earlier that different degrees of radicalism were possible within any given health education/promotion programme and the term 'agenda setting' was employed to refer to reformist possibilities. In relation to smoking, *Health of the Nation* recognised the need for using price controls on smoking in public places and controls on advertising and promotion. It also adopted a strategy of *at least maintaining the real level of taxes on tobacco products* both in Britain and within the context of the European Union. On the other hand, it affirmed that the decision whether or not to smoke was a matter of individual choice. Moreover, a complete ban on advertising tobacco products – directly or indirectly through 'brand stretching' – was still ideologically unthinkable!

These observations reinforce earlier points about the primacy of ideology in determining the meaning of success. Success according to the *Preventive Model* and *Health of the Nation* is simple to illustrate. For instance, in order to achieve the 40% reduction in CHD and stroke in people under 65 by the year 2000, health education would be expected to contribute to a reduction in prevalence of cigarette smoking in men and women aged 16 and over to no more than 20% by the year 2000. Evidence from educationally sound programmes such as the North Karelia Pro-

ject would seem to indicate that this kind of success can be achieved. Puska *et al.* (1985) reported a net change in the amount of daily smoking reported by men in North Karelia of 28% and by women of 14% over a 6 year period. Schwartz (1987), in a comparative report of the results of a number of community projects, recorded a decline in the number of male smokers in North Karelia from 44% to 31%, compared with only a 4% reduction in the rest of Finland.

*Health of the Nation* also established a series of objectives for dealing with another important set of preventive targets concerned with reducing the incidence of accidents. One of these specified a one-third reduction in road casualties by the year 2000 and this may serve as a second illustration of a major focus for a *Preventive Model* of health education. First we should note that a good deal of progress has been made in reducing accidental injuries: a fall of 23% has been observed between 1981 and 1991. It would not be unreasonable to suppose that health education had made some real contribution to that success – even though it may not be possible to specify the precise pathways from intervention to outcome (a problem which will receive further attention in Chapter 2). We do, however, have some more tangible evidence of the potential of safety education for influencing health behaviour.

Levens and Rodnight (1973) assembled evidence of the effectiveness of a series of carefully controlled area experiments in the use of mass media to promote the wearing of seat belts by car drivers and front seat passengers in Britain. They calculated that an appropriately structured mass media campaign could raise the level of seat belt use by a maximum of 16% from an initial 15% start point and do so within a period of 3 weeks. This result clearly demonstrates effectiveness; whether it demonstrates efficiency depends on what might be achieved by competing measures. In the case in point a much better result was achieved by legislation, i.e. by implementing healthy public policy. It is now rare in Britain for drivers not to wear seat belts. However, as was suggested earlier in the chapter, policy change would have been unlikely without the incidental agenda setting effect of individually directed campaigns. In fact, this provides an excellent example of the interaction of education and policy. It also gives an indication of the potential of mass media in health education, something which will later receive detailed analysis.

**Box 20** *Preventive Model*: Evidence of Effectiveness

- *Asthma:* significant improvements in knowledge, beliefs, attitudes, skills and morbidity sustained over 1 year (Colland, 1993).
- *Dental health:* decline in frequency of sugar consumption as between meal sweet consumption (Holund, 1990); changes in legislation and adoption of water fluoridation after programme of mass media and social action (Smith and Christen, 1990).
- *Childhood accidents:* significant rise in rate of use of car seats after counselling of mothers in hospital and paediatrician's office (Reisinger et al., 1981); fall in accidents of 28% after community mobilisation programme (Schelp, 1988).
- *Breast feeding:* 93% start breast feeding (70% controls) and maintain for 12 weeks (44%, compared with 12% controls) (Kistin et al., 1994).
- *Nutrition:* mothers in Head Start pre-school programme give their children a more varied and high quality diet and more servings of nutritious foods than controls (Koblinsky et al., 1994).
- *Sexual health:* significant changes in knowledge about AIDS, beliefs about benefits of prevention, susceptibility, self efficacy and self reported risk-related sexual behaviours (Walter and Vaughan, 1993).
- *Child abuse:* significant reduction in morbidity; lower incidence of physical abuse in population of 30,000 parents and children – largely from low s.e.s. group (Barker et al., 1992).

See Tones (1997) for further details.

Turning now to England's most recent national health policy *Saving Lives: Our Healthier Nation* (Department of Health, 1999b), the preventive imperative is still clearly (and not unreasonably) discernible. Those diseases which account for 75% of deaths in UK by the age of 75 are specifically targeted. Success will have been achieved, therefore, if the following goals have been achieved.

- The death rate from cancer in people under 75 has been reduced by at least a fifth.
- The death rate from coronary heart disease and stroke and related diseases in people under 75 have been reduced by at least two-fifths.
- The death rate from accidents has been reduced by at least one fifth and the rate of serious injury has been reduced by at least one-tenth.
- The death rate from suicide and undetermined injury has been reduced by at least a fifth.

However, in relation to its stated intentions, *Saving Lives* has a much more radical and broad-based agenda. In short, it not only explicitly acknowledges the existence of health inequalities but identifies the following ... *key developments to target those most likely to experience health inequalities.*

- National Minimum Wage.
- New Deals for Employment.
- Working Families Tax Credit.
- Sure Start (provision of child care, early education an play facilities, etc.).
- Capital Receipts Initiative (provision of additional social housing).
- Proposals for a Programme to Tackle Fuel Poverty.
- White Paper on Transport.

Unlike the previous governmental health policy, rather more than lip-service is paid to intersectoral working. Moreover, following the precept of 'health impact assessment' (i.e. the analysis of the impact of *all* policy decisions on health), it will be apparent from the policies listed above that there is a commitment to coordinated work between different government departments.

In short, many of the targets identified by *Saving Lives* are more consistent with an *Empowerment Model* than a *Preventive Model*. We should bear in mind though – as we have been at some pains to point out elsewhere in this chapter – the *Empowerment Model* ultimately will be more effective in preventing disease than working within the confines of a narrower *Preventive Model*.

**Box 21**  A Mental Health Programme

> *Intervention in a whole school district using group discussion/workshops/role play/games/ one-to-one counselling/booklets and video; staff training; organisational change to school ethos and national policy measures: resulted in 50% reduction in bullying at 8 and 12 months both in and out of school. Incidence of victimisation falls from 2.6% to 0.6% in boys and from 1.7% to 0.59% in girls. Reduction in truanting and anti-social behaviour. Dose–response relationship established.*
>
> (Olweus, 1992)

See also Tones (1997) for further details.

## Effectiveness and the radical imperative

In this chapter we have incorporated so-called radical models of health promotion into the *Empowerment Model* described in Figure 1.7. It will, however, be useful to consider separately the meaning of success for the radical imperative *per se*. Radical health education has one significant feature in common with the *Preventive Model* discussed above. It is concerned with action outcomes. A preventive approach looks for indicators of success in the adoption of behaviours and in the medical or epidemiological outcomes which are considered to result from such behaviours. On the other hand, success for a radical model would be measured in terms of social action. Again, this action is not necessarily an end in itself but would be seen as a means of achieving healthy public policy in order to achieve the kinds of health promotion goals discussed previously, such as a redistribution of power and resources. We will consider here two examples of what proponents

of a radical model might judge to be success. The first example concerns healthy diet.

A 'standard' *Preventive Model* would seek to persuade individuals to adopt a prudent diet in order to minimise the likelihood of their falling prey to a number of dietary-related diseases. The classic victim blaming approach would, while exhorting people to eat wisely, ignore the environmental circumstances which either promoted the consumption of unhealthy food or prevented people from adopting a healthy diet. A radical approach would, on the other hand, set out to tackle those unhealthy environmental determinants of poor nutritional status. As Charles and Kerr (1986) have demonstrated in their research into the experience of 200 British women acting as nutritional gatekeepers for their families, ignorance of what constitutes healthy food is not the problem. Real barriers to choice included one or more of the following: accessibility and cost of healthy food; problems with food labelling or lack of it; relegation of the importance of providing healthy foods in the context of other social and domestic pressures; feelings of powerlessness. Effective radical nutrition education would, therefore, be judged by such measures as (in descending order of radicalism): decrease in poverty; successful battle with food manufacturers seeking to promote junk food and empty calories in Western countries and formula baby milk and diarrhoea medicines in developing countries; providing a full range of healthy foods (preferably subsidised) at retail outlets and in the context of institutional catering; proper food labelling. It is interesting to note that variations on the last two (relatively) radical proposals figured in *Health of the Nation*, indicating perhaps that reformist compromise is a real possibility!

Freudenberg (1981) provides our second exemplification of effectiveness in radical health education. The cases he cites include a range of intermediate and outcome indicators. Three examples are listed below.

- In the context of critical consciousness raising about environmental issues, mothers in New Jersey were alerted to a cluster of child cancer deaths in an industrial area. As a result they formed an organisation which exerted pressure on the state and, ultimately, forced it to undertake an epidemiological investigation.

- In the context of occupational safety and health, the Carolina Brown Lung Association was formed. This set out to explain safety procedures to textile workers and taught them how to monitor dust levels in the workplace. They were also shown how to take action when legal standards were violated.
- In the context of the women's health movement, groups of women were taught how to write papers and develop these as a course for women about women and their bodies. A Committee Against Sterilization Abuse was also formed. This action group resulted in the implementation of 'healthy public policy' in the form of new legislation requiring the provision of mandatory counselling and a 30 day waiting period between decisions about sterilisation and performing the surgery.

Consideration of these examples of radical health promotion will reveal that a variety of different kinds of learning had taken place in addition to consciousness raising. Indeed, it seems clear that empowerment figured prominently in all three instances and we will finally consider what success might mean for an *Empowerment Model*.

**Box 22**   Contribution to a Virtuous Circle

---

*In a quasi experimental evaluation study, the Perry Pre-School Programme provided 58 black children aged 3 from low s.e.s. backgrounds) with 5 _ 30 minute sessions; their parents received one 90 minute home visit. At age 19, 59% of the intervention group were employed (32% control); 38% had a college education (21% control); 16% experienced special education (28% controls); there were 64 pregnancies (117 control); 31% arrest/detections for criminal activity (51% controls). Cost benefit ratio calculated at 9:1.*

(Berrueta-Clement *et al.*, 1984)

---

See Tones (1997) for further details.

## Effectiveness and empowerment

We have already noticed that CCR and, indeed, the radical model form an integral part of the *Empowerment Model* described earlier. It will also be recalled that the main difference between this and the radical model was the extent of the emphasis placed on the process of self-empowerment and community empowerment. Not only was it argued that this process needed to be defined in terms of precise operations, but we also sought to address some of the dilemmas associated with the principle of voluntarism. The implications for evaluation can be stated quite simply as follows. The ultimate indicator of success will be the extent to which it is genuinely possible for individuals (and the communities of which they are a part) to make decisions about their lives and their health 'without let or hindrance' but within the limits imposed by the overriding need to ensure that their choice does not damage other people's health and their capacity for such decision making.

More particularly, the effectiveness of empowerment strategies would be revealed by:

- the removal or minimisation of social and environmental barriers to choice;
- the creation and strengthening of active participating communities, e.g. by increasing social capital;
- the strengthening of individuals' capacity to take action.

Accordingly, one of the most significant pieces of evidence of successful empowering strategies would be the extent to which 'healthy public policy' has been adopted and implemented in order to manage the social and environmental determinants of health and overcome the barriers mentioned above. We earlier pointed out that the policy document *Saving Lives* (Department of Health, 1999b) incorporated measures which were entirely consistent with the *Empowerment Model* of health promotion. We also observed that, since health problems cut right across interdepartmental boundaries, cooperation is essential to the adoption of health promoting policy. The UK Social Exclusion Unit's (1999) approach to addressing the problems associated with teenage pregnancy acknowledges this fact and, while noting the strategy on sexual health, offers an interesting list of other government programmes which impact on teenage parenthood. This is reproduced in Appendix 4 and summarised in Box 23.

**Box 23**   Government Programmes Which Impact on Teenage Parenthood

---

Programme and possible applications to teenage health

- *Health improvement programmes*: include teenage pregnancies as local priorities for action.
- *Health Action Zones*: focus on areas of deprivation and high health need.
- *Primary Care Groups*: targeted incentives to improve access for young people to contraceptive advice in primary care.
- *Sexwise*: free confidential telephone advice about sex and personal relationships (currently receiving 2500 calls/day).
- *NHS Direct*: telephone advice line.
- *Quality Protects programme*: focus on children in need.
- *Healthy Living Centres*: possible reproductive health groups and parenting classes as part of general collaborative health promotion programme.
- *Education Action Zones*: partnership of local schools with community coalition. Focus on disadvantage.
- *New Start:* focus on 14–17 year olds who have dropped out of learning or are at risk of doing so; multi-agency partnership.
- *Excellence in Cities*: secondary schools have access to a learning mentor who will identify vulnerable or disaffected pupils; including helping young mothers to return to school.
- *Education Maintenance Allowance*: provides weekly allowance to increase participation and achievement in education by 16–19 year olds.

- *Student Support*: access to funds to help students with the cost of further education.
- *Further Education Funding Council*: allows colleges to provide free child care to students.
- *New Deal for Lone Parents*: personal advisory service provides help and financial support with search for jobs, training and child support.
- *New Deal for Communities*: aims to tackle multiple deprivation and provide resources and support.
- *New Deal for 18–24 Year Olds*: helps young people who have been unemployed.
- *ONE*: people of working age given support in removing barriers to work.
- *Working Families Tax Credit*: paid to working families on low or middle incomes, including Child Care Tax Credit.
- *National Childcare Strategy and Early Years Development and Child Care Partnerships*: focus on good quality child care for all children 0–14.
- *Sure Start*: coordinates help for families in need.
- *National Family and Parenting Institute*: advice and information on all aspects of family life.
- *Child Support Scheme*: helping young people understand responsibilities of parenthood.
- *Housing Investment Programme*: capital funding to local authorities to build new housing.

---

Apart from the extent to which the policies outlined in Box 23 have been implemented – or measurable progress has been made towards implementation – there are a number of often well-validated measures to assess the success of initiatives associated with the *Empowerment Model*. At the individual level these measures might, for instance, include beliefs about control, enhanced self-esteem or the acquisition of self-regulatory skills. The dynamics of empowerment and the interaction of these various measures will be discussed in Chapter 2, but we might usefully note here one appropriate piece of evidence that an empowerment strategy had been successful might be an increase in internal locus of control. In actual fact, a variety of researchers have reported correlations between perceived locus of control and a number of health- and illness-related outcomes, suggesting that internality might well be a desirable goal for empowerment education. For instance, Strickland (1978), in a review of published work, made the following observation:

> *... the bulk of research is consistent in implying that when faced with health problems, internal individuals do appear to engage in more generally adaptive responses than do externals .... . Findings suggest that the development of an internal orientation could lead to improved health practices for some individuals who have been inclined to believe that life events are beyond their responsibility and more a function of external control.*

(p1205)

At first glance, then, it would seem that we might use measures of internality to assess the effectiveness of programmes of empowerment education, especially since we have a number of more or less standardised psychometric scales at our disposal. Indeed, this might well be a feasible strategy, provided that we also take account of the many other factors which also contribute to empowerment – a point which will be made more explicitly in a later chapter. We would in addition need to have a substantial and long-lasting programme if we were to seriously expect a shift from externality to internality, given that locus of control results from a long period of socialisation. A more realistic strategy might be to gauge effectiveness by looking for changes in self-efficacy beliefs and/or the acquisition of a set of competencies and skills which are central to assertiveness. Both of these might ultimately be expected to make significant contributions to internality and empowerment more generally.

A review of the effectiveness of assertiveness training or of attempts to enhance self-efficacy is not appropriate at this point. However, by way of further exemplifying the nature of success for an *Empowerment Model*, we will comment on the effectiveness of providing anticipatory guidance in a clinical context and of enhancing feelings of control in institutionalised elderly people.

A large number of studies have provided an indication of the beneficial effects of providing patients with health education prior to their undergoing some more or less traumatic experience such as surgery. Arguably, the beneficial effects of the education or counselling derive in large part from the enhanced feelings of control they experience. One of the most impressive results of such 'empowerment' education is provided by an early and classic study by Egbert *et al.* (1964) in which an experimental group receiving anticipatory guidance required a significantly lower dosage of analgesics post-operatively and were discharged from hospital on average 2.7 days earlier than the control group. We might note here that the selected measures of success were in fact those associated with a *Preventive Model* rather than an *Empowerment Model*, which serves to make a point which will receive further consideration later: what might be considered to be appropriate outcome measures for one particular model will be regarded as intermediate indicators of performance for another model.

The final example selected to illustrate how the success of empowerment education within a general *Empowerment Model* might be judged concerns the significance of control in the institutionalised elderly. Unlike the previously reported study of Egbert *et al.*, the prime concern was to enhance quality of life: perceived, existential and actual control were all extremely important contributory factors. The research in question is, additionally, of interest in that it provides a nice illustration of a small-scale health promotion programme, i.e. one which involved policy, environmental change and education.

Langer (1983) has provided an insightful review of the psychological dimensions of control and describes interventions designed to empower individuals in various circumstances. For instance, Langer and Rodin (1976) deliberately attempted to enhance the independence and personal control of a group of nursing home residents. The elderly people concerned lived on one floor of what was described as a 'modern, high quality nursing home'. The residents were counselled about their existing opportunities to influence the ways in which the home was run – for instance, how they might influence menus – and, perhaps more importantly, given particular responsibilities. They were, for example, encouraged to arrange the furniture in their rooms and were given potted plants to care for. By comparison, a control group occupying a different but similar floor in the home was merely provided with the plants and told that the nursing staff would look after them. Measures of activity levels and general happiness of the two groups revealed that the 'responsibility' group was more alert, active and contented than their counterparts. Moreover, a year and a half later the experimental group had maintained their gain in quality of life (Rodin and Langer, 1977). Similar results were recorded by Ryden (1984), who demonstrated that the morale of a group of institutionalised elderly was significantly related to perception of situational control.

However, one of the most intriguing features of Rodin and Langer's research was the improvement in physical health of the 'empowered' elderly group compared with the control group: one of the more dramatic findings was that the death rate of the empowered group was half that of the residents who lacked the benefits of actual and perceived control over their lives.

## CONCLUSIONS

In this first section of the book we have discussed in some detail the meaning of health and, above all, explanations of the different factors contributing to health and illness. We have, in particular, explored the ethical dimension associated with health and equity and incorporated this in a discussion of the victim blaming tendency – which we have categorically rejected as inconsistent with the ideological stance underpinning WHO's conceptualisation of health promotion. We have considered the relationship of health education to this conceptualisation and encapsulated it in a simple assertion that health promotion involves a synergistic relationship between health education and health policy. Above all, we have provided a quite detailed analysis of empowerment, viewing this as a central element in health education and health promotion.

We have, additionally, reviewed a number of so-called 'models' of health education and, in doing so, have sought to compare and contrast differentiation made on the basis of ideology with more 'technological' distinctions. We have questioned the utility and, indeed, the reality of distinctions popularly made between models and noted areas of overlap and even false dichotomies. In practice many features of the different models may be reconciled. On the other hand, it is hopefully clear that there are genuine differences in ideology inherent in this 'model making'; practitioners who opt for one or other model are, consciously or unconsciously, revealing what for them are important values and/or different ways of constructing their personal realities. In particular we have noted real differences associated with commitment to one or more features of a *Medical Model*; we have observed commitment to the principle of voluntarism; we have even speculated on the influence of personality in respect of people's location on tenderminded–toughminded and radical–conservative continua.

In this last section we have explored the implications of subscribing to one or other model of health education for the evaluation of success. We have emphasised that, in seeking to answer questions about the effectiveness and efficiency to health education, we must first of all take account of these ideological and value considerations.

In the next section our concern will be rather more technological than ideological. We will be seeking to examine the essential role played by theory in explaining how communities and individuals come to adopt, sustain or reject particular courses of action leading to health- and illness-related outcomes. We will also demonstrate the links between this 'technological' analysis and the construction of effective health education interventions. We will also argue that competent decisions about evaluation cannot be made without having an effective theoretical framework which helps us understand how people come to make health- and illness-related decisions. We will consider the ways in which various indicators may be selected to demonstrate the success or failure of programmes designed to achieve valued goals. In other words, we will argue that a careful selection of indicators based on sound theory is essential if the various ideological thrusts discussed in this chapter are to be operationalised and evaluated.

## REFERENCES

Anderson, R. (1984) *Health promotion: an overview.* In L. Baric (Ed.) *European Monographs in Health Education Research,* no. 6, pp. 4–126. Scottish Health Education Group, Edinburgh.

Anderson, V. and Draper, P. (1991) *Economics and hostile environments.* In P. Draper (Ed.) *Health Through Public Policy.* Merlin Press, London.

Antonovsky, A. (1979) *Health, Stress and Coping.* Jossey-Bass, San Francisco, CA.

Antonovsky, A (1984) *The sense of coherence as a determinant of health.* In J. D. Matarazzo, S. M. Weiss and J. A. Herd (Eds) *Behavioral Health.* John Wiley, New York, NY.

Barker, W., Anderson, R. and Chalmers, C. (1992) *Child Protection: the Impact of the Child Development Programme.* University of Bristol Child Development Unit, Bristol.

Baric, L. (1988). *The new public health and the concept of advocacy. Journal of the Institute of Health Education,* 26 (2), 49–55.

Beattie, A. (1991) *Knowledge and control in health promotion: a test case for social policy and social theory.* In J. Gabe, M. Calnan and M. Bury (Eds) *The Sociology of the Health Service.* Routledge and Kegan Paul, London.

Berruetea-Clement, J.R., Schweinhaert, L.J., Barnett, W.S., Epstein, A.S. and Weikart, D.P. (1984) *Changed Lives: the Effects of the Perry Preschool Preogram on Youths Through Age 19.* High/Scope Press, MI.

Blane, D, Brunner, E. and Wilkinson, R. (Eds) (1996) *Health and Social Organization: Towards a Health Policy for the 21st Century.* Routledge, London.

*British Medical Journal* (1986) *Whatever happened to the Black Report? British Medical Journal,* 293, 91–92.

Brown, R. E. and Margo, G. E. (1978) *Health education, can the reformers be reformed? International Journal of Health Services,* 8 (1), 3–23.

Brunner, E. (1996) *The social and biological basis of cardiovascular disease in office workers.* In D. Blane, E. Brunner and R. Wilkinson (Eds) *Health and Social Organization: Towards a Health Policy for the 21st Century.* Routledge, London.

Buckingham, A. (1996) *A statistical update.* In R. Lister (Ed.) *Charles Murray and the Underclass: the Developing Debate.* IEA Health and Welfare Unit, London.

Bunker, J. P., Frazier, H. S. and Mosteller, F. (1994) *Improving health: measuring effects of medical care. Millbank Quarterly,* 72, 225–258.

Bury, M. and Gabe, J. (1994) *Television and medicine: medical dominance or trial by media?* In J. Gabe, D. Kelleher and G. Williams (Eds) *Challenging Medicine.* Routledge, London.

Caldwell, J. C. (1986) *Routes to low mortality in poor countries. Population and Development Review,* 2, 171–220.

Campbell, C., Wood, R. and Kelly, M. (1999) *Social Capital and Health.* HEA, London.

Canterbury (1985) *Faith in the City: Report of the Archbishop of Canterbury's Commission on Urban Priority Areas.* Lambeth Palace, London.

Carstairs, V. and Morris, R. (1989) *Deprivation and mortality: an alternative to social class? Community Medicine,* 11, 210–219.

Cassell, E. J. (1991) *The Nature of Suffering and the Goals of Medicine.* Oxford University Press, Oxford.

Cattell, R. B. (1965) *The Scientific Analysis of Personality.* Penguin, Harmondsworth.

Charles, N. and Kerr, M. (1986) *Issues of responsibility and control in the feeding of families.* In S. Rodmell and A. Watt (Eds) *The Politics of Health Education: Raising the Issues.* Routledge and Kegan Paul, London.

Chanan, G. (1997) *Active citizenship and community involvement: 'Getting to the Roots',* a discussion paper. European Foundation for the Improvement of Living and Working Conditions: Dublin.

Cochrane, A. L. (1972) *Effectiveness and Efficiency,* Rock Carling Monograph. Nuffield Provincial Hospitals Trust, Oxford.

Colland, V. T. (1993) *Learning to cope with asthma: a behavioural self-management program for children.*

*Patient Education and Counselling*, 22, 141–152.

Constantino-David, K. (1982) *Issues in community organization. Community Development Journal*, 17, 190–201.

Coreil, J. and Levin, J. S. (1985) *A critique of the lifestyle concept in public health education. International Quarterly of Community Health Education*, 5 (2), 103–114.

Crawford, R. (1980) *Healthism and the medicalization of everyday life. International Journal of Health Services*, 10, 365–388.

Dahlgren, G. and Whitehead, M. (1991) *Tackling inequalities: a review of policy initiatives.* In M. Benzeval, K. Judge and M. Whitehead (Eds) *Tackling Inequalities in Health; an Agenda for Action.* Kings Fund Institute, London.

Davie, R., Butler, N. and Goldstein, H. (1972) *From Birth to Seven.* Longman, London.

De Kadt, E. (1982) *Ideology, social policy, health and health services: a field of complex interactions. Social Science and Medicine*, 16, 741–752.

Department of Health (1992) *The Health of the Nation: A Strategy for Health in England.* HMSO, London.

Department of Health (1998) *Independent Inquiry into Inequalities in Health: Report* (chairman, Sir Donald Acheson). HMSO, London.

Department of Health (1999a) *Reducing Health Inequalities: an Action Report. Our Healthier Nation.* HMSO, London.

Department of Health (1999b) *Saving Lives: Our Healthier Nation.* HMSO, London.

DiMatteo, M. R. and DiNicola, D. D. (1982) *Achieving Patient Compliance: the Psychology of the Medical Practitioner's Role.* Pergamon, New York, NY.

Dingwall, R. (1994) *Litigation and the threat to medicine.* In J. Gabe, D. Kelleher and G. Williams (Eds) *Challenging Medicine.* Routledge, London.

Doll, R. (1992) *Health and the environment in the 1990s. American Journal of Public Health*, 82 (7), 933–941.

Downie, R. S., Fyfe, C. and Tannahill, A. (1992) *Health Promotion: Models and Values.* Oxford University Press, Oxford.

Doyal, L. (1981) *The Political Economy of Health.* Pluto Press, London.

Doyal, L. (1994) *Challenging medicine? Gender and the politics of health care.* In J. Gabe, D. Kelleher and G. Williams (eds) *Challenging Medicine.* Routledge, London.

Draper, P. (1983) *Tackling the disease of ignorance. Self Health*, 1, 23–25.

Draper, P., Best, G. and Dennis, J. (1977) *Health and wealth. Royal Society of Health Journal*, 97, 121–127.

Draper, P., Griffiths, J., Dennis, J. and Popay, J. (1980) *Three types of health education. British Medical Journal*, 281, 493–495.

Dubos, R. (1959) *The Mirage of Health.* Harper and Row, New York, NY.

Dubos, R. (1965) *Man Adapting.* Yale University Press, London.

Durrant, K. (1993) *The creative arts and the promotion of health in community settings.* Unpublished MSc dissertation, Leeds Metropolitan University.

Eagleton, T. (1991) *Ideology: An Introduction.* Verso, London.

Egbert, J. A., Battit, G. E., Welch, C. E. and Bartlett, M. K. (1964) *Reduction of postoperative pain by encouragement and instruction of patients. New England Journal of Medicine*, 270, 825–827.

Elston, M. A. (1994) *The anti-vivisectionist movement and the science of medicine.* In J. Gabe, D. Kelleher and G. Williams (Eds) *Challenging Medicine.* Routledge, London.

Eysenck, H. J. (1960) *The Structure of Human Personality.* Methuen, London.

Field, F. (1996) *Britain's underclass: countering the growth.* In R. Lister (Ed.) *Charles Murray and the Underclass: the Developing Debate.* IEA Health and Welfare Unit, London.

Forcinelli, O. (1974) *Values education in the public school. Thrust*, 2, 81–84.

Freire, P. (1974) *Education and the Practice of Freedom.* Writers and Readers Publishing Cooperative, London (originally published in Portuguese, 1967).

French, J. and Adams, L. (1986) *From analysis to synthesis: theories of health education. Health Education Journal*, 45 (2), 71–74.

Freudenberg, N. (1981) *Health education for social change: a strategy for public health in the US. International Journal of Health Education*, 24 (3), 1–8.

Fryer, P. (1988) *A health city strategy three years on – the case of Oxford City Council. Health Promotion*, 3 (2), 213–218.

Gabe. J., Kelleher, D. and Williams, G. (Eds) (1994) *Challenging Medicine.* Routledge, London.

Galbraith, J. K. (1992a) *The Culture of Contentment*. Penguin, Harmondsworth.

Galbraith, J. K. (1992b) *Shifting gear, not direction*. *The Guardian*, 25 November.

Goffman, E. (1961) *Asylums*. Doubleday Anchor, New York, NY.

Green, L. W. and Kreuter, M. W. (1991) *Health Promotion Planning: An Educational and Environmental Approach*. Mayfield Publishing, CA.

Green, L. W. and Raeburn, J. M. (1988) *Health promotion. What is it? What will it become? Health Promotion*, 3 (2), 151–159.

Haglund, B. J. A., Pettersson, B., Finer, D. and Tillgren, P. (1993) *We Can Do It. Sundsvall Handbook*. Karolinska Institute, Sweden.

Harre, R. and Lamb, R. (Eds) (1983) *The Encyclopedic Dictionary of Psychology*. Blackwell, Oxford.

*Health Promotion* (1986) *Health Promotion*, 1 (4), whole issue.

*Health Promotion* (1988) *The Adelaide recommendations: healthy public policy. Health Promotion*, 3 (2), 183–186.

Hirst, P. (1969) *The logic of the curriculum. Journal of Curriculum Studies*, 1 (2), 142.

Holund, U. (1990) *Promoting change of adolescents' sugar consumption: the 'Learning by Teaching' study. Health Education Research*, 5, 451–458.

Hunter, D. (1994) *From tribalism to corporatism: the managerial challenge to medical dominance*. In J. Gabe, D. Kelleher and G. Williams (Eds) *Challenging Medicine*. Routledge, London.

Illich, I. (1976) *The Limits of Medicine – Medical Nemesis: the Expropriation of Health*, Marion Boyars, London.

Jaco, E. G. (1979) *Patients, Physicians and Illness: a Source Book in Behavioral Science and Health, 3rd edn*. Free Press, New York, NY.

Jarman, B. (1984) *Underprivileged areas: validation and distribution of scores. British Medical Journal*, 289, 1587–1592.

Karasek, R. and Theorell, T. (1990) *Healthy Work: Stress, Productivity, and the Reconstruction of Working Life*. Basic Books, New York, NY.

Keillor, G. (1989) *We Are Still Married*. Faber and Faber, London.

Kelleher, D., Gabe, J. and Williams, G. (1994) *Understanding medical dominance in the modern world*. In J. Gabe, D. Kelleher and G. Williams (Eds) *Challenging Medicine*. Routledge, London.

Kempson, E. (1996) *Life on a Low Income*. Joseph Rowntree Foundation/York Publishing Services, York.

Kickbusch, I. (1986) *Issues in health promotion. Health Promotion*, 1 (4), 437–442.

Kickbusch, I. (1989) Healthy cities: a working project and a growing movement. *Health Promotion*, 4 (2), 77–82.

Kistin, N., Abramson, M. S. and Dublin, P. (1994) *Effect of peer counselors on breastfeeding initiation, exclusivity, and duration among low-income urban women. Journal of Human Lactation*, 10, 11–16.

Koblinsky, S. A., Guthrie, J. F. and Lynch, L. (1992) *Evaluation of a nutrition education program for Head Start parents. Journal of Nutrition Education*, 24, 4–13.

Labonte, R. and Penfold, S. (1981) *Canadian perspectives in health promotion: a critique. Health Education*, April, 4–9.

LaFramboise, H. (1973) Health policy: breaking the problem down into more manageable segments. *Canadian Medical Association Journal*, 108, 388–391.

Lalonde, M. (1974) *A New Perspective on the Health of Canadians*. Government of Canada, Ottawa.

*Lancet* (1990) *The Underclass. Lancet*, 335, 1312–1315.

Lang, T., Andrews, H., Bedale, C. and Hannan, E. (1984) *Jam Tomorrow: A Report of the First Findings of a Pilot Study of the Food Circumstances, Attitudes and Consumption of 1000 People on Low Incomes in the North of England*. Food Policy Unit, Manchester Polytechnic.

Langer, E. J. (1983) *The Psychology of Control*. Sage Publications, Beverly Hills, CA.

Langer, E. J. and Rodin, J. (1976) *The effects of enhanced personal responsibility for the aged. Journal of Personality and Social Psychology*, 34 (2), 191–198.

Lefanu, J. (Ed.) (1994) *Preventionitis: the Exaggerated Claims of Health Promotion*. The Social Affairs Unit, London.

Levens, G. E. and Rodnight, E. (1973) *The Application of Research in the Planning and Evaluation of Road Safety Publicity. Proceedings of the European Society for Opinion in Marketing (Budapest) Conference*, pp. 197–227.

Lister, R. (Ed.) (1996) *Charles Murray and the Underclass: the Developing Debate*. IEA Health and Welfare Unit, London.

Luck, G. M. and Luckman, J. (1974) *Patients, Hospitals and Operational Research*. Tavistock, London.

Macdonald, J. J. and Warren, W. H. (1991) *Primary health care as an educational process: a model and a Frierean perspective. International Quarterly of Community Health Education*, 12 (1), 35–50.

Mackenback, J. P., Bouvier-Colle, M. H. and Jougla, E. (1990) *'Avoidable' mortality and health services: a review of aggregate data studies. Journal of Epidemiology and Community Health*, 44, 106–111.

McMillan, D. W. and Chavis, D. M. (1986) *Sense of community: a definition and theory. Journal of Community Psyhchology,* 14, 6–23.

Mahler, H. (1986) *Towards a new public health. Health Promotion*, 1 (1), 1.

Marmot, M. G. (1986) *Social inequalities in mortality: the social environment*. In R. G. Wilkinson (Ed.) *Class and Health*. Tavistock, London.

Marmot, M. G. (1996) *The social pattern of health and disease*. In D. Blane, E. Brunner and R. Wilkinson (Eds) *Health and Social Organization: Towards a Health Policy for the 21st Century*. Routledge, London.

Marmot, M. G., Shipley, M. J. and Rose, G. (1984) *Inequalities in death: specific explanations of a general pattern. Lancet*, 1, 514–525.

Maslow, A. H. (1967) *Self-actualization and beyond*. In J. F. T. Bugental (Ed.) *Challenges of Humanistic Psychology*. McGraw-Hill, New York, NY.

Maslow, A. H. (1970) *Motivation and Personality, 2nd edn*. Harper and Row, New York, NY.

Maton, K. I. and Rappaport, J. (1981) *Empowerment in a religious setting: a multivariate investigation*. in *Studies in Empowerment: Steps Toward Understanding and Action*, (eds J. Rappaport, C. Swift and R. Hess), Haworth Press, New York.

McGregor, D.M. (1966) *The human side of enterprise*. in H. L. Leavitt and L. R. Pondy (Eds) *Readings in Managerial Psychology*. University of Chicago Press, Chicago, IL.

McKeown, T. (1979) *The Role of Medicine: Dream, Mirage or Nemesis?* Blackwell, Oxford.

McKinlay, J. B. (1979) A case for refocusing upstream: the political economy of illness. In E. G. Jaco (Ed.) *Patients, Physicians and Illness*. The Free Press, New York, NY.

McPhail, P. (1977) *Living Well, Health Education Council Project 12–18*. Cambridge University Press, Cambridge.

Milio, N. (1986) *Promoting Health Through Public Policy*. Canadian Public Health Association, Ottawa.

Mill, J. S. (1961) *On Liberty* (reprinted in *Essential Works of John Stuart Mill*). Bantam Books, New York, NY.

Minkler, M. (1989) *Health education, health promotion and the open society: an historical perspective. Health Education Quarterly*, 16, 17–30.

Minkler, M. and Cox, K. (1980) *Creating critical consciousness in health: applications of Freire's philosophy and methods to the health care setting. International Journal of Health Services*, 10 (2), 311–322.

Mitford, N. (1969) *The Sun King*. Sphere Books, London.

Morris, D. (1987) *Healthy cities: self reliant cities. Health Promotion*, 2 (2), 169–176.

National Consumer Council (1992) *Your Food: Whose Choice?* HMSO, London.

MRFFIT (1982) *The Multiple risk Factor Intervention Trial – risk factor changes and mortality results. Journal of the American Medical Association*, 248, 1465–1476.

Mustard, J. F. (1996) *Health and social capital*. In D. Blane, E. Brunner and R. Wilkinson (Eds) *Health and Social Organization: Towards a Health Policy for the 21st Century*. Routledge, London.

Navarro, V. (1976) *The underdevelopment of health of working America: causes, consequences and possible solutions. American Journal of Public Health*, 66, 538–547.

Olweus, D. (1992) Bullying among schoolchildren: intervention and prevention. In V. Peters, R. J. McMahon and V. L. Quinsey (Eds) *Aggression and Violence Throughout the Life Span*. Sage, Newbury Park.

Parsons, T (1951) *The Social system*. Free Press, New York, NY.

Parsons, T. (1979) *Definitions of health and illness in the light of American values and social structure*. In E. G. Jaco (Ed.) *Patients, Physicians and Illness, 3rd edn*. Free Press, New York, NY.

Phillips, M. (1996) *Where are the New Victorians?* In R. Lister (Ed.) *Charles Murray and the Underclass: the Developing Debate*. IEA Health and Welfare Unit, London.

Preston, S. (1976) *Mortality Patterns in National Populations*. Academic Press, London.

Puska, P. *et al.* (1985) *The community-based strategy of preventing coronary heart disease: conclusions* from the ten years of the North Karelia Project. *Annual Review of Public Health*, 6, 147–193.

Putnam, R. D. (1993a) *Making Democracy Work: Civic Tradition in Modern Italy*. Princeton University Press, Princeton, NJ.

Putnam, R. D. (1993b) *The prosperous community: social capital and public life. American Prospect*, 13, 35–42.

Putnam, R. D. (1995) *Bowling alone: America's declining social capital. Journal of Democracy*, 6 (1), 65–79.

Putnam, R. D., Leonardi, R. and Nanetti, R. Y. (1993) *Making Democracy Work: Civic Traditions in Modern Italy*. Princeton University Press, Princeton, NJ.

Reisinger, K. D., Wells, A. F., John, C. E., Roberts, T. R. and Podgainy, H. J. (1981) *Effect of paediatrician's counselling on infant restraint use. Pediatrics*, 67, 201–206.

Rodin, J. and Langer, E. J. (1977) *Long-term effects of a control-relevant intervention with the institutionalized aged. Journal of Personality and Social Psychology*, 35, 897–902.

Rodmell, S. and Watt, A. (Eds) (1986) *The Politics of Health Education: Raising the Issues*. Routledge and Kegan Paul, London.

Ryan, W. (1976) *Blaming the Victim*. Vintage Books, New York, NY.

Ryden, M. B. (1984) *Morale and perceived control in institutionalized elderly. Nursing Research*, 33 (3), 130–136.

Schelp, L. (1987) *Community intervention and changes in accident pattern in a rural Swedish municipality. Health Promotion*, 2, 109–125.

Schwartz, J. L. (1987) *Smoking Cessation Methods: The United States and Canada, 1978–1985*, pp. 62–71. US Department of Health and Human Services, Washington, DC.

SOPHE (Society for Public Health Education) (1976) *Code of Ethics*. SOPHE, San Francisco, CA.

Social Exclusion Unit (1999) *Preventing Teenage Pregnancies*. Cabinet Office, TSO.

Smith, K. G. and Christen, K. A. (1990) *A fluoridation campaign: the Phoenix experience. Journal of Public Health Dentistry*, 50, 126–135.

Stark, E. (1977) *Introduction. Review of Radical Political Economics*, 9 (1), 45–59.

Stenhouse, L. (1969) *Handling controversial issues in the classroom. Education Canada*, December.

Strickland, B. R. (1978) *Internal-external expectancies and health-related behaviours. Journal of*

Consulting and Clinical Psychology, 46 (6), 1192–1211.

Sweeney, B. (1998) *The place of the humanities in the education of a doctor. British Journal of General Practice*, 48, 998–1102.

Syme, S. L. (1989) *Control and health: a personal perspective*. In A. Steptoe and A. Appels (Eds) *Stress, Personal Control and Health*. Wiley, New York, NY.

Syme, S. L. (1996) *To prevent disease: the need for a new approach*. In D. Blane, E. Brunner and R. Wilkinson (Eds) *Health and Social Organization: Towards a Health Policy for the 21st Century*. Routledge, London.

Sutherland, I. (1979) *Health Education: Perspectives and Choices*. Allen and Unwin, London.

Tarlov, A. R. (1996) Social determinants of health: the sociobiological translation. In D. Blane, E. Brunner and R. Wilkinson (Eds) *Health and Social Organization: Towards a Health Policy for the 21st Century*. Routledge, London.

Taylor, S. E. (1979) *Hospital patient behavior: reactance, helplessness, or control? Journal of Social Issues*, 35 (1), 156–184.

Tones, B. K. (1985) *Health promotion – a new panacea? Journal of the Institute of Health Education*, 23, 16–21.

Tones, B. K. (1987) *Health promotion, affective education and personal-social development of young people*. In K. David and T. Williams (Eds) *Health Education in Schools, 2nd edn*. Harper and Row, London.

Tones, B. K. (1992) *Health promotion, self-empowerment and the concept of control*. In *Health Education: Politics and Practice*. Deakin University Press, Victoria.

Tones, B. K. (1997) *Health education: evidence of effectiveness. Archives of Disease in Childhood*, 77, 189–195.

Tones, B. K. (1998) *Health promotion: empowering choice*. In L. B. Myers and K. Midence (Eds) *Adherence to Treatment in Medical Conditions*. Harwood, Amsterdam.

Tones, B. K. and Green, J. (1999) *A Case Study of Withymoor Village Surgery – A Health Hive*. Health Promotion Design, Leeds.

Townsend, P. and Davidson, N. (1992) *Inequalities in Health: The Black Report*. Penguin, Harmondsworth.

Townsend, P., Whitehead, M. and Davidson, M. (1992) *Introduction*. In P. Townsend and N.

Davidson (Eds) *Inequalities in Health: The Black Report*. Penguin, Harmondsworth.

United Nations Development Programme (1994) *Human Development Report*. Oxford University Press, New York, NY.

US Department of Health, Education and Welfare (1978) *Disease Prevention and Health Promotion*. US Department of Health, Education and Welfare, Washington, DC.

US Department of Health, Education and Welfare (1979) *Healthy People*. US Department of Health, Education and Welfare, Washington, DC.

US Department of Health and Human Services (1980) *Promoting Health, Preventing Disease: Objectives for the Nation*. US Department of Health, Education and Welfare, Washington, DC.

Vuori, H. (1980) The medical model and the objectives of health education. *International Journal of Health Education*, 23, 1–8.

Walter, H. and Vaughan, R. (1993) *AIDS risk reduction among a multiethnic sample of urban high school students. Journal of the American Medical Association*, 270, 725–730.

Whitehead, M (1990) *The Concept and Principles of Equity and Health*. WHO, Copenhagen.

Whitehead, M. (1992) *The Health Divide*. Penguin, Harmondsworth.

Wilkinson, R. G. (1992) *National mortality rates: the impact of inequality? American Journal of Public Health*, 82 (8), 1082–1084.

Wilkinson, R. G. (1994) *The epidemiological transition: from material scarcity to social disadvantage? Daedalus*, 123 (4), 71–77.

Wilkinson, R (1996) *How can secular improvements in life expectancy be explained?* In D. Blane, E. Brunner and R. Wilkinson (Eds) *Health and Social Organization: Towards a Health Policy for the 21st Century*. Routledge, London.

Willetts, D. (1992) In D. Smith (Ed.) *Understanding the Underclass*. Policy Studies Institute, London.

Wilson, J. (1987) *The Truly Disadvantaged: the Inner City, the Underclass, and Public Policy*. University of Chicago Press, Chicago, IL.

Witz, A. (1994) *The challenge of nursing*. In J. Gabe. D. Kelleher and G. Williams (eds) *Challenging Medicine*. Routledge, London.

World Bank (1993) *World Development Report 1993, Investing in Health*. Oxford University Press, New York, NY.

World Health Organization (1946) *Constitution*. WHO, Geneva.

World Health Organization (1978) *Report on the International Conference on Primary Health Care*, Alma Ata, 6–12 September. WHO, Geneva.

World Health Organization (1984) *Health Promotion: A Discussion Document on the Concepts and Principles*. WHO Regional Office for Europe, Copenhagen.

World Health Organization (1985) *Targets for Health for All*. WHO Regional Office for Europe, Copenhagen.

World Health Organization (1986) *Ottawa Charter for Health Promotion, An International Conference on Health Promotion, November 17–21*. WHO Regional Office for Europe, Copenhagen.

World Health Organization (1991) *Sundsvall Declaration*. WHO, Geneva.

World Health Organization (1992) *Health Dimensions of Economic Reform*. WHO, Geneva.

World Health Organization (1997) *The Jakarta Declaration on Leading Health Promotion into the 21st Century*. WHO, Geneva.

World Health Organization (1998) *Health for All in the Twenty-first Century*. WHO, Geneva.

Zola, I. K. (1970) *Helping – does it matter? The problems and prospects of mutual aid groups*. Address to United Ostomy Association.

# 2 SELECTING INDICATORS OF SUCCESS: THE IMPORTANCE OF THEORIES OF CHANGE

In Chapter 1 we argued that the meaning of success in health education is dependent on the values and philosophies of practitioners. The measures used to indicate a successful outcome will in turn depend on the model of health promotion which is guiding practice – for instance, indicators of the effectiveness of a preventive model will often provide evidence of the adoption of appropriate behaviours and, arguably, the medical or epidemiological outcomes assumed to result from such behaviours. Indicators of the effectiveness of an *Empowerment Model*, on the other hand, might provide evidence of communities taking action or changes in public policy. At the micro level, appropriate measures of a self-empowerment model might include enhanced self-esteem, increased 'internality' and the acquisition of certain key social skills. Again, an essentially salutogenic approach would formulate indicators to serve as evidence that some positive state of health had been attained. This might include an individual sense of meaningfulness or broader social outcomes, such as those associated with the development of 'social capital'.

We will, later in the chapter, pay particular attention to the choice of appropriate indicators of success. However, since we will emphasise the importance of theory in the development and selection of indicators, we will first consider the availability of those theoretical models, at the macro and micro levels, that are particularly suitable for this particular task and for efficient evaluation in general.

## THE IMPORTANCE OF THEORY

As we will see in our later discussion of indicators, there is a wide range of measures which might and should be used to evaluate any given health promotion programme. Obviously such measures should not be selected randomly and it is perhaps

the main contention in this chapter that in order to make a judicious selection of indirect, intermediate and outcome indicators, we must have a sound theoretical framework. Apart from any other more technical reason, we need such a framework to enable us to justify our choice with confidence when confronted with the often unreasonable demands of managers and politicians!

A sound theoretical framework will, then, provide a substantial basis for practice. The main requirement for such a framework is that it should help explain how people make health-related decisions, individually or *en masse*. It will attempt to define the ways in which social and environmental factors influence these decisions and will provide insight into the nature of both inter- and intra-personal dynamics governing behaviours. If we have some understanding of the constellation of factors influencing human behaviour in health and illness we will be in a better position to devise strategies and formulate methods which will achieve our health promotion goals – no matter what our philosophy or what model we choose to follow. Again, if we understand the existing relationships between, for example, knowledge, beliefs, skills, attitudes, social pressures and environmental constraints we should have some insight into the likely effects of a given educational programme and might thus select our indicators of success in a more rational and meaningful way. For instance, we might on the basis of theoretical understanding expect a conventionally taught and essentially didactic lesson on drugs to produce an increase in knowledge but little else. We would not expect it to affect attitudes or any of the other several psychosocial and environmental factors that may influence drug misuse. We would therefore have a limited expectation of what the lesson might achieve and what it might contribute to a more comprehensive drug education programme. We would also know that it would be pointless to use any indicator other than one which measured recall of information.

Before proceeding further it is important to observe that theories and models that aim to identify and explain the factors influencing behaviour – at the macro or micro levels – are significantly different from the 'ideological models' that we described in Chapter 1. Indeed, as Figure 2.1 seeks to demonstrate, there is (or should be) a kind of logical progression from models that focus on ideological issues to models that provide an explanation of different approaches to evaluation. For instance, an *Empowerment Model* indicates the values position on which practice should be based – if the health promoter acts consistently. The theoretical approach which is represented by the model is related to Morrow and Brown's (1994) conceptualisation of '*normative theory*' which the authors describe as ... *modes of theorizing that legitimate different ethical, ideological, or policy positions with respect to what ought to be. The authors remind us that claims that there should be more social justice or less inequality are value judgements or "normative statements"*. The similarities between this latter statement and the emphasis we placed on the centrality of equity in Chapter 1 is doubtless obvious.

Morrow and Brown contrast '*normative theory*' with '*empirical theory*' (alternatively described as '*analytical*' or '*substantive*' theory), which is concerned with the systematic organisation of concepts and principles in order to provide an explanation and interpretation of social phenomena.

Accordingly, in Figure 2.1 a number of different 'empirical models' derive from and are influenced by the basic philosophical and ideological 'doctrines' and commitment associated with empowerment. Therefore, if the process of planning health promotion activities is to be successful, action must be based on a sound understanding of the many and various factors influencing health choices. In Figure 2.1 two models are presented by way of example. The first of these, *Communication of Innovations Theory* seeks to explain macro level choices relating to the adoption of innovations at the population level. The second example is provided by the *Health Action Model* (HAM). This seeks to explain individual health- and illness-related decision making. Both models will be discussed in greater detail below.

Assuming that the factors influencing health choices have been adequately identified, the next logical step is to work out ways of actually influencing those choices – at the individual or community level. A number of examples of related sets of activity are shown in Figure 2.1. At the strategic level it is argued that certain 'interventions' will benefit from the use of mass media – perhaps associated with 'community coalitions'. However, successful deployment of mass media and coalitions is more likely to be achieved if a realistic model of mass media use has been adopted and, for instance, the theoretical underpinning of inter-sectoral working has been understood. Again, more specific techniques will be employed within the broader strategic arena; for example, counselling and group work will frequently be used within a health care setting which is, itself, part of a community coalition. Critical consciousness-raising (CCR) might form part of a community development (CD) approach (depending on whether CD is considered to be a strategy or a process) which also utilises group work.

Of course, no model can be entirely values free: they are all social constructions and the very act of model building typically derives from some values base or other. An *Empowerment Model* might, on ethical grounds, restrict consideration of explanatory models to those focusing on voluntaristic choices: models which provide an account of those factors that result in individuals being conditioned and coerced would be excluded as irrelevant to ethical practice.

Again, the development or use of an empirical model to guide health promotion practice would also depend to some extent on an ideological imperative. For example, the insights gained from a model explaining 'irrational' behaviours might lead logically to intervention techniques such as those encapsulated in the 'persuasive communication' formulations originally associated with Hovland and collaborators at Yale University, i.e. the deliberate selection of communicators having high credibility and attractiveness; the structuring of message style to arouse particular emotions, such as fear; the use of particular methods, such as group discussion–decision to gain commitment to particular causes; the careful analysis of audience characteristics in order to select the best intervention tactics to persuade them to adopt the beliefs, attitudes or behaviours advocated by the persuader (Hovland *et al.*, 1949; McGuire, 1981).

On the other hand, a model such as the HAM might lead to advocacy of a particular community development strategy based on client felt needs and designed to facilitate rather than manipulate choice.

Finally, while the model of evaluation utilised by the health promoter has a major empirical and technical dimension, it is also very much driven by

philosophy and ideology – a point that will be discussed at some length in Chapter 3. For instance, epistemological concerns (i.e. matters to do with explaining the nature of knowledge and how we come to know our worlds) might lead to a rejection of conventional and much-hallowed 'scientific' research methodologies associated with logical positivism. Again, genuine commitment to the empowerment criteria of WHO would proscribe the use of research methods which did not routinely involve clients: in other words any research which was carried out on people rather than with people would be ideologically unacceptable.

## PROGRAMME PLANNING: THE PLACE OF RESEARCH

It is self-evidently the case that health promotion programmes are more likely to be efficient if they are based on a systematic plan. There are, in fact, a number of systematic guidelines readily available for the practitioner to use. They range from short, but often useful, lists to elaborate and well-researched models – of which the PRECEDE–PROCEED Model (Green and Kreuter, 1999) is a case in point. Any such plans must include at least the following elements:

- identification of a need or problem in respect of an individual, target group or population;
- statement of aim and objectives;
- a 'diagnosis' of important characteristics of individuals, groups and organisations; identification of contexts or settings and broad intervention strategies and their inter-relationship;
- identification of specific intervention methods and associated resources;
- evaluation.

Research must figure prominently in the systematic planning model – as indicated in Figure 2.2.

Research is involved in the systematic assessment of need and in the analysis of individuals' characteristics relevant to programme development and the situation in which they find themselves. *Evaluation* research is involved in assessing the effectiveness and efficiency of the programme.

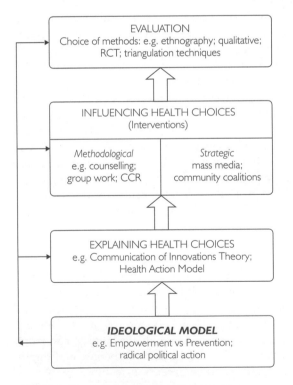

**Figure 2.1** Ideological and Empirical Models in Programme Planning

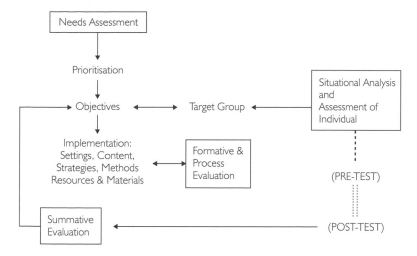

**Figure 2.2**  The Place of Research in Programme Planning

*Summative* evaluation assesses effectiveness at the end of the programme – often by checking the extent to which objectives have been achieved and/or by measuring the difference between pre-test and post-test measures. *Formative* and *process* evaluation, on the other hand, is concerned to use information acquired *during* the programme in order to monitor developments. The information thus acquired may be used at the end of the programme to provide *illumination*, i.e. to provide insights into why the programme was a success or failure. Alternatively, or additionally, it may be used to modify the programme itself to maximise the chance of success. Some further consideration of these terms will be provided later in this book.

### Gaining insight into client characteristics

Returning to the matter of assessing individual and group characteristics, it is an obvious truism to state that an efficient programme will depend on the extent to which the planner understands those features of the target group/client population that are needed to construct a sensitive and appropriate programme and, of course, to evaluate the extent to which it has achieved its valued goals and objectives. In this endeavour it is possible to construct an *ad hoc* list or model of characteristics – based on research or practical experience and common sense

– or both. The number and variety of characteristics may be extensive – especially in community-wide initiatives – and include not only individual attributes, such as knowledge or attitude, but also details of the social and material circumstances in which the individual lives and works. This will be apparent from the complex of psychosocial and environmental influences on the adoption of drug use illustrated in Figure 2.3 (Tones, 1986).

Clearly there are many indicators that might be extracted from Figure 2.3 in order to assess the effectiveness of any programme designed to influence the drug-taking outcome. They include 'indirect' and more 'distal' influences, such as extent of unemployment in a particular neighbourhood, as well as individual, 'intermediate' level indicators, such as knowledge about the negative effects of drugs and the level of social skills possessed by a young person who might be exposed to pressure from peers. However, the 'model' illustrated by Figure 2.3 is an *ad hoc* assemblage of items which – although doubtless having some relevance – is, as it stands, atheoretical. It is our contention that the analysis of client characteristics will be more useful for both structuring and evaluating programmes if it is derived from theoretically constructed models. Such models will, ideally, use research evidence in order to ensure that only the

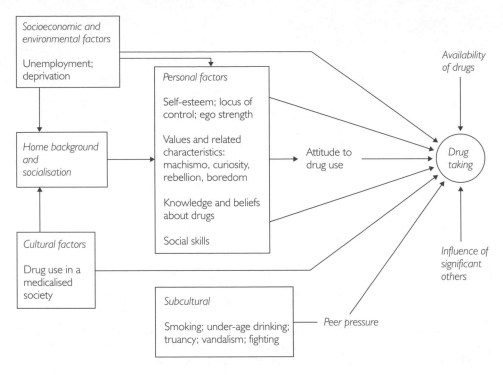

**Figure 2.3** Misuse of Drugs: Psychosocial and Environmental Influences

most important variables from a plethora of *possible* variables are specified together with their inter-relationship. We will, therefore, now consider a number of potentially useful theories and models which have been used to design and evaluate health promotion initiatives. We will first consider a theory that seeks to explain the factors influencing whole social systems and then consider a number of models centring on the individual and the factors influencing his or her health-related decision making.

## Macro level theory: the *Communication of Innovations Theory*

It is a truism that health promotion is concerned to promote change. In the last analysis health education, as pointed out earlier, seeks to promote health- and illness-related learning, i.e. a relatively permanent change in disposition or

capability. The implementation of healthy public policy involves, for instance, change in legislation, fiscal and economic measures and in the material environment. Change can usefully be categorised in terms of macro, meso and micro. As used here, 'macro' refers to large-scale developments, e.g. at the national level. 'Micro' level work happens at the level of interaction between individuals, e.g. between teacher and class or doctor and patient. The 'meso' level is somewhere in between these two and would be nicely exemplified by 'health promoting school' or 'health promoting hospital' initiatives. From among a number of alternative empirical macro level models we have chosen by way of example one of the best researched and most frequently used explanatory systems, *Communication of Innovations Theory* (Rogers and Shoemaker, 1971; Rogers 1995).

This approach seeks to describe the ways in which large numbers of people forming a 'social system' (i.e. populations or communities) come to change their customary practices and adopt new behaviours. It has a particular appeal in that it has been used for the analysis of the factors governing the adoption of health-related innovations.

According to the authors, it is based on seven major research traditions and, at the time of publication, drew upon 1084 publications in anthropology, sociology, education, communication and marketing.

Rogers and Shoemaker (1971) define an innovation as:

*... an idea, practice, or object perceived as new by an individual. It matters little, so far as human behavior is concerned, whether or not an idea is 'objectively' new as measured by the lapse of time since its first use or discovery. It is the perceived or subjective newness of the idea for the individual that determines his reaction to it. If the idea seems new to the individual, it is an innovation.*

(p19)

Self-evidently, our concern here is with health innovations.

A community (or, more accurately, a social system) may be geographic, i.e. a group of people in a defined place, or less typically 'relational' or 'virtual'. In the latter instance the social system will be defined in terms of interactions which are not geographically rooted; for instance, a 'population' of doctors, teachers or nurses may be widely distributed throughout a relatively large area and, accordingly, not having an opportunity for face-to-face primary contact. Further consideration will be given to the notion of community in a later chapter.

Six major generalisations may be made from the findings of communication of innovations theory. They are concerned, primarily, with the rate of adoption of innovations and with the impact of certain important variables on the rate of adoption. These variables include:

- the characteristics of potential adopters;
- the rate of adoption;
- the nature of the social system;
- the characteristics of the innovation;
- the characteristics of 'change agents';
- community participation.

## Characteristics of the adopters

All adopters of an innovation are presumed to move through a series of stages before adopting (or rejecting) new ideas and practices. However, some people move through these stages more rapidly than others. In other words, potential adopters first become aware of the existence of the innovation (clearly if this does not happen, the innovation will not be adopted no matter how beneficial it might be); this may then be followed by arousal of interest prior to trying out the new practice; ultimately, after the trial phase, the new practice will either be adopted or rejected. Rogers and Shoemaker hypothesised the existence of five types of individual to explain this differential progress. Accordingly, they used the term '*laggards*' to describe those individuals who take an inordinate amount of time before committing themselves to action, whereas, on the other hand, '*innovators*', were presumed to have greater exposure to communications and for some reason tend to express immediate interest; they might even have a general tendency to espouse novelty – perhaps even novelty for novelty's sake. Table 2.1 lists these different adopter categories.

As may be seen, those who adopt first of all are labelled innovators; they are closely followed by early adopters who are in turn succeeded by the early majority. Bringing up the rear are the late majority and, last of all, the laggards.

## Rate of adoption: the 'S-shaped' curve

When the proportion of those who adopt the innovation is plotted against time, a characteristically 'S-shaped' curve results. The shape is determined by the differential rate of adoption of the population and reflects the different adopter characteristics mentioned above and other facilitating factors described below. A steep curve indicates a rapid rate of adoption; a flattened curve shows a slow rate of adoption. This is shown graphically in Figure 2.4.

**Table 2.1**  The Communication of Innovations: Major Adopter Categories (adapted from Rogers and Shoemaker, 1971)

| Adopter category | Characteristics |
|---|---|
| Innovator | 2.5% of population: eager but a 'deviant'; probably mistrusted by the safe majority |
| Early adopter | 13.5% of population: respectable but amenable to change; good candidate for opinion leader or community aide |
| Early majority | 34% of population: according to Rogers and Shoemaker their motto might be *Be not the last to lay the old aside, nor the first by which the new is tried!* |
| Late majority | 34% of population: the sceptics reluctant to change until benefits of innovation have been clearly proved |
| Laggards | 16% of population: the diehard conservatives; will doubtless incorporate a sub-group who will never change and appear to be against everything most of the time |

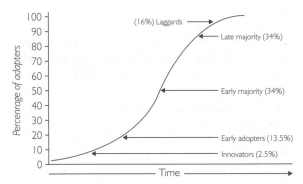

**Figure 2.4**  The S-shaped Diffusin Curve and Adopter Categories (after Rogers and Shoemaker, 1971)

There are two key points worthy of note by programme evaluators. The first lesson to be learned from communication of innovations theory is that it can take a very long time before the last laggard has yielded to the force of change! Indeed, Rogers and Shoemaker cite early examples of diffusion time lag and readers may be interested in the following somewhat esoteric facts. It apparently took some 40 years before the tunnel oven was adopted in the English pottery industry, 14 years for the adoption of hybrid seed corn in Iowa, 50 years before US schools adopted the idea of the kindergarten and 5 or 6 years to adopt modern mathematics in the 1960s (Rogers and Shoemaker, 1971 p16). Rogers (1995) provides telling examples of recent successes and failures of innovations including the dramatic rise in use of the Internet (paralleled doubtless by the escalating use of mobile phones!). Particularly

interesting is the failure of the DVORAK keyboard to replace the traditional QWERTY keyboard.

**Box 1**  A Tale of Two Keyboards

Since the first typewriters tended to jam fairly readily, the QWERTY keyboard was originally designed to curb the enthusiasms of early typists and avoid a cluster of mangled levers. In other words, the keys were arranged in a deliberately inefficient manner. With the improvement in typewriter mechanics, the ergonomically designed DVORAK keyboard was introduced; it could reputedly increase speed by some 20%. It was spectacularly unsuccessful!

It is clearly wise not to expect instant success and, more technically, to take account of the fact that it will be increasingly difficult to influence later adopters and shift a residual hard core within the broader category of laggards. In other words, a law of diminishing returns will operate in health promotion programmes seeking to influence large groups of people. As we will note later, evaluators should, on that account, build some form of compensation into their calculations.

### The social system

Three further general influences on the adoption of new ideas and practices will be made here. The first of these is concerned with the nature of the social system itself and in this respect it seems reasonable to accept Rogers and Shoemaker's view that certain 'traditional' communities will take longer to adopt *any* innovation whereas, on the other hand, a 'cosmopolitan' social system will be more open to change, perhaps because it lacks the culturally created caution of the former or has better communication systems, or both. Although conservatism is a quite common characteristic, some communities and professional groups, for example, are more conservative than others!

**Box 2**  The Painful Nature of Change

> *One of the greatest pains to human nature is the pain of a new idea. It is, as common people say, so upsetting, it makes you think that after all, your favorite notions may be wrong, your firmest beliefs ill-founded... . Naturally, therefore, common men hate a new idea, and are disposed more or less to ill treat the original man (sic) who brings it.*
>
> Bagehot (1873)

## Characteristics of the innovation

We may paraphrase Rogers and Shoemaker's list of the features which maximise an innovation's likelihood of adoption. Ideally the innovation should have the following perceived characteristics:

- relative advantage compared with practices to be replaced;
- compatibility with practices and structures that will remain;
- simplicity rather than complexity;
- the possibility for trying the innovation without permanent commitment ('trialability');
- observability, i.e. it should be possible to observe the effects of the innovation – preferably in a relatively short period of time.

By way of example, if a community perceives that a recommended dietary change has benefits for them by comparison with their existing diet; if the proposed change is compatible with lifestyle and culture; if it is not too complicated, e.g. to grow, collect and cook; if it is relatively easy to try out without making a full commitment; if the community can readily and rapidly observe the benefits – then the innovation stands a pretty good chance of being adopted!

**Box 3**  An Educational Innovation Doomed to Fail

The headteacher has been pressured by her governing body to address the apparently escalating problem of unwanted teenage pregnancies. The local advisor has sent the head details of a new (and rather expensive) teaching package designed to be used in the school science curriculum with details of the training needed to implement it. The head of biology has been charged with appraising this curriculum package. She discusses it with colleagues. The new sex education curriculum appears decidedly complicated to biology department staff who will have to implement it. It would be rather difficult to try it out since it involves quite a heavy commitment of staff training time and expensive materials: if it does not work the resources will be lost. It looks as though it will involve a reorganisation of the present tutor system and will involve collaboration with those teachers involved in personal and social education. A major shift in timetabling would be needed. As with many health education programmes, success would not be immediate! It would not be apparent for some time whether or not the programme would actually reduce the teenage pregnancy rate. Although the headteacher appears to be committed (she thinks she ought to be!), senior staff have their doubts and junior staff in the department are decidedly anxious at the prospect of tackling a sensitive subject like sex education – for which they have had no training. The educational supplier and advisor have made it clear that the programme must be implemented fully and the recommended teaching methods must be used if success is to be achieved.

In other words, it looks as if it will be difficult to adapt the programme to the needs of the children and within the constraints of the overstretched timetable. As a matter of principle, the teachers object to such efforts to 'teacher-proof' packages. Apart from being seen to do something about the problem of teenage pregnancies, satisfy the governors and gain some 'brownie points' at the next inspection, there seem to be very few gains for school and staff and a plethora of costs: it is expensive and the tuck shop budget has already been allocated for new reading schemes; it will involve the staff in a heavy commitment of time; the personal and social education staff will be reluctant to hand over responsibility to their biology colleagues (and collaboration is always a problem!); the subject matter and the (new) experiential teaching methods appear rather threatening.

## Change agent characteristics

The penultimate facet of *Communication of Innovations Theory* of interest to us has to do with the characteristics of the change agent, e.g. the health educator working with a community or group of people.

It is, of course, a matter of common sense to note that whether or not people are persuaded to modify their lifestyle may very well hinge on the repertoire of skills possessed by the health educator. However, Rogers and Shoemaker additionally remind us that the change agent must be acceptable to the community (or be sufficiently cunning to employ those people who are acceptable). This notion is elaborated in the principle of 'homophily'. Before commenting further on its significance, it is worth asserting a commonly held dictum of *Communication of Innovations Theory*: innovators are deviants! It would be extremely unwise for change agents to recruit them as 'lay leaders'!

**Box 4** The Concept of Homophily

> *Homophily is the degree to which pairs of individuals who interact are similar in certain attributes, such as beliefs, values, education, social status and the like.*
>
> *A further refinement of this proposition includes the concept of empathy ... the ability of an individual to project himself into the role of another.*
>
> Rogers and Shoemaker (1971)

It is a truism to say that there are different kinds of leader and, while acknowledging that different leaders having different kinds of credibility may stimulate community action, the principle of homophily places special emphasis on the fact that people are more likely to be influenced by those with whom they can identify. They tend to identify with those whom they perceive to have certain attributes in common – such as similar beliefs, values, education and shared social circumstances generally. By definition, 'opinion leaders' are homophilous – whether they enjoy popularity in their village or are respected doctors in a medical community. Taken at face value, the outlook for professionals (who, by definition, are dissimilar – or 'heterophilous' – to their clients) is pessimistic. However, the 'refinement to the proposition' notes that professionals who have empathy – a social skill which can be learned – can have a similar effect to the genuinely homophilous individual. And so, a judicious mix of empathic change agents in alliance with 'opinion leaders' would form an essential feature of a macro intervention developed in accordance with '*Communication of Innovations Theory*.

## Community participation

The importance of community participation was highlighted in Chapter 1, where it was asserted that the involvement of clients and community was a *sine qua non* for ideologically sound health promotion. *Communication of Innovations Theory* supports this contention – but from a technical, 'empirical' perspective.

**Box 5**   Chinese Wisdom

> *Go to the people*
> *Live among them*
> *Love them*
> *Start with what they know*
> *Build on what they have*
> *But of the best leaders*
> *When their task is accomplished*
> *Their work is done*
> *The people all remark*
> *We have done it ourselves.*
>
> (Chabot, 1976)

Clearly, communities change frequently without any apparently deliberate intervention from health or other professionals. However, health promotion or any other deliberate effort to improve the welfare of social groups typically seeks to facilitate change in communities. If the advice embodied in the Chinese poem in Box 5 is to be heeded, the process of facilitation must be unobtrusive and subtle – and will typically take a long time. Figure 2.5 examines the relationship between the nature and extent of community participation in relation to the ease of difficulty with which an innovation is adopted.

When a community itself recognises it has a 'felt need' and identifies the ways of achieving that need without any external intervention, change will happen rapidly. On the other hand, the worst possible scenario occurs when an external agency (for instance a district health authority) has concluded that a community has a problem and then proceeds to prescribe a solution to that problem, the chances of the innovation being adopted are indeed slight. As we will see later in this book, the process of community development adopts an approach in which the external agency employs a sensitive and skilled change agent to help the community recognise its needs and difficulties and then supplies the assistance necessary for community members themselves to solve the problems they have identified.

| Level of Community Participation | Anticipated rate of adoption of the innovation |
|---|---|
| Community spontaneously recognises it has a problem<br><br>Community identifies solution to problem | VERY RAPID CHANGE |
| External agency considers that community has a problem<br><br>Prescribes solution | VERY SLOW – OR NEVER! |

**Figure 2.5**   Level of Community Participation by Anticipated Rate of Adoption

## THEORY AT THE MICRO LEVEL

Having considered the usefulness of macro level theory in the form of Rogers and Shoemaker's formulation, we will now continue with the general assertion that 'there is nothing so practical as a good theory'. This time we will be operating at the micro level and will consider how an understanding of psychological social and environmental factors may influence individual decision making and subsequent choices and behaviours.

As Green (1984) has pointed out, there is a wide range of theoretical models at the disposal of health educators and we might reasonably ask why one particular model should be selected at the expense of any other. We discussed the nature and purpose of models in Chapter 1, noting how they are derived from theory and thus seek to provide an explanation of some feature of our world. Models do not provide a detailed replica of reality but rather they offer a partial and simplified representation of whatever aspect of the real world is of interest to the theoretician or practitioner. The process of simplification is necessary because it allows us to concentrate on what is most important for particular needs while excluding irrelevancies and unnecessary detail. A good model will achieve this goal of simplification while including all key elements. Following the nomenclature adopted earlier, 'empirical' models seeking to provide a coherent but concise account of the factors influencing health choices should incorporate the various components which are essential to human decision making and explain their inter-relationships. A better model might quantify those relationships or provide a more sophisticated explanation of the relationship between the various components within a system. It might also facilitate predictions about the likelihood of individuals – or, more problematically, groups of individuals – adopting and sustaining a particular course of action under given circumstances.

Some so-called models offer no more than a useful but limited formula that may provide a rough guide for practice and the evaluation of practice. For instance, the 'K-A-P' formula – possibly because of its simplicity – enjoyed wide currency a few years ago (and in some quarters still appears to be alive and well!). It derived from the fairly obvious assumption that knowledge (K) might be necessary for the adoption of particular practices (P) but were certainly not sufficient. As a consequence, it was assumed that A for attitude should be inserted to fill the conceptual gap. Since the concept of attitude is rather vague and research has indicated that the adoption of practices can lead to attitude change rather than vice versa, this addition often did little to explain the complexities of human behaviour. A somewhat more elaborate formula was used by the seminal North Karelia Heart Disease Prevention Project – a successful, community-wide Finnish programme designed to reduce the high rate of heart disease in that country. Although the authors would not consider it a model as such, it was deemed useful to develop a *...framework of general goals and theoretical principles...* consisting of five programme elements which were thought to be the minimum necessary for coherent programme design. They were:

- improved preventive services;
- information (*'to educate people about their health'*);
- persuasion (*'to motivate people'*);
- training (*'to increase skills of self-control, environmental management and social action'*);
- community organization (*'to create social support'*).

(McAlister *et al.*, 1982)

Whilst an improvement on the simplistic 'K-A-P' formulation , the five point plan refers to interventions rather than to explanation of the influences on health-related choices. It would therefore appear at a later stage in the succession of models listed in Figure 2.1. There is, however, no shortage of models that seek to provide insights into human health- and illness-related behaviour and several authors have provided details of the most common of these (see for instance Conner and Norman, 1996; Bennett and Murphy, 1997; Glanz *et al.*, 1997; Nutbeam and Harris, 1998). Reviews and applications of individualistic, decision making models may also be found nested within broader, ecological models and planning models – of which the prime example is the PRECEDE–PROCEED model (Green and Kreuter, 1999).

*Box 6*   Some Common Theories and Models of Health-
Related Decision Making

- *Health Belief Model*
- *Theory of Reasoned Action*
- *Theory of Planned Behaviour*
- *Social Learning/Social Cognitive Theory*
- *Trans-theoretical Model*
- *Protection Motivation Theory*

## The *Health Belief Model*

Rather more refined theoretical models provide a narrower and sharper focus. Probably the best known of these is the *Health Belief Model* (HBM) – originally developed to explain why people failed to utilise health services (Hochbaum, 1958; Rosenstock, 1966), it has undergone various revisions (Becker, 1984; Janz and Becker, 1984). Its main contribution to programme planning has been the way it has highlighted the role of certain beliefs in stimulating preventive health actions. In short, the central tenets of the HBM are that individuals will not adopt health behaviours designed to prevent specific diseases unless they believe they are susceptible to the disease or disorder in question, they believe it is serious, they accept that the recommended preventive actions will be effective and that the benefits accruing from their actions will outweigh any costs or disadvantages that they believe will be incurred as a result. It was also acknowledged that some trigger might be necessary before the individual's intention was translated into practice.

*Box 7*   The *Health Belief Model*

Adoption of preventive practices will depend on:

- Beliefs about susceptibility
- Beliefs about seriousness
- Beliefs about benefits
- Beliefs about costs

... and, in addition, may require the presence of a trigger.

There is always a danger in judging the value of a model on the basis of the shorthand version which is commonly used. For instance, it is quite evident that beliefs about seriousness, costs and benefits will only be useful as indicators of likelihood of action if the motivation they engendered is assessed. The more complete version of the model does in fact incorporate a motivational element in that beliefs about susceptibility and seriousness are considered to generate a level of 'perceived threat' which in turn contributes ultimately to health choices – together with beliefs about cost and benefit. Moreover, a later version of the model argued that predictions about the adoption of behaviours would be enhanced if the individual had a generally positive attitude to health (often measured by totting up the number of preventive measures already undertaken by the individual in addition to the preventive action currently under consideration). However, the HBM is undoubtedly weak in relation to precise examination of social influences and also emotional aspects of human behaviour. For instance, although 'perceived threat' is considered to mediate the effect of beliefs, the effect of fear and arousal on decision making is by no means simple and, according to Prentice-Dunn and Rogers (1986), requires a particular focus and the development of particular theory (in this instance *Protection Motivation Theory*, which, in the author's words, takes us **beyond the health belief model** in its capacity to explain the effect of these important variables.

It is, of course, an easy matter to generate indicators of success from the HBM. It is assumed that health promotion would seek to influence beliefs and provide triggers for action. Success would, therefore, depend on the extent to which individuals, after the intervention, now believed they were susceptible to the disease, considered the disease serious and accepted that the benefits of the action outweighed the costs. We will later describe such indicators as intermediate indicators, since the outcomes of a successful programme would be measured in terms of actual behaviour change, such as use of a cancer screening service, or even (inappropriately!) by changes in the incidence of the disease in question. The provision of effective triggers, on the other hand, will be defined as indirect indicators of process.

### The *Theory of Reasoned Action* – and *Planned Behaviour*

A comprehensive account of micro level models is patently beyond the scope of this book. The main purpose of our discussion here is to reiterate the importance of using theoretical models, both for effective practice and for evaluating the results of that practice. It is also a concern of this chapter to demonstrate that certain models are superior to others in the sophistication and comprehensiveness of the explanations they provide. It is also our concern to recommend a 'horses for courses' approach in selecting models. On occasions a relatively limited model may be appropriate because of its simplicity or because its central element is consonant with the particular programme that is being evaluated. In the light of these comments, it is important to refer to one of the models most frequently used in assessing the characteristics of client groups and evaluating the interventions resulting from that analysis. First, though, it should be noted that the term model and theory are being used almost interchangeably in this section of the chapter – for sake of convenience. The characteristics of models and theories were, however, discussed more completely in Chapter 1 and will not be repeated here.

The model under discussion now is the *Theory of Reasoned Action* (TRA) developed by Fishbein and his colleague Ajzen (Ajzen and Fishbein, 1980; Fishbein and Ajzen, 1985; Schifter and Ajzen, 1985) Fishbein and Ajzen complement and improve on aspects of an HBM analysis of health decision making by separating belief from attitude and emphasising the paramount importance of the influence of '*significant others*' on an individual's '*intention to act*'. The often substantial gap between intention and practice is acknowledged and the relationship between beliefs, attitudes, normative factors, intention and practice is expressed in mathematical terms. For a recent application of the theory to the prevention of AIDS see Terry, Gallois and McCamish (1993) and for further discussion of TRA and its variants – and other 'Social Cognition' models – see Conner and Norman (1996).

As good model builders, Fishbein and Ajzen developed their model to take account of additional demands for explanation deriving from work in new areas of investigation – such as the health domain. The *Theory of Planned Behaviour* was the result. This involved the construction of an extension (architecturally speaking) – i.e. the addition of the notion of *perceived behavioural control* (Ajzen, 1985, 1991; Ajzen and Madden, 1986; Montano *et al.*, 1997).

**Box 8** A Formula for Predicting Health Choices

response efficacy × self-efficacy
= health choices

The concept of behavioural control, in turn, could be said to derive from *Social Learning Theory* and the seminal work of Bandura (1986). Bearing in mind an earlier reference to simple but useful 'models', it is worth noting the especially simple but useful formula derived from social learning theory which rivals the K-A-P formula in its brevity but outstrips it completely in its explanatory value. In short, two complementary notions are considered to operate multiplicatively in influencing any behavioural outcome – including health outcomes. They are, first, '*response efficacy*', i.e. the belief that a given course of action will lead to some desirable result (or avoid some negative or unwanted consequence). Incidentally, this important belief formed the basis for a much earlier theoretical canon of behaviourist psychology, the '*Law of Effect*'. This, so-called, law argued that behaviours were shaped by individuals' learning which actions resulted in the achievement of some positive state of affairs or the avoidance of some unpleasant outcome (Thorndike, 1905).

**Box 9** The 'Law of Effect'

> *... any act which in a given situation produces satisfaction becomes associated with the situation, so that when the situation recurs, the act is more likely than ever before to recur also. Conversely, any act which in a given situation produces discomfort becomes disassociated from that situation, so that when the situation recurs, the act is less likely than before to recur.*

The second complementary construct in Bandura's formulation is that of '*self-efficacy*', i.e. the extent to which an individual accepts that (s)he is actually capable of achieving the desired result. The concept of self-efficacy will be re-examined later in the chapter in the context of an analysis of the dynamics of self-empowerment. For now, it is worth signalling the relevance of self-efficacy and '*perceived behavioural control*' in operationalising the ideologically based commitment to empowerment.

The *Theory of Planned Behaviour* is outlined in Figure 2.6. The 'extension' which converts the *Theory of Reasoned Action* (TRA) is shown in bold.

A major feature of the TRA is its conceptualisation of intention to act as a product of beliefs about the health action and evaluation of those beliefs. In other words, a given belief will only have an effect on intention to act if the outcome associated with that belief is valued. As noted above, a second key dimension of the model is the emphasis it places on the influence of other people on a given individual's intentions. Again, the multiplicative relationship between belief and attitude is apparent: not only must individuals believe that a given significant other will react positively or negatively to a proposed action but they must be motivated to comply with the wishes of that particular 'referent'. The conversion of TRA to the *Theory of Planned Behaviour* is achieved by recognising that predictions are improved if a self-efficacy dimension is added. This describes the extent to which an individual believes that he or she is capable of achieving the desired goal – taking account of the power relationship involved between that individual and either environmental circumstances or other people.

Indicators of success can readily be generated by the TRA and, of course, the *Theory of Planned Behaviour*. Typically these would include evidence that a number of relevant beliefs about the health action had been acquired

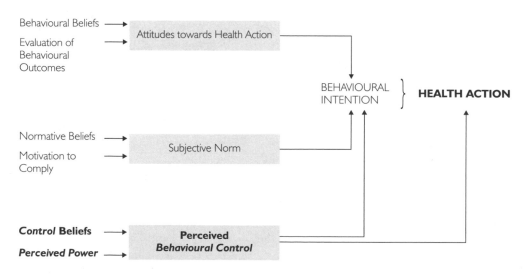

**Figure 2.6** The Theory of Planned Behaviour

since the intervention and that these beliefs had a 'motivational charge' converting them to positive attitudes to the health action. Ajzen and Fishbein's formulation recommends the use of rating scales which measure not only attitude strength but the degree of certainty attached to the beliefs. Similarly, a successful programme might be expected to influence beliefs about the likely reaction of other people and this too could be measured. Again, health promoters seeking to reduce the 'unhealthy' impact of, say, peer groups might also hope to record a shift in motivation to comply! Clearly, it would also be possible to measure the effects of changed beliefs and attitudes in respect of the health action together with influence of significant others in a global measure of intention to act or, indeed, with the adoption of the recommended health action.

## The *Trans-theoretical Model*

One of the models most commonly used as a basis for health promotion is the *Trans-theoretical Model*, more popularly known as the *Stages of Change Model*. It is due, primarily, to Prochaska and DiClemente (Prochaska and DiClemente, 1984; Breteler *et al.*, 1990; DiClemente, 1991; Prochaska, 1992; Prochaska *et al.*, 1997). This model is usually applied to inter-personal encounters – particularly the face-to-face relationship between health professional and client (Miller and Rollnick, 1991; Lawrence, 1999). Its major contention is that individuals typically move through a series of stages before they actually adopt a new practice or quit an existing health damaging practice. This observation has two particular implications that are especially useful for health promoters: first, health education should be tailored to the client's readiness to change and, second, practitioners should acknowledge that relapse is likely but the client who has relapsed will, in all probability, re-enter the 'revolving door' of the change process at a later date. Additionally, of course, it is important to anticipate the possibility of relapse by providing anticipatory guidance and skills – a point to which we will return in our discussion of the HAM.

**Box 10**  Stages of Change

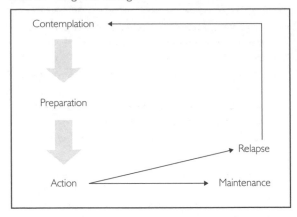

Within the context of programme planning, the stages of change analysis is particularly relevant to the process of needs assessment. In relation to evaluation, success could be measured by the extent to which an individual had moved from one stage to another (an outcome indicator) and the appropriateness of the counselling or education provided by the practitioner to facilitate that transition (i.e. a process indicator).

## The work of Triandis

Before discussing the HAM reference will be made to a sophisticated model which lacks the popularity of HBM or TRA but which nonetheless has much greater relevance for health education. It is interesting to speculate why this should be so. Is the model too complex or has it, by pure chance, not received the publicity associated with other models? The model was developed by Triandis (1980) and two equations from the model will be provided below so that readers may judge for themselves the relevance of the constructs used.

*Equation 1*

$$P_a = (w_H H + w_I I) \, P.F.$$

where: $P_a$ is the probability of the (health-related) act occurring – indexed by a number between 0 and 1; $w$ signifies a weight to be attached to the construct to which it is attached; $I$ refers to the behavioural intentions or self-instruction to perform the act; $H$ refers to habits, i.e. those automatic behaviour tendencies developed during the past history of the individual; $F$ describes the facilitating conditions that increase (or decrease) the probability of the act occurring.

*Equation 2*

$$I = w_s S + w_A A + w_C C$$

where: $I$ is behavioural intention; $S$ is the individual's self-instruction to do what is viewed as correct from the point of view of the individual's moral code and to do what has been previously agreed with others; $A$ is the affect (i.e. 'the general motivational charge' attached to the behaviour); $C$ is the value of the number of perceived consequences of the behaviour. Again, $w$ is a weight to be assigned to each factor.

In order to facilitate appraisal of the constructs which should be incorporated into an efficient explanatory model for health education practice, readers might care to compare and contrast the components within Triandis' system with the HAM. Before explaining the HAM, we would like to reiterate the point that although models should be judged on the basis of their sophistication and applicability, personal predilection should legitimately play a part in selection. Alternatively, practitioners may prefer to build their own model. Whatever the choice, a theoretical framework is a *sine qua non* for professional decision making.

## THE 'HEALTH ACTION MODEL'

The HAM was developed in an attempt to provide a comprehensive framework which would incorporate the major variables influencing health choices and actions (Tones, 1979, 1981, 1987). Although its original concern was with health education, it proved to be compatible with the formulation of health promotion described in Chapter 1.

### Overview

Figure 2.7 provides an overview of key system components.

It will be seen that there are two major sections to the HAM. The first of these contributes to an individual's intention to act, or *behavioural intention* (BI), and comprises an interacting system having three parts: cognitive, affective and normative. Central to the cognitive dimension is a belief system which interfaces with an *'information processor'* which incorporates the various psychological factors associated with the reception of information and associated with effective communication. It therefore includes the processes of attention and perception. In addition, the information processor includes important cognitive skills typically associated with efficient decision making and problem solving (see for instance Janis and Mann, 1977) and needed to make 'rational' choices between incoming data.

A two-way interaction exists between the *belief system* and the information handled by the 'processor'. On the one hand, the information input can create new beliefs and modify existing beliefs; on the other hand, existing beliefs may distort or even block incoming information – for instance as part of the phenomenon of defensive avoidance.

***Box 11*** The Information Processor

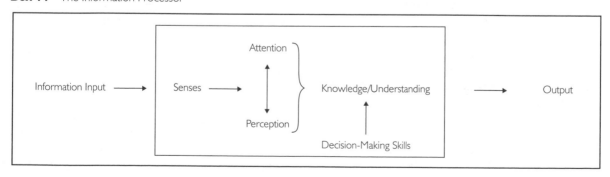

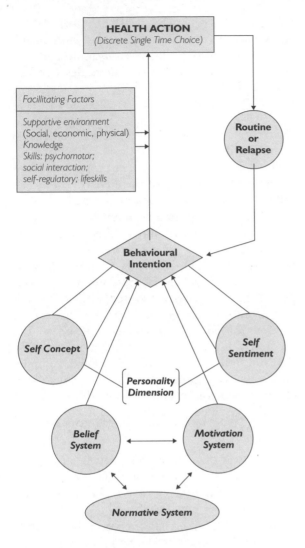

**Figure 2.7** The *Health Action Model:* An Overview

cerned with whatever factors make it likely that an action will be sustained or become routinised or, on the other hand, lead to relapse or rejection of a previously made decision.

In terms of health promotion goals, the first section (belief system; motivation system; normative system) relates to the motivation of individuals to act; the second section is concerned with the analysis of barriers to implementing intentions and, conversely, with providing post-decisional support.

It is not, of course, assumed that behavioural intention is necessarily a conscious state; an individual will frequently make a decision in a choice situation without any conscious calculation of the costs and benefits and without weighing up alternatives. The decision is, however, influenced by a peculiar cluster of beliefs, motives and social pressures which have created a state of readiness for action when the appropriate circumstances arise. Clearly, efficient decision making will in fact require conscious calculations and many health education approaches will incorporate that goal into their rationale.

The term 'discrete single time choice' refers to a single specific decision. The goals of most health promotion programmes may include a large number of such decisions – although programme planners are more likely to hope that these choices will be translated into enduring 'routines'.

Once the choice has been made there are two possibilities: the decision may become part of an individual's behavioural repertoire or it may be reversed. For instance, purchase and preparation of a high fibre meal may result in a firm commitment never to try it again or, alternatively, the experience may prove enjoyable and subsequently may be incorporated into habitual dietary practice. Routines may be established in the way described above or may result from an often protracted process of socialisation. Children do not routinely brush their teeth after meals as a result of a process of 'vigilant decision making' based on appraisal of costs and benefit. They do it as a result of Skinnerian conditioning in which parents shape their behaviour through the application of reward (and sometimes punishment). The whole procedure would typically be supported by the use of 'modelling' in accordance with the dictates of social learning theory.

The affective dimension is defined by the *motivation system*. This has a reciprocal relationship with the *belief system* and is the repository of many and various elements comprised by an individual's motivational state. The *normative system*, on the other hand, incorporates both cognitive and affective aspects and signals the importance of different kinds of social pressure on people's intention to act.

The second major section is concerned with all those factors which determine whether or not an intention is translated into practice; it is also con-

Routine practices of any kind are not under direct conscious control and do not therefore require a conscious decision, except perhaps when they are becoming established, when they are disrupted or when attempts are made to change them. For example, drivers need to make a deliberate choice once they have formed an intention to wear seat belts, however, once the choice has become routine, it will recur automatically.

The notion of routine shares many of the characteristics of the concept of 'habit' as used by Triandis and mentioned earlier.

**Box 12** In Praise of Habit (!)

> *Habit simplifies the movements required to achieve given results, makes them more accurate and diminishes fatigue.*
>
> *Habit is the enormous flywheel of society, its most precious conservative agent. It alone is what keeps us all within the bounds of ordinance, and saves the children of fortune from the envious uprisings of the poor.*
>
> *In most of us, by the age of thirty, the character has set like plaster, and will never soften again.*
>
> *The great thing, in all education, is to make our nervous system our ally instead of our enemy. We must make automatic and habitual, as early as possible, as many useful actions as we can.*
>
> *In the acquisition of a new habit, or the leaving off of an old one, we must take care to launch ourselves with as strong and decided an initiative as possible. Never suffer an exception to occur until the new habit is securely rooted in your life.*
>
> *Seize the very first possible opportunity to act on every resolution you make, and on every emotional prompting you may experience in the direction of the habits you aspire to gain.*
>
> *Keep the faculty of effort alive in you by a little gratuitous exercise every day.*
>
> (James, 1890)

Figure 2.7, accordingly, shows a feedback process. This indicates how the experience of performing a particular health action, a break in a routine or other related event can either consolidate action or, as it were, 'switch it off'. For instance, a negative experience at an antenatal clinic may cause a woman to modify her previous beliefs about the costs and benefits of attending. A woman who has been persuaded to breast feed her children may experience discomfort and pain from sore nipples and start to bottle feed; a man who has succeeded in quitting smoking for several days may no longer be able to cope with the feelings of anxiety and irritability – and relapses. On the other hand, someone who has reluctantly decided to use a condom to assuage a sense of apprehension about risk of HIV infection may discover the experience is quite colourful and exciting!

Of course, even relatively well established health actions may be discarded. When this involves a return to previous behaviours judged to be health damaging (and/or morally reprehensible) the term 'relapse' is typically used.

### Barriers to action, facilitating factors and the provision of support

Bearing in mind the importance attached by health promotion and the empowerment model to the provision of support to facilitate genuine decision making, it is essential to take account of those barriers or inhibiting factors which may be interposed between intention and action. Conversely, we might say that the identification of appropriate facilitating factors is an essential feature of effective health promotion. In Figure 2.7 two varieties of factor are depicted. The first of these is the physical, cultural and socio-economic environment: following the extensive discussion of this set of influences in Chapter 1, this factor must be regarded as the most important. The second set of factors are 'personal' in the sense that they refer to the knowledge and skills which the individual needs to ensure that the health action will actually be adopted and sustained. Skills may include psychomotor competences, such as the dexterity needed for the proper use of a condom or for the efficient practice of first aid techniques. They will also include social interaction skills – for instance, the capacity to communicate assertively with a partner about safer sex practices. Less obvious, perhaps, is a need for self-regulatory skills.

As observed above in connection with discussion of the problem of relapse, sustaining behaviours that involve loss of gratification is one of the most difficult of the tasks which health education seeks to facilitate. Again as noted earlier, the difficulties involved in controlling 'addictive behaviours' are well documented. Accordingly, a variety of techniques associated with behaviour modification have been evolved to help people monitor their behaviours and environmental circumstances, avoid temptation and discover substitute gratification and rewards for successful maintenance of the healthy activities they have chosen to adopt. These various techniques are here referred to as '*self-regulatory skills*' (Kanfer and Karoly, 1972).

While on the subject of gaining control over addictive behaviours, we might note how the *Stages of Change Model* or *Trans-theoretical Model* is conceptualised in HAM. In the HAM the stages of pre-contemplation and contemplation relate to the changing dynamic within the belief, motivation and normative systems that results from individuals' experience or follows one or more of a number of health education encounters. The effects of the experience or the education will impact on behavioural intention, leading individuals to formulate a new and previously unconsidered course of action or increasing the strength of an existing intention to act. The strength of the intention may or may not be sufficient to lead to the 'action stage'. If, however, it does, the kind of support mentioned above will be required to ensure transition to the 'maintenance stage' and 'immunise' the individual against the alternative final stage of 'relapse'.

## The belief system

Some indication of the importance of health beliefs has already been provided in the earlier discussion of the 'Health Belief Model'. However, although the notions of susceptibility, seriousness and beliefs about costs and benefits are useful, an alternative formulation is preferred in the 'Health Action Model'. This alternative view is summarised below.

- The notion of susceptibility is incorporated into the self-concept.
- Beliefs about costs, benefits and seriousness are only useful if the nature of their relationship with the affective dimension is clear. In HAM this relationship is explained as a multiplicative interaction between the belief system and the motivation system. For example, the extent to which people believe that a disease or condition is serious and the proposed health actions will incur costs and/or benefits will depend on an individual's value system, emotional state, gratifications and addictions and, to some extent, aspects of their personality – in other words, their general motivational system.
- All of the beliefs emphasised in the HBM ultimately derive from and depend upon 'subordinate beliefs' which are frequently the main target of health promotion interventions. They must, therefore, be specified.

It will doubtless be apparent that beliefs are defined in the HAM as cognitive rather than affective constructs. In this we follow Fishbein's (1976) formulation, namely

*A belief is a probability judgement that links some object or concept to some attribute. (The terms 'object' and 'attribute' are used in a generic sense and both terms may refer to any discriminable aspect of an individual's world.) For example, I may believe that PILL (an object) is a DEPRESSANT (an attribute). The content of the belief is defined by the person's subjective probability that the object–attribute relationship exists (or is true).*

The importance of subordinate beliefs and the hierarchical nature of beliefs in general, can be illustrated by considering the ways in which a number of beliefs may contribute to a hypothetical individual's decision to seek early medical advice in relation to a skin lesion which might prove to be skin cancer.

Before seeking medical assistance, the individual must first recognise that (s)he has a skin lesion. She must then believe it might be skin cancer, i.e. she must form a level of subjective probability that justifies a visit to her doctor. For reasons to be stated below, it may indeed facilitate her medical consultation if she believes that it is unlikely that the lesion is in fact skin cancer but, nonetheless, feels it is worth checking it out.

The individual's belief about the likelihood of the sore on her hand being skin cancer will be influenced by her pre-existing belief about her susceptibility to that disease (which, in turn, will depend on her understanding and beliefs about the risk factors). Her intention to visit her doctor will also be influenced by her belief about the seriousness of the disease. Now, according to the HBM the product of susceptibility and seriousness is a particular level of perceived threat. However, as we indicated earlier, this HBM formulation is problematic since too high a level of fear generated by that perception of threat may give rise to defensive avoidance rather than 'rational' action. For that reason, it may be better if the individual in question should have only a moderate level of conviction about the likelihood of her particular lesion being cancer: a very high level of certainty may create too high a level of arousal and give rise to a delay in taking action.

The limitations of the HBM notion of beliefs about seriousness as necessary precursors to preventive action are particularly well illustrated by cancer. Indeed, one of the major goals of cancer education is to reduce cancerophobia – an inappropriately high level of fear of the disease – and so rather than enhancing beliefs about seriousness it may be necessary to reduce their potency. Cancerophobia (which derives from the general belief system that we label 'pessimism') is a significant barrier to action. It will also be apparent that this barrier derives from a number of subordinate beliefs, one of which is the belief that treatment for cancer is (i) generally ineffective and (ii) painful or distressing (in popular parlance, the treatment is worse than the disease).

Again, we need to probe further before structuring our education programme. We need to ask about the origin of these 'higher order' beliefs. If we do so, we realise that we must consider beliefs about the nature of cancer and its causes. For instance, it has been well documented that people may have a variety of 'theories' about the cause of cancer. A so-called 'retribution theory' centres on a belief that cancer has been visited on the individual as a punishment for past moral transgressions. The 'seed and trigger' theory posits that we all have cancer within us in a dormant form, like a kind of seed, which is merely waiting for some event (almost any event – a knock, death in the family, work stress) to trigger it.

More recently, according to audience research by the BBC (British Broadcasting Corporation, 1983), it appears that many people consider that cancer is one single undifferentiated disease. This can lead to an often fatal confusion – for instance, people may believe that smoking causes all cancers. More importantly, the belief about its intrinsic nature will in turn affect the higher order belief that cancer may not be curable. After all, if people know that in many cases treatment fails and they believe that all cancers are the same, they may reasonably suspect that all treatment will be ineffective (and traumatic). Similarly, if you cannot prevent one cancer, you will not be able to prevent any. Figure 2.8 summarises this dynamic interaction of lower and higher order beliefs and their relationship with motivation – especially that most powerful motivator, fear.

The hierarchical nature of beliefs demonstrated in Figure 2.8 acknowledges the importance of identifying beliefs about causal factors that ultimately determine the nature and strength of the various main beliefs central to the 'Health Belief Model'. Such beliefs in mainstream psychology are typically defined as *attributional beliefs* – and the theory of attribution in general may provide valuable insights for health promotion. Although a more complete further discussion is not feasible here (see Kelley, 1967), it will probably be enlightening at this point to observe the importance of one particular application of attribution theory in relation to individuals' perception of and beliefs about risk and risk-related behaviours.

The interpretation of risk has clear relevance to the HBM variable of susceptibility. Individuals' beliefs about their susceptibility to negative outcomes depend on the way in which they process information about objective risk. As with any set of beliefs (i.e. subjective probabilities), their accuracy will depend on the degree of correspondence with objective probabilities (i.e. objective risk). It is possible to accurately calculate many risks, i.e. the real probability of occurrence of some negatively valued event – and especially so in respect of health risk (British Medical Association, 1990). League tables of such risk are frequently published and one such table showing the likelihood of any one individual succumbing to various negative events is shown in Box 13.

Clearly the same calculations can be applied to the attainment of *valued* outcomes. For instance the chance of wining the UK National Lottery is 1 in 14,000,000 – rather less than being struck by lightning!

**Box 13**  The Likelihood of an Individual Dying in any One Year from Different Negative Events

| | |
|---|---|
| • being struck by lightning | 1 in 10,000,000 |
| • drowning in the bath | 1 in 800,000 |
| • homicide | 1 in 100,00 |
| • playing soccer | 1 in 25,000 |
| • in a plane crash | 1 in 20,000 |
| • an asteroid colliding with the Earth | 1 in 20,000 |
| • being involved in a road accident | 1 in 8000 |
| • influenza | 1 in 5000 |
| • smoking 10 cigarettes a day | 1 in 200 |

As noted earlier, one of the major purposes of health education is to ensure that, as far as possible, subjective probabilities match objective reality. In the situation under discussion here it is manifestly

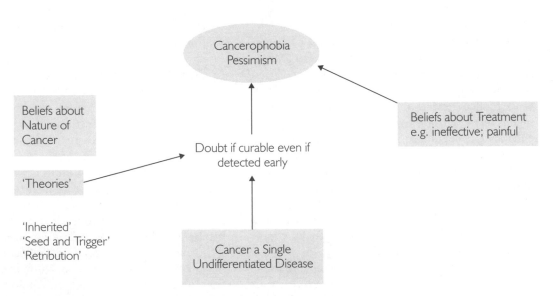

**Seaking Early Medical Advice**

Cancerophobia Pessimism

Beliefs about Nature of Cancer

'Theories'

'Inherited'
'Seed and Trigger'
'Retribution'

Doubt if curable even if detected early

Beliefs about Treatment e.g. ineffective; painful

Cancer a Single Undifferentiated Disease

***Figure 2.8***  Hierarchy of Beliefs and Secondary Prevention of Cancers

important that people's health choices should be based on realistically held beliefs. However, considerable research demonstrates that beliefs about susceptibility are rarely based on reality: people may not accept the level of risk to which their behaviour exposes them. There is often a tendency to overestimate the likelihood of the unlikely and underestimate the real frequency of relatively common threats (Lichtenstein *et al.*, 1978; Weinstein, 1982, 1984; Slovic *et al.*, 1982; Kasperson *et al.*, 1988). One broad set of factors contributing to these misperceptions of threat has to do with faulty information processing and a lack of decision making skills (Janis and Mann, 1977). For instance, the so-called 'availability heuristic' results in risk appraisal being biased by frequently reported but not necessarily frequently occurring events. Again, affective factors often influence the interpretation or risk and the 'availability heuristic' is accompanied by the '*dread factor*'. A useful basis for analysing beliefs about risk and susceptibility is to be found in *Social Amplification of Risk Theory* (Kasperson *et al.*, 1988). We might also note at this juncture a point that will be considered in discussion of the *motivation system* of HAM below. The mere perception of risk (and therefore susceptibility) may increase the probability of some individuals adopting that risky behaviour. Naïve subscription to the HBM might, therefore, be unwise!

A particularly important application of *Attribution Theory* centres on how people explain the various vicissitudes which they experience during their lives and the extent to which they believe they can control these. This will be further examined, in some depth, later in this chapter.

## The *motivation system*

The *motivation system* describes a complex of affective elements which ultimately determines the individual's attitude to the specific action and his or her intention of adopting it. Part of this complex is the individual's value system. Values are acquired through socialisation; they are affectively charged sets of beliefs referring to particular aspects of experience (for more detailed discussions see Rokeach, 1973; Horley, 1991).

Religious and moral issues relate to all-embracing values; the feelings one has for a career or in relation to family or spouse may be important in underpinning many health related actions.

Attitudes, on the other hand, are more specific than values. They describe feelings towards particular issues. Fishbein and Ajzen (1985) provide a definition which is both congruent with the HAM perspective and which shows how attitudes relate to beliefs:

> *... an attitude (refers) solely to a person's location on a bipolar evaluative or affective dimension with respect to some object, action or event. An attitude represents a person's general feeling of favourableness or unfavourableness towards some stimulus object ... .*
>
> *Each belief links the object to some attribute; the person's attitude toward the object is a function of his evaluations of these attributes.*

Each value will thus produce a large number of attitudes. For instance, the value associated with sex and gender roles will give rise to a series of attitudes towards, say, the employment of women, the nature of the marriage contract, the role of women in trade unions, the adequacy of medical care for female maladies and so on. The acquisition of new beliefs will, in turn, generate new attitudes energised by the value systems. For example, a belief that breast feeding would militate against full sharing of the parental role might lead to a negative attitude to breast feeding derived originally from the gender value mentioned above.

Obviously several values may conspire to produce one single attitude and this situation is illustrated in Figure 2.9.

It is apparent from this analysis – indeed, it is a truism – that it will be much more difficult to change an attitude which derives its motivational force from several values, especially where such values are deep-seated and salient. Given our emphasis so far on the importance of recognising the hierarchical nature of beliefs and the fact that

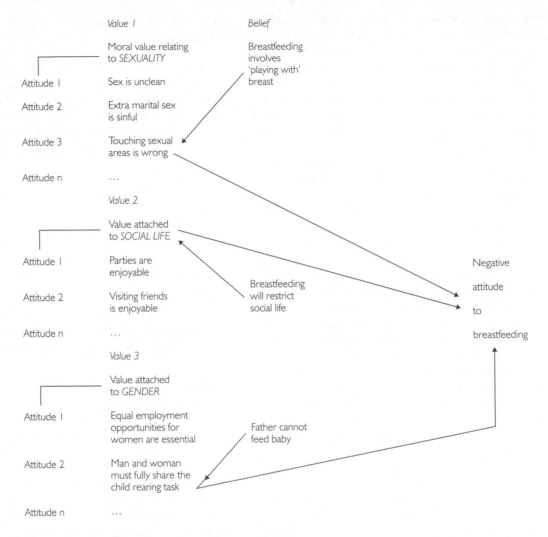

**Figure 2.9** The Contribution of Values to Attitude to Breast Feeding

belief strength may vary from doubt and uncertainty to absolute conviction, it is enlightening to note the possibility of a hierarchical categorisation of values. Simon (1974) was a leading figure in the US 'values clarification movement' and he viewed values clarification as moving through a seven stage process as follows:

1 prizing and cherishing;
2 publicly affirming;
3 choosing from alternatives;
4 choosing after consideration of consequences;
5 choosing freely;
6 acting;
7 acting with pattern, consistency and repetition.

Arguably, those individuals who have clarified their values successfully and who have developed a fully integrated system, which is always consistently applied in their everyday life, will be much more resistant to change than those at an earlier stage of development. In relation to performance indicators we are presented with a ready made 'scale' allowing us to measure the effectiveness of the values clarification (or values promotion) exercise.

In addition to values and attitudes, the motivation system incorporates 'drives'. The *Health Action Model* differs from some of the approaches already mentioned in that it recognises the fact that certain basic and powerful influences may override socially acquired values and attitudes. The term drive is therefore used to describe largely inherited, species-specific motivational factors such as hunger, sex and pain. It is also used here to refer to those acquired motivators having drive-like qualities, such as addictions to drugs. The importance of drives is obvious at the common sense level of explanation. For instance, a teenager might believe in the benefits of contraception and have acquired the appropriate techniques in using them; he or she may also have a well-developed moral sense but congruent beliefs, values and attitudes may yield to the pressures of sexual passion! Similarly, alcoholics may well know the harm they are inflicting on their families and may value children and spouse highly but it is the drive-like influence of the addiction which may determine behaviour.

Frequently, however, there may be no obvious drive influencing intention to act. Nonetheless, the presence of certain emotional states may signify the existence of motivational factors derived from drives. For instance, guilt and anxiety may usefully be considered a fractionated or 'watered down' version of pain or fear. Again at a common sense level it is apparent that nagging feelings of anxiety at the prospect of a spouse's disapproval may prevent a person undertaking some otherwise valued healthy action.

According to the HAM the classic notion of dissonance (Festinger, 1957) is best explained functionally in terms of derived drive rather than an all-embracing theory of attitude change. The state of dissonance is thus viewed as a feeling akin to that of guilt but created by perceptions of inconsistency between beliefs, attitudes and behaviours. As with other drive-like states, it is 'negatively reinforcing', i.e. it creates a state of discomfort which individuals are motivated to reduce by whatever means they have at their disposal. Dissonance reduction techniques may be 'rational', as for instance when a smoker who values his health stops smoking. Alternatively, dissonance may be reduced by denying the evidence that smoking causes disease and/or studiously avoiding any anti-smoking 'propaganda'.

Following our discussion of the most appropriate way of conceptualising the HBM notion of perceived susceptibility and our comments on risk taking, it would be remiss not to comment on the *positive* reinforcement which risk taking provides for many people. Of equal interest is the argument that some individuals actively pursue risk for the sake of its physiological effects. To put it somewhat crudely, it would seem that they become 'addicted'. Lyng (1990) discusses a number of reasons why people indulge in high risk behaviour and cites Delk (1980) who describes high risk behaviour as ... *a form of tension-reduction behavior with addictive qualities related to the build-up of intoxicating stress hormones.*

Lyng's own preferred explanation is in terms of 'edgework', which is seen as a way of handling ... *the problem of negotiating the boundary between chaos and order.* Lyng's analysis could be said to have a certain authority since it was based on participant observation as a jump pilot! He asserts that all edgework involves:

> ... *a clearly observable threat to one's physical or mental well-being or one's sense of an ordered existence. The archetypical edgework experience is one in which the individual's failure to meet the challenge at hand will result in death or, at the very least, debilitating injury.*

He also argues that many features of drug taking and even 'binge drinking' do not involve self-destructive behaviour as such but rather an attempt to demonstrate mastery and control, i.e. both concepts that are central to the notion of empowerment – as we will demonstrate later.

Clearly, both categories of risk taking render the notion of susceptibility irrelevant in predicting likely behaviour. Indeed, in relation to edgework, an activity in which there is no susceptibility to danger would cease to be attractive. Whatever the explanation, it is the *motivation system* which incorporates the relevant constructs. In the first instance we are dealing with the drive-like 'addictive' motives; in the case of Lyng's explanation we are concerned with a mix of beliefs about control, the associated notion of self-esteem and, perhaps primarily, a particular value in relation to the meaning of life and living.

Needless to say, the various drive-like states described above may pose a substantial challenge to the metacognitive and self-referent processes involved in self-regulation – as is apparent in health educators' often desperate attempts to find competing but healthy alternative reinforcers!

A final point should be made about the *motivation system* and its reciprocal relationship with the *belief system*. It will be seen in Figure 2.7 that a potentially significant influence may be exerted on behavioural intention not only by any given drive or emotional state but also by *beliefs* about these. This is shown as 'beliefs about affect'. The point may be illustrated by the fact that many smokers may never form an intention to quit despite believing in the benefits of doing so and the costs of continuing smoking. The reason is perhaps obvious: they believe that they would be unable to cope with either the loss of gratification from smoking or/and the negative affect they would experience from withdrawal (Marsh and Matheson, 1983). In HAM terms, this belief about affect would contribute *inter alia* to a 'belief about self' in the form of a negative 'self-efficacy' belief.

The *motivation system* is, then, a composite of different drives, values and attitudes having different emotional charges and giving rise to a particular level of arousal – or a 'push' to take action. Drawing on the experience of those enthusiasts who observed the behavioural minutiae of the white rat's maze learning skills, we might reasonably expect that a 'goal gradient' effect will operate. In other words, whatever the initial level of arousal in relation to a given goal (for example a sexual encounter), that level will increase proportionately as the individual approaches the desired stimulus object. The significance for the prevention of HIV and other STIs by avoiding unprotected sexual activity will doubtless be self-evident!

The *normative system* also contributes to the level of arousal mentioned above in the form of an individual's motivation to conform to pressures from other people. We will now consider this.

## The *normative system*

The term 'norm' describes cultural, sub-cultural and group behaviours together with the various values, beliefs and routines associated with such behaviours. The actual observable behaviours may be termed statistical norms while the beliefs held by the relevant population about such behaviours may be called social norms. Current figures on the prevalence of smoking in, for example, the UK and USA would indicate that the smoker is a deviant in higher social class groups. The notion of deviance underlines the importance of the coercive power of norms and their influence on behavioural intentions and decision making. The effect of the social norm is clearly most important here, for although it would often be correlated with the statistical norm, it is an individual's belief about other people's activities which is influential rather than the extent of the activities themselves.

Norms do not only operate within relatively large cultural units. The influence of norms within a small group on its individual members may be very powerful indeed and has been widely documented; the effect does of course depend on the extent to which the group member values membership of the group in question. Again, the norms of a reference group, i.e. a group to which an individual does not belong but for which (s)he has membership aspirations, may also be influential in determining attitudes and behaviours.

The *Health Action Model* describes the *normative system* from an individual and therefore psychological perspective (for a functionalist sociological point of view of normative influences see Baric, 1978). This individual perspective includes not only a person's belief about normal practices in the local or national community but also beliefs about the likely reaction of significant others, as described earlier in the discussion of Fishbein's model. It is, however, obvious – again as Fishbein indicated – that such beliefs will only influence behaviour where the individual is motivated to comply with the wishes of significant others or to conform to what (s)he perceives as acceptable norms.

One further normative phenomenon merits some explanation. It has to do with what Baric (1978) termed a 'quasi routine'. This term describes a situation in which a particular practice (healthy or unhealthy) is so pervasive in a given culture or social group that the existence of choice is purely notional and decisions may be reduced in practice to the status of 'quasi routines'. In other words, individuals are effectively unaware that a choice is really possible. They are, as it were, blind to the possibilities. A particular course of action may be so unusual or reprehensible that only the most reckless of deviants would ever contemplate the action in question. Note, for instance, Harfouche's (1965) description of the normative expectations of the maternal role regarding breast feeding:

> *Nursing is a duty; a mother who does not nurse denies her baby's right ... she is stingy, lazy, negligent, lacks affection like a step-mother ... no lactation, no affection.*

In a case of this kind, although there would appear to be an alternative of artificial feeding, the only real choice is breast feeding, i.e. a *'quasi routine'*. The phenomenon is related to the process of 'inferior' decision making which Janis and Mann (1977) labelled *'quasi-satisficing'*.

One further observation might be made in relation to the restriction of genuine freedom of choice. The 'quasi-routine' might usefully be viewed as the psychological equivalent of the sociological construct of *'false consciousness'*.

To sum up, then, it is assumed that, in addition to the *belief system* and *motivation system*, one of the major influences on an individual's intention to adopt any health action is the sum of normative and other inter-personal pressures. It is further assumed that more distal pressures will be less powerful than pressures 'closer to home'. Accordingly, an individual's perception of national norms and his or her motivation to conform to these will be much less significant than the pressures exerted by beliefs about what are normal practices in his or her local community or neighbourhood and the corresponding motivation to conform. More powerful still is the influence of peer groups – friends, classmates or workmates, for example – and, even more so, of family and close friends. One of the most powerful prescriptions for smoking cessation is a zealous non-smoking lover!

The differential effect of social pressures is illustrated in Figure 2.10.

It is apparent that the normative system generates an additional set of variables which might be used as diagnostic measures and indicators of success. These will include a description of the actual normative status quo (statistical norms), e.g. the prevalence of a particular practice in a given community; the 'norm sending' aspects of the environment, such as the advertising of unhealthy products or the availability of smoke-free places; the nature of the 'lay referral system'(Freidson, 1961); the nature of social support networks; group behaviours; the actions and attitudes of significant others. The catalogue of normative indicators would also incorporate individual perceptions and beliefs about all of the aforementioned measures, such as people's interpretations of the significance of the presence or absence of healthy foods in works canteens, their awareness of prevalent lay constructions of illness, their beliefs about the level of peer smoking and the likely reaction of their friends to their proposed membership of a health and fitness club. These indicators, incidentally, might be used in an evaluation of a health promotion programme having as its main goal either a change in the normative status quo or a change in people's beliefs about the normative situation.

## The personality dimension

In addition to proclaiming the importance of the psychological constructs featured in the *belief system*, *motivation system* and *normative system*, the *Health Action Model* draws attention to the relevance of some of those relatively enduring individual characteristics that are commonly described as personality traits or types. In Figure 2.7 these are shown as the joint effect of *self-concept* and *self-sentiment*. As with other personality traits, they differ from other beliefs and values in that they are relatively constant, consistent and long lasting. The *self-concept* (or self-image) is located within the cognitive domain and refers to the whole set of understandings and beliefs that are held by an individual about himself or herself. On the other hand, *self-sentiment*

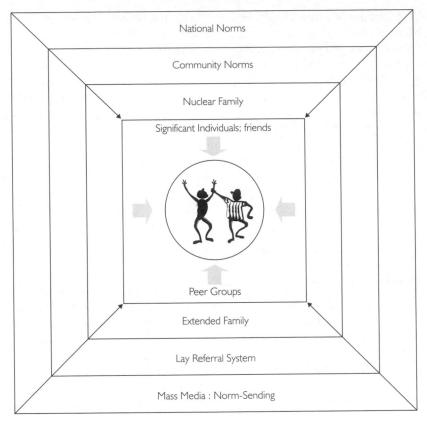

National Norms

Community Norms

Nuclear Family

Significant Individuals; friends

Peer Groups

Extended Family

Lay Referral System

Mass Media : Norm-Sending

**Figure 2.10**   Normative Influences on Individual Health Choices

is an affective construct associated with individual temperament and various enduring clusters of core values and persistent orientation to certain gratifications. For instance, one such affectively charged personality trait has been described as '*sensation seeking*': some individuals appear to have a particular predilection for risk taking – which can of course lead to health damaging behaviours. The sample items listed in Box 14 are derived from a 40 item validated scale (Zuckerman, 1979) and were applied by Kraft and Rise (1994) to smoking, alcohol consumption and sexual behaviour in a sample of Norwegian adolescents.

One of the most common core personality values that has been consistently associated with health and health promotion is self-esteem. In HAM this is considered to complement the *self-concept* and refers to the extent to which an indi-

vidual values himself or herself. However, the term '*self-sentiment*' is preferred to describe the sum total of personality traits associated with all kinds of motivation. This concept has been borrowed from Cattell's (1965) classic analysis of personality.

The conceptualising of *self-concept* in HAM also incorporates those beliefs about self associated with self-empowerment, such as '*self-efficacy*' and '*perceived locus of control*' – and these will be further discussed below. The HBM notion of perceived susceptibility is also contained under the general rubric of *self-concept*.

Both *self-concept* and *self-sentiment* are assumed to make a combined though separately identifiable contribution to the formation of *behavioural intention*.

However, because of the importance of the ideological dimension of empowerment that was explored in Chapter 1, it is worth reviewing and developing some of the aspects of *self-concept* and *self-sentiment* within the general concept of empowerment and relating these more specifically to HAM.

**Box 14**  Some Measures of Sensation Seeking

---

*Thrill and Adventure Seeking*
- I like to dive off the high board *versus* I don't like the feeling I get standing on the high board.

*Experience Seeking*
- I would like to take off on a trip with no pre-planned or definite routes or timetable *versus* when I go on a trip I like to plan my route and timetable fairly carefully.

*Disinhibition*
- A person should have considerable sexual experience before marriage *versus* it's better if two married people begin their sexual experience with each other.

*Boredom Susceptibility*
- I prefer friends who are excitingly unpredictable *versus* I prefer friends who are reliable and predictable.

---

## THE DYNAMICS OF SELF-EMPOWERMENT

In Chapter 1 we noted two perspectives on empowerment: individual or self-empowerment and community empowerment. We will give further consideration to aspects of community empowerment in a later chapter when we consider the 'strategy' of community development. At this juncture we will focus on individual empowerment but it is useful to include Wallerstein and Bernstein's (1994) definition of community empowerment which is not only particularly apposite, but also signals the inter-relationship between community empowerment and self-empowerment (a point that was noted in Chapter 1).

**Box 15**  Community Empowerment

---

*The popular use of empowerment has unfortunately been appropriated by politicians and management...*

*Community empowerment is defined as a social-action process in which individuals and groups act to gain mastery over their lives in the context of changing their social and political environment.*

*... (it) embodies an interactive process of change, where institutions and communities become transformed as people who participate in changing them become transformed. Rather than pitting individuals against community and overall societal needs, the community empowerment construct focuses on both individual and community change.*

*Brazilian educator Paulo Freire has brought us this dialectical understanding of individual and social empowerment, by sharing lessons learned from liberation movements in developing countries. He advocates a participatory education process in which people are not objects or recipients of political and educational projects, but actors in history, able to name their problems and their solutions to transform themselves in the process of changing oppressive circumstances.*

(Wallerstein and Bernstein, 1994 p142.)

---

Figure 2.11 identifies the major components of individual or self-empowerment. Embedded in this representation is the triangular relationship between humans and their environment which figures prominently in social learning theory (and, subsequently, social cognitive theory) and, as we noted earlier, is associated with the work of Bandura (1977, 1982, 1986). One of these components is the environment itself – and the reciprocal relationship between the individual and the environment has already been mentioned. The second key element consists of a cluster of significant psychological characteristics. These are in turn related to the third element – the behaviours which act as a kind of interface between personality and the environment. These behaviours are described in Figure 2.11 as health and life skills. They comprise a wide variety of competencies which facilitate environmental control, both directly and indirectly. A full discussion of life skills is not appropriate here but the list in Box 16 will serve to illustrate their nature.

**Box 16**  Selected Lifeskills

> - How to communicate effectively.
> - How to make relationships.
> - How to manage conflict.
> - How to be assertive.
> - How to work in groups.
> - How to build strengths in others.
> - How to influence people and systems.
>
> (Hopson and Scally, 1980)

The term 'health skill' is used here to refer to the application of life skills to specific health-related situations; for instance, stress management skills or the use of assertiveness techniques to resist pressures to take drugs or to demand proper medical care from practitioners.

Although not normally used in this sense, life skills are also considered to incorporate 'self-regulatory' skills, i.e., as noted earlier, techniques to help clients control various drives and urges or, more technically, to put them in charge of their own reinforcement (Kanfer and Karoly, 1972).

Central to the state of self-empowerment is a set of psychological attributes of which perhaps the most significant are beliefs about control. Langer (1983) provides a succinct definition of control as ... *the active belief that one has a choice among responses that are differentially effective in achieving the desired outcome.* Various typologies of control have been provided by a number of authors and are discussed in further detail elsewhere (Tones, 1992). For instance, Sarafino (1990) compares 'informational control' (the possession of an opportunity to acquire information about, say, an aversive event) with 'decisional control' (the opportunity to make actual choice). Lewis (1986), in the context of providing anticipatory guidance for patients, refers to 'cognitive control' (the capacity intellectually to manage an event and thus reduce its threatening characteristics). This may be compared with 'behavioural control' in which the individual actually possesses some skill (e.g. a motor skill or health skill) which can provide some real, tangible control over events.

The notion of *perceived locus of control* (PLC) is perhaps the most widely known of the psychological constructs associated with beliefs about control. This key conceptualisation is described by Rotter (1966) in a seminal article; the essence of the concept is clearly stated in Rotter's original definition. Inspection of the definition (in Box 17) will serve to indicate the origins of the theoretical basis in behaviourist psychology.

**Box 17**  Perceived Locus of Control: the Definition

> *When a reinforcement is perceived by the subject as following some action of his own but not being entirely contingent upon his action, then, in our (US) culture, it is typically perceived as the result of luck, chance, fate, as under the control of powerful others, or as unpredictable because of the great complexity of the forces surrounding him. When the event is interpreted in this way by an individual, we have labeled this a belief in external control. If the person perceives that the event is contingent upon his own behavior or his own relatively permanent characteristics, we have termed this a belief in internal control.*
>
> (Rotter, 1966 p1)

It is worth noting that the emphasis is on *perceived* locus of control, i.e. a *belief* in capacity to control rather than actual possession of control capabilities. Moreover, these beliefs about control refer to reinforcement, i.e. reward and/or punishment. For instance, an 'internal' differs from an 'external' in that (s)he is more inclined to believe

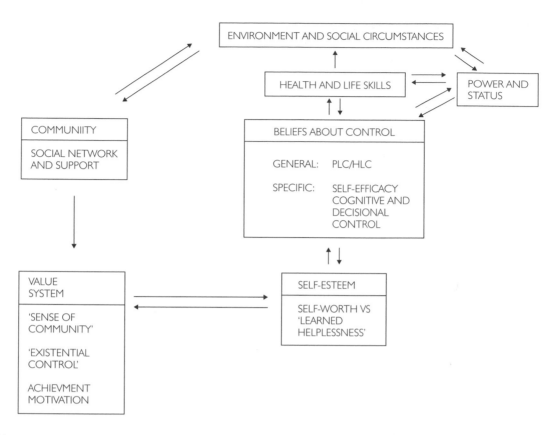

*Figure 2.11* The Dynamics of Self-empowerment

that both the pleasant and unpleasant occurrences in life result from his or her own efforts. It is also important to note that these individual beliefs or expectancies are *generalised*: they refer to a general tendency to feel in control or, conversely, to feel powerless. They might therefore, consistent with an earlier definition, be usefully viewed as a personality trait or attribute.

The construct of locus of control merits a central place in any discussion of an *Empowerment Model* of health education; this is not only because of the pivotal role of control in empowered decision making but also because of its direct and indirect relationship to health. As indicated earlier, it is clearly possible to argue that a state of

empowerment is *ipso facto* a state of health. It is equally clear that this assertion may be contested! However, it is much less contentious to argue that a complete feeling of powerlessness is unhealthy. Indeed, Seligman's (1975) notion of '*learned help-lessness*' could be described as the very antithesis of self-empowerment. In fact, Seligman provided a convincing argument that six major symptoms of learned helplessness had almost exact parallels in clinical depression.

More commonly, the relationship between locus of control and health is deemed to be mediated and investigation into the relationship between PLC and a number of health- or illness-related outcomes has been facilitated by the development of a number of psychometric scales. Rotter's (1966) original I-E Scale was later refined by Levenson (1973). It was not long before health locus of control (HLC) scales were also devised, largely by Wallston *et al.* (1976) and Wallston and Wallston (1978). We will continue our review of key dynamics of self-empowerment by recording the importance of another significant control concept – that of 'self-efficacy'.

As we noted earlier in the context of presenting a simple model for predicting health-related actions (self-efficacy × response efficacy), the construct of self-efficacy is associated with Albert Bandura (1977, 1982). Self-efficacy (or 'self-perceptions of efficacy') is, in effect, a belief. People who have self-efficacy expectations believe that they are capable of performing a given activity. The similarity of this concept to locus of control will be evident; the difference lies in the specificity of the former notion. Bandura's own elaboration of the concept is worthy of report:

> *Perceived self-efficacy is concerned with judgements of how well one can execute courses of action required to deal with prospective situations .... Self-percepts of efficacy are not simply inert estimates of future action. Self-appraisals of operative capabilities function as one set of proximal determinants of how people behave, their thought patterns, and the emotional reactions they experience in taxing situations. In their daily lives people continuously make decisions about what course of action to pursue and how long to continue those they have undertaken. Because acting on misjudgements of personal efficacy can produce adverse consequences, accurate appraisal of one's own capabilities has considerable functional value.*

> *Self-efficacy judgements, whether accurate or faulty, influence choice of activities and environmental settings. People avoid activities that they believe exceed their coping capabilities, but they undertake and perform assuredly those that they judge themselves capable of managing.*

(1982 pp122–3)

This relatively simple idea of self-efficacy is of especial importance to our analysis of control and empowerment. For instance, overestimates of capability will lead to failure and, if repeated, will limit future effort and damage self-esteem. Underestimates will, on the other hand, generally limit the potential for learning and personal growth. Again, the stronger the perceived self-efficacy, the greater the level of perseverance and persistence and, typically, the greater the feeling of control. In contrast, low perceptions of self-efficacy are likely to produce negative self-evaluations, leading to lower self-esteem.

Self-efficacy has additional value for health promotion planning: it is not only a readily usable concept but also its very tangibility suggests techniques for enhancing beliefs about control. The prospect of changing deficits in global attributes such as self-esteem is at the very least rather complex; similarly, it would be difficult to provide an easy prescription for shunting 'externals' on to an 'internal' health career. On the other hand, creating a self-efficacy belief in one's capacity to purchase condoms, for instance, is more readily achieved by, for example, situation-specific assertiveness training. It would also not be unreasonable to assume that 'internality' represents the sum total of a lifetime's self-efficacy beliefs. Therefore, insofar as internality constitutes a desirable health promotion goal, it is potentially achievable by a consistent, continuing and coherent set of experiences designed to create experience of success.

Reference to Figure 2.11 will reveal the existence of a reciprocal relationship between the beliefs about control which we have outlined above and that cluster of feelings about self which is typically referred to as self-esteem. It will also be apparent that 'learned helplessness' has been included as a bipolar opposite of self-esteem. Earlier we suggested that it was the antithesis of self-empowerment. It would, however, be more accurate – given its association with the negative affective state of depression – to contrast it with (high) self-esteem. This latter concept itself is often employed in rather cavalier fashion and, given its frequent association with empowerment, it merits some further brief comment.

The empowered person, it is said, enjoys high self-esteem whereas learned helplessness is characterised by a sense of worthlessness. Coopersmith (1967), one of the earliest writers on self-esteem, quotes an even earlier observation by William James about the negative effects of low self-esteem.

*A man ... with powers that have uniformly brought him success with place and wealth and friends and fame, is not likely to be visited by the morbid differences and doubts about himself which he had when he was a boy, whereas he who has made one blunder after another and still lies in middle life among the failures at the foot of the hill is liable to grow all sicklied o'er with self-distrust, and to shrink from trials with which his powers can really cope.*

(p2)

It is therefore clear that a good level of self-esteem is considered to be healthy, in several ways. First, it may with some justification be argued that realistically based high self-esteem is a significant feature of mental health. It may, in this context, be viewed as the obverse of learned helplessness and, thus, as a desirable 'medical' state. Alternatively, it provides a relatively tangible example of well-being and is worth pursuing in its own right.

Second, it would seem reasonable to assume that persons who value themselves are more likely to respond to the health educators' traditional 'look after yourself' message. After all, if you value yourself you will presumably believe you are worth looking after!

**Box 18**  Self-esteem and Control

*The apprentice human being must act to affect the world around him. The exercise of power is a condition for self esteem and full humanity.*
Bettelheim (1967)

Less obviously, self-esteem is presumed to promote health in an indirect way. For instance, it is commonly assumed that people high in self-esteem are less likely to succumb to pressures to conform (Aronson, 1976) and more likely to have the courage of their convictions. There is also evidence to support the contention that self-esteem is positively associated with the ability to handle fear. This is not, of course, to argue for the use of fear appeal but merely to note that individuals frequently have to respond to communications which are intrinsically threatening. The 'approved' response is to deal vigilantly with the threat, seek out information and adopt an empowered decision. This somewhat idealistic strategy is, it appears, more likely to be pursued by those having a high level of self-esteem.

For instance, Dabbs (1964) showed that high self-esteem was significantly related to 'coping' and 'copers' tended to respond to fear in a realistic rather than a defensive way. Moreover, self-esteem was itself related to subjects' response to different levels of fear appeal designed to promote adoption of tetanus injections. Whereas low self-esteem subjects showed high compliance in both high and low fear of conditions, high self-esteem subjects showed compliance only in high fear conditions. The researchers presumed that high self-esteem people are more active and vigorous in dealing with their environments and more skilful in meeting danger. They were thus only motivated to take action when the threat was perceived to be very high. At first glance it might appear that conformity shown by low self-esteem persons is actually desirable since the robust independence of those enjoying high self-esteem would not necessarily lead to compliance! It perhaps hardly needs saying that only convinced advocates of the preventive model should experience dismay at results such as these. It is one of life's little paradoxes that empowered people do not necessarily follow what educators feel is good advice!

There is, however, a further and perhaps more important set of observations about the indirect relationship between self-esteem and health choices. These centre on the fact that people having high self-esteem will experience greater dissonance (Festinger, 1957) if they fail to live up to their own expectations and moral imperatives (Aronson and Mettee, 1968). If someone believes that high fat consumption is unhealthy, values health and acknowledges that he or she consumes a good deal of fat, then dissonance will be experienced. Those having a high level of self-esteem will experience more discomfort than those having little self-respect. After all, people with low self-esteem will accept that such inconsistency is consistent with their normal behaviour. We should, however, not expect too much from these feelings of dissonance. As we have already noted, there are many more psychological and social factors governing behaviour: in the last analysis the likelihood of action may depend on the outcome of conflict between dissonance and taste buds!

Two main inter-related factors appear important in determining self-esteem: one of these is the reaction of significant others to the individual; the other is the individual's success in achieving goals which are valued not only by self but by the social group.

A comprehensive discussion of tactics designed to enhance self-esteem is not possible here. We might observe that a judicious mix of appropriate socialisation and life skills training would be central to the successful promotion of positive self-esteem. In the context of Figure 2.11 we should merely note that influencing the whole range of beliefs about control – especially by the provision of skills which enable individuals to control their environments – provides the most likely avenue to success. However, Figure 2.11 again reminds us of the potentially inhibiting or facilitating effect of the environment. In particular, we should note how people's actual power and status in a given social system can substantially influence their beliefs about control and their associated self-esteem. On the other hand, the reciprocity intrinsic to this analysis is again revealed in individuals' potential for acquiring status and power by means of both their belief in their capacity to do so and the possession of a number of necessary skills and competencies.

Apart from self-esteem (i.e. the value we attach to ourselves), two other values-related constructs may figure prominently in the model of self-empowerment portrayed in Figure 2.11. The first of these is nicely described by Lewis' (1986) term 'existential control'.

It is apparent to the casual observer that there are many people (perhaps even cultures) who clearly are not in control of their lives nor do they believe they are. Paradoxically, they appear to exhibit equanimity in this situation and, arguably, good levels of self-esteem. It would appear that the sense of well-being which is enjoyed is due to their capacity to impose meaning on their existence: even if they are not in control, they believe that someone or something is in control and they are happy with that arrangement. This somewhat Panglossian notion is closely related to Antonovsky's (1979) concept of a 'sense of coherence', i.e.

> *... a global orientation that expresses the extent to which one has a pervasive, enduring though dynamic feeling of confidence that one's internal and external environments are predictable and that there is a high probability that things will work out as well as can reasonably be expected.*
>
> (p123)

The nature of coherence was discussed in Chapter 1. By way of reminder, it consists of three components: 'comprehensibility, manageability and meaningfulness'. The first of these describes the extent to which people consider that their worlds are predictable and make sense; the second refers to their perception that they have resources available to meet environmental demands. The meaningfulness component provides the closest parallel with Lewis' concept indicating the extent to which people's lives make sense emotionally – and for this reason it has been included in Figure 2.11 as part of the *value system*. On the other hand, it has been incorporated in the list of beliefs in Box 19. This seems reasonable as it clearly fits Antonovsky's conceptualisation of the *sense of coherence* being '*negentropic*', i.e. in imposing meaning on life and thus reducing perceptions that the world is chaotic.

We should perhaps draw attention in passing to the relationship between the micro level notion of an individual sense of coherence and the meso level concept of 'sense of community' – a key feature of social capital.

The beliefs in Box 19 additionally reflect different degrees of belief strength and actual control over circumstances.

**Box 19**   A Typology of Control

*Cognitive Control*
Acquisition of information allows intellectual management of an event and may, thus, reduce its threatening properties.

*Decisional Control*
Individual has opportunity to make actual choices.

*Contingency Control*
Individuals believe that outcomes (positive or negative) are under their own control (cf. self-efficacy and perceived locus of control).

*Behavioural Control*
Individuals possess skills enabling them to exercise control over events.

*Existential Control*
Particular 'Panglossian' belief/value system allows individual to impose meaning on events and thus accept them.

## Social and environmental limitations to choice

A quite extensive discussion of the environmental determinants of health was initiated in Chapter 1 – particularly those relating to inequity. In the light of Wallerstein and Bernstein's observations above we might reiterate this importance here. We should also recall that social support has been consistently associated with not only empowered communities but also with better health. As Mittelmark (2000) reminds us,

> *A large literature has now developed from epidemiological research on the negative relationship between social integration and perceived availability of social support, on the one hand, and morbidity and mortality, on the other.*
>
> (p101)

## The *Health Action Model* and empowerment

Since it is the kind of model described earlier as an empirical or explanatory model (rather than a normative or ideological model), HAM can be pressed into service to explain 'victim blaming', preventive actions (admittedly by ignoring some of its component parts) or, alternatively, it can readily serve to translate ideology into practice. In relation to empowerment, this would involve identifying those values, personality states and beliefs – especially beliefs about control – that contribute to behavioural intention. It would also highlight the limitations imposed on empowered choice by various social pressures. Above all, it would emphasise the knowledge, skills and environmental circumstances that either limit or facilitate the translation of intention into practice and minimise the likelihood of relapse into various 'addictive' states that, by definition, reduce the addict's freedom of action.

## HEALTH PROMOTION INTERVENTIONS

Earlier in this chapter a sequential series of models was identified. This ranged from ideological models to evaluation models. It was noted how an empirical model offering explanations of influences on behaviours, such as HAM, would lead logically on to the specification of educational or other health promotion programmes. It was also observed that the ideological model underpinning this sequence would impinge on the various models leading to the ultimate evaluation model. Ideology, therefore, determines what might legitimately be included in specifications for interventions. In fact the very term 'intervention' would not be acceptable to those who argue that all health promotion must involve community participation. Now, as we noted in earlier considerations of *Communication of Innovations Theory*, there are many cases where change appears to happen spontaneously – or at any rate without intervention from an outside agency. However, by definition, any health promotion programme involves some kind of intervention from someone somewhere. These interventions may not be intrusive and, certainly, may be empowering where, for instance, a community worker helps a group identify its 'felt needs' and then facilitates its achievement of the goals arising from those needs. We can, though, clearly identify different types of intervention and many of the techniques and psychosocial processes will be peculiar to those interventions. For instance, an authoritarian preventive approach will operate differently from an empowerment approach. Figure 2.12a and b makes this distinction.

## HAM: implications for interventions

As already argued, health promotion is viewed as a synergistic combination of education and 'healthy public policy'. Any consideration of HAM would suggest that there might be two policy 'inputs'. First, and most important, policy measures would be essential if environmental barriers to choice are to be removed and/or healthy choices are to be encouraged. These measures might range from substantial financial and legislative effects to handle disadvantage, unemployment and more general 'social pathogens'. More particularly, specific measures such as food labelling and ready access to condoms would be needed to facilitate healthy dietary choice and safer sex practices respectively.

Less obviously perhaps, policy measures may be needed to counter 'norm sending' features of the environment (which therefore influence indi-

vidual intentions to act via the *normative system*). For instance, the most cogent argument against refusal to ban direct and indirect promotions of tobacco products is its norm sending effect, i.e. the way in which advertising signals a degree of approval of smoking and legitimises individuals' doubts about its health damaging effects.

In relation to health education, it is important to make a distinction between 'supportive' health education, which seeks to facilitate people's intentions to act, and education which operates at an earlier stage and contributes to the formation of those intentions. Supportive health education, therefore, provides the knowledge and skills an individual needs in order to translate intention into practice – for instance, knowing where to apply for welfare benefits and having the psychomotor skills needed to use a condom in the approved manner and the social interaction skills to negotiate its use with a partner. It is self-evidently much easier for health promotion to achieve a successful outcome by providing people with the knowledge and skills they need to do something they really want to do than to struggle to influence beliefs and intentions of individuals who are not committed to the health action.

If we consider the ways in which health educa-

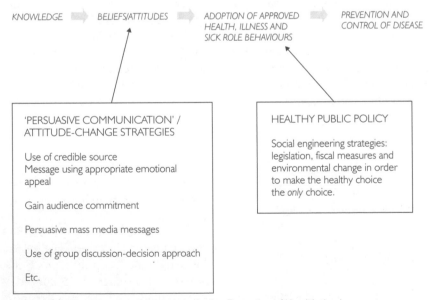

*Figure 2.12* (a) Prevention: the Educational Process Including Examples of Key Methods

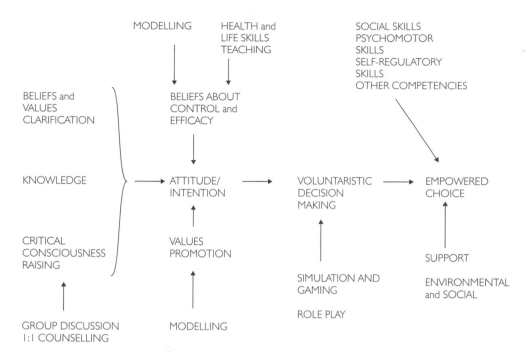

**Figure 2.12** (b) Empowerment: the Educational Process Including Examples of Key Methods

tion might influence behavioural intention we can identify from Figure 2.7 two possible sources of input. One of these influences the *belief system* while the other, as it were, feeds into the *motivation system*.

The most common way in which health education operates is via the *belief system*. Three major 'inputs' designed to influence beliefs can be identified. These are, in ascending order of general effectiveness, supplying information, the use of inter-personal persuasion and actual experience. The provision of information has traditionally been a stock in trade of health educators and takes many forms. These include the use of a variety of media – including written materials – and, usually more effectively, inter-personal communication. As we noted earlier when referring to the K-A-P 'formula', the provision of information is rarely sufficient to achieve action – even when the information has been understood. Individuals who have been exposed to the information must actually believe it if they are to develop a positive attitude to the adoption of the health practice. The

use of effective inter-personal persuasion has, therefore, been widely advocated as a strategy for influencing beliefs and attitudes. The strategy has been subjected to substantial and extensive research and various techniques for achieving belief and attitude change have been recommended. For instance, traditional *Attitude Theory* has demonstrated that people may be influenced not so much by the message but by the person delivering it – as we pointed out earlier in our reference to the importance of communicator credibility in the context of *Communication of Innovations Theory*. Accordingly the input category of 'inter-personal persuasion' should include the careful consideration of the credibility and general characteristics of those who seek to communicate, teach, train or persuade (e.g. levels of confidence, perceived expertise, trustworthiness and attributes associated with the notion of 'homophily'). However, of the three strategies for influencing beliefs, personal experience is undoubtedly the most powerful. We are, in short, most likely to believe what we actually experience

– whether this be at first hand or vicariously. Indeed, one of the central tenets of *Social Learning Theory* is based on this fact and has been incorporated into recommended health promotion practice. *Social Learning Theory* demonstrates that perhaps the most common way that people gain experience and understanding of their world is merely by observing. Accordingly, 'modelling' may be deliberately used to facilitate 'observational learning', e.g. by seeking to provide a model of good practice from which observers can learn and, on occasions, with which they can identify.

We might recall, at this juncture, that different ideologies would determine whether or not particular intervention strategies are acceptable. For instance, there is a clear difference in intent between those interventions that use observational learning to provide information and empower choice from those deliberate attempts to persuade, manipulate and generally appeal to the emotions by using prestigious or otherwise attractive personalities as models for imitation or identification.

Although the information processor, described in Box 11, is shown as being attached to the *belief system*, the three inputs – experience, information and inter-personal persuasion – might impact directly on the *motivation system* (rather than influencing it less directly via the *belief system*). The result might be to generate a greater or lesser degree of emotional arousal – either incidentally or by means of deliberate attitude change measures. Again, a particular communicator may have a direct effect on an audience's or a client's feelings. There could, therefore, be a significant distinction between a situation in which an audience or client merely accepts the message delivered by communicators who are credible and a situation in which a client's beliefs and attitudes are largely influenced by the direct emotional impact arising from, say, sexual attraction or identification with a model's perceived power.

Again, in relation to the ways in which persuasive communications may influence intentions by the *motivation system* route, classic *Attitude Change Theory* shows how deliberate attempts

may be made to separate the cognitive substance of message from its style: the most controversial and notorious of these is the deliberate use of fear appeal. Messages might be deliberately designed to create either positive or negative affect. Typically pictures would be used – for example, to arouse disgust or anxiety or, alternatively, to trigger nostalgia or feelings of parental warmth.

Once more, experience is likely to have the most powerful impact, although on this occasion it would exert its effects directly on the emotions. For example, the deliberate use of role play in which smokers underwent the unpleasant vicarious experience of having lung cancer diagnosed from X-rays provides a prime example of such a technique. Those who subscribe to such ethically dubious methods might be interested to learn that, according to Janis and Mann (1965), the technique *had a marked influence on smoking habits and attitudes!*

## The importance of horizontal programmes

We have considered the relevance of HAM for health promotion programmes and we will now turn to the penultimate kind of model in the sequence described earlier. In other words, theories or models that purport to explain how best to apply understandings such as those provided by HAM to strategic interventions and the choice of specific methods.

A little consideration of the complexity and multifactorial nature of the influences on the choices of both individuals and social groups and the sometimes labyrinthine pathways between health promotion inputs and health outcomes should lead inexorably to the conclusion that designing a programme that has a narrow focus on a specific behaviour (or *a fortiori* a disease) will typically not be the best way of achieving success. In other words, it is often more productive (although politically more problematic) to develop '*horizontal*' programmes rather than '*vertical*', disease-centred interventions.

For instance, let us consider the five key areas targeted in the UK government's strategy for health in England (Department of Health, 1992). These five key areas (selected on the basis of ... *both the greatest need and greatest scope for making cost-effective improvements* …) comprised coronary heart disease and stroke, cancers, mental illness, HIV/AIDS and sexual health and accidents. Each of them might be the focus of a health promotion programme; each programme might be evaluated in terms of outcome measures such as a reduction in the incidence of accidents among children under 15 or by a decline in the overall suicide rate. However, to develop five separate 'vertical' programmes would not necessarily be the most efficient or the most economical strategy, since a number of 'horizontal' influences underpin some or all of the five disease-related outcomes. The five key vertical areas are shown in Figure 2.13 together with these underlying 'strata'.

First of all, it is clear that some of the five key areas have risk factors in common (for example, diet and smoking in the case of cancers and cardiovascular disease). At a more fundamental level, certain attributes of the at-risk population predispose them to adopt a lifestyle which puts them at risk from the diseases and disorders defined by the five key areas. A 'horizontal' health and life skills programme which addresses this underlying lifestyle is more efficient because it is literally more radical, i.e. it gets to the roots of the situation. A yet more radical programme consonant with the philosophy of health promotion will also seek to tackle the environmental and socio-structural factors underpinning lifestyle by incorporating healthy public policy.

Figure 2.13 also reminds us of the reciprocal determinism of environment and life skills: healthy public policy facilitates healthy lifestyles; life skills are needed to influence the implementation of healthy public policy. Additionally, this conceptualisation alerts us to the importance of looking for different kinds of 'intermediate indicator' of success at each horizontal layer.

As a passing note, the most recent English government strategy, *Saving Lives: Our Healthier Nation* (Department of Health, 1999), has placed much greater emphasis on the underlying, horizontal influences on health – although five vertical health problems have again been identified, namely cancer, coronary heart disease, stroke, accidents and mental health.

Jessor and Jessor's (1977) work on 'problem behaviour' in adolescents provide a further instance of the importance of not being seduced by superficial manifestations of deep-seated health problems. Adolescence is widely recognised as a period of transition, which is likely to be more or less problematic. However, it is not uncommon to concentrate on the 'symptoms' of adolescents' attempts to cope with the developmental tasks imposed on them by the culture in which they live. Quite frequently we ignore the fact that what are superficial behaviours – healthy or unhealthy – derive from more fundamental developmental pressures. Figure 2.14 is a simplified version of Jessor's model of problem behaviour.

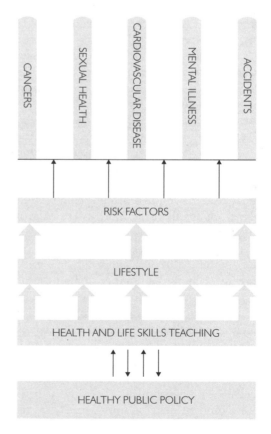

**Figure 2.13** A Horizontal Approach to Vertical Problems

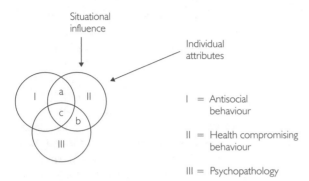

**Figure 2.14**  Problem Behaviour in Adolescence (after Jessor and Jessor, 1977).

Figure 2.14 shows three overlapping varieties of dysfunctional behaviour. Segment I has been labelled antisocial behaviour, such as vandalism and taking vehicles without the owner's consent. Segment II relates to activities which are traditionally the main concern of health educators. These health compromising behaviours would include sexual behaviours leading to sexually transmitted infection or unwanted pregnancy, substance misuse and a variety of other 'risky' behaviours. Segment III is concerned with 'psychopathology' – for instance, depression or suicide.

Overlap in the categories can be readily identified. Area a in the Venn diagram could include car theft and drunk driving; area b might be illustrated by dietary disorders such as anorexia and bulimia; area c would represent some awesome combination of all three, perhaps suicidal ramraiding while under the influence of hallucinogens and without wearing seat belts.

Clearly these different problem behaviours can be directly related to a number of medical or disease problems and Jessor's analysis reveals the wisdom of avoiding the vertical programmes which might result from too narrow a response to difficulties rooted in human behaviour and the social and economic infrastructure.

Figure 2.14 provides yet another reminder of the reciprocal determinism of the individual and the environment. This is not untimely, as in the recent past we have frequently witnessed attempts to explain antisocial and 'delinquent' behaviour either in terms of broader social factors, such as

poverty or unemployment, or in terms of individual 'lack of responsibility', often allegedly due to failures of parenting. Preference for one of other stance seems to be determined by ideological orientation or even narrow party political preference.

As with our analysis of the vertical programme areas, indicators of effectiveness are stratified in that we might identify ways of measuring broader social factors or, more superficially, individual attributes. For instance, it seems probable that a strong network of community control and social support (i.e. 'social capital') might minimise the likelihood of problem behaviours. We would, therefore, need to employ indicators of inter-sectoral working and community perception of control in addition to treading the more familiar terrain of measuring knowledge, beliefs, attitudes and even coping skills in order to gauge the effectiveness of our anticipatory guidance or life skills teaching.

## Mass media and community development

One of the most common intervention strategies for health promotion and health education over many years is the use of mass media. We will say no more about this strategy here since it will be the subject of a later chapter – except that it can be usefully compared and contrasted with the horizontal approach mentioned above, which centres on the use of inter-personal methods. Again, mass media programmes can be contrasted with the intensely interactive approach of community development – which will also merit separate consideration later. However, the essential components of a 'non-formal' community development approach to working with the community are described in Figure 2.15.

The main features of Figure 2.15 relate to our earlier discussions of both empowerment, with special reference to the work of Paulo Freire (1972), and *Communication of Innovations Theory*. The particular Freirean processes have, however, been augmented by the addition of supportive life skills (in accordance with our earlier discussion of self-empowerment) and with an endorsement of the importance of remedying the

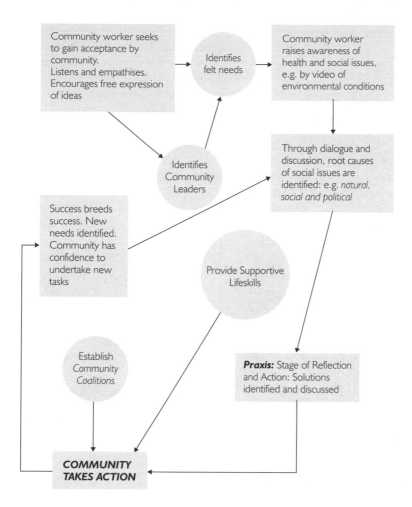

**Figure 2.15** Praxis and Community Action

power imbalance existing between disadvantaged communities and the wider social and political system by incorporating '*community coalitions*' of the great, the good and, above all, the powerful!

This model of community-based working provides immediate guidance for devising indicators of success. For instance: how effective are the community worker's listening skills; are community leaders identified; how do they rate on homophily; to what extent are the criteria for effective collaboration met in respect of establishing community coalitions?

## EVALUATION

The final model in the sequence – starting from the ideological base – centres on evaluation. As was indicated earlier, evaluation models are both technical and ideological. They specify strategies and techniques for action but, at the same time, these techniques may or may not be ethically acceptable depending on the values stance underpinning health promotion in general and evaluation in particular. Such matters will receive detailed consideration in Chapter 3. For the present we might usefully reflect again on the nature of *evaluation research* in the context of the contribution of research in general to programme planning. Figure 2.2 represents the relationship diagrammatically.

As Figure 2.2 demonstrates, research into health needs should precede the construction of any health promotion intervention. Although a discussion of health needs assessment is beyond the scope of this book, we should note its importance and, indeed, the importance of a related 'diagnostic' function. Prior to the implementation of the programme it is essential not just to identify the 'target' population or client group but to develop a detailed profile of their characteristics. In part this would include the construction of a community or organisational profile – which might, for instance, refer to the prevalence of certain norms or to the availability of resources – e.g. local media and/or potential members of a 'community coalition'. It would also require a detailed assessment of individual characteristics, e.g. knowledge deficits, prevailing beliefs and attitudes and lack of key skills. The result of this latter analysis has, of course, a direct relevance for evaluation in that it may generate baseline data that may act as a kind of 'pre-test' to serve as benchmarks against which to judge programme success. The analysis of individual situations will also lead to the formulation of *appropriate* programme objectives – an important issue which will be further discussed below.

As for evaluation research, at this juncture it is useful to distinguish three kinds of evaluation: summative evaluation, process evaluation and formative evaluation.

## Evaluation: summative and process

*Summative evaluation* occurs at the end of a programme and describes the extent of the programme's success – or failure – after the event. It frequently consists of checking the degree of difference between pre-test and post-test and deciding whether any apparent change is: (i) a genuine effect; (ii) big enough to have any significance. Clearly, lessons can be learned for future programmes from the results of summative evaluation. However, the data cannot be used to improve the *current* programme.

*Process evaluation* takes place during the programme and provides 'documentary evidence' of accompanying processes. There are two situations. Firstly, process indicators can serve as a form of milestone or benchmark that will signal whether important conditions for a successful intervention have taken place. For example, a number of key characteristics have been deemed to be necessary for effective sex education programmes (Kirby, 1995) and are listed in Box 20.

**Box 20** Key Features of Successful Sex Education Programmes

- They should be based on social learning theory;
- they should focus on sexual risk taking;
- a minimum of 14 hours teaching/small group teaching should be supplied;
- active learning methods should be used;
- basic information on sex and reproduction must be available;
- the issue of social pressure should be addressed;
- clear messages must be provided and reinforced;
- modelling should be included;
- teachers should be trained to deliver the programme.

Process indicators would be used to demonstrate how many of these key components had in fact been included. In the event of significant omissions less than adequate results revealed by *summative evaluation* could then be at least partially explained. Clearly, if important processes have not benefited from such benchmarks, any explanation will be limited.

A second and more important situation is where programme processes are not just presented as a kind of check-list but rather recorded in sufficient detail that insights may be gained into key features of programme delivery and dynamics together with client responses to the programme. In this way, light may be shed on strengths and weaknesses and a superior kind of explanation created. This use of *process evaluation* may thus, with reason, be categorised as '*illuminative evaluation*'.

**Box 21**

> *As with the lamp post and the drunk, summative evaluation may be used for support rather than illumination!*
>
> *(Green and Tones, 1999a)*

The value of *illuminative evaluation* is admirably illustrated by an extract from Labonte *et al.* (1999) and appears at Appendix 2.1.

## Formative evaluation: research into action?

*Formative evaluation* is a procedure that also assembles information as the programme unfolds. However, unlike *process evaluation*, it then translates the information into action. The origins of *formative evaluation* can be found in 1960s and 1970s attempts to improve the efficiency of training. Briefly, instead of using a pre- and post-test to assess the success of the course summatively, formatively evaluated training makes a series of assessments at regular intervals and utilises the resulting measures of success (or failure) to modify training inputs. If an individual trainee makes insufficient progress, the assessment is used diagnostically and remedial training is provided. Conversely, those who perform better than the norm are promoted to a fast track. All trainees should, therefore, ultimately achieve the same degree of success – although some may take longer than others.

We commented earlier that even technical procedures and models may have an ideological twist to them and the approach just described has a value position which should be congenial to those involved in health promotion. In short, it adopts a principle of 'mastery learning' – assuming that trainees have been appropriately selected for the course, they should all – or very nearly all – achieve success. Since health promotion specialists spend a good deal of their time conducting various training activities, the mastery learning approach fits particularly well with their presumed ideological commitment to empowerment and the enhancement of self-esteem! There is, inevitably, still room for conflict: the use of mastery learning can wreak havoc with the Gaussian curve and the normal distribution of marks. It may thus offend more conventional psychometricians!

The procedure is illustrated in Figure 2.16.

Regrettably mastery learning is difficult to implement – substantially due to its focus on individual learning and the associated demands on staff time. On the other hand, automated systems of instruction – such as programmed learning and, more recently, computer assisted learning – can be constructed to provide individually tailored, learning experiences.

## Participation and action research

One particular and important version of *formative evaluation* has a peculiar relevance for health promotion which, on ideological grounds, is expected to routinely involve clients in the evalu-

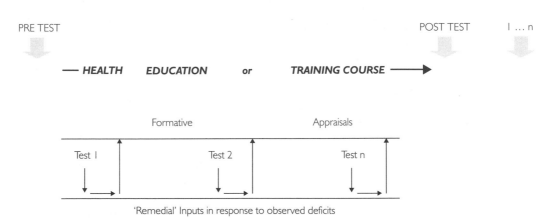

**Figure 2.16**  Mastery Learning and Formative Evaluation

ative process. As the WHO has observed, participatory research should characterise health promotion work. Macaulay *et al.* (1999) provide insight into the nature and importance of the process of participation.

> *Participatory research attempts to negotiate a balance between developing valid generalisable knowledge and benefiting the community that is being researched and to improve research protocols by incorporating the knowledge and expertise of community members ... these goals can best be met by the community and researcher collaborating in the research as equals.*

The authors continue:

> *Participatory research began as a movement for social justice in international development settings. It was developed to help improve social and economic conditions, to effect change, and to reduce the distrust of the people being studied. Although different applications and labels include 'action research' and 'participatory action research', all provide a framework to respond to health issues within a social and historical context.*
>
> (p774)

Cohen and Manion (1994) also provide an authoritative definition of action research which is described as:

> *... an on the spot procedure designed to deal with a concrete problem located in an immediate situation. This means that the step by step process is constantly monitored (ideally that is) over varying periods of time and by a variety of mechanisms (questionnaires, diaries, interviews and case studies, for example) so that the ensuing feedback may be translated into modifications, adjustments, directional changes, redefinitions, as necessary so as to bring about lasting benefit to the ongoing process itself rather than to some future occasion as is the purpose of more traditionally orientated research.*
>
> (p192)

As we will observe later, formative research in general poses certain problems for the specification of precise objectives which – as observed earlier – should be an essential feature of effective programmes.

## Effectiveness and efficiency: costs and benefits

The term *effectiveness* is concerned with whether or not an intervention has 'worked' and is commonly used to denote the extent to which programme objectives have been achieved. The term *efficiency* normally refers to relative effectiveness, i.e. how well a programme has done by comparison with actual or potential competing programmes and strategies – or specific methods within programmes. For instance, a school-based initiative designed to reduce recruitment to smoking might have achieved a degree of effectiveness – such as delaying the onset of smoking by 2 years (a not uncommon finding). On the other hand, legal and fiscal measures might possibly achieve a greater reduction in recruitment by substantially increasing the tax on cigarettes and vigorously prosecuting the sale of cigarettes to minors. If this were to be the case, the latter programme would be more efficient. Since, other things (such as ethical considerations) being equal, efficiency centres on programme costs, it is appropriate at this juncture to give some due consideration to issues of cost and benefit.

## Some reflections on cost effectiveness

In a very real sense, economics is the ultimate arbiter of programme implementation even if, on occasions, it is not the primary concern. In other words, health promotion cannot avoid confronting some of the thorny issues raised by cost effectiveness and cost–benefit analysis. All programmes must take account of cost since all programmes consume resources and resources are finite. The most obvious situation where economic analysis is viewed as an essential part of programme planning and evaluation is where the major purpose of health education and health promotion generally has been one of creating savings on expensive health care costs so that money may be spent on other and presumably better things. However, even where a health education model of choice is, say, to create a sense of wonder at the marvellous workings of the human body, resources are necessary. Even where society values knowledge for its own sake (currently a somewhat eccentric view), it is manifestly better to create such knowledge efficiently, i.e. with minimal rather than profligate use of resources.

We can therefore argue that whatever the precision of the objectives set or the sophistication of the criteria of success adopted by a programme, some measure of efficiency should be considered. As we will see, certain 'tough' behavioural objectives have, of course, an in-built measure of efficiency in the form of conditions and standards. Health economics seeks to quantify efficiency by expressing it in monetary terms.

Three common analytical tools are employed in health economics:

- cost analysis – which merely indicates the financial cost of competing programmes or other initiatives;
- cost effectiveness analysis (CEA) – which compares the efficiency of competing interventions in achieving a given goal by stating the relative financial costs involved;
- cost–benefit analysis (CBA) – which, unlike CEA, not only states the costs in monetary terms but also seeks to fix a price tag on the benefits accruing from the programme; a calculation of the cost per given benefit is then possible (typically expressed as a cost–benefit ratio).

It is important to note the difference between CBA and CEA. CEA seeks only to state the cost involved in, say, using smoking cessation clinics compared with family doctors providing routine advice on giving up smoking. On the basis of reported research, GP involvement would seem to be more cost effective.

CBA, on the other hand, would not necessarily assume that smoking cessation was a worthwhile goal under any circumstances and would compare the financial costs of delivering the programme with the financial costs of the benefits resulting from smoking cessation. It is therefore controver-

sial insofar as many people will fundamentally question the morality of attaching a financial label to human life and health; others will merely question the feasibility of doing so. The arguments used here are somewhat similar to those involved in the debate about behavioural objectives. The objection on grounds of ethical principle suggests that cherished human values are somehow demeaned by the process of subjecting them to critical analysis. The second category of objection is manifestly different: its criticism is based on accusations of incompleteness or naïveté.

The fact is, however, that just as behavioural objectives clarify goals through their precision and specificity, CBA and CEA may provide useful information to help decision making under conditions of resource limitation. They may also be politically useful for health promoters who, in the face of criticism of the costs of proposed programmes and demands for proof of efficiency, may be able to point out the relative cost of routinely accepted medical practices and non-educational preventive procedures. It is clear that the amount of money spent on different lifesaving interventions varies enormously in relation to the pay-off in terms of lives saved, as may be seen in Table 2.2.

**Table 2.2** Cost Per Life Saved for Various Preventive Measures.

| Preventive measure | Cost per life saved (£) |
| --- | --- |
| Screening for stillbirth | 50 |
| Childproof containers | 1000 |
| Department of the Environment (road safety) | 39,300 |
| Screening for cervical cancer | 10,000–41,700 |
| Trawler safety | 1,000,000 |
| Alterations to high rise flats after Ronan Point disaster | 20,000,000 |

Derived from Mooney (1977)

An important health economics concept is that of opportunity cost. Any service expenditure involves not only the cost of delivering that service but also the loss of some other facility which might have been financed by the money spent on that service provision. Thus while it might be argued that the money spent on prevention and health education could have been spent on curative services, it would seem equally reasonable to stand the argument on its head and assert that the resources used in high technology acute medicine might be better spent on health education and preventive services. Cochrane's (1972) classic *Random reflections on the health service* showed how many routinely practised medical procedures had never been evaluated. Townsend (1986), in discussing cost effectiveness, cites Bodmer (1985), who commented on the escalating cost of chemotherapies in the treatment of cancers and asserted that despite *... very serious side effects ... these had ... no more than a marginal effect at the present time on increased survival*. Again, if we were to take account of evaluations of coronary care units (Mather *et al.*, 1971; Colling *et al.*, 1976) we would conclude that the prospect of surviving an acute myocardial infarction would be enhanced by being nursed at home or in a general hospital ward rather than in a coronary care unit.

It is certainly not the intention of this book even to begin to explore the intricacies of CEA and CBA and interested readers are referred to authoritative discussions (Windsor *et al.*, 1984; Green and Lewis, 1987). Two points are worth making, however. First there is evidence that health promotion has been both effective and efficient, even when judged by the rigorous criteria of CBA. Second, despite such evidence of success, we should be very careful before allowing ourselves to be seduced into making such analyses routinely. Prevention in general and health promotion in particular may prove to be eminently worthwhile but intrinsically expensive!

Let us, nonetheless, consider an example where on the basis of existing theory a health promotion intervention could be expected to be cost effective. Townsend (1986) considered how a hypothetical mass media anti-smoking campaign costing £250,000 might be judged in a CEA. Assuming that 1000 people gave up smoking permanently, 10,000 gave up temporarily, 2000 cut down temporarily and 15,000 seriously considered giving up, then 2991 life years would be saved at a cost of £84 per life. The cost would appear to be reasonable by comparison with Table 2.2. The reader will be better able to judge whether, on the basis of historical, normative and theoretical standards, such a campaign could be expected to deliver these results after referring to Chapter 8, which discusses the effectiveness and efficiency of mass media.

Terris (1981) has enthusiastically argued the cost effectiveness case for prevention, estimating that a moderately effective programme in the USA might save each year at least 400,000 lives, 6,000,000 person-years of life and $5,000,000,000 worth of medical costs. Green (1974) has provided several much more closely argued examples of favourable cost–benefit ratios for specific health education programmes. One of these demonstrates a saving of $7.81 per dollar invested in a hypertension screening and education programme; the other, which analysed the impact of using group discussion techniques to modify unnecessary use of emergency rooms for asthma patients, notched up a cost–benefit ratio of 1:5.

A British study by the Policy Studies Institute (Laing, 1982) on the benefits and costs of family planning identified conservative benefit to cost ratios of 1.3:1 for the typical prevented unplanned pregnancy, a ratio of 4.5:1 for prevented pregnancies among mothers of three or more children and a 5.3:1 ratio for unplanned, premarital conceptions. In other words, ... *for every £100 spent on family planning services, the public sector can expect a benefit of £130, £450 and £530 respectively*. Although this illustration does not refer to a health education programme *per se*, it is clear that family planning, like other health promotion initiatives, cannot be achieved without an educational component.

A more recent example of CBA (ASH, 2000) was provided by the UK Health and Safety Executive in its draft Approved Code of Practice for control of smoking in the hospitality sector (public bars, restaurants, etc.). It concludes that, in March, 2000, the costs of implementing protective measures were between £2,800,000,000 and £3,300,000,000; on the other hand, it was calculated that the benefits amounted to between £12,500,000,000 and £23,400,000,000. A major boost for the development of healthy public policy!

There is, then, clear evidence that health promotion may not only be effective but its benefits can outweigh programme costs. However, as indicated above, we must strike a cautionary note. We will argue later that health promoters should resist attempts to cajole them into using medical or epidemiological indicators of success; it should also be wary of adopting CBA too enthusiastically. While a favourable cost–benefit ratio is possible, there will be many instances where health education may in the long run prove expensive. For example, the cost of successful alcohol and smoking programmes in terms of lost employment in those industries and lost government revenues is well known and although many if not all of these costs can be offset by savings on health service treatment costs, the balance sheet is still complex. The longer people live, the more demands they make on the welfare state. As Smith (1977) elegantly reminded us:

*Various kinds of false optimism are invoked by many doctors. … First, they argue that preventive and curative medicine may one day be as successful with diseases that are currently chronic and incurable as it has been in the past with those acute diseases that relatively speaking no longer trouble us. But unless we succeed in abolishing death we shall always have to treat the dying. The optimists sometimes seem to look forward to a time when most people will make their exit from this world without causing inconvenience to doctors. The evidence provides little ground for any such hope. In general, the older we are when we die the longer the period of alleviative care we require before death. Since it seems reasonable to suppose that the older we are when we die the more likely it is that we have died of old age, it follows that when most people die of old age rather than intercurrent disease, the demands they make on medical care are greater. When we all die of old age, after a lifetime of health, the main task of the health service will be with the alleviative care of terminal illness. If we should succeed in abol-ishing death the main preoccupation of the health service will be with contraception.*

Although health economists may offset some of the costs of future health care by the process of 'discounting' – so that future costs are rated as less important than current costs – or by resorting to the somewhat casuistic notion of 'merit good' (Cohen, 1981), which appears to acknowledge that some social benefits are so intrinsically meritorious that financial costs are deemed irrelevant, nonetheless and in the last analysis we have to be prepared to pay for health.

If the entire focus of our evaluation is, however, to be on achieving favourable cost–benefit ratios, presumably the ideal intervention is one which ensures that individuals achieve a level of health which is just sufficient to enable them to carry out an approved social role while indulging themselves in unhealthy activities to the extent that they avoid sickness absence, are vigorous and productive but manage to inflict sufficient damage on their constitution that they die as soon as possible after they reach pensionable age. In reality, though, Draper's observations are nearer the mark: health promotion, he argues, is inherently inconsistent with the goal of economic productivity. In which case we are more likely to have to choose health or wealth (Draper *et al.*, 1977).

## The notion of efficacy

While 'effectiveness' and 'efficiency' are readily used in common research parlance, the notion of '*efficacy*' appears less frequently. It is, nevertheless, of great importance in developing and assessing the effectiveness of health promotion programmes. The term is used here following Brook and Lohr's (1985) usage and refers to the effectiveness of performance *under ideal conditions*. In other words, there is an implication that it is inappropriate to assess the effectiveness or efficiency of interventions that do not meet all of the known requirements for a successful outcome.

If all of the known requirements have been met, e.g. an appropriate educational strategy utilising state-of-the-art methodology and supported by 'healthy public policy', then it can rightly be presumed that the programme is not merely ineffective but lacks efficacy and should not misuse resources (at least until some better intervention strategies have been discovered!). As will be emphasised later, it is more common for health promotion initiatives to be judged as more or less ineffective despite the fact that the conditions under which they are delivered are far from ideal. Furthermore, it would be inappropriate at this point not to mention a common and persistent paradox: even when the ideal conditions for an intervention can be specified – and would presumably lead to successful outcomes – the cost implications are often such that ideal conditions cannot be met. For instance, it might be possible to create a substantial change in dietary patterns in a community provided that a small army of dieticians could provide virtually round-the-clock advice and support. Such a venture would clearly outstrip the resources of most health services and must be the preserve of the wealthy – together with their personal trainers! Accordingly, the question must be asked – what kind of intervention will be good enough to achieve an *acceptable* level of success? This is an issue which will be addressed below in relation to the development of programme objectives.

## Aims, objectives and standard setting

There is some degree of terminological confusion between various statements of educational intent. Reference is made to aims, goals, targets and objectives almost interchangeably and indiscriminately. While there may be no universal agreement about the meaning of all of the above terms, there is general agreement about the difference between two of them: aims and objectives. An aim would normally describe a general statement of intent; it would usually provide an indication of the value underpinning a given health education programme – but little else. For instance, an aim for a nutrition education programme might be to improve the nutritional status of the nation. The implicit assumption is that this is worth doing, but because of the generality of the aim and the value position embodied within it, it is difficult to challenge its appropriateness (as opposed, say, to its

practicability). On the other hand, objectives are much more specific and precise. Any one aim might generate a large number of objectives. The nutritional aim referred to above might be translated into dozens of objectives including, for example, that a target group should reduce *average saturated fatty acids (SFA) intake from 59 g (18% of total energy) to 50 g (15% of total); i.e. a 15% reduction* (NACNE, 1983).

The specificity of objectives is now widely recognised and the use of the acronym 'SMART' to encourage people to be precise is now quite widespread.

***Box 22*** SMART Objectives

| |
|---|
| • S – specific<br>• M – measurable<br>• A – achievable<br>• R – realistic<br>• T – timescale stated |

Two observations may be made about the term objective: first, an objective is likely to generate more controversy than an aim – because it provides specific details of what is intended; second, it is considerably easier to measure (for the same reason). Objectives have an especially important part to play in evaluation. On the one hand, it has been argued that evaluation designs derived from objectives may well corrupt the educational programme while, on the other hand, it has been stated with equal vigour that the attainment of properly constructed objectives provides the best of all possible indicators of programme success. For the present, however, we will merely consider the objective as a guide for providing indicators of performance. Before doing so, we need to give some further thought to the question of specificity.

It is possible to envisage a spectrum of specificity ranging from the delightfully vague to the almost pedantically precise. An aim would be located at the general end of this spectrum while the other pole would be occupied by a particularly specific variety of goal statement generally known as a behavioural objective. This highly refined statement describes the behaviours which a learner (as opposed to a teacher, educator or instructor) will produce in order to demonstrate that the desired terminal outcome has been achieved. The behavioural objective will, moreover, specify the conditions under which the learned outcome will emerge and criteria (or standards of acceptable performance) which will be used to signal success. Figure 2.17 illustrates this specificity spectrum as a goal continuum.

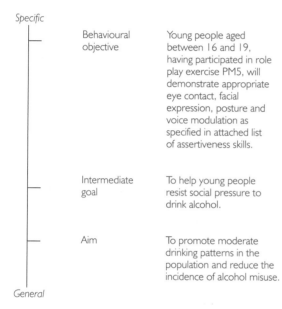

**Figure 2.17** A Goal Continuum. An Example from Alcohol Education

In accordance with standard practice, an aim is positioned at the general end of the continuum while a behavioural objective is located at the other end in acknowledgement of its high degree of specificity. While a properly constructed behavioural objective could hardly be rendered more specific – being, as it were, at a pinnacle of precision – other health promotion goals could be placed at virtually any point on the continuum. Their location would depend entirely on how general or specific they were. The example of alcohol education has been used to illustrate the potential variation in specificity and it can imme-

diately be seen that the general aim of promoting moderate drinking could be translated into literally hundreds of more specific goals. The intermediate goal of helping young people to resist social pressure represents one of these and, in turn, could be translated into a much more limited number of more detailed, precise objectives. The term behavioural objective has traditionally been associated with learning and is, therefore, applicable to health education rather than to, say, the achievement of policy goals.

**Box 23**  A Social Interaction Objective

In addition to recalling three key principles of verbal assertiveness, the learner will make appropriate use of non-verbal communication as follows.

When saying, 'No thanks, I don't want another drink' (s)he will:

- smile;
- maintain steady eye contact;
- use a firm tone of voice;
- use supportive gestures.

It is not the purpose of this book to explore the merits and demerits of using behavioural objectives. However, the interested reader should consult an amusing article by Popham (1978) in which he describes the rise and fall of the 'behavioural objectives movement'. The zenith of this quest for precision and specificity in his own personal position is symbolised by a 1962 bumper sticker which read 'Help stamp out non-behavioural objectives' and which indicates the degree of emotional involvement which curriculum design can inspire in its devotees. Since that high point there has been a move away from what Parlett and Hamilton (1978) have called the 'agricultural botany paradigm' of educational evaluation and this has been accompanied by a demise in the popularity of the behavioural objective – certainly among educationalists (Popham modified his position to the point at which his bumper sticker read 'Help stamp out some non-behavioural objectives!').

It will also be recalled that commitment to formative evaluation centring on community participation would seem to question the possibility of specifying objectives since a programme's goals may shift from time to time in response to the results of community action. However, this does not pose a serious threat to the value of utilising specific objectives since it is possible and, indeed, desirable for the community itself, in collaboration with the community worker, to set agreed objectives which may be modified almost *ad infinitum* according to the results of intervention and community action.

In fact, whatever the fashion, the advantages of the behavioural objective are very real. Once the objective has been constructed, the success of the related educational programme can be determined in a reliable and observable way by merely noting whether or not the objective has been attained – in other words, by means of a simple yes/no decision. It is worth adding here the observation made by a doyen of the behavioural objective movement, ... *if you give each learner a copy of your objectives, you may not have to do much else* (Mager, 1962). This somewhat cryptic statement makes the entirely justifiable assertion that in many instances the specificity and clarity of the goal statement embodied in behavioural objectives are sufficient to generate learning. Unfortunately, one of the main difficulties in constructing this kind of goal statement stems from the fact that many educators and health promoters are insufficiently clear about their goals! Without such clarity a behavioural objective cannot be produced.

It is worth commenting that the behaviour to which reference is made in the appellation 'behavioural objective' refers to concrete actions produced by the learner to demonstrate that learning has indeed taken place. Accordingly, objectives can not only refer to the ultimate outcome of an intervention – such as attending a clinic for immunisation – but can also generate 'indirect' and 'intermediate' indicators of success – such as the acquisition of knowledge or attitude change. A behaviour in the sense used above, therefore, refers to any observable act: for instance a behavioural indication of successful learning about the

involvement of fats in coronary heart disease might include producing a list (verbally or in writing) of various cooking oils which correctly indicated which of these were saturated and which were polyunsaturated.

Apart from the advantages of specificity, behavioural objectives have two further benefits to offer evaluators. These derive from their emphasis on the importance of including the conditions under which a given learned outcome is to be demonstrated and the standards which have to be met if the learning is to be adjudged successful. The former requirement serves as a useful reminder that a given learning outcome will only be achieved if the conditions necessary for any learning situation are fulfilled. For instance, the acquisition of social interaction skills (Box 23) requires repeated practice and feedback, perhaps using a role play technique; attitude change, on the other hand, might require the use of 'group discussion-decision' (Bond, 1958) or some other appropriate methodological tactic. The matter of standards merits rather more detailed consideration since it has an important bearing on the politics of evaluation.

## Standards of achievement

Green and Lewis (1986) identify four kinds of standard that might be used to determine the relative success of any given intervention. The results of a health education programme might simply be compared with the degree of success achieved in previous ventures of a similar kind (*historical standards*) or, alternatively, a comparison might be made with the level of performance produced by other workers in programmes of a similar nature designed for similar target groups (*normative standards*). A third kind of yardstick is provided by 'theoretical standards', in which the criteria of success are derived from a knowledge of relevant theory – which indicates what one might reasonably expect on the basis of a conceptual analysis which is ultimately derived from all previous research in a given area. Green and Lewis contrast these with a fourth level of expectation based on 'absolute standards' which demands nothing less than perfection, i.e. 100% success!

The reference to absolute standards should remind us of the important political dimension to evaluation – a dimension which we ignore at our peril. While our political paymasters may not really be so naive as to expect complete success, they frequently appear to have entirely unrealistic expectations of what health education might achieve, both in general and in relation to particular programmes. It is an interesting paradox that these same politicians – whose whole experience in politics will typically have led them to redefine the ambitious and idealistic goals of their youth so that their expectations have come to be more consistent with the 'art of the possible' – may expect health education to achieve substantial switches in public opinion and the deep-seated values which frequently underpin these attitudes. For instance, a mass media campaign might be expected significantly to shift lifestyles in a way which is largely inconsistent with existing social norms. If such a change were to happen in the political arena, it would be akin to achieving a dramatic reversal of political allegiance in large sectors of the population as a result of a series of party political broadcasts. It would rightly be viewed as little short of miraculous!

More commonly, perhaps, political goals for a programme may differ, consciously or unconsciously, from overt health education goals. On the surface a hypothetical media-based drug education programme might be seeking to harden attitudes against heroin use or even to reduce the proportion of the population misusing that substance. However, the hidden agenda may well be to demonstrate governmental concern to an irrationally anxious public and to placate vocal and influential party supporters who have been outraged at what they perceive to be a major social and moral problem. In such cases it is essential that this hidden agenda be explored with the paymasters so that false expectations are not established and the subsequent and often inevitable failure of the programme is not used as evidence of the ineffectual nature of health education. Logically, the purpose of evaluation in these circumstances should be to provide a kind of performance indicator which will record activity, energy and perhaps enthusiasm! It should not seek to measure changes in the stated target population, i.e. drug abusers or those at high risk of misusing drugs; only minimal change would be set as a theoretical standard in a programme of this sort.

While it may not be possible to specify standards of success precisely, a sound understanding of existing theory in health education should allow us to establish criteria for programme evaluation and to indicate what we might expect from any given intervention. Clearly, past experience and specific *ad hoc* research will sharpen our predictions, but even where such prior knowledge is limited, our understanding of health-related behaviour and educational theory should enable us to make realistic estimations of likely success. For example, we should be able to comment on the very best standard we could hope to achieve (a theory-based *'absolute standard'*). Reference was made above to the use of formative evaluation in achieving 'mastery learning'. Accordingly, we might expect from both theory and experience that a high level of success would be achieved provided that the health promoter adhered to the criteria associated with the formative process. In fact, expectations of success from mastery learning created the so-called 90/90 rule, which was used as a rough guide in developing linear teaching programmes in the heyday of programmed learning. In other words, programme developers and trainers would attempt to achieve a success rate of 90% in 90% of a relatively homogeneous and appropriately selected target group. This is sometimes expressed as a 90/90/90 criterion (Davies, 1981), i.e. 90% of students will achieve 90% of the objectives 90% of the time. Further attempts at refining programmes would be subject to a law of diminishing returns and not be cost effective. One might therefore say that a properly structured and essentially cognitive programme which has been pre-tested on a homogeneous target group might hope to achieve a comparable 90% success rate but no more.

Let us consider a second hypothetical example, this time in the affective area. Let us assume that a vaccine has been developed to immunise against AIDS. The vaccine can be administered in a one-shot, once-for-all form on a lump of sugar at any doctor's surgery, outpatient department, health centre or chemist. There are no side effects and effectiveness has been proven. Little knowledge of attitude change theory is required to predict the success rate of a properly pre-tested mass media-based programme which utilises all appropriate channels to deliver the message and which provides specific information about where to obtain the vaccine – and, of course, uses minimal fear appeal! The 90/90/90 criterion mentioned above might even be surpassed in certain high risk groups!

Finally, reference should be made to *Communication of Innovations Theory*. It will be recalled that an S-shaped curve describes the rate of adoption of innovations and once a majority of the population in question has adopted the innovation, a law of diminishing returns operates; in other words, 'laggards' are exceedingly difficult to influence! Evaluators should, therefore, build in some form of compensation into their calculations. In fact, Green and Lewis (1986) have argued that this 'ceiling effect', originally noted by Hovland *et al.* (1949) in the field of mass communications, may be countered by means of an 'effectiveness index' (see Box 24).

**Box 24**  An Effectiveness Index

$$EI = (P2 - P1) \div (100 - P1)$$

where *EI* is the effectiveness index, *P1* is the percentage of the population adopting the innovation prior to the intervention and *P2* is the percentage adopting at a given time after the intervention.

Thus, a relatively small change in the group of die-hard 'resistants' might be a cause for congratulation whereas a similar or even greater degree of change in an unexposed and virgin population might well require a change of programme and personnel!

## INDICATORS AND THE PROXIMAL–DISTAL CHAIN OF EFFECTS

Throughout this chapter reference has frequently been made to the nature and importance of indi-

cators and some particular examples have been provided of the criteria that might be used to assess success. In this final section we discuss a rationale for selecting indicators and, above all, try to demonstrate how different kinds of indicators could and should be used as part of programme evaluation. More particularly, we will identify outcome indicators and compare these with 'intermediate' and 'indirect indicators' of performance. We will locate these on a continuum that we will call a 'proximal–distal chain' that *inter alia* demonstrates graphically the complexity of health promotion programmes – and the associated implications for developing criteria for effectiveness and efficiency. First, though, we will comment on a late 1980s vogue for '*performance indicators*' which will allow us to make comparisons with the way in which the notion of indicator is employed here. We will then consider indicators for programme outcomes, commenting on one particular kind of outcome – the achievement of well-being. This will lead us to comment briefly on what will be called 'epidemiological indicators' and their misuse in evaluation of health promotion initiatives.

### Performance indicators

As part of a general strategy to encourage more efficient use of resources, performance indicators (PIs) were introduced to monitor performance within health and medical services. They were essentially attempts to introduce more central control of health expenditure and effective scrutiny of performance (Small, 1989). PIs were intended to be practical and useful tools for management. The original approach was to develop a range of crude indicators of performance from routinely collected data on the basis of which comparisons could be made between districts, between types of service and between specialisms. PIs can be of three types: clinical; manpower; financial and estate management. Examples of PIs are: length of stay in hospital; annual throughput per hospital bed; cost per day; ratio of trained to untrained staff. The first set of indicators was used in the UK on a trial basis in 1982 and the complete set published in 1983 and revised in 1985.

By comparison with the indicators to be discussed below, PIs, as conceptualised in the 1980s, were indicators of input and overall levels of activity: they might have had a bearing on the structure and process elements of quality assurance but did not actually measure the impact of inputs on the health of populations. There have also been criticisms of the number of indicators and their comprehensibility as well as questions about the accuracy of summary statistics resulting from their use (Allen *et al.*, 1987).

However, of much greater importance was this underlying assumption that indicators are in some way related to positive health outcomes. Indeed, it was hoped that the focus on inputs and levels of activity might encourage reduction of costs and increased productivity without at the same time requiring related assessments of impacts on health and other outcome indicators. This was clearly a major flaw in a policy that led to an unbridled pursuit of PIs. Health educators were also subjected to demands to produce PIs. Ironically, perhaps, instead of judging the quality of health education by the level of activity or checking the existence of a critical mass of health education personnel and resourcing, there was frequently an expectation that while input indicators were appropriate for clinical services, output indicators were appropriate for health education. The inequity of expecting health educators to demonstrate that they had had a major impact on a reduction in smoking or an increase in health might well be imagined!

It is, of course, possible to develop PIs for health education which are comparable with clinical service measures. For example, as will be seen in a later chapter, there is evidence that more effective patient education is achieved in hospitals which have trained coordinators (Pack *et al.*, 1983). Accordingly, an easy-to-measure PI for a health district might be the number of hospitals with patient education coordinators. There is evidence that written material in booklet form is an effective way to reinforce education in hospital settings and is associated with patient satisfaction. A simple indicator would record the percentage of patients who had received such booklets.

In the last analysis, though, input measures of performance are only as good as the evidence linking them to important outcomes. In the formulation adopted here and discussed below the 'traditional' PI is seen as an 'indirect' indicator of eventual success.

Interestingly, at the time of writing, the UK National Health Service Executive launched a new initiative entitled *Quality and Performance in the NHS: High Level Performance Indicators and Clinical Indicators* (NHSE, 2000). The Secretary of State observed that

> *... it is not possible to raise standards unless we have the right information to start with. In the past, there was too much meaningless bean-counting combined with a narrow focus on efficiency. Now ... we have made a start in assessing the outcome of treatment and the effectiveness of services.*

(p2)

## Outcomes: indicators of well-being

Three types of indicator were mentioned above. The most obvious of these relate to outcomes. Outcome is used here to refer to a particular end-point and, therefore, an ultimate measure of success. However, the definition of outcome is not as clear-cut as might at first be imagined. As we will see, an outcome for one kind of programme might well be only an intermediate indicator for another. Moreover, there are at least two different kinds of outcome that are worth consideration here. The first may be said to define successful end-points for programmes committed to enhance well-being and achieve more holistic, positive goals. The second concerns traditional 'epidemiological' outcomes, i.e. those typically concerned with mortality and morbidity or other 'medical' measures. First, though, the question of indicators of well-being.

In Chapter 1 we noted how one school of thought argued that the prime concern for the emergent health promotion movement should be the resurrection of WHO's 1946 clarion call for a holistic and positive approach to the definition of health. This view has certainly persisted – if not as the major concern of health promotion, then certainly as a significant component. Insofar as this more 'salutogenic' goal remains a major or minor component of a health promotion programme, reliable and valid indicators must be developed to assess that programme's efficiency. Indeed, since the aims of interventions designed to achieve holistic and positive outcomes are more likely to be vague, relevant and precise indicators are more rather than less important.

Even before the shift from health education to health promotion Hunt and McEwen (1980) had argued, in their rationale for the development of the Nottingham Health Profile, that the philosophical shift from logical positivism and empiricism, combined with the changing nature of disease and disability in contemporary society, had resulted in a need to devise more subjective measures of well-being and quality of life. In the context of this book such indicators are the positive analogues of the traditional medical outcome measures mentioned above. A brief comment will therefore be made about the kinds of subjective indicator which have been used and are available to the evaluator.

Briscoe (1982), writing from a social work perspective, commented that ... *subjective measures of well-being are therefore needed in order adequately to assess – and hence treat – a wide spectrum of psychosocial dysfunction*. The reference to 'dysfunction' and 'psychosocial' should incidentally remind us that it is difficult to completely distance oneself from negative aspects of health. Hall (1976) underlined this point in his observation that two of the best buys in subjective indicators were the *Housing Nuisance Index* and the *Health Symptom Index*!

Hall also described the development of a variety of subjective measures of quality of life in Britain between 1971 and 1975. Clearly the most problematic aspect of measuring quality of life is defining it. Hall cited Tom Harrisson, the founder of '*Mass Observation*', who said *You cannot, yet, take a census of love in Liverpool or random sample the effect that fear of the future has on the total pattern of contemporary life in Leeds*. Researchers of an ethnographic orientation

would, of course, challenge this pessimistic statement and, in fact, Hall describes the result of the Social Science Research Council's 1975 survey in which respondents were asked to define '*quality of life*'. The results are particularly revealing – not only for the construction of subjective indicators but also for the way they provide an insight into perceptions of health and well-being. For instance, 23% of the sample of 932 people of all social groups referred to 'family, home life, marriage' while 19% made rather more vague references to being contented or happy. A further 17 and 18% valued decent living conditions and money, respectively. Health was relegated to a 10% response rate while more abstract and altruistic aspects of quality of life, such as equality and justice, were mentioned by only 2% of the sample. These findings confirm the view that many people's notion of positive health or well-being derived from whatever happens to be their salient value system and/or from a meaning of health which is consistent with the medical model perspective – lack of disease or social impairment.

Measures of quality of life, therefore, included people's level of satisfaction with the various 'life domains' mentioned above: more particularly, housing, health, standard of living, etc. In addition, more global measures of well-being have been used. These have attempted to measure personal competence and trust in others and positive and negative affect [using, for example, Bradburn's (1969) *Affect Balance Scale*].

In contrast, the Nottingham Health Profile (Hunt and McEwen, 1980) adopted an approach which focused more on personal than social well-being. The Profile consists of six sections referring to: emotional life; experience of pain; energy levels; social integration; physical mobility; sleep patterns.

Although positive health indicators may be more appealing to health educators than illness-related measures, they may prove to be equally, if not more, problematic. Like mortality and morbidity, quality of life will be affected by a wide variety of social and environmental influences beyond the control of even the most thorough programme.

## Outcomes: social health

The positive health indicators above are essentially individualistic – and we must recognise that the concerns of contemporary health promotion are also with positive social outcomes. For instance, we argued in Chapter 1 that the overriding goal of health promotion is with the achievement of equity and social justice. Now while it is possible to specify distal outcomes of this social goal – for instance the distribution of income within and between nations – it is not practicable to assess programme effectiveness and efficiency using such measures. This is quite clearly because such a dramatic change in individuals and political and social structures would require a long-term programme of stunning complexity. The best we might aim for would, for example, be a demonstration that national literacy had increased and female literacy matched that of males – or, on a smaller scale, that levels of social capital had increased in a region with a consequent reduction in social exclusion.

It is not, of course, even as straightforward as depicted above since the achievement of equity, or at any rate a reduction in inequalities, might be seen by those whose professional concern is with preventive medicine, as an intermediate step in making progress towards the ultimate target of preventing disease and disability. In which case, markers of the end-point would be expressed in terms of epidemiological or medical indicators.

## Outcomes: epidemiological and medical

As we will demonstrate below, the use of any outcome indicator of achievements may often be less useful than various 'intermediate' indicators; the use of traditional epidemiological indicators are rarely if ever appropriate for the task of assessing the effectiveness and efficiency of health promotion programmes. Hopefully the reason for this sweeping statement will become apparent when we consider the nature of the proximal–distal chain of events that intervene between health promotion inputs and final end-points. For now, we can assert that epidemiological indicators are too blunt a tool to assess the effects of complex concatenations of health promotion inputs delivered over a relatively long timescale.

**Box 25**  Beware the Epidemiological Indicator!

> *Traditional epidemiological indicators – such as measures of the incidence and prevalence of coronary heart disease or the decayed missing or filled (DMF) index employed by dental researchers – should not be used to assess the success or failure of health promotion interventions. Epidemiological data should be used to provide justification for launching health promotion initiatives not for evaluating them.*
>
> Green and Tones (1999a)

The argument against epidemiological indicators is succinctly stated below.

- As with broad social goals, such as the achievement of equity, a considerable number of integrated programme inputs – often operating over quite a long period of time – will have to be in place before a reduction in, say, mortality or morbidity can be achieved. Each programme element may be necessary but not sufficient for achievement of the final outcome.
- The time lag between a programme element and the behaviour that is considered to affect epidemiological outcomes may be so great that it would require a substantial cohort study to establish the links between input and outcome.
- The relationship between risk factors and the incidence and prevalence of disease in populations is by no means isomorphic – as Dale Groom's ironic review of CHD risk factors circa 1960 demonstrates (Box 26). Even though Dale Groom's list has been reduced to cardinal risk factors, our comments in Chapter 1 about the percentage of variance remaining unexplained by those risk factors demonstrates that there is still a substantial problem. If a link has, in fact, been demonstrated, there is no need to use epidemiological indicators to assess success: a change in behaviour or risk factor will suffice. Clearly, if there is no link between behaviour and disease it is not only inefficient, it is unethical for health promotion to try to change the behaviours in question [unless, of

course, the behaviours are worthwhile in their own right – for instance, the (arguable!) joy of exercise – or because they are implicated in the aetiology of some other disease].

Patently, these remarks do not question epidemiological research *per se*. However the purpose of the research is – as observed elsewhere (Green and Tones, 199a) – to provide *justification* for health promotion programmes not to evaluate them.

**Box 26** A Thumbnail Sketch of the Man Least Likely to Have Coronary Heart Disease

> *An effeminate municipal worker or embalmer, completely lacking in physical or mental alertness and without drive, ambition or competitive spirit who has never attempted to meet a deadline of any kind. A man with poor appetite, subsisting on fruit and vegetables laced with corn and whale oils, detesting tobacco, spurning ownership of radio, TV, or motor-car, with full head of hair and scrawny unathletic appearance, yet constantly straining his puny muscles by exercise; low in income, B.P., blood sugar, uric acid, and cholesterol, who has been taking nicotinic acid, pyridoxine, and long term anticoagulant therapy ever since his prophylactic castration.*
>
> Groom, in Tilford and Tones (1977)

## The temporal relationship between programme effects and indicators of success

As noted above, there is, inevitably, a time lag between a given health promotion input and its outcome. Quite frequently there is more than one particular input and these multiple inputs may operate not just at one point in time but over a quite considerable period of time. The complex interactions between these various inputs and the time lag itself pose problems for evaluation and account for the need for different kinds of indicator other than those that signal the achievement of outcomes. There is another especially important implication deriving from both the gap between

input and output and the complex interactions between the different inputs characteristic of all but the smallest and simplest health promotion programmes. In short, insofar as all of the various programme inputs are necessary for the achievement of the final goal – and may even act synergistically – a good deal of care must be exercised in determining the standards of levels of success to be expected from any single input. Caution needs to be exercised even for an apparently straightforward persuasive communication using mass media. Consider, for instance, Figure 2.18, which describes the psychological changes that must occur in individuals exposed to the media messages before they subscribe to a recommended course of action (in the case described below, the adoption of the 'slip, slap, slop' prescription for the avoidance of skin cancer: 'slip' on a t-shirt; 'slap' on a hat; 'slop' on the sun cream!

The first barrier to be overcome is to ensure that the target population becomes aware of the skin cancer message and pays attention to it; this, in turn, depends on a sufficient level of media exposure. Assuming that the audience has become aware of the message, is not threatened by it and, therefore, does not indulge in defensive avoidance behaviour, they must correctly interpret the information provided and understand it. The assumption is made that 30% of the audience has become aware of the message and 85% of that 30% actually understand it. They must subsequently accept the truth of the message and have a positive attitude toward adoption of the recommended slip/slap/slop action. It is assumed that some 31% have done so. However, before that proportion of the audience actually progresses to adoption, it will be necessary that they have the skills and other supportive factors necessary to translate positive attitude into practice. It is assumed that some 40% are in such a position. The assumptions, incidentally, are not completely hypothetical, but are consistent with empirically based media research on what might be expected (for the marketing of commercial products) when communications have been properly pre-tested. By performing the appropriate multiplication, it will be seen that we might expect approximately

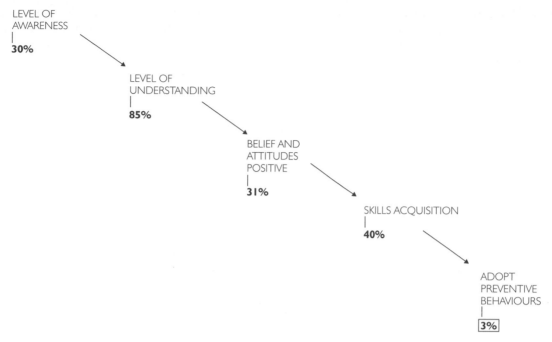

**Figure 2.18** A Hierarchy of Communication Effects

3% of the audience to actually adopt the recommended preventive behaviour (though not necessarily sustain it).

Apart from illustrating the sequential process involved in even the simplest health promotion programme, the presentation in Figure 2.19 provides reinforcement for earlier comments about the importance of setting realistic objectives and standards.

McGuire (1981) provided a more detailed analysis of the various steps and associated pitfalls in the 'marketing' process – and this will receive further explication in a later chapter. McGuire, for instance, refers to a number of 'fallacies' arising when communicators fail to acknowledge the various hurdles to be overcome on the road to media success! For example, he describes what he calls an *'attenuated effects fallacy'* where the evaluator fails to take account of the various links in the input–output chain and refuses to acknowledge that the probability of achieving all of them is a function of the probability of achieving step 1 multiplied by the probability of achieving step 2 and so on until the final step is reached. In other words,

the chances of success are relatively small and, in accordance with the calculation shown in Figure 2.18, it would be unwise to write a programme objective having an anticipated standard of success greater than 1 or 2%. He also refers to the *'distal measure fallacy'* when a decision is made to evaluate the ultimate outcome or end-point of a campaign solely on the basis of the early indicators.

### Indicators and community-wide programmes

The media-based programme described in Figure 2.19 would normally be 'nested' in a much broader community programme. Indeed, as we shall see in our later chapter on mass media in health promotion, the use of unsupported mass media interventions is considered to be fundamentally unsound. Moreover, given the emphasis on the importance of multi-agency, collaborative working across large sections of a population, many health promotion ventures will be both complex and extensive in both space and time. Figure 2.19 provides a simplified analysis of a health promotion programme that might be expected to ultimately influence the early detection and, therefore, reduce the incidence of cervical cancer. It will be seen that it does in fact contain a small mass media component relating to the importance of taking a smear test.

Let us, however, consider Figure 2.19 from the perspective of a school-based cancer education programme that emerged from negotiations with a cancer charity and involved the free provision of a package of teaching materials together with a training course for teachers. The programme had a dual function. First, it was concerned with primary prevention and aimed to raise awareness of the importance of avoiding unprotected exposure to the sun and of responding to invitations by GPs to take a smear test. It also had a secondary preventive goal, namely to encourage early diagnosis

and thus attempting to persuade individuals to seek early medical advice whenever one of the classic early warning signs and symptoms of cancer might present (cough or hoarseness, change in appearance of wart or mole, etc.). Now clearly the students would not receive an invitation to have a smear test for several years after they had left school. Similarly, potential cancer symptoms would be unlikely to occur and require attention for perhaps 20 or 30 years or more after the teaching had taken place. Any evaluation of the school programme based on behavioural outcomes (let alone epidemiological evidence) would require a cohort study if the causal chain between education and behavioural outcome were to be established. Such a study would be too costly to contemplate even if all the extraneous inputs of

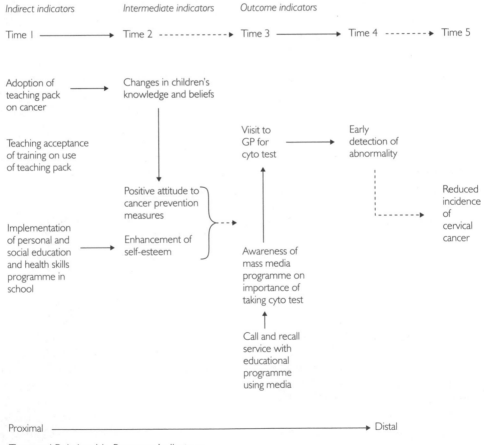

**Figure 2.19** Temporal Relationship Between Indicators

information and influences occurring over 20 years or more could be controlled. *Intermediate indicators* – i.e. proxy measures of success – would have to suffice.

The kind of time lag examined above is perhaps self-evident. Less obvious is the time lag imposed by the dictates of sound educational theory and practice. For instance, educational planners would hopefully recognise that various processes of socialisation (e.g. early family influences on attitudes to cancer) contribute to an individual's health career – i.e. the development over an individual's lifespan of health-related behaviours and the psychosocial factors underpinning these. Professional educators would be expected to think in terms of a '*spiral curriculum*'. This seeks to ensure that appropriate teaching occurs at the right time and in the right way at significant points on the health career such that a topic is not merely taught at only one point in time but is rather revisited and handled in a manner appropriate to the developmental requirements of the student. The adoption of a health career approach should thus ensure that a planned and cumulative series of educational inputs has been provided prior to the moment when an individual is expected to make a given health choice. The concept of a smoking career exemplifies this process since research on the natural history of smoking has made it clear that a single lesson or even a series of lessons on smoking will neither prevent recruitment nor facilitate genuine decision making about whether to smoke or not. A programme must be started long before early secondary school age and the time when experimentation starts in earnest. Such a programme will require not only differential provision of biological and social knowledge related to the children's developmental age but also expert teaching which will equip young people with social interaction skills so that they might be '*inoculated*' against various pressures to smoke. Each element in the smoking career is necessary and thus intermediate indicators are needed *en route* to check that each stage of the programme has been effective. (This should, ideally, be part of the process of *formative evaluation*, to which reference was made earlier in the chapter.)

A sound programme of health education will thus require not only coordination of inputs *during* the health career but also coordination across the range of inputs provided at any one time. In other words, both longitudinal and cross-sectional integration are a prerequisite for most complex programmes since the influences of health-related behaviours are many and varied and are brought to bear in a cumulative way over time.

Inspection of Figure 2.19 will reveal two unacceptable indicators of effectiveness (following the discussion above about medical and epidemiological indicators). The first of these is a reduced incidence of cervical cancer while the second refers to the actual detection of abnormality in individuals having precursor pathology – and thus refers to the effectiveness of screening. Clearly, a positive response to an invitation to attend the GP's surgery to undergo the screening procedure is a perfectly respectable *outcome indicator* of the sub-programme relating to the use of mass media and the associated service provision. However, a number of intermediate indicators will be needed to provide evidence of the effectiveness of the various programmes, past and present, that ultimately contribute to the outcome in question. In short, moving from proximal to distal, these might be:

- knowledge and beliefs about cancer;
- attitudes to cancer and its prevention;
- the empowering personal characteristic of self-esteem;
- awareness of mass media and other indicators of the kind listed in Figure 2.19.

### Indirect indicators

The term intermediate indicator has been used here to describe individual characteristics that result from programme inputs and which may demonstrate a change that will act as a mediator between input and outcome. Since these indicators can reveal the direct effect of programme inputs, the term 'impact' evaluation may thus be used to describe the effectiveness or otherwise of those inputs. There are, however, other different kinds of input that have an indirect impact: in other words, these inputs make it possible for different aspects of a programme to create the kinds of change signalled by intermediate indicators. For instance, in Figure 2.19 it is presumed that teachers will be more successful in producing changes in children's knowledge, beliefs, attitudes and levels of self-esteem if they have been trained to use the cancer education teaching package and then actually use it in class. Prior to this the teaching pack and the training should have been pre-tested to ensure that they were appropriate for the needs of children and teachers, respectively. Again, the enhancement of children's self-esteem (which in turn is presumed to contribute to self-empowerment and a commitment to look after themselves) will depend on effective teaching. Accordingly, the success of the teaching will depend on teachers having the necessary competencies to manage informal and possibly unconventional teaching methods. Both the pre-testing and the teacher training should, therefore, be evaluated. The evaluation will, in turn, generate *indirect indicators* of success.

Again, effective health education interventions may either be dependent on or at least facilitated by various policy measures – including availability of and access to relevant services. In Figure 2.19 the existence of a properly funded and designed call and recall service would be an important prerequisite for a satisfactory outcome. The existence of such a service and its quality would, therefore, also exemplify the importance of using indirect indicators.

Bearing in mind earlier observations about evaluation generally, the assessment of the existence and quality of the policy provision would constitute the kind of *process evaluation* that checks whether or not key programme elements are in place. Clearly, if this also involves the use of that information to make immediate changes to training or other aspects of service provision, we can with justification describe this as *formative evaluation*.

It is appropriate at this point to make what is doubtless a fairly obvious statement: apparently identical indicators can serve to indicate *indirect* achievements, the achievement of *intermediate*

goals or even *outcomes*. This changing identity will often reflect the ideological purpose of the programme. For instance, the attainment of a raft of capabilities and dispositions associated with assertiveness might be considered a desirable goal in its own right – just as the attainment of self-esteem might be considered as an *outcome indicator* of mental health. On the other hand, if a salutogenic or empowerment model is not adopted, these very same measures might be categorised as *intermediate indicators* of success along the route towards the achievement of behavioural outcomes relating to the prevention and management of disease. Again, the purpose of a programme might be primarily to achieve inter-sectoral working and evidence of having achieved this goal would serve as an outcome measure. More typically, though, collaborative working might be seen as a means to an end – either empowerment or the prevention of disease. It would, therefore, be signalled by *indirect indicators* (which, of course, might provide appropriate fodder for process evaluation).

## HAM and the selection of indicators

The various empirical models discussed above can provide guidelines for the logical and comprehensive selection of indicators. For instance, the *Health Action Model* readily helps us identify indirect, intermediate and outcome indicators and Box 27 offers an example related to the adoption of regular condom use as part of a programme designed to promote safer sex.

**Box 27**  HAM Indicators for the Evaluation of a Safer Sex Programme

---

*Outcome Indicators*
- Routine use of condom.
- Uses condom for first time.

*Intermediate Indicators*
- Strength of intention to use condoms.
- Beliefs about susceptibility to AIDS and STIs.
- Beliefs about the nature of AIDS and its transmission leading to beliefs about the

---

effectiveness of condoms and benefits of their use.

- Beliefs about costs associated with condom use: embarrassing, messy, interrupts love making, etc.
- 'Normative' beliefs about use of condoms by peers and other significant people; beliefs about reaction of parents and significant others to intention to use condoms.
- Motivation to comply with/conform to norms and wishes of other people.
- Beliefs about gender: beliefs about responsibility for use of contraception and protection.
- Self-efficacy beliefs: beliefs about capability of negotiating condom use and using them.
- Perceived locus of control: general level of internality.
- Extent to which health is valued and level of concern for other people, especially actual or potential partners.
- Values associated with morality and consequent beliefs about what is appropriate/inappropriate sexual behaviour.
- Level of self-esteem.
- Degree of concern, anxiety or fear derived from threat of AIDS.
- Degree of sensation seeking.
- Level of psychomotor skill in using and disposing of condoms.
- Level of assertiveness and communication skills needed to negotiate use with partner.

*Indirect Indicators*

- Environmental support: availability of condoms.
- Availability of advice, counselling and training.
- General level of community empowerment/alienation/helplessness.

Clearly, various instruments, devices and approaches might be used to provide a valid measure of the different indicators. For instance, a scale of self-efficacy might be employed (see Box 28).

**Box 28**  Example of a Self-Efficacy Scale

*Scene 1 (of three)*

*You have just finished a hectic week, and want to forget about all your problems for a while. You find yourself walking around one of your favourite areas and talking to people. You've had one drink to unwind. Even though you have had only one drink, you feel it affecting you a little bit. Someone that you've met once or twice before, and that you are very attracted to, has been flirting with you. This person makes it clear that (he/she) wants to have sex with you. You are interested.*

Q.1 How confident are you that you could bring up the issue of condoms in a conversation in the situation described above ?

0_____10

Not at all confident          Extremely confident

Q.3 How confident are you that you would leave this situation if (he/she) refused to use a condom?

0_____10

Not at all confident          Extremely confident

(from Maibach and Murphy, 1995 p46)

### Indicators at the macro, meso and micro levels

It is useful to contemplate the way in which health promotion indicators may operate at different levels – levels often described as *macro*, *meso* and *micro*. Figure 2.20 describes part of a school-centred programme designed to reduce the rate of unwanted pregnancies in a local community. Clearly, it could be viewed as but one element in a much broader community-wide development which, in turn, might be embedded in a national programme which would probably include government policy initiatives.

Developments at the national level would, accordingly, yield potential macro level indicators of effectiveness and efficiency. Insofar as they contributed to the success of the community level programme, they would also be operating as indirect indicators.

Micro level activities refer mainly to interpersonal interactions, e.g. as characterised by teachers working with their classes or teacher trainers running courses for teachers.

Meso level work is more difficult to define precisely as it operates at some point between macro and micro. It would certainly include health promotion within specific organisations and settings – for instance, the health promoting school illustrated in Figure 2.20. Of course, *within* a given organisation it is possible to identify different levels of action – such as top management's policy development, middle management communication and, at the micro level, the health education encounters between occupational health nurse and worker.

In fact, it is more appropriate to think of a continuum extending from micro to macro.

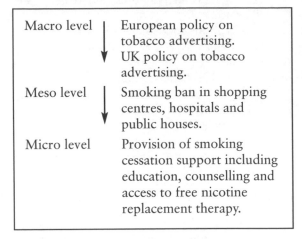

**Box 29** A Macro–Micro Continuum

| | |
|---|---|
| Macro level | European policy on tobacco advertising. UK policy on tobacco advertising. |
| Meso level | Smoking ban in shopping centres, hospitals and public houses. |
| Micro level | Provision of smoking cessation support including education, counselling and access to free nicotine replacement therapy. |

As Box 29 demonstrates, there are also different levels of macro influences – most obviously apparent in the relative influence of international policies on national policies. For example, the UK

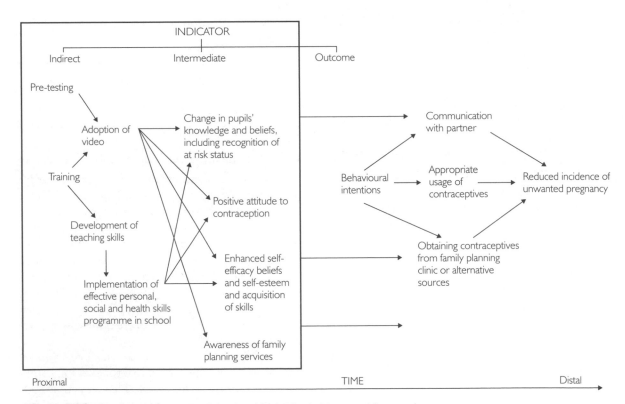

**Figure 2.20** The Health Promoting School and Reduction in Unwanted Pregnancies

government's initial failure to implement a total tobacco advertising ban was due to the tobacco industry's successful legal challenge based on the assertion that the UK should not anticipate the agreed implementation of a Europe-wide ban. Again, it is generally accepted that the effectiveness of national policies on the control of illegal drugs frequently depend on controlling supplies from 'third world' countries; the control of supply in those countries would, in turn, typically require changes in economic and agricultural policy before production could be stopped.

Although, at first glance, the programmes portrayed schematically in Figures 2.20 and 2.21 appear quite complex, they would typically be mere windows providing a limited and simplistic view of more sophisticated and broad-based interventions. A more comprehensive perspective would reveal that major national or community-wide collaborative ventures are composed of a complicated network of interacting agencies, professionals and lay people. Not surprisingly then, the indicators needed to reveal the degrees of success or failure of those ventures would be many, varied and, above all, sophisticated. Moreover, as we will reiterate later, the act of selecting from the armamentarium of potential indicators requires a high level of discrimination derived from theoretical insights. These observations will be examined by considering the features of a strategy that emphasises inter-sectoral working.

## Inter-sectoral working and indicators of success: the example of a healthy living centre

*Healthy Living Centres* (HLCs) are, at the time of writing, UK government projects funded by the National Lottery. Together with other related developments, such as *Health Action Zones* (HAZs), they seek to tackle some of the social and economic determinants of ill health and social malaise that were discussed at length in Chapter 1.

Their main, stated intentions are as follows:

- to address inequalities;
- to support other local health goals;

- to achieve community participation;
- to work collaboratively;
- to ensure 'additionality';
- to ensure sustainability.

Since these general aims differ qualitatively one from another and operate at different levels, indicators of effectiveness and efficiency of the HLCs will equally differ in terms of type and level. By way of example, the social and ethical goal of reducing inequalities and achieving equity defines the ultimate outcome of the programme: it is the be-all and end-all. Accordingly, measures of success would be categorised as outcome indicators. However, from the perspective of a preventive medical model they would be viewed as indirect indicators, since the achievement of equity in its various forms would give rise to a series of intermediate effects (such as a reduction in learned helplessness and enhanced self-efficacy and self-esteem) which might subsequently contribute to health enhancing action outcomes and, finally, have an impact on the prevalence and incidence of disease at a population level or yield parallel medical benefits at an individual level. Our earlier strong assertion, it should be recalled, was that this latter kind of indicator should not be used by health promoters!

Again, community participation might be considered either as a desirable outcome in its own right or as a means for achieving more 'distal' goals. For instance, community participation might be considered an instrumental strategy for generating an 'active participating community' (to use the parlance of the Ottawa Charter) which might result in individuals developing a 'sense of coherence' (Antonovsky, 1979) or, at the macro level, in the attainment of a 'sense of community'.

Similarly, 'working in partnership' (also known as inter-sectoral collaboration or 'healthy alliances') is both a means and an end. Together with community participation, it forms part of the desirable outcome of accumulating a healthy stock of 'social capital' and/or it may be conceptualised as a 'community coalition' (*Health Education Research*, 1993) that maximises the chance of achieving preventive goals in the context of community wide programmes epitomised by the various heart disease prevention programmes such as North Karelia (Puska *et al.*, 1985) and Minnesota, (Jacobs *et al.*, 1985).

The effectiveness of 'additionality' would be appraised by using indirect indicators since it is effectively an efficiency device that signals (1) the avoidance of duplicated efforts (essentially an economic goal) and (2) the enhancement of existing ventures. Similarly, evidence of 'sustainability' would demonstrate a 'value-added' element in that programme effects are demonstrably enduring. Sustainability criteria might also be incorporated as standards of anticipated excellence when programme objectives are constructed.

This hierarchy of interacting programme effects is summarised in Figure 2.21. It should be noted that the various programme components are at the macro or meso levels. Micro level effects on individuals and indicators of these have been excluded to avoid confusion, but can be assumed to be embedded within the schematic overview.

## Some problems of evaluation

It is, typically, difficult to maintain conceptual (and practical) control over programmes generated by initiatives such as HLCs. Each programme would normally produce multiple levels of effect and those effects would emerge over an often quite lengthy timescale; moreover, as discussed earlier, the effects may either comprise outcomes in their own right – depending on the 'normative' philosophy underpinning the initiative – or, alternatively, may provide 'benchmarks' along the route to some more distant goal. And, what is more, programmes often appear to acquire a life of their own as one initiative triggers one or more successive or parallel initiatives that had not been originally foreseen but which seemed to meet the overall programme aims – or even suggested additional, unanticipated but worthy goals.

The programme described in Box 30 is hypothetical but derived from elements of real life developments. It seeks to illustrate the complex interactions described above.

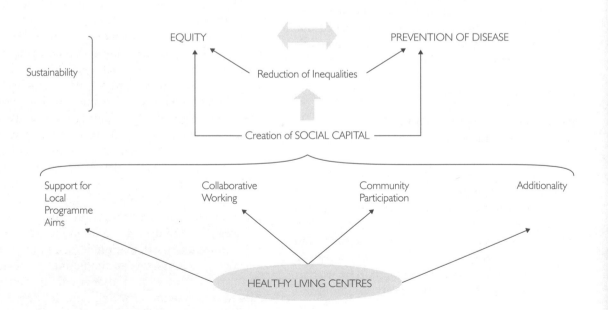

***Figure 2.21*** Different Goal Levels: Healthy Living Centres

**Box 30**  A Healthy Living Centre Takes Shape

A community development project was initiated in a disadvantaged, urban housing estate [1]. It was an outreach programme based in a local school and two community workers set up a toy library and delivered toys in their van to mothers in the neighbourhood. It was assumed that their children lacked stimulation and the women needed to learn how to play with them. Having discovered that the base in the school intimidated local inhabitants, the team moved into a vacant maisonette on the estate and based many activities there. They discovered a good deal of latent talent in the women and took advantage of Health Education Council funding to enrol a number of them on an Open University diploma course in childcare. Successful completion of the course, not surprisingly, boosted levels of self-esteem in this group of 'uneducated' women having very limited aspirations. Problems with looking after and feeding children were discussed and the oft-quoted difficulties of providing healthy food for families soon emerged as a significant 'felt need'. Accordingly, the community workers established a food cooperative, using their 'toy' van to fetch cheap but fresh food from the market several miles away. Since they felt that it was uneconomical to use their valuable time by acting as delivery drivers, the workers took the unprecedented and radical step of using some of their project money to pay for a number of the women to learn to drive – so they could collect and deliver the food.

Naturally, establishment of the food cooperative led to a most effective and practically-based form of nutrition education.

Somewhat later the health authority, working in partnership with the local authority, were successful in gaining funding to establish a HLC. Their main initial focus was on the problem of

unwanted teenage pregnancies and they immediately collaborated with the local education authority and worked with a school that had recently joined the regional health promoting school network. Figure 2.20 describes their strategy. The school had already established a link with the local general practitioner that centred on the use of creative arts in defining local felt needs, fostering inter-sectoral working and providing user-friendly health education [2]. An attempt was made to widen the approach by negotiating with the health promotion adviser in the newly established Primary Care Group and this resulted in contacts with the Home-Link scheme and extending work into the prevention of childhood disorders and child care generally. Three developments occurred quite rapidly. First, advice was sought from creative arts workers who had helped the local community establish a lantern festival as part of a plan to generate a 'sense of community' and the arts were used as a trigger for raising critical consciousness about the problem of child accidents in the housing estate. A national pharmacy chain had established a community 'drop-in' centre in its local premises and this was used to plan strategies. The use of creative arts proved particularly attractive to local media and press; local radio and television gave valuable coverage. Strong pressure was exerted on the local authority...

*Notes*

[1] *This element of the hypothetical tale is based on the Home-Link Project* (Bell *et al.,* 1978).

[2] *See Green and Tones (1999b) for a description of such an initiative in Withymoor, West Midlands.*

Hopefully the extract from the hypothetical case study introduced in Box 30 will emphasise both the complexity and fluidity of collaborative initiatives and demonstrate the plethora of indica-

tors of success that might be generated. These might range from the success of collaborative action in achieving a sense of community to the enhancement of self-esteem in those women who successfully passed their driving tests; they might include indirect indicators such as the establishment of committees to formalise joint working or access to a maisonette on the housing estate. Table 2.3 provides a *sample* of indicators derived from Meyrick and Sinkler's (1999) concise review of the evaluation of HLCs. The indicators are categorised with respect to level ('individual level, community level and project level') and in terms of process, outcome and impact. Impact indicators refer to what we have defined elsewhere as 'intermediate indicators'.

***Table 2.3*** Sample Indicators for a Healthy Living Centre Project

**Individual level**

*Outcomes*
- Adoption of healthy lifestyle and behaviours, e.g. emotional health and well-being; enhanced physical activity; sexual health.
- Taking 'political' action, e.g. join lantern procession; complain to council about housing.

*Intermediate*
- Knowledge and understanding of health issues.
- Increased feeling of responsibility for own health.
- Accurate beliefs about how to improve health.
- Development of a sense of common identity/sense of connection with place and people.

*Process*
- Level of attendance at project meetings.
- Number of volunteers for project tasks.
- Perceptions of ease of access to project.

**Project level**

*Outcomes*
- Project responds to changing needs of community.
- A majority of people consider the project is worthwhile.
- The project demonstrates an ability to respond to crisis.

*Intermediate*
- Increased representation of the project on decision making bodies.
- Increased political visibility of the project.
- Evidence of money moving from short-term funding to longer term contracting of services.

*Process*
- Extent to which local people were involved in evaluation.
- Number and variety of partnerships developed with private, voluntary and public sectors.
- Additionality: uniqueness of the project's contribution to promotion of health.

**Community level**

*Outcomes*
- Increased access to affordable/appropriate housing; user participation in housing management; home ownership.
- Environmental development: recycling systems established; provision of public transport at low cost; traffic management; recreational facilities and green spaces.
- Level of policing: adequacy, fairness and effectiveness.

*Intermediate*
- Changes in local laws and resources; reduction in incidence of problems.
- Community's feeling about how their community stands relative to other communities.
- Civic engagement: amount of time devoted to participation in voting; community views on power and control of state/local government

*Process*
- Equitable involvement of different community groups in HLC management.
- Representation of the HLC at local forums.
- Regular consultation with the community.

*Derived from Meyrick and Sinkler (1999).*

## SELECTING INDICATORS: THE IMPORTANCE OF THEORY

It is hopefully self-evident by now that even the simpler health promotion programmes can generate a plethora of indicators of effectiveness and efficiency. Which to choose ? While never simple, the task of selecting indicators is considerably facilitated by the judicious use of theory. Existing theories will not only suggest the appropriate strategies and methods to use in designing and running programmes, they may also be employed to quite precisely specify requirements for successful health promotion interventions. The following examples at the micro level will illustrate this observation and include reference to indirect, intermediate and outcome indicators – following the parlance used so far in this chapter.

### Community development theory and indicators of progress in group thinking

Box 31 summarises Batten's (1967) analysis of a community group moving from an initial stage of relative helplessness to a more empowered state.

The column headed 'Community worker' describes the ways in which the community worker asks questions to raise awareness in the community group with which (s)he is working. The descriptions of the worker task at each of the six stages, therefore, serve as indirect indicators of effective working: it is assumed that, on the basis of community development theory, the worker should provide this input and lead the community group through each successive stage.

On the other hand, the column headed 'Reactions of members of the group' provides a series of intermediate indicators of success. If the worker has employed the approved strategy, community group members should move from feelings of dissatisfaction through a process of motivated decision making until they eventually take action.

This latter action can be considered as an outcome indicator together with the feeling of satisfaction at having achieved their objective. The ultimate goal would be the attainment of that complex of psychosocial and environmental outcomes characterising empowerment – and described by both the *Health Action Model* and the 'normative' *Empowerment Model* of health promotion.

### Brief interventions in primary care

An example will now be provided of the ways in which theory-based courses of action in health promotion in primary care can show how realistic and appropriate indicators might be selected to assess the effectiveness and efficiency of the interventions discussed.

***Box 31***    Stages in the Thinking Process Leading to Action by a Group

| Stage | Community worker | Reactions of members of the group |
|-------|------------------|-----------------------------------|
| One | Stimulates people to think why they are dissatisfied and with what | Vaguely dissatisfied but passive |
| Two | Stimulates people to think about what specific changes would result in these needs being met | Now aware of certain needs |
| Three | Stimulates people to consider what they might do to bring such changes about by taking action themselves | Now aware of wanting changes of some specific kinds |
| Four | If necessary, stimulates people to consider how best they can organize themselves | Decide for, or against, trying to meet to do what they now want to do for themselves |
| Five | Stimulates people to consider and decide in detail just what to do, who will do it, and when and how they will do it | Plan what to do and how they will do it |
| Six | Stimulates people to think through any unforeseen difficulties or problems they may encounter in the course of what they do | Act according to their planning |
| Seven | Satisfied with result of what they have achieved? | |

(After Tones, 1992)

First, let us consider an educational programme in which family doctors routinely provide their patients with advice about smoking cessation as part of opportunistic health promotion during the consultation. As Russel *et al.* (1979) have demonstrated, the provision of such advice can produce a smoking cessation rate of 5.1% after 1 year when supportive leaflets are given to patients. This compares with a rate of 0.3% in a control group and, as the authors have argued, if all 20,000 general practitioners in UK were to adopt this approach as a matter of course then there would be 500,000 fewer smokers in the first year. This level of success could only be matched by developing 10,000 special smoking cessation clinics! Having demonstrated this cost effective result – and in the absence of unlimited resources – it would make sense to assume that such a programme would be at least as effective in future and would continue to reduce smoking in a practice population. An indirect measure of effectiveness might then legitimately be used to monitor the extent to which doctors delivered the service – for instance, by recording the number of practitioners who requested dispensers of leaflets designed to be used as a support for the inter-personal advice on smoking cessation.

The above observations may remind us that judgements of effectiveness and efficiency depend on the expected standards built into programme objectives. Decisions about what counts as a good enough result is a policy decision. The results recorded by Russel *et al.* are certainly good enough in cost–benefit terms. The real problem, as we noted earlier, is when unrealistic expectations lead to rejection not only of particular strategies but, occasionally, to the whole health promotion venture itself! At all events, it is important to use the results of research not only to judge effectiveness but to determine how levels of effectiveness might be improved with 'superior input'. As Box 32 demonstrates, there is wide acceptance within the smoking cessation field that different levels of success can be achieved with different methods (although, as noted above, some methods my produce quantitatively superior results but not be as cost effective as alternatives that yield lower percentage success rates but at low cost and with larger numbers of clients.

***Box 32***  Effectiveness of Different Smoking Cessation Strategies

| Method | Success (%)[a] |
|---|---|
| 'Spontaneous' cessation (without professional assistance) | 1–2 |
| Advice from doctor (with supportive leaflet) | 5–6 |
| Smoking cessation 'clinic' | 15–20 |
| Cessation 'clinic' plus nicotine replacement[b] | 25–30 |

[a]*Criterion, quit smoking for 1 year.*
[b]*Nicotine replacement can enhance all of the listed methods.*

## Taking account of *Stages of Change Theory*

A second example – again at the micro level – provides a more detailed illustration of the way in which theory can and should inform the selection of particular methods. The theory in question is the *Stages of Change* or *Trans-theoretical Theory* mentioned in our earlier discussions. Rollnick *et al.* (1992) provide a detailed description of the application of this theory to the face-to-face method of '*Brief Motivational Interviewing*' (see also Diclemente and Prochaska, 1982; Diclemente, 1991). The method is considered to be particularly appropriate to behaviours related to 'addiction' and the not unreasonable assumption is made that health promotion input will have greater success if it is precisely tailored to the particular motivation state of readiness of the client. The authors identify the following 'menu' of eight change strategies.

- Opening strategy: lifestyle, stresses and substance use.
- Opening strategy: health and substance use.
- A typical day/session.
- The good things and the less good things.
- Providing information.
- The future and the present.
- Exploring concerns.
- Helping with decision making.

(Rollnick *et al.*, 1992 p29)

The authors also provide specific examples of each strategy and Table 2.4 details opening strategy 1.

Box 33 provides an example of the particular counselling tactics 'prescribed' for use in strategy number 8, 'helping with decision making'.

**Box 33**  Helping with Decision Making

> - *Do not rush patients into decision-making.*
> - *Present options for the future rather than a single course of action.*
> - *Describe what other patients have done in a similar situation.*
> - *Emphasize that 'you are the best judge of what will be best for you'.*
> - *Provide information in a neutral, non-personal manner.*
> - *Failure to reach a decision to change is not a failed consultation.*
> - *Resolutions to change often break down. Make sure that patients understand this and do not avoid future contact if things go wrong.*
> - *Commitment to change is likely to fluctuate. Expect this to happen and empathize with the patient's predicament.*
>
> (Rollnick *et al.*, 1992 p35)

The various 'strategies' identified by Rollnick *et al.* may readily be used as indirect indicators of the effectiveness of the client–practitioner encounter since they ask whether the practitioner has accepted certain beliefs, holds certain attitudes and adopts the recommended counselling practices.

## An empowering encounter

The final example of the indicators that might be generated at the level of encounters between health professionals/counsellors/teachers and their clients derives from a 'blueprint' designed to lead to any 'empowered' health-related decision making by an individual (or, indeed, a small group of individual clients). Unlike the previous examples it yields the three categories of indicators examined here: indirect, intermediate and outcome.

It would, of course, be cumbersome to provide a complete prescription for micro level health promotion that incorporates all of the minutiae of successful inter-personal health promotion. In any case, detailed guidelines for efficient counselling already exist and training in generic skills associated with counselling (such as active listening and providing reflexive feedback) is presumed to have been provided for the practitioner involved in the procedure outlined below.

Table 2.5 (Tones, 1996) seeks to identify the key features characterising an *empowering* and specific *health-related* encounter. These features derive from both the 'normative' *Empowerment Model* and the 'empirical' models, such as the *Health Action Model*, which incorporate notions of self-empowerment and take account of environmental constraints and facilitating factors.

It will be observed from Table 2.4 that the encounter is described in terms of the '*health promotion task*' (for the practitioner) and the '*client task*'. The health promotion task provides an extensive number of key indirect indicators (defining the extent to which 'process' is satisfactory); these indicators can be used if necessary as pre-determined benchmarks to guide the practitioner. The practitioner should of course utilise the reaction of the client or client group at each 'benchmarked' stage to assess the effectiveness of the health promotion input and modify it as and when necessary (it thus comprises *formative evaluation*). The 'blueprint' for action does not necessarily apply only to practitioners and describes an appropriate interaction between lay people – whether in the context of 'co-counselling' or merely when they act as friends and good neighbours providing help and support – as specified by the 'lifeskills' philosophy espoused by authors such as Hopson and Scally (1981).

## Complexity, efficacy and avoiding Type 3 error

Hopefully, one of the most powerful messages emerging from the discussion in this chapter is that even relatively unambitious health promotion programmes are complex and, if properly designed, must be sophisticated in their theory and practice.

**Table 2.4** Strategy Outline for Negotiating Behaviour Change

| | |
|---|---|
| *Aim* | To explore patients' feelings about the behaviour in question, without imposing on them any assumptions about it being problematical. They, rather than you, identify problem areas or reasons for concern. |
| *Functions* | Often used soon after first raising the subject, this strategy serves the following functions. |

1. Useful for building rapport and for understanding context of substance use.
2. Useful with patients who seem unconcerned or when you are unsure about what they feel about their substance use. Resistance is minimised because:
   - You start with the positive things about person's substance use.
   - You talk about 'less good things' rather than 'concerns'. This allows the patient to identify problem areas without feeling that these are being labelled as problematical.

*How to do it*

1. Ask the key question: ***What are some of the good things about your use of ...?*** These usually emerge quite quickly. Summarise them, if necessary.
2. Ask: ***What are some of the less good things about your use of ...?*** Elicit these one by one, with the aim of finding out why this patient thinks these are 'less good things'. Open questions are useful here, for example, How does this affect you? or What don't you like about it?
3. Summarise the good things and the less good things, in 'you' language, as succinctly as possible and leave the person time to react. For example: ***So, using alcohol helps you relax ... you enjoy doing this with friends, and it helps when you are really feeling fed-up. On the other hand, you say you sometimes feel controlled by the stuff and that on Monday mornings you find it difficult to do anything at work.***

*Note*

- Avoid using words like 'problem' or 'concern', unless the patient does. If this happens, consider soon moving on to the 'Exploring concerns' strategy. Don't assume that 'a less good thing' is a cause for concern to patient.
- Keep to task at hand, and avoid raising new topics or hypotheses of your own.
- An alternative format is to ask, What do you like/dislike about your use of ...?

*After Rollnick et al. (1992), reproduced with permission from Carfax Publishing Co.*

**Table 2.5** An Empowering Encounter

| **Educational task** | **Client task** |
|---|---|
| *Communication* | |
| Check felt needs/need for information | |
| Establish rapport using counselling skills: active listening, etc. | |
| Take account of non-verbal communication | Receive message: pay attention |
| Check for understanding | Interpret message correctly |
| Check intelligibility of any written information provided | |
| Take steps to maximise recall and provide aide memoire if necessary | |
| *Motivation: facilitating decision making* | |
| Explore existing beliefs, attitudes skills; seek to modify beliefs and attitudes where appropriate | Form appropriate beliefs (e.g. about causes and nature of disease and health issues; about susceptibility, seriousness, costs and benefits of recommended actions) |
| Provide information; provide skills: decision making, psychomotor, social and life skills | Develop self-efficacy beliefs<br>Acquire skills |
| Check learning and recall | Agree 'contract' |
| Analyse environmental circumstances | ↓ |
| Negotiate and agree contract | POSITIVE ATTITUDE/INTENTION TO ACT |
| | ↓ |
| *Provide support* | |
| Provide opportunity for acquiring supportive knowledge, social and self-regulatory skills | Acquire new information and skills |
| | ↓ |
| Help mobilise social and environmental support | ADOPT AND SUSTAIN HEALTH ACTION |
| Act as advocate for social and environmental change | ↓ |
| Check client's progress | IMPROVED HEALTH |

Consideration of the portrayal of the intricate chains of indicators illustrated in Figures 2.20, 2.21 and 2.22 underlines the challenge of providing meaningful evaluations of such programmes.

One of the most important lessons to be learned from various attempts to evaluate health promotion initiatives is the ever-present tendency to underestimate complexity, design naïve evaluations and then draw inappropriate conclusions. The term Type 3 error has been applied to situations where incorrect conclusions are, in fact, reached about the effectiveness and efficiency of health promotion due to limited appreciation of the sometimes labyrinthine inter-connections of programme inputs together with flawed assumptions about the appropriateness of outcomes. This chapter will conclude by seeking to locate Type 3 error within the four (or arguably five) sources of error to which health-related interventions are prone (for further discussion see Tones, 2000). All three types of error will be further discussed in Chapter 3 in the context of reviewing the design of evaluations.

**Box 34**  Five Types of Error

Type 1 error: refers to an erroneous conclusion that an intervention has achieved significant change when, in fact, it has failed to do so.

Type 2 error: refers to an erroneous conclusion that an intervention has failed to have a significant impact when in fact it has actually done so.

Type 3 error: asserts that an intervention has failed to achieve successful results when it was so poorly designed that it could not possibly have had a desired effect.

Type 4 error: this is … *defined as the conduct of an evaluation of a program that no one cares about and is irrelevant to decision makers. Evaluation for the sake of evaluation is central to this error.*

Type 5 error: an intervention has been shown to produce a real effect that is statistically significant, however, the change is so slight as to have no practical significance.

The definition of Type 4 error shown in italics in Box 34 above is due to Basch and Gold (1986), who cited Scanlon (1977) and who also added Type 5 error to the list of pitfalls awaiting the unwary evaluator. Bearing in mind current interest in effectiveness reviews, managers and those responsible for commissioning services frequently face a dilemma in deciding what action to take when those effectiveness reviews suggest that there are minimal or uncertain effects from the health promotion initiatives under investigation. It is, therefore, a matter of some importance to use theoretical understanding (and common sense) in subjecting not only the design and results of health promotion evaluations to critical scrutiny but also to examine even more critically the pretensions and adequacy of the programmes that have been evaluated.

## REFERENCES

Ajzen, I. (1985) *From intention to actions: a theory of planned behaviour.* In J. Kuhl and J. Beckman (Eds) *Action Control: From Cognition to Behaviour.* Prentice-Hall, Englewood Cliffs, NJ.

Ajzen, I. (1991) *The theory of planned behavior. Organizational Behavior and Human Decision Processes,* 50, 179–211.

Ajzen, I. and Fishbein, M. (1980) *Understanding Attitudes and Predicting Social Behavior.* Prentice-Hall, Englewood Cliffs, NJ.

Ajzen, I. and Madden, T. J. (1986) *Prediction of goal-directed behavior: attitudes, intentions and perceived behavioral control. Journal of Experimental Social Psychology,* 22, 453–474.

Allen, D., Harley, M. and Makinson, G. T. (1987) *Performance indicators in the National Health Service. Social Policy and Administration,* 21 (1), 70–84.

Antonovsky, A. (1979) *Health, Stress and Coping.* Jossey-Bass, San Francisco, CA.

Aronson, E. (1976) *The Social Animal, 2nd edn.* W.H. Freeman, San Francisco, CA.

Aronson, E. and Mettee, D. (1968) *Dishonest behaviour as a function of different levels of self esteem. Journal of Personality and Social Psychology,* 9, 121–127.

ASH (2000) *Comments on draft AcOP.* Action on Smoking and Health, London.

Bagehot, W. (1873) *Physics and Politics*. Appleton-Century, New York, NY.

Bandura, A. (1977) *Self-efficacy toward a unifying theory of behavioural change. Psychological Review*, 64 (2), 191–225.

Bandura, A. (1982) *Self-efficacy mechanism in human agency. American Psychologist*, 37 (2), 122–47.

Bandura, A. (1986) *Social Foundations of Thought and Action: A Social Cognitive Theory*. Prentice-Hall, Englewood Cliffs, NJ.

Baric, L. (1978) *Health education and the smoking habit. Health Education Journal*, 37, 132–137.

Basch, C. E. and Gold, R. S. (1986) *Type V errors in hypothesis testing. Health Education Research*, 1 (4), 299–305.

Batten, T. R. (1967) *The Non-Directive Approach in Group and Community Work*. Oxford University Press, Oxford.

Becker, M. H. (Ed.) (1984) *The Health Belief Model and Personal Health Behavior*. Charles B. Slack, Thorofare, NJ.

Bell, S., Burn, C. and Quiery, M. (1978) *Homelink* (Newsletter), Liverpool (mimeo).

Bennett, P. and Murphy, S. (1997) *Psychology and Health Promotion*. Open University Press, Buckingham.

Bodmer, W. F. (1985) *Understanding statistics. Journal of Royal Statistical Society*, 148, 69–81.

Bond, B. W. (1958) *A study in health education methods. International Journal of Health Education*, 1, 41–46.

Bradburn, N. (1969) *The Structure of Psychological Well-being*. Aldine, New York, NY.

Breteler, R. H., Mertens, N. H. M. and Rombouts, R. (1990) *Motivation to change smoking behaviour: determinants in the contemplation stage*. In L. R. Schmidt *et al.* (Eds) *Theoretical and Applied Aspects of Health Psychology*. Harwood Academic, London.

Briscoe, M. E. (1982) *Subjective measures of well-being, differences in the perception of health and social problems. British Journal of Social Work*, 12, 137–147.

British Broadcasting Corporation (1983) *Understanding Cancer*, BBC Broadcasting Research Special Report. BBC Research Information Desk, London.

British Medical Association (1990) *BMA Guide to Living with Risk*. Penguin, London.

Brook, R. and Lohr, K. (1985) *Efficiency, effectiveness, variations and quality. Medical Care*, 23, 710–722.

Cattell, R. B. (1965) *The Scientific Analysis of Personality*. Penguin, Harmondsworth.

Chabot, J. H. T. (1976) *The Chinese system of health care. Tropical Geographical Medicine*, 28, 87–134.

Cochrane, A. C. L. (1972) *Effectiveness and Efficiency: Random Reflections on the Heath Service*, Rock Carling Lecture 1971. Nuffield Provincial Hospitals Trust, London.

Cohen, D. (1981) *Prevention as an Economic Good*. Health Economics Research Unit, University of Aberdeen.

Cohen, L. and Manion, L. (1994) *Research Methods in Education, 4th edn*. Routledge, London.

Colling A., Dellipiani A. W., Donaldson, R. J. and McCormack, R. (1976) *Teesside coronary survey: an epidemiological study of acute attacks of myocardial infarction. British Medical Journal*, 2, 1169–1172.

Conner, M. and Norman, P. (Eds) (1996) *Predicting Health Behaviour: Research and Practice with Social Cognition Models*. Open University Press, Buckingham.

Coopersmith, S. (1967) *The Antecedents of Self Esteem*. W.H. Freeman, New York, NY.

Dabbs, J. W. (1964) *Self-esteem, communicator characteristics and attitude change. Journal of Abnormal and Social Psychology*, 69, 173–181.

Davies, I. K. (1981) *Instructional Technique*. McGraw-Hill, New York, NY.

Delk, J. L. (1980) *High-risk sports as indirect self-destructive behavior*. In N. L. Farberow (Ed.) *The Many Faces of Suicide*. McGraw-Hill, New York, NY.

Department of Health (1992) *Health of the Nation*. HMSO, London.

Department of Health (1999) *Saving Lives: Our Healthier Nation*. HMSO, London.

DiClemente, C. C. (1991) *Motivational interviewing and the stages of change*. In W. R. Miller and S. Rollnick (Eds) *Motivational Interviewing: Preparing People to Change Addictive Behavior*. Guilford Press, New York, NY.

DiClemente, C. C. and Prochaska, J. O. (1982) *Self change and therapy change of smoking behaviour: a comparison of processes of change in cessation and maintenance. Addictive Behaviours*, 7, 133–142.

Draper, P., Best, G. and Dennis, J. (1977) *Health and wealth. Royal Society of Health Journal*, 97, 121–127.

Festinger, L. (1957) *A Theory of Cognitive Dissonance*. Row Peterson, Evanston, IL.

Fishbein, M. (1976) *Persuasive communication*. In A. E. Bennet (Ed.) *Communication Between Doctors and Patients*. Oxford University Press, Oxford.

Fishbein, M. and Ajzen, I. (1985) *Belief Attitude, Intention and Behavior: An Introduction to Theory and Research*. Addison-Wesley, Reading, MA.

Freidson, E. (1961) *Patients' Views of Medical Practice*, pp. 146–147. Russell Sage, New York, NY.

Freire, P (1972) *Pedagogy of the Oppressed*. Penguin, Harmondsworth.

Glanz, K., Lewis, F. M. and Rimer, B. K. (Eds) (1997) *Health Behavior and Health Education, 2nd edn*. Jossey-Bass, San Francisco, CA.

Green, J. and Tones, K. (1999a) *Towards a secure evidence base for health promotion. Journal of Public Health Medicine*, 21 (2), 133–139.

Green, J. and Tones, K. (1999b) *The health promoting school general practice and the creative arts: an example of inter sectoral collaboration. Health Education*, 100 (3), 124–130.

Green, L. W. (1974) *Toward cost-benefit evaluations of health education: some concepts, methods, and examples. Health Education Monographs*, 2, 34–64.

Green, L. W. (1984) *Health education models*. In J. D. Matarazzo, S. M. Weiss, J. A. Herd, N. E. Miller and S. M. Weiss (Eds) *Behavioural Health: A Handbook of Health Enhancement and Disease Prevention*. John Wiley, New York, NY.

Green, L. W. and Kreuter, M. W. (1999) *Health Promotion Planning: An Educational and Ecological Approach, 3rd edn*. Mayfield, Mountain View, CA.

Green, L. W. and Lewis, F. M. (1986) *Measurement and Evaluation in Health Education and Health Promotion*, pp. 174–176. Mayfield, Palo Alto, CA.

Groom, D. In Tilford, S. and Tones, B. K. (1977) *Workshop on Health Education and the Prevention of CHD*. Leeds Polytechnic, unpublished mimeo.

Hall, J. (1976) *Subjective measures of quality of life in Britain: 1971 to 1975: some developments and trends. Social Trends*, 7, 47–60.

Harfouche, J. K. (1965) *Infant Health in Lebanon: Customs and Taboos*. Khayats, Beirut.

*Health Education Research* (1993) *Special issue on community coalitions. Health Education Research*, 8 (3).

Hochbaum, G. M. (1958) *Public Participation in Medical Screening Programs: A Sociopsychological Study*, PHS Publication no. 572. US Government Printing Office, Washington, DC.

Hopson, B. and Scally, M. (1981) *Lifeskills Teaching*. McGraw-Hill, London.

Horley, J. (1991) *Values and beliefs as personal constructs. International Journal of Personal Construct Psychology*, 4, 1–14.

Hovland, C., Lumsdaine, A. and Sheffield, F. (1949) *Experiments on Mass Communication*. Princeton University Press, Princeton, NJ.

Hunt, S. M. and McEwen, J. (1980) *The development of a subjective health indicator. Sociology of Health and Illness*, 2, 231–246.

Jacobs, D. R, Luepker, R. V., Mittelmark, M. B. *et al.* (1985) *Community-Wide Prevention Strategies: Evaluation Design of the Minnesota Heart Health Program*. University of Minnesota, Minneapolis, MN.

James, W (1890) The *Principles of Psychology*. Henry Holt and Co., New York, NY.

Janis, I. L. and Mann, L. (1965) *Effectiveness of emotional role playing in modifying smoking habits and attitudes. Journal of Experimental Research in Personality*, 1, 84–90.

Janis, I. L. and Mann, L. (1977) *Decision Making*. The Free Press, New York, NY.

Janz, N. K. and Becker, M. H. (1984) *The Health Belief Model: a decade later. Health Education Quarterly*, 11, 1–47.

Jessor, R. and Jessor, S. L. (1977) *Problem Behavior and Psychosocial Development: A Longitudinal Study of Youth,*. Academic Press, New York, NY.

Kanfer, F. H. and Karoly, P. (1972) *Self-control: a behavioristic excursion into the lion's den. Behavior Therapy*, 3, 398–416.

Kasperson, R. E., Renn, O., Slovic, P., Brown, H. S. *et al.* (1988) *The social amplification of risk: a conceptual framework. Risk Analysis*, 8, 177–187.

Kelley, H.H. (1967) *Attribution theory in social psychology*. In D. Levine (Ed.) *Nebraska Symposium on Motivation, 1967*. University of Nebraska Press, Lincoln, NE.

Kirby, D. (1995) *A Review of Educational Programmes Designed to Reduce Sexual Risk-taking Behaviors Among School-aged Youth in the United States*. US Congress Office of Technology Assessment and the National Technical Information Service, Washington, DC.

Kraft, P. and Rise, J. (1994) *The relationship between sensation seeking and smoking, alcohol consumption and sexual behavior among Norwegian adolescents. Health Education Research*, 9 (2), 193–200.

Labonte, R., Feather, J. and Hills, M. (1999) *A story/dialogue method for health promotion knowledge development and evaluation. Health Education Research*, 14 (1), 39–50.

Laing, W. A. (1982) *Family Planning: The Benefits and Costs*, no. 607. Policy Studies Institute, London.

Langer, E. J. (1983) *The Psychology of Control*. Sage, Beverly Hills, CA.

Lawrence, T. (1999) *A stage-based approach to behaviour change*. In E. R. Perkins, I. Simnett and L. Wright (Eds) *Evidence-Based Health Promotion*. John Wiley, Chichester.

Levenson, H. (1973) *Multidimensional locus of control in psychiatric patients. Journal of Consulting and Clinical Psychology*, 41, 397–404.

Lewis, F. M. (1987) *The concept of control: a typology and health-related variables. Advances in Health Education and Promotion*, 2, 227–309.

Lichtenstein, S., Slovic, P., Fischoff, B., Layman, M. and Combs, B. (1978) *Judged frequency of lethal events. Journal of Experimental Psychology: Human Learning and Memory*, 4 (6), 551–578.

Lyng, S. (1990) *Edgework: a social psychological analysis of voluntary risk taking. American Journal of Sociology*, 95 (4), 851–886.

Macaulay, A. C., Commanda, L. E., Freeman, W. L., Gibson, N., McCabe, L., Robbins, C. M. and Twohig, L. (1999) *Participatory research maximises community and lay involvement. British Medical Journal*, 319, 774–778.

Mager, R. F. (1962) *Preparing Instructional Objectives*. Fearon, Belmont, CA.

Maibach, E. and Murphy, D. A. (1995) *Self-efficacy in health promotion research and practice: conceptualization and measurement. Health Education Research*, 10 (1), 37–50.

Marsh, A. and Matheson, J. (1983) *Smoking Attitudes and Behaviour*. HMSO, London.

Mather, H. G., Morgan, D. C., Pearson, N. G. *et al.* (1971) *Acute myocardial infarction: home and hospital treatment. British Medical Journal*, 3, 334–338.

McAlister, A., Puska, P., Salonen, J. T., Tuomilehto, J, and Koskela, K. (1982) *Theory and action for health promotion: illustrations from the North Karelia Project. American Journal of Public Health*, 72, 43–53.

McGuire, W. J. (1981) *Theoretical foundations of campaigns*. In R. E. Rice and W. J. Paisley (Eds) *Public Communication Campaigns*. Sage, Beverly Hills, CA.

Meyrick, J and Sinkler, P (1999) *An Evaluation Resource for Healthy Living Centres*. Health Education Authority, London.

Miller, W. R. and Rollnick, S. (1991) *Motivational Interviewing: Preparing People to Change Addictive Behavior*. Guildford Press, New York, NY.

Mittelmark, M. B. (2000) *Social ties and health promotion: suggestions for population-based research* (editorial). *Health Education Research*, 15 (2), 101–105.

Montano, D. E., Kasprzyk, D. and Taplin, S. H. (1997) *The theory of reasoned action and theory of planned behaviour*. In K. Glanz, F. M. Lewis and B. K. Rimer (Eds) *Health Behaviour and Health Education: Theory, Research and Practice*. Jossey-Bass, San Francisco, CA.

Mooney, G. H. (1977) *The Valuation of Human Life*, Appendix C. Macmillan, London.

Morrow, R. A. and Brown, D. D. (1994) *Critical Theory and Methodology*. Sage, Thousand Oaks, CA.

NACNE (1983) *A Discussion Paper on Proposals for Nutritional Guidelines for Health Education in Britain*. Health Education Council, London.

NHS Executive (2000) *Quality and Performance in the NHS: High Level Performance Indicators and Clinical Indicators*. HMSO, London.

Nutbeam, D. and Harris, E (1998) *Theory in a Nutshell. A Practitioner's Guide to Commonly Used Theories and Models in Health Promotion*. National Centre for Health Promotion, University of Sydney, Sydney.

Pack, B. E., Hendrick, R. M., Murdock, R. B. and Palma, L. M. (1983) *Factors affecting criteria met by hospital based patient education programmes. Patient Education and Counselling*, 5, 76–84.

Parlett, M. and Hamilton, D. (1978) *Evaluation as illumination: a new approach to the study of innovatory programmes*. In D. Hamilton *et al.* (Eds) *Beyond the Numbers Game*. Macmillan, London.

Popham, W. J. (1978) *Must all objectives be behavioural?* In D. Hamilton *et al.* (Eds) *Beyond the Numbers Game*. Macmillan, London.

Prentice-Dunn, S. and Rogers, R. W. (1986) *Protection motivation theory and preventive health: beyond the Health Belief Model. Health Education Research*, 1 (3), 153–162.

Prochaska, J. O. (1992) *What causes people to change from unhealthy to health enhancing behaviour?* In T. Heller, L. Bailey and S. Pattison (Eds) *Preventing Cancers*. Open University Press, Milton Keynes.

Prochaska, J. O. and DiClimente, C. C. (1984) *The Transtheoretical Approach: Crossing Traditional Boundaries of Therapy*. Dow Jones Irwin, Homewood, IL.

Prochaska, J. O., Redding, C. A. and Evers, K. E. (1997) *The transtheoretical model and stages of change*. In K. Glanz *et al.* (Eds) *Health Behaviour and Health Education: Theory, Research and Practice*. Jossey-Bass, San Francisco, CA.

Puska, P., Nissinen, A., Tuomilehto, J., Koskela, K., McAlister, A., Kottke, T. E., Maccoby, N. and Farquhar, J. W. (1985) *The community-based strategy to prevent coronary heart disease: conclusions from the ten years of the North Karelia Project. Annual Review of Public Health*, 6, 147–193.

Rogers, E. M. (1995) *The Diffusion of Innovations, 4th edn*. The Free Press, New York, NY.

Rogers, E. M. and Shoemaker, F. F. (1971) *Communication of Innovations*. The Free Press, New York, NY.

Rogers, R. W. (1975) *A protection motivation theory of fear appeals and attitude change. Journal of Psychology*, 91, 93–114.

Rokeach, M. (1973) *The Nature of Human Values*. The Free Press, New York, NY.

Rollnick, S., Heather, N. and Bell, A. (1992) *Negotiating behaviour change in medical settings: the development of brief motivational interviewing. Journal of Mental Health*, 1, 25–37.

Rosenstock, I. M. (1966) *Why people use health services. Milbank Memorial Fund Quarterly*, 44, 94–124.

Rotter, J. B. (1966) *Generalized expectancies for internal versus external control of reinforcement. Psychological Monographs*, 80 (1), 1–28.

Russel, M. A. H., Wilson, C., Taylor, C. and Baker, C. D. (1979) *Effect of general practitioners' advice against smoking. British Medical Journal*, 2, 231–235.

Sarafino, E. P. (1990) *Health Psychology: Biopsycho-social Interactions*, Ch. 10. John Wiley, New York, NY.

Scanlon, J. W. *et al.* (1977) *Evaluability assessment: avoiding Type II or Type IV errors*. In G. R. Gilbert and P. J. Conklin (Eds) *Evaluation Management: Source Book of Readings*. US Civil Service Commission, Charlottesville.

Schifter, D. B. and Ajzen, I. (1985) *Intention, perceived control and weight loss: an application of the theory of planned behavior. Journal of Personality and Social Psychology*, 49, 843–851.

Seligman, M. E. P. (1975) *Helplessness: On Depression, Development and Death*. W.H. Freeman, New York, NY.

Simon, S. B. (1974) *Meeting Yourself Halfway*. Argos, Niles, IL.

Slovic, P., Fischoff, B. and Lichtenstein, S. (1982) *Why study risk perception? Risk Analysis*, 2 (2), 83–93.

Small, N. (1989) *Politics and Planning in the National Health Service*. Open University Press, Milton Keynes.

Smith, A. (1977) *The unfaced facts. New Universities Quarterly*, Spring, 133–145.

Terris, M. (1981) *The primacy of prevention. Preventive Medicine*, 10, 689–699.

Terry, D. J., Gallois, C. and McCamish, M. (1993) *The Theory of Reasoned Action: Its Application to AIDS-Preventive Behaviour*. Pergamon, Oxford.

Thorndike, E. L. (1905) *The Elements of Psychology*. Seiler, New York, NY.

Tilford, S. and Tones, B. K. (1977) *Workshop on Prevention of CHD*. Leeds Polytechnic (unpublished mimeo).

Tones, B. K. (1979) *Past achievement, future success*. In I. Sutherland (Ed.) *Health Education Perspectives and Choices*. Allen and Unwin, London.

Tones, B. K. (1981) *Affective education and health*. In J. Cowley, K. David and T. Williams (Eds) *Health Education in Schools*. Harper and Row, London.

Tones, B. K. (1986) *Preventing drug misuse: the case for breadth, balance and coherence. Health Education Journal*, 45, 197–203.

Tones, B. K. (1987) *Devising strategies for preventing drug misuse: the role of the health action model. Health Education Research*, 2, 305–318.

Tones, B. K. (1992) *Measuring success in health promotion: selecting indicators of performance. Hygie*, XI (4) 10–14.

Tones, B. K. (1996) *Health education, behaviour change, and the public health*. In R. Dettels, J. McEwen and G. Omenn (Eds) *Oxford Textbook of Public Health, 3rd edn*. Oxford University Press, Oxford.

Tones, B. K. (2000) *Evaluating health promotion: a tale of three errors. Patient Education and Counseling*, 39, 227–236.

Townsend, J. (1986) *Cost effectiveness*. In J. Crofton and M. Wood (Eds) *Smoking Control: Strategies and Evaluation in Community and Mass Media Programmes, Report of a Workshop*. Health Education Council, London.

Triandis, H. C. (1980) *Values, attitudes, and interpersonal behavior*. In H. E. Howe (Ed.)

*Nebraska Symposium on Motivation, 1980.* University of Nebraska Press, Lincoln, NE.

Wallston, B. S., Wallston, K. A., Kaplan, G. D. and Maides, S. A. (1976) *A development and validation of the health locus of control (HLC) scale. Journal of Consulting and Clinical Psychology,* 44, 580–585.

Wallston, K. A. and Wallston, B. S. (Eds) (1978) *Health locus of control. Health Education Monographs,* 6 (2).

Wallerstein, N. and Bernstein, E. (1994) *Introduction to community empowerment, participatory education, and health. Health Education Quarterly,* 21 (2), 141–148.

Weinstein, N. D. (1982) *Unrealistic optimism about susceptibility to health problems. Journal of Behavioral Medicine,* 5 (4), 441–460.

Weinstein, N. D. (1984) *Why it won't happen to me: perceptions of risk factors and susceptibility. Health Psychology,* 3 (5), 431–457.

Windsor, R. A., Baranowski, T., Clark, N. and Cutler, G. (1984) *Evaluation of Health Promotion and Education Programs,* Appendix C. Mayfield, Palo Alto, CA.

Zuckerman, M. (1979) *Sensation Seeking. Beyond the Optimal Level of Arousal.* Lawrence Earlbaum, London.

# 3 EVALUATION RESEARCH

## INTRODUCTION

This chapter discusses the nature of evaluation research, the debates about methodologies for health promotion evaluation and considers technical aspects of carrying out evaluations. While there was an established history of addressing evaluation issues in health education the emergence of health promotion has stimulated considerable critical reflection on evaluation. There have been a number of reasons for this. In some of the key institutional sectors in which health promotion is provided – particularly health and education – questions of effectiveness, efficiency and quality have become increasingly important, in parallel with an emphasis on achieving evidence-based practice. The accumulation of evidence in the health care sector has been facilitated by the increasing number of systematic reviews and the production and dissemination of meta analyses of evidence. There has been extensive discussion of these techniques in health promotion and reactions, both negative and positive. The nature of the evidence brought together in systematic reviews and the types of studies through which it is acquired has been challenged (Kippax and Van de Ven, 1998). Others have defended such techniques (Oakley, 1990, 1998; Oakley and Fullerton, 1996). Such discussions have been in the context of an ongoing assessment of alternative and competing methodologies for evaluation and consideration of what is appropriate for health promotion. In particular, the evolution of health promotion from health education has been associated with thinking about its purposes, the processes it should adopt in its activities and the nature of evidence to be generated in evaluating its activities. Health promotion, in drawing concepts and theories from a wide range of disciplines, has also been influenced by thinking about research in these disciplines. Health promotion is still in the process of debating its paradigm status, in establishing its credibility as an activity and defining appropriate ways of practice. This devel-opment has been associated with adoption of differing standpoints on evaluation and energetic dismissal of positions which may be at variance with preferred ones. While debate about health promotion research and evaluation is necessary and can be creative and energising, it can also generate confusion. There are signs, however, that there is some degree of consensus emerging about evaluation in health promotion.

The chapter will begin with a brief consideration of evaluation research and the ways in which it is seen to differ from other areas of research prior to providing a brief general background on the developments in evaluation of social programmes. The debates about methodologies for evaluation in health promotion will then be considered and brief consideration of differing approaches will be provided. The second part of the chapter will provide discussion of the stages of the evaluation process. We will not be providing detailed consideration of specific research designs and data collection methods, for which readers are referred to standard research texts. Currently there is considerable emphasis within health promotion on the importance of participatory approaches and the place for these in research evaluation will be assessed. The chapter will conclude with brief comments on the dissemination of evaluation findings.

## What is evaluation research and why is it carried out?

From the earlier chapters it will be clear that evaluation is undertaken for a range of reasons:

- to assess the outcomes of a programme and measure its success using a variety of indicators;
- to review the process of programmes and enhance understanding of how effects are achieved;
- to generate information which can be used as a basis for improving programmes;
- to assess satisfaction with programmes;

- to identify efficient ways of achieving desired outcomes;
- to account for resources received and make a case for their continuation;
- to generate knowledge for use in influencing policy makers;
- to contribute to the development of the broad knowledge and theory base within a discipline, including its evidence base;
- in the case of *formative evaluation* to provide information to a project during its progress which can be used to make modifications and enhance the achievement of aims; the early identification of any harmful effects is particularly important.

Not all of the above will be relevant to each and every evaluation study.

A number of terms which are widely used in discussing research are variously understood and evaluation research is no exception. Two fairly typical definitions can be offered:

*Evaluation is the systematic examination and assessment of an initiative and its effects in order to produce information that can be used by those who have an interest in its improvement or effectiveness.*

(WHO, 1998a)

*The systematic application of social research procedures for assessing the conceptualisation, design, implementation and utility of social intervention and social service programmes. It is used for assessing program effectiveness and/or efficiency, for improving programs and service delivery, and for guiding resource allocation and policy development.*

(Thompson, 1992)

Both definitions make reference to systematic activities, indicate some of the key areas on which there is focus and the purposes for which evaluation is undertaken. Neither definition makes explicit reference to assessing the process as well as the outcomes of activities. It is useful to bear these definitions in mind when considering methodologies for evaluation research and in assessing whether alternative approaches are equally suited to achieving evaluation goals.

Distinctions are often made between evaluation research and what may be described as pure or basic research. On occasion there are implications that the latter activity is somewhat superior to the former. Some of the characteristics of evaluation research which are said to make it distinctive include the following.

- The research is carried out with the purpose of generating information that can be used for the specific purpose of improvement of programmes rather than the development of the knowledge base of a discipline.
- Where evaluation is a commissioned process rather than an internal programme activity the research questions and the methodology may be prescribed by the sponsor. The constraints on the evaluator may, therefore, be greater than in general research.
- Where evaluation is an externally managed process research may not be a priority for participants and conflicts of interests can arise between the interests of the programme and the interests of the evaluation research. The methodology adopted will have a significant bearing on the extent to which these can become difficulties.
- The implementation of evaluation activities can be seen as threatening by the participants in a programme and this poses particular demands on aspects of data collection and reporting of findings.
- While most funded research is time bound, constraints of time can be particularly acute in evaluation research where the results often have to be available for policy decisions at specific times.
- Given the purposes for which evaluation research is undertaken some might argue that there are limitations on the types of evidence to be sought and, consequently, for the ways of acquiring it. For example, if it is planned to implement a progamme on a large scale, after gaining evidence of effectiveness from small-scale implementation, the nature of evidence

acquired would need to permit generalisation.

- A difference is often drawn about the use of findings from evaluation and general research. The former is intended to be used to inform decision making and the latter to enhance knowledge and understanding within particular disciplines.

While the differences specified are legitimate ones, we would argue that in most cases they do not add up to a basis for making a distinct demarcation between evaluation and other types of research. Taken as a whole they are differences in emphasis rather than clear qualitative differences. For example, while the prime purpose of evaluation may not be knowledge building within a discipline, findings from evaluations clearly contribute to the knowledge base. We would continue to concur with Finch (1986 p158), who observed that evaluation, insofar as it involved empirical research, entailed the same kind of methodological issues as other research, although the particular blend of issues may be unique to evaluative studies. McQueen (1986) also commented on the distinction with reference to health education:

> *For many years now health education (and other) researchers have carried forth the myth of 'evaluation research' as a special field requiring its own peculiar jargon and literature. In reality there is little distinction about evaluation research except perhaps the fact that the research 'questions' are usually not set by the researchers and that all too often the findings are foreseen by other interested parties.*

Others will wish to disagree and maintain a clear distinction between research and evaluation (Scott, 1998). There is evidence from a recent study that the differing views in the literature about the relationship between evaluation and other research are reflected in health promotion practice – with some people making clear distinctions, others seeing overlap between the two and some people being unclear about the relationships (South and Tilford, 2000). The existence of differing views may only be important if these impact on the confidence and readiness to take on evaluation research as a part of professional practice.

### Development of evaluation research in health education and promotion

Health promotion is a relatively new activity and still debating its own nature and the way its activities should be pursued, but health education, as it developed throughout the last century, regularly addressed matters of evaluation. Progress, globally, was reviewed for the WHO as early as 1968 by Roberts and Green (Green and Lewis, 1986). They drew the following conclusions:

- the majority of evaluation projects were being carried out in the USA;
- most evaluation in developing countries was descriptive, using survey methods, rather than experimental ones;
- taken as a whole there had been little experimental evaluation except in a few projects.

These conclusions implied, of course, that experimental evaluation was to be preferred and this view has been challenged strongly in the interim period. Green and Lewis (1986) marked the early 1970s as a turning point in the evaluation of health education, both with respect to the methods adopted and improvements in training for evaluation. Other disciplines have longer histories of evaluation and have been instructive reference points for health education and promotion.

From the time of the development of modern systems of education, social care and health care in the late 19th century there were activities designed to monitor and assess these areas of provision. Evaluation activities have been central to modern societies and described as part of the 'surveillance' associated with modernity by Foucault and others (Armstrong, 1983; Rabinow, 1984 p201). It was not, however, until the 20th century that such activities came to be more systematically research driven. In the USA evaluation developed particularly rapidly during the 1960s, when there were major efforts to reform educational curricula and also to deal with pressing social issues. There were political pressures to document the effectiveness of the major investments in educational and social initiatives and rapid developments in thinking and practice around evaluation occurred. Health education – and more recently health promotion – developed its own thinking about evaluation partly in response to the developments in its contributory disciplines. Most recently evaluation in health promotion has been reviewed in the context of a maturing sense of its own nature.

Within the health care field the push to evaluation has largely been within a classic experimental style. In the early part of the last century controlled clinical trials began to be more widely used and the process of randomisation was introduced into medical research in 1946 in assessing the use of streptomycin in treating tuberculosis. The credit for the importance given to randomised controlled trials (RCTs) in acquiring evidence of effectiveness is attributed to Cochrane (1972). He advocated the use of RCTs for assessing the effectiveness of new treatments and for treatments already in use where the evidence of effectiveness had not been established. There has been a rapid growth in the use of RCTs in the intervening period.

In education and social care, although there is a well-documented history of support for experimental styles of evaluation (Oakley, 1998), the methodological situation has been more complex than in the health sector. In education, for example, while there was early domination by strongly positivistic styles of evaluation there was at the same time a use of models informed by alternative methodologies (Lawton, 1980). In much the same way, experimental and survey models of evaluation predominated in health education before the 1970s but other models also came to be adopted, as will be discussed below. We will now examine the methodologies which have underpinned evaluation activity.

## METHODOLOGIES OF EVALUATION

In the last edition we referred to the debates about evaluation methodology and these have continued with great energy and the term 'paradigm wars' has been used to describe the situation (Pawson and Tilley, 1997 p2). Increasingly there are efforts to reflect more calmly on the diverse contributions to the debates and to develop constructive, if differing, ways forward. Recently in health promotion there have been clear normative statements from the WHO about evaluation which are being widely disseminated and are likely to be influential (WHO, 1998a). Given, however, that the debates do still figure strongly in the literature and, as yet, there is no fully supported consensus about approaches to evaluation we will review the issues that are being discussed.

Much of the discussion has focused at the epistemological level on what are typically presented, somewhat over simplistically, as the opposing positions of positivism and interpretivism and, at the data level, on quantitative and qualitative data. There are other related positions which also need to be considered since they are influential within health promotion at the present time or appear likely to inform evaluation work in the future. The two main positions will be addressed and the evaluation methods associated with them described prior to examining alternatives. The implications of the methodological debates for evaluation research in health promotion will then be discussed.

### The positivist tradition

It continues to be relevant to comment on the key elements of positivist philosophy and the research methods informed by it. While there is considerable opposition within health promotion to the ideas associated with the tradition there is much activity which has been, and continues to be, informed by it. Positivist principles have a long history, have underpinned the natural sciences and were adopted by the social sciences from the 19th century. Within the former the experiment has been the dominant research design for answering questions but was extended to the social sciences by the use of surveys. As a philosophical position positivism has various strands but there are a set of assumptions that are broadly held in common:

- objective accounts of the world can be generated and causal patterns and general theories about phenomena can be produced and theories are tested through the application of scientific method;

- explanations of phenomena consist of showing that they are instances of general laws;
- there is a unity of methods between natural and social sciences and the natural sciences are taken as a model for all sciences;
- sciences study external realities, there is a correspondence between the truths of science and actual realities;
- science is a neutral activity free of social and ethical values.

Positivism needs to be distinguished from empiricism. Both share the view that there are facts about the world that can be gathered but differ in the place given to theory in this process. In positivism the collection of data is driven by theory while empiricism lacks this and is explained by Bulmer (1982 p31) as:

*a conception of social research involving the production of accurate data – meticulous, precise, generalisable – in which the data themselves constitute the end for the research. It is summed up by the catch phrase 'the facts speak for themselves'.*

Positivism has been critiqued extensively both from within and from outside the tradition and post-positivist positions have emerged. There has been challenge to the ideas of correspondence and to the claims for objectivity and the value-free nature of inquiry. Examination of these critiques are widely available and we will comment only briefly on selected well-known ones (Chalmers, 1980). Within the positivist tradition significant challenges have come from Popper and Kuhn.

Popper (1959) challenged the way that positivism, in some versions, presented the development of theory as an inductive process, building from data to theory construction, and argued that observation and observation statements are theory dependent. He also contested the notion of confirmation of theory, arguing that however many times a theory was tested and supported there was always the possibility that it could be

falsified. He proposed, therefore, that science should be viewed as progressing through attempts to falsify theories with theories being maintained until such falsification occurs. Scientific truths, therefore, were to be viewed as provisional and not open to verification.

Kuhn's (1970) work came from a different perspective. He built on observations of how science took place as a social activity and he, in turn, challenged the propositions of Popper. He claimed that the scientific community does not progress its work through the falsification of hypotheses derived from theory but through working consistently over a period of time within scientific paradigms. Work is undertaken within a set of concepts and practices, described as a paradigm, and facts which emerge that do not conform to theory do not immediately lead to rejection of the theory. What he describes as 'normal science' continues until some point when 'revolutions' occur, there is a paradigm shift and reunification occurs around a new set of practices. In turn, Kuhn's work has also been criticised as too simplistic when viewed from a historical perspective (Chalmers, 1980). Kuhn illustrated his proposals with references to shifts in thinking in the natural sciences, but similar ideas have been applied to health education and health promotion where Rawson has discussed whether the move from health education to promotion constituted a Kuhnian paradigm shift (Rawson, 1992). Critiques of positivism originating from the differing traditions of interpretivism will be discussed below after commenting on the main designs used in evaluations informed by the positivist tradition.

### Experimental design

Experimental studies in medicine are typically described, as noted earlier, as RCTs and this term has been adopted widely in health promotion. Experiments introduce a planned change and study its outcomes. Their objective is to establish causal relationships between interventions and outcomes, described as independent and dependent variables. The relationship between variables is expressed in advance in the form of a null hypothesis, i.e. that the independent variable has no association with or effect on the dependent variable. If the hypothesis is rejected there is evidence, therefore, that the proposed relationship does exist. There are a number of designs for experimental studies and these are described fully in general research texts. In its simplest form an experiment randomly assigns individuals to one of two groups, experimental and control, a process designed to minimise bias in the composition of the groups. Confounding factors (those other than the intervention which could influence the outcome) are assumed to be distributed equally across the two groups as a result of randomisation. One group receives the intervention to be tested and the other, the control group, does not. The control group may experience, for the same length of time, an existing activity against which the new one is to be compared, an activity unrelated to the experimental intervention or no activity at all. Baseline measures are typically carried out for both groups followed by outcome measures – both immediately and as follow-ups over varying periods of time (Box 1)

**Box 1**   Simple Experimental Design

RO1   ×   RO2   Experimental group
RO3   –   RO4   Control group

where R is randomisation, O is measurement and × is intervention

Randomisation of individuals is the defining characteristic of a true experiment. In some situations it may not be practically possible or ethically appropriate to randomise individuals and in these cases matched groups may be randomised to the experimental or control conditions. Experimental style studies in schools and community settings have adopted such procedures and they are described as quasi-experimental (Campbell and Stanley, 1963). Their design looks like a classic 'true' experiment except for the absence of individual randomisation. It should be noted that some discussions of experimental design and some published systematic reviews do not draw a clear distinction between true and quasi-experimental studies of the type referred to above. In this book we will use true experiment to refer to those studies where the individual is exposed to randomisation. Examples of evaluation studies which conformed to a true or a quasi-experimental design are summarised in Box 2

**Box 2**   True Experimental Design

Evaluation in a primary care setting of nicotine gum-assisted group therapy with smokers with an increased risk of coronary heart disease (Basler *et al.*, 1991).

*Design*
Randomisation to intervention or control groups with controls receiving intervention at a later date.

*Intervention*
Use of gum together with nutritional information, behavioural training for the promotion of self-management techniques and the prescription of a quit smoking date.

*Control*
Individuals received no specific intervention but were offered the programme after the conclusion of the programme with those in the experimental group.

*Results*
At a 3 month follow-up 63.9% of the experimental group were abstaining from smoking, in comparison with 3.3% of the control group.

Quasi-experimental Design

Class of 89 Study (Perry *et al.*, 1994)

*Design*
Two communities matched for size and socio-economic factors – one intervention and the other the control. Eleven year olds in schools as target group.

*Intervention*
School programme, public commitment not to smoke, population-wide community programme including risk factor screening, community organisation, health education, media campaigns and continuing education for health professionals. Lasted 5 years.

*Control*
No intervention.

*Results*
Weekly smoking prevalence lower in intervention community than in control; 14.6% versus 24.1%.

The major strength of an experimental design is its capacity to establish causal relationships. The experimental and control groups are set up with the intention that they will be identical at the outset and will differ subsequently in whether or not they receive an intervention. Differences in impact and outcome can, therefore, be attributed to the intervention. There are, however, a number of technical problems associated with experimental design that have a bearing on the conclusions that can be drawn. These will be discussed prior to assessing the relevance of experimental studies in health promotion.

## Type errors

For supporters of experimental design a key problem is presented by what are described as Type 1 and Type 2 errors, referred to in an earlier chapter. Type 1 error occurs when it is concluded, wrongly, on the basis of outcome data that the null hypothesis is false. In other words, it is claimed that there is a significant difference between experimental and control groups and the intervention has been successful when, in reality, this is not the case. The probability of committing Type 1 errors depends on the levels of significance that we set. If the null hypothesis is rejected when the chance of it being true is less than 0.05 we shall be wrong in 5% of cases. We can guard against Type 1 error by setting a more stringent level of significance of 0.01 or even 0.001. If we do so we risk, as a consequence, Type 2 error, where we accept the null hypothesis of no difference when there is, in fact, a real difference. In effect we conclude that the intervention has not had an effect when it actually has had some impact. A significance level of 0.05 is typically taken as a value which gives a balance between Type 1 and Type 2. Type 1 and 2 errors can occur for a number of reasons. The process of randomisation may still create groups that are different. Possible confounding factors are not evenly distributed and the impacts of intervention are obscured. Studies may have included sample sizes which were too low to detect the change expected and adequate sample size is necessary to minimise Type 2 error. Errors may also arise from measurement problems where, for example, measurement tools may have been insufficiently sensitive or inappropriate for the measures required. Researcher knowledge of the intervention and control groups can also contribute to measurement bias. Procedures to obscure the groups to which research participants belong may be impractical or undesirable. The timing of measures may also be inappropriate – they may come too soon before an intervention has had an impact or, conversely, when effects have died away. Commenting on such limitations in relation to educational evaluation Eisner (1985) observed:

*A (fifth) characteristic of experimental research which filters into evaluation practices is the extreme brevity of the treatment that is provided. Making important and enduring differences in people either requires a great deal of time or a very powerful treatment. Neither peak experiences nor traumas are typical of our experiments; thus, time is required to bring about changes of a significant and enduring variety. Yet the average duration of experimental treatment time per subject reported in 2 volumes of a recent educational research journal is about 40 minutes – 40 minutes to bring about a change that has educational significance.*

(p76)

155

Green and Lewis (1986 p264) have described a number of timing problems related to measurement that can contribute to Type errors (Box 3)

**Box 3**  Timing of Measurement and Effects

---

*Sleeper Effect*

The impact of an intervention may appear after the period during which the intervention comes under observation. Green proposes that the effect is especially important in the evaluation of school health education.

*Decay of Impact*

An intervention may have a short impact which rapidly declines. The times of measurement might miss the impact altogether or overestimate the impact if the subsequent rapid decline is not picked up through follow-up measures. This problem can often emerge when measures are taken shortly after the completion of an intervention but follow-up is too short term to pick up the decline in impact.

*Borrowing From the Future*

Some educational programmes are triggers for changes that would have occurred anyway. They may bring earlier action but longer term gains do not occur.

*Contrast Effect*

Premature termination of a programme can have a negative impact on the experimental group and lead to a reduction or a reversal of desired behaviours. There is a real risk of such an effect where funding is not continued or the demands of research programmes dominate those of the needs of the people experiencing the intervention.

---

The nature of the control activity in experimental studies can also create difficulties. If the control group has no activity any gains in the intervention group originating from the Hawthorne effect – the impact of attention rather than the specifics of the intervention – will be obscured. There are many situations where contamination between experimental and control groups is difficult to avoid and this has been reported as a problem in several of the major heart disease prevention studies (Nutbeam *et al.*, 1993).

There is a particular contribution to Type 2 error that is often described separately as Type 3. This describes those situations where the null hypothesis may have been accepted but where the intervention was, in actual fact, inadequately implemented and no gain could reasonably have been expected. This is particularly relevant in health promotion critiques of experimentation and has been discussed fully elsewhere (Tones, 2000). This error will be discussed further in considering the quality of interventions.

**Ethical issues in experimentation**

Experiments which involve people rather than inanimate objects generate ethical concerns. They include the need to be clear about the situations when it is ethical to conduct an experiment, the mechanisms for recruitment of people into studies and obtaining consent for participation. The ethical position in the case of the first issue is that experimental studies should only be conducted when there is no clear indication of which is the better of two interventions. For example, in developing a new drug if a RCT is not undertaken before the drug is made available, there is the risk that negative consequences will come to light after the drug is already in widespread use. The completion of reputable trials does not obviate such problems but it is generally accepted that they are likely to be reduced. Health education (where experimental studies are more likely to take place than in health promotion) tends to present situations that on the surface are less problematic ethically than in clinical settings but interventions have regularly been introduced in the absence of any assessment of their potential harm or, alternatively, of their effectiveness.

There are a number of issues surrounding recruitment to experimental studies. Concerns about putting people under pressure to participate arise where payments are made and the amounts offered are sufficiently large to make it difficult to resist, particularly for people who are economically disadvantaged. This has tended to be more of a concern in clinical trials than in mainstream health promotion where, in the former, payments can be offered by drug companies to participants. A further issue arises when requests to participate are made to patients in health care institutions. There may be a reluctance to refuse in case treatment is, in some way, compromised. The issue of securing consent for participation in experimental studies has received considerable attention in medical contexts and such consent was not routinely sought until relatively recently. The difficulties of explaining the principle of randomisation and patient acceptance of the idea that treatment has been decided through such a process has been given as a reason for not including consent procedures in some clinical trials. Where informed consent is required it may be difficult to recruit enough participants to generate valid findings. With a much greater acceptance of consent as a key principle of trials there remains the difficult question of ensuring that fully informed consent is achieved. There are further issues of consent when children are involved in experimental studies in school settings. Traditionally children have not been asked for their consent.

### Responses to the use of experimental studies in health promotion

In health promotion there are concerns raised about the use of experimentation, some of which are related to the technical and ethical problems associated with design and implementation but increasingly there are fundamental challenges at the epistemological level.

As we have already noted, there has been a history in health education of adopting experimental designs in evaluating interventions. True experimental designs have been used most frequently in patient education (which some might wish to argue is not strictly health promotion) but they have also been used in assessing interventions in schools and in other contexts. Quasi-experimental studies have been widely used in school- and community-based interventions. Within the broad mix of people involved in health promotion research and evaluation there are many who recognise and acknowledge the difficulties in undertaking experimental studies but, at the same time, remain committed to their use in establishing the evidence of effectiveness base of the discipline. One particular factor which influences the attitudes towards and the use of experimentation in health promotion derives from the nature and variety of its interventions Some narrowly focused small-scale health education interventions can be evaluated through the use of true experimental designs. The majority of health promotion interventions, however, are more complex and not readily amenable to such designs, although a number of complex multi-component interventions, implemented in community settings, have adopted quasi-experimental designs. It should be noted that a great deal of the critique of experimentation in health promotion focuses on the true experimental design – the RCT.

A particular difficulty identified with experimentation is its 'black box' nature. This term refers to the attention to input – the intervention – and to impact and outcomes but general neglect of the intervening processes by which the variables are related. This is a particular issue for many health promotion interventions where differing levels of fidelity in implementation of interventions can occur. Interventions can be complex and not easily provided in a uniform way, even if it is desirable for the purposes of assessing effectiveness that they should be. Interventions can also be actively modified by implementers. For example, evidence from evaluations of school-based health education projects in the 1980s demonstrated that teachers were reluctant to use curriculum materials exactly as provided (Tilford, 1982). It was seen as a part of professional practice to modify such materials in line with the context and the young people who were worked with. Publications, in drawing conclusions on the effectiveness of studies, can often be relatively silent on the matter of implementation and the risk of Type 3 error can be overlooked.

The question of costs of experimental studies has been raised as an objection to their use in health promotion. This can be a legitimate observation if large trials of the heart disease prevention type are planned, but many studies which have adopted an experimental approach have not been of this size. There is also questioning of the wider relevance of small studies, especially where these are undertaken in artificial experimental conditions. Even when demonstrable successes are achieved, whether these can be achieved in the everyday contexts of practice is questionable and replication in real life situations is required. Concerns have also been expressed about the differing results that can arise in multi-centre interventions as a result of context variables. Where results are aggregated the differences can be obscured. A useful discussion of this has been provided by Kaneko (1999), focusing on the Community Intervention Trial for Smoking Cessation (COMMIT) which used a quasi-experimental approach incorporating 11 pairs of matched communities with one in each pair randomly assigned as the experimental condition and the other as the comparison. Wide differences between the 11 matched pairs were found, with marked success in some and failure in others. Kaneko notes that in spite of such crucial differences the research group apparently paid no attention to them.

A major concern in health promotion is about the relevance of experimental studies, however well they may be conducted (WHO, 1998a; Van de Ven and Aggleton, 1999). The holistic nature of health promotion interventions and the values of participation, collaboration and empowerment which are, for many, integral to health promotion are seen to be incompatible with experimentation. The WHO in its recent guide to policy makers has offered as one of its conclusions:

> *The use of randomised controlled trials to evaluate health promotion initiatives is, in most cases, inappropriate, misleading and unnecessarily expensive.*

(WHO, 1998a)

To summarise, there are a number of possible views about the use of experimental designs in health promotion. These can be presented as positions on a continuum progressing from the wholly negative through to the positive.

NEGATIVE

Total rejection of the use of experimental designs in any evaluation of activities designated as health promotion since they are incompatible with the values and principles of health promotion.

Experimental designs are unethical in many areas of health promotion and also impracticable for evaluating many health promotion interventions but they have limited usefulness in specific cases. Examples could include true experimental studies of small-scale health education interventions and quasi-experimental studies in some settings.

Acknowledgement that experimental designs have limitations but they can still have an important place in establishing the evidence base in health promotion. Advocates of this position would place emphasis on the achievement of the ultimate goals of health promotion of promoting health and reducing inequalities and would be ready to use evidence that may help achieve such goals. At times the evidence required to persuade decision makers may need to be obtained from experimental studies.

Experimental evaluation designs in health promotion pose challenges but overcoming these are seen as technical questions and support is given to the use of experimentation as long as it is carried out within a commitment to ethical practice. The adoption of experimental designs is essentially unproblematic and necessary if the health promotion evidence base is to be strengthened.

POSITIVE

Given the diversity of people involved in health promotion, the scope of evaluation questions and the contexts in which health promotion is practised, with their attendant constraints and demands, examples of all the above positions on the use of experimentation are likely to be found. While we broadly endorse the reservations about the use of true experimental designs in health promotion we also recognise that they can have a measure of usefulness, especially in evaluating some focused health education interventions. Quasi-experimental designs, carefully executed, can be used rather more extensively. In reviewing evidence of effectiveness of health promotion in later chapters we will be drawing on all types of study including experimental and quasi-experimental ones.

## Observational studies

While experimental studies are frequently held up as the gold standard in evaluation there are situations where they are not feasible or desirable and where studies which are more susceptible to bias are more appropriate. A substantial amount of evaluation work uses designs which are based on survey models, the strongest being those which include measures prior to implementation of a project, measures at points during a project and measures of impact and longer term outcomes. Examples of evaluation studies using a survey approach will be drawn on in subsequent chapters.

We have previously noted the early dominance of experimental and survey approaches in health education evaluation. Given that these approaches, properly implemented, can claim to develop generalisable findings designed to be of value to policy makers, a case can be made for their use. Nonetheless, the lack of information on the process of implementation in many studies and, more importantly, the growing challenge to positivist approaches within social science has steadily influenced thinking in evaluation research. The lack of incorporation of qualitative data as a component in evaluation was, for example, noted by Campbell in 1979:

> *It is with regret that we report that in US programme evaluations the sensible joint use of quantitative and qualitative modes of knowing is not yet practiced.*
>
> (cited in Green and Lewis, 1986 p149)

Broughton (1991) marked the early 1980s as the point at which dissatisfaction with experimental designs and quantitative methods in evaluation emerged clearly:

> *Spurred by the seemingly frequent failure of policy makers to incorporate evaluation research findings in their decisions, frustrated by the oft reported difficulties of executing a conventional research design under field conditions, and aware that conventional evaluation methodologies were failing all too often to detect positive program outcomes many began to look to the traditions of qualitative research methods for appropriate new techniques.*

Various ways of incorporating qualitative data into studies developed – these ranged from adding in data to describe process issues in what continued to be broadly positivistic studies through to the full adoption of non-positivist approaches. We will now consider such alternative interpretivist approaches.

## Interpretivist approaches

There are a number of related and overlapping intellectual traditions that can be brought together under this heading, the main ones being hermeneutics and phenomenology. Within these traditions social reality is conceived as a meaningful construction rather than, as described within positivism, as an objective reality. Individuals routinely interpret and make sense of their worlds and knowledge comes from gaining access to these subjective meanings. The data acquired from research is typically qualitative rather than quantitative. Interpretivist enquiry is essentially inductive and, where theory is concerned, research is oriented towards the generation of theory from data rather than the testing of existing theory. Sampling of people for participation in studies is theoretical rather than random – those who are thought to have contributions to make to understanding of the subject in question are selected for participation. The main methods used in data collection are the interactive ones of one-to-one interviews, focus groups and participant observation or there may be analysis of existing documentation and artefacts. The relationship between a researcher and participants is seen to be a crucial one and the reactivity of the researcher is integral to the process, and there is an expectation that this will be acknowledged and discussed in the writing up of projects. Within the approach there is also explicit attention to issues of power in the research context and the impact that these can have on the process. The findings of research are viewed as specific to the context from which they were generated and generalisability, as understood within quantitative research, is not the goal. Interpretivist research is, therefore, described as relativist, although some would argue that limited transferability of findings beyond the research setting is possible (Mason, 1996).

Research in this tradition presents its own challenges and concerns, including:

- the drawing of boundaries around a specific study and reaching agreements about who should define what is or is not relevant to a specific piece of research;
- the maintenance of an open-ended approach in data collection;
- ensuring sensitivity to power considerations and generating appropriate responses;
- the procedures for the analysis and validation of data and the presentation of findings.

Feminist researchers have made important contributions to thinking about the processes in qualitative inquiry, particularly in the use of interviewing (Oakley, 1981 p30). Beneath the rhetoric about redressing imbalances of power in research relationships there is seen to be the potential in interviews for the exploitation of weaker people – who may reveal aspects of their lives that they would not otherwise choose to do under the influence of the interview and the skills of the interviewer (Finch, 1984). The importance of giving, as well as taking, information within the interview context has also been addressed and the need identified for providing opportunities for answering interviewees' questions at the end of an interview (Hobson, cited in Oakley, 1981 p80).

There are various ways of undertaking analysis of qualitative data and quite often in published papers there is relatively little detail of how analysis has been undertaken; this raises questions about the quality of the analysis. While it is an axiom of the approach that various analyses of the same data can be provided, there can be concerns about the prioritisation of a researcher's analysis over that of respondents. Techniques of respondent validation involve taking research back to interviewees to seek their responses to the analysis. Whether or not analyses should be modified in the light of this is open to debate, although inclusion of the different perceptions in a report and leaving it to others to adjudicate would be appropriate. The lack of rigid procedures in carrying out qualitative research leads critics to describe such research as 'sloppy' and emphasis has been placed on establishing rigour.

### Establishing the rigour of qualitative research

The different approaches to establishing the rigour and quality of this style of research have been outlined by Popay *et al.* (1998):

> *On one side there are those who argue that there is nothing unique about qualitative research and that traditional definitions of reliability, validity, objectivity and generalisability apply across quantitative and qualitative approaches. On the other hand there are those post modernists who contend that there can be no criteria for judging qualitative research outcomes … The third approach accepts that some criteria may be equally applicable to the evaluation of any research product regardless of the methods but also acknowledges the differences.*

We would support the view that assessments of the quality of interpretivist research should acknowledge its epistemological basis and be clear about the type of knowledge that qualitative research generates. Discussions of establishing rigour have addressed all stages of the qualitative research process, including the extent to which some generalisation, in a theoretical sense, can be made of the findings of studies (Mason, 1996; Mays and Pope, 1996; Popay *et al.*, 1998). Essentially, a rigorous study is one which is carried out with reference to the quality of the process at each stage of the study from the setting of research questions through to the writing up stage. Mason has questioned any transfer to qualitative research of the concept of reliability as it is understood within positivist research. She has summarised the attention to rigour in qualitative enquiry:

> It is important to emphasise that qualitative researchers must be concerned with overall questions of reliability and accuracy in their methods and research practice, albeit in a rather different way. I think this concern should be expressed in terms of ensuring – and demonstrating to others, that your data generation and analysis have been not only appropriate to the research questions, but also thorough, careful, honest and accurate (as distinct from true or correct – terms which many qualitative researchers would, of course, wish to reject). At the very least this means you must satisfy yourself and others that you have not invented or misrepresented your data, or been careless and slipshod in your recording and analysis of data. In order to convince others, you must provide some account of exactly how you achieved the degree of accuracy and reliability you claim to be providing. The presentation of your analysis therefore includes an explanation of why it is that the audience should believe it to be reliable and accurate.

> (p146)

The criteria suggested by Popay *et al.* for assessing qualitative research are given in Box 4.

**Box 4**  Criteria for Assessing Qualitative Research and Key Questions

*Evidence of Responsiveness to Social Context and Flexibility of Design*
Is there evidence of the adaptation and responsiveness of the research design to the circumstances and issues of real life social settings met during the course of the study?

*Evidence of Theoretical or Purposeful Sampling*
Does the sample produce the type of knowledge necessary to understand the structures and processes within which the individuals of situations are located?

*Evidence of Adequate Description*
Is the description provided detailed enough to allow the researcher or reader to interpret the meaning and context of what is being researched?

*Evidence of Data Quality*
How are different sources of knowledge about the same issue compared and contrasted?

Are subjective perceptions and experience treated as knowledge in their own right?

*Evidence of Theoretical and Conceptual Adequacy*
How does the research move from a description of the data, through quotations and examples, to an analysis and interpretation of the meaning and significance of it?

*Potential for Assessing Typicality*
What claims are being made for the generalisability of the findings either to other bodies of knowledge or to other populations or groups?

The aim is to make logical generalisations to a theoretical understanding of a similar class of phenomena rather than probabilistic generalisations to a population.

Mason also offers a careful discussion of activities which can ensure rigour in terms of reliability and accuracy of method, data analysis and use of findings (Mason, 1986 pp135–163) and Guba and Lincoln (1989 p213) provide five criteria for judging the trustworthiness of quality of enquiry together with their parallels in positivist research:

- credibility (paralleling internal validity);
- transferability (paralleling external validity);
- dependability (paralleling reliability);

- confirmability (paralleling objectivity);
- authenticity.

Finally, criteria for quality in using qualitative methods in health promotion research have also been discussed by Secker *et al.* (1995) and their paper reports on evidence of good practice in health promotion research papers.

### Interpretivist approaches to evaluation

These were developed in education with Parlett and Hamilton's (1972) critique of the experimental paradigm and the promotion of what they described as *'illuminative evaluation'* They argued that evaluation should be concerned to generate in-depth understanding through description and interpretation rather than focus on measurement and prediction. A major contribution to interpretivist evaluation in health promotion – under the terms constructivism and fourth generation evaluation – has been made by Guba and Lincoln (1989, 1998). Guba and Lincoln acknowledge that constructivist, interpretive, naturalistic and hermeneutic are all similar notions but propose that constructivism has its own particular emphases. They describe constructivist enquiry as aiming to achieve a consensus or, failing that, an agenda for negotiation on issues and concerns that define the nature of an enquiry (see Box 5). They stress that there are multiple, often conflicting constructions of an evaluation situation and all are, potentially, meaningful. For them truth is a matter of the best informed and most sophisticated construction on which there is consensus at a given time. Any act of inquiry begins with the issues and concerns of participants and is developed through iteration, analysis, critique, reiteration and, eventually, a joint construction of the subject in question. There is, therefore, a strong emphasis on interactions between investigators and respondents and joint production of findings. The joint constructions (Schwandt, 1998) can be evaluated for their fit with data and information, the extent to which they work in offering a credible level of understanding and the extent to which they have relevance and are modifiable. Constructions are not seen to be more or less 'true' in any absolute sense but simply more or less informed or sophisticated at a point in time. Constructions are alterable, as are their associated realities. We can, therefore, have pluralist accounts of any situation and they are also relativist, i.e. local and specific constructed realities. Guba and Lincoln (1998) use the term *'hermeneutic dialectic'* to describe their process of enquiry:

> *It is hermeneutic because it is interpretive in character and dialectic because it represents a comparison and contrast of divergent views with a view to achieving a higher synthesis of them all, in the Hegelian sense.*

The constructivist position, also described as fourth generation evaluation, is portrayed as more wholeheartedly relativist than some other interpretivist positions on evaluation.

**Box 5** The Stages of a Process of Fourth Generation Evaluation

1. Identify the full array of stakeholders in the projected evaluation.
2. Elicit from each stakeholder group their constructions about the evaluand and the range and claims, concerns and issues they wish to raise in relation to it.
3. Provide a context and a methodology (the hermeneutic/dialectic through which different constructions and different claims, concerns and issues can be understood, critiqued and taken into account).
4. Generate consensus with respect to as many constructions and their related claims, concerns and issues as possible.
5. Prepare an agenda on items about which there is no, or incomplete, consensus.
6. Collect and provide the information called for in the agenda for negotiation.
7. Establish and mediate a forum of stakeholder representatives in which negotiation can take place.
8. Develop a report (probably several reports) that communicate to each stakeholder group any consensus on constructions and resolutions.
9. Recycle the evaluation once again to take up still unresolved constructions and their attendant claims, concerns and issues.

Interpretivist approaches, taken as a whole, have been of particular importance in shifting attention away from inputs and outputs towards processes in the evaluation of programmes. Many health promotion programmes entail complex social interactions and they work, or do not work, because of processes of reasoning, negotiation, persuasion, advocacy and so on. Interpretivist approaches enable evaluators to generate insights into these processes.

Those who look at interpretivist evaluation from a sceptical standpoint raise a number of issues. Although a case for limited transferability of findings to similar situations can be made, the fact that findings are mostly relative to one situation or group of people is a serious shortcoming when there is a demand for evidence which can be generalised to other equivalent situations or used to inform the development of policy. Where constructivist approaches are concerned the nature of the power relationships that are contained within most social programmes are also presented as a barrier to successful implementation, and Pawson and Tilley (1997 p20) are particularly critical on this matter. Achieving consensus about constructions is likely to be easier in some situations than others. Where major conflicting viewpoints are to be expected, even where adequate time and resources are available, achieving consensus may be an unrealistic goal.

Although, as we have indicated above, there continues to be support for health promotion evaluation informed by the positivist and post-positivist tradition, there has been a growing ground swell in support of the use of approaches informed by interpretivism either as the sole approach in an evaluation or as part of a pluralist approach (House, 1993 p4). As with experimental design we can identify a continuum of responses to evaluation informed by interpretivist approaches ranging from the wholly positive to the largely negative.

## POSITIVE

Interpretivist research should be the dominant, if not the sole, approach to use in evaluating health promotion programmes. Such approaches are in harmony with health promotion values and goals.

Interpretivist research approaches are of major importance in evaluating health promotion research but they must be practiced with due reference to establishing the rigour of the findings. They may be used together with some limited use of methods which generate quantitative data.

Interpretivist approaches are best used in the context of a full embrace of methodological pluralism. Qualitative data contribute to 'illumination' and understanding of the process of interventions. Triangulation of data from a number of sources adds to the strength of findings.

Interpretivist approaches have little to offer to the project of establishing a strong evidence base in health promotion because of the relativism of studies. They should be confined to limited use in commenting on process issues.

## NEGATIVE

We noted earlier that the tension between positivist and interpretivist positions has underpinned much of the methodology debate. Other traditions, related in differing ways to those already discussed and increasingly drawn on in health promotion include critical theory, feminist research practice and critical realism

### Critical Theory

This tradition is of particular relevance to health promotion when it is conceived as committed to specific values and oriented towards achieving change in order to develop health and to reduce inequalities. In contrast to positivism no clear distinction is made in critical research between facts and values and there is no concern to maintain a position of value neutrality. While sharing much of the thinking that informs interpretivist research critical theorists note the lack of attention in interpretivist research to the structures and processes through which subjectivities are shaped and maintained (Everitt and Hardiker, 1996). The *Critical Theory* tradition is a complex one and elucidation is beyond the scope of this chapter, but differing contributors include the Frankfurt School (Habermas, 1972), Freire (1972) and Lyotard (1984). Research in the tradition has been explained by Harvey (1990) as follows:

> *At the heart of critical social research is the idea that knowledge is structured by existing sets of social relations. The aim of a critical methodology is to provide knowledge which engages the prevailing social structures. These social structures are seen by critical social researchers as oppressive structures.*
>
> (p2)

Research as an activity is directed, therefore, towards addressing the oppressive social structures, initially through understanding them using a process of dialectical enquiry as discussed in earlier chapters and, ultimately, using findings to secure changes. In dialectical inquiry the researcher and the subjects of the inquiry engage in a dialogue designed to achieve critical consciousness and, it is hoped, eventual emancipation. The enquiry does not claim to be value neutral – quite the contrary, in that particular values are fully engaged. Research is often seen as a first step towards political action which can lead to the redress of injustices. The adoption of a critical approach to health promotion was examined some years ago (Poland, 1992). In seeking to develop a new research methodology for health promotion he proposed that:

> *health promotion in its articulation of a new holistic and ecological stance has reached a turning point in its evolution that must be accompanied by the adoption of a more explicitly critical and interpretive research methodology.*

Vanderplaat (1995) has also provided a detailed discussion of a critical approach to evaluation in social programmes. She argues that the emancipatory potential of an empowerment approach to social intervention is extremely constrained if not accompanied by supportive evalua-

tion practices. Much current thinking in health promotion is influenced by writing in the critical tradition and the 'emancipatory' *Action Research* model of evaluation, to be discussed later, is a good example of a critical approach.

### Feminist research

There are differing traditions within contemporary feminism, but all branches can be said to be unified in a concern for the position of women, for promoting research which leads to greater understanding of women's position and a goal of using knowledge to bring about change. Feminist research practice has increased understanding about women's health and health-related experiences, about women's positions in societies and the role of male power in the social construction of knowledge. There are very close links with critical research and many would argue that feminist research is contained fully within the critical tradition. However, not all feminist researchers would necessarily ally themselves fully with the critical tradition and it is for this reason that the traditions are addressed separately. There have been similar debates about epistemology and methodology in feminist research as in other areas of social science and branches of feminism have taken distinctive positions on research issues. While there has been strong advocacy for working within the interpretivist traditions and significant contributions to the practice of qualitative inquiry by feminist researchers, as noted earlier, there are also feminist researchers who accept the adoption of pluralist approaches. Where the key purpose of research is to establish the basis for achieving change in women's positions in society there can be a pragmatic acceptance to the use of methods which will generate data most appropriate to achieving this goal. The feminist research tradition is an important point of reference for health promotion where there is concern to understand issues of women's health and aspirations to reduce inequalities of health related either to gender or to those arising from the interactions of gender with age and/or ethnicity. Health promotion research has been as vulnerable as other areas of health and social care to the criticism that gender has been insufficiently addressed in enquiries and feminist researchers are making important contributions to redressing this lack.

### Realist approaches and critical realism

The realist tradition has been evident in the philosophy of science for some 30 years or more (Keat and Urry, 1975; Bhaskar, 1975; Harre, 1986) but has only recently been given much attention in health promotion. Realist ideas have been presented in a lively and influential book (Pawson and Tilley, 1997) which has attracted notice in health promotion and is informing approaches to evaluation in the English *Health Action Zones*.

The approach, which can be described as a post-positivist one, has a number of important features. In common with positivism there is an acceptance of the existence of reality but with the modifying claim that this reality can only be apprehended imperfectly. The social world is seen as an objective material structure of relations which is not accessible to direct observation. Blaikie (1991) describes the aims of realist science as explaining phenomena with reference to the underlying structures and mechanisms which make up reality. Models of mechanisms are built up which, if they were to exist and act in the postulated way, would account for the phenomenon being investigated. Such models:

> constitute hypothetical descriptions which, it is hoped, will reveal reality; reality can only be known by constructing ideas about it.
>
> (Blaikie, 1991)

The term 'critical realism' derives from an emphasis on subjecting claims about reality to the widest possible critical examination in seeking to apprehend such reality as closely as possible. Knowledge is said to consist of non-falsified hypotheses. There is an acceptance within this approach that the clear separation between researcher and researched as presented in positivism cannot be maintained but a commitment to objectivity is, nonetheless, retained. Where methodology is concerned a modified experimental approach is used and is applied in natu-

ralistic rather than artificial experimental situations. The approach addresses the lack of attention to process noted earlier in consideration of experimental designs. The methods used are mixed and there is a willingness to draw on qualitative as well as quantitative data. Scientific realism uses what is described as a 'generative' logic of causation – this addresses the underlying events between events and causes and proposes that it is these underlying mechanisms that cause the relations between surface events. This is in contrast to what is described as the successionist cause–effect logic of experimentation. The realist approach to evaluation focuses on social programmes within their social contexts and examines the ways that the social contexts into which interventions are introduced facilitate or inhibit underlying mechanisms. Evaluations, while focusing on outcomes, equally need to address the contexts of interventions and the underlying mechanisms which mediate between events and outcomes. The design for realist and related *'theory of change'* evaluations will be discussed further in the second part of the chapter.

## Methodological pluralism and the triangulation of data

There are frequently comments that it is time to stop debating the merits of alternative methodologies for research and to move on constructively. The commonest response has been an espousal of methodological pluralism and it is probably fair to say that this has become a mantra in health promotion and is promoted with relatively little expressed reservation. By methodological pluralism we are describing the combination of methods of enquiry that derive from what are widely portrayed as differing epistemologies. Pluralism is often used interchangeably with the term triangulation but not all triangulation would involve a combination of methodologies, in contrast to the combination of methods informed by a single methodological tradition. Triangulation is a term taken over from surveying where accurate location of a position can be achieved by taking a bearing from two or, even better, three positions. Applied to research, triangulation has been used in a number of ways, as indicated in Box 6.

**Box 6**  Types of Triangulation

- Data triangulation: collection of data at various times, in different locations and from a range of people or groups.
- Investigator triangulation: using multiple rather than single researchers.
- Theory triangulation: using more than one approach to generate categories of analysis.
- Methodological triangulation: use of more than one method.

(after Denzin, 1970)

Superficially, where two contrasting types of data appear to provide similar findings it can be tempting to conclude that they are correct but, equally, both could be incorrect. If, on the other hand, different findings emerge, this may be important and illuminating and acceptance of both sets of data may be more relevant than seeking to adjudicate between one and the other. Where more than one researcher comes up with similar accounts this again does not necessarily support the view that two are more correct than one – they may be coming with equivalent preconceptions while a third researcher could come up with different conclusions. Methodological triangulation as described by Denzin (1970) can include the combination of methods within one epistemological tradition or across traditions. It is better, however, to differentiate method from methodological triangulation. At times the combination of methodologies appears to be the pragmatic response to answering research questions in a specific study and there is little or no reference to epistemological questions. In other cases the epistemological differences are discounted and pluralism is not seen to pose difficulties. Methodological pluralism was debated fully in sociology and, subsequently, in health promotion – for many it is a tired debate and one that should be

left behind. Pluralist approaches are clearly popular with evaluators and widely adopted. Nonetheless, various cautions have been expressed about the adoption of methodological pluralism and the uncritical acceptance of triangulation (Blaikie, 1991; Tilford and Delaney, 1992; Milburn *et al.*, 1995). Blaikie has produced a sustained analysis of this topic while Milburn *et al.* have focused specifically on triangulation in health promotion research. While the latter writers welcome the growing trend to acknowledge the usefulness and limitations of the two main approaches to research they suggest that one result of the trend is that:

*it has become axiomatic that a combination of quantitative and qualitative methods should produce the most reliable and valid research results. Indeed, matters have moved at such a pace that research involving combined methods may now be felt to demonstrate greater skill and sophistication and thus be more likely to attract funding.*

Given the pressures to adopt pluralism it is relevant to comment a little further on the practice. It is necessary to ask why pluralism is being adopted and also, at the same time, why the practice might be conceived as problematic.

Methodological pluralism occurs in studies in different ways:

- some qualitative data collection is added into a largely quantitative study because this 'illuminates' the process and the final study provides a more complete account of the implementation and impact of an intervention;
- there is limited quantification and some use of quasi-statistics in what is predominantly a qualitative study;
- parity is given to quantitative and qualitative approaches as most appropriate in providing a comprehensive evaluation.

Given the wide variety of research questions addressed within the rubric of health promotion, methodological pluralism in the discipline as a whole makes good sense. Whether or not the process is problematic within a single study depends, to a large extent, on responses to the epistemological questions. If it is claimed that there are distinct and contradictory positions on ontological and epistemological matters the combining of research methods which stem from competing positions in answering a research problem would, at the very least, seem to be questionable. This position has been summarised by Bednarz:

> *there is reason to believe that quantitative and qualitative approaches cannot be synthesised because they occupy alternative – rather than complementary – philosophical spaces. Any synthesis must necessarily adopt the perspective of one or the other, so that any effort to reach a middle ground does so only in terms of a single perspective.*
>
> (cited in Blaikie, 1991)

Blaikie viewed methodological triangulation as particularly problematic for interpretivist researchers and has criticised Denzin for abdicating the interpretivist concern for the primacy of meaning in favour of a positivist concern for validity and bias. Silverman (1985) has also commented on Denzin's methodological triangulation:

> *underlying this suggestion is, ironically ... elements of a positivist frame of reference which assumes a single (undefined) reality and treats accounts as multiple mappings of this reality.*
>
> (p105)

If, on the other hand, the polarisation between approaches is seen to be artificial and any distinctions are more of degree than of type, to take a strong line on the adoption of pluralism would seem to be unnecessary. The arguments to support the latter view refer to the use of theory in the two approaches and to the quantification of data. It is claimed that it is virtually impossible to approach a qualitative research study devoid of the use of some theoretical ideas that have already been developed and to avoid drawing on these in framing interviews. Where quantity in the two approaches is concerned much qualitative data analysis, while not moving to the point of infer-

ential statistics, quite often uses some descriptive statistics or some notions of quantification in discussing findings, even if this is restricted to the use of 'some', 'most', 'few' and so on. McQueen (1986) proposed the view that it was more helpful to use the idea of a continuum of approaches rather than to draw on the notion of competing positions and also argued that it was 'necessary' to combine quantitative and qualitative techniques in health promotion research to achieve meaningful and adequate accounts of phenomena.

Blaikie (1991) suggested from his review of triangulation that there was a need:

- for a moratorium on its use in social research;
- to identify appropriate and also inappropriate combinations of methods and data sources, in light of the incommensurability of ontological and epistemological perspectives;
- to develop new labels for appropriate combinations.

There is little evidence that his proposals have been responded to actively in health promotion research, since triangulation becomes increasingly more popular.

While differing conclusions can be drawn about the merits of methodological pluralism the reality is that it is widely adopted in evaluation studies, as will become apparent in referring to studies in later chapters. A recent example of a small evaluation adopting a pluralist approach is provided in Box 7. In this project it was agreed by commissioners of the evaluation and by the researchers that in order to provide answers to the questions proposed within the resources available a pluralistic approach was preferred.

What does seem important to stress is that the reasons for adopting a pluralistic approach within an evaluation study need to explained and justified. It has been apparent for some time that most justification, if actually provided, is pragmatic. This observation is endorsed by Milburn *et al.* (1995), who examined a sample of health promotion studies where combined methods were used and identified any questions which were raised about such usage. They concluded:

**Box 7** Evaluation of a City-wide Evaluation of an
Occupational Health Project

The project worked across an English city. In common with a small number of equivalent projects in the UK it adopted an *Empowerment Model* and was designed to promote positive health at work and prevent work-related ill health. Project activities included:

- interviews by an occupational health advisor with patients in primary care; information and counselling were provided designed to enable workers to make changes in their workplace;
- work in community settings with employees in small and medium enterprises with the same aims as above;
- self-referral and drop-in activities in a city centre location for people wanting information and advice on occupational health issues;
- the maintenance of databases on work-related ill health;
- city-wide and national activities to publicise issues of work-related ill health and to advocate for changes.

The evaluation was designed to record activity over the whole period of the project's history, to gain some in-depth insights of the project held by key stakeholders and to ascertain users views of the project. The methods of data collection appropriate to addressing the commissioners questions within the resources available were:

- quantitative analysis of work-related health statistics;
- focused interviews with representative stakeholders to generate qualitative data;
- surveys of primary care users of the project to generate quantitative data;
- surveys of general practitioners in primary care practices where the project worked;
- quantitative and qualitative analysis of project documentation.

(after Tilford *et al.*, 2000)

*We found that such questions were rarely addressed and that the use of combined methods was usually pragmatic and unreflective. Often the approach was presented as a fait accompli, a solution to a problem. In such instances, the value of quantitative and qualitative methods independently of each other tended to be given as a rationale for the approach. Methods were seen simply as research tools or techniques and little attention was paid to issues involved in the act of combining them.*

Evaluators will need to come to their own conclusions about what to do in practice, but what does seem important is the need to be explicit about the possible limitations of triangulation and to justify its use in specific situations. The decisions made in the evaluation described in Box 7 were largely made for pragmatic reasons, within the prevailing constraints, and the study would be vulnerable to any critique of pluralist evaluation. As discussed by Milburn *et al.* (1995), there is less of a need to make a case that triangulation is right or wrong than to be explicit about how and why it is being undertaken.

Finally, in this first part of the chapter we will provide a brief discussion of a process which has been referred to earlier, that of the systematic review of existing evidence. As already noted, strong feelings have been generated about such reviews in health promotion. We will make reference to a number of such reviews in later chapters. At this stage we will outline the review processes and comment on some of the reactions to systematic reviews in health promotion.

### Systematic reviews

In areas of any discipline where there are a large number of studies on which to draw it has been customary for commentators to seek to summarise the evidence from existing studies. Commentary reviews have typically brought together those studies which could be acquired and were dependent on the capacities to access literature and the idiosyncracies of selection and interpretation of particular reviewers. Systematic reviews seek to bring together *all* the material, published or unpublished, on interventions for a particular subject and to draw conclusions from the evidence which can be drawn on by decision makers. In contrast to commentary reviews, the intention is to secure all available evidence and to make the criteria fully explicit for searching for and selection of studies included in a review. Full replication of such a review should, therefore, be possible. Systematic reviews are intended to reduce, as far as possible, subjective bias in the reviewing process by bringing together all available literature and extracting the same type of information from each study which meets inclusion criteria, using a standard proforma. The recent rapid development of such reviews has been in the context of the evidence-based medicine movement. Professionals have been under pressure to adopt practices which have been demonstrably effective and, wherever possible, cost effective. It should be noted that evidence has not been presented as the sole criterion on which decisions should be made. For example, the definition of evidence-based medicine from Sackett *et al.* (1996) is:

> *the integration of individual clinical expertise with the best available external clinical evidence from systematic research.*

Applied to health promotion evidence-based practice has been defined as:

> *the systematic integration of research evidence into the planning and implementation of health promotion activities.*
>
> (Wiggers and Sanson-Fisher, 1998)

Systematic reviews aim to bring together the strongest possible evidence and the strength of evidence is related to the type of study from which it was generated. Study designs are presented hierarchically in accordance with their susceptibility to bias (Box 8).

Where the results from several studies on the same subject are pooled and brought together and analysed a meta-analysis is being carried out. Meta-analysis aims to provide an integrated and

**Box 8**   Hierarchy of Research Evidence Quality

| Level | Source of research evidence |
|-------|------------------------------|
| I | At least one properly designed randomised controlled trial |
| II.i | Well-designed controlled trials without randomisation. Quasi-experimental studies |
| II.ii | Well-designed cohort (prospective) studies, preferably from more than one centre or research group |
| II.iii | Well-designed case control studies, preferably from more than one centre or research group |
| III | Large differences in comparisons between times and/or locations, with or without interventions |
| IV | Opinions of respected authorities, based on clinical experience, descriptive studies or reports of expert committees |

*(after NHS Centre for Reviews and Dissemination, 1996)*

quantified summary of research results on a specific question with particular reference to statistical significance and effect size. Evidence derived from a systematic review of multiple well-designed RCTs is stated to provide the strongest basis of evidence on which to base practice (Muir Gray, 1997). In most areas of health promotion there are, to date, insufficient studies available on any specific subject to make such meta analyses feasible. The stages of a systematic review process are described in Box 9.

**Box 9**   Stages of a Systematic Review

1 Define subject for review and research questions and consult end users.
2 Establish methodological criteria for inclusion.
3 Develop a search strategy and acquire literature.
4 Extract data.
5 Summarise findings and develop conclusions.
6 Disseminate.

We will comment briefly on the stages of the review process particularly as they relate to systematic reviews in health promotion. Reviews typically use two reviewers for all key stages of a review as a quality procedure.

### Setting the boundaries

These include both content and methodological boundaries. Specifying content boundaries superficially appears to be simple. For highly specific types of interventions, such as drug or treatment interventions, this can be the case, but many areas of health promotion are not so specific. Different reviewers working on systematic reviews of the same subject can come to differing decisions about boundaries, thus generating some difficulties in making comparisons between the completed reviews. An example of this was provided in the case of reviews of mental health promotion (Hosman and Veltman, 1994; Hodgson and Abbasi, 1995; Tilford *et al.*, 1997). There is an expectation that end users of a review are fully consulted at the outset and at points throughout the process. Not all end users are fully aware of the nature and the particular strengths and limitations of systematic reviews and careful dialogue is needed in the early review phases if later disappointments are to be avoided.

Methodological criteria for the inclusion of studies prioritise RCTs, although in those areas of medicine which, like health promotion, are characterised by more complex interventions other types of studies lower down the hierarchy may also be included. A recent review of interventions aimed at preventing the uptake of smoking in young people contained almost entirely quasi-experimental designs, as defined earlier, rather than classic RCTs. (NHS Centre for Reviews and Dissemination, 1999). Given the concerns in health promotion about experimental studies it is the RCT as a gold standard in selecting review studies which generates the most objections.

### Acquiring literature

The objective of a review is to bring together all literature, published and unpublished, on the review subject, using both electronic and paper-based databases, and this is where systematic reviews do not necessarily deliver on their promises. Some electronic databases are more difficult to search for experimental studies than others and relevant studies can be difficult to locate (Dickerson *et al.*, 1994). Even in Pubmed (previously Medline) it has been stated that only about 50% of relevant studies can be identified through a computerised search (Muir Gray, 1997 p62). By using the bibliographies in papers and through other hand searching the percentage can, however, be raised to 94%. There are variations in the extent to which reviews complete such full procedures for searching. Not many reviews include papers in more than one language – predominantly English – even though it cannot be assumed that all important literature necessarily appears in English language publications. Acquiring the unpublished 'grey' literature is time consuming and few reviews have the resources to do this comprehensively. It is unlikely that the grey literature will provide many examples of RCTs not known about from other sources but promising directions for future work can be identified. In making recommendations at the end of a review it is helpful to be able to set these within a context of familiarity with the full range of interventions in any specific area and knowledge of the grey literature supports this process. This literature may also include studies using methods not acceptable in a review but which generate findings that can be of interest to a wide audience. Some reviewers have recommended undertaking subsidiary analyses of the grey literature and disseminating these in addition to a systematic review report.

### Inclusion and exclusion of papers in the review

When all literature has been brought together decisions have to be made about the papers to include in the data extraction and summarising of data phases. Papers can be rejected on methodological or on substantive grounds. Reviews are expected to report fully on exclusion processes.

### Extracting data

Information is drawn from reviews according to the criteria specified on an agreed data extraction form. Such forms have generally focused on various aspects of the design of the evaluation studies bearing on the reliability and validity of evidence generated. Health promotion reviewers have increasingly pointed to the equal importance of providing a full documentation of the nature of the interventions being assessed and their theoretical underpinnings. In addition to extracting quantitative evidence on impacts and outcomes the importance of extracting process information which may be qualitative has also been emphasised and recent reviews have begun to respond to these proposals.

## Summarising evidence and implications for practice

The final stage is to summarise evidence and to draw implications for practice and subsequently to disseminate the evidence to where it is most needed. While many studies can generate results which are of statistical significance, particularly where extensive analyses are undertaken, it is also important to be able to comment on practical significance. Effect size can provide a more useful basis for making decisions about practice. This is discussed further in Chapter 6. Further details for undertaking systematic reviews can be found elsewhere (Oxman, 1994; NHS Centre for Reviews and Dissemination, 1996) and, in addition, published health promotion reviews often contain useful reflections on the processes.

## Systematic reviews and health promotion

While some systematic reviews have been undertaken in health education for a relatively long time, especially in the areas of prevention of substance misuse and in patient education, the evidence-based health care movement triggered off a particular interest in applying such techniques more fully. A number of reviews in the UK have been undertaken by the NHS Centre For Reviews and Dissemination and the Social Science Research Unit, University of London, following the model established by the Cochrane Collaboration (Cochrane Collaboration, 1993; NHS Centre for Reviews and Dissemination, 1996). Some of these reviews were restricted to RCTs but in oth-

ers arguments were made for the inclusion of a wider range of studies. The dilemmas presented to reviewers were numerous. For example, where reviews were expected to include RCTs only it was often difficult to find suitable studies for inclusion for many areas of health promotion. The studies that could be included were evaluating interventions which were unrepresentative of those taking place in practice. If methodologically weaker studies formed a large part of reviews the logic of the systematic review process was being undermined, although the final review might appear to be more relevant to end users. A recently published paper has cast some doubts on the conventional wisdom that RCTs are to be preferred to observational studies on the grounds that the latter are more open to confounding factors which may distort results (Benson and Hartz, 2000). The writers compared observational studies with RCTs where two or more treatments or interventions for the same condition were evaluated. They found little evidence that estimates of treatment effects reported in observational studies were either consistently larger (as is usually claimed) or qualitatively different from those obtained in RCTs. They concluded that observational studies do provide valid information.

Systematic reviewers in health promotion across a number of subject areas have come to a number of similar conclusions:

- in many areas there are relatively few studies of the RCT type and many of the RCTs that are available have methodological weaknesses;
- in many review areas there are insufficient studies to undertake meta-analysis;
- the majority of studies eligible for inclusion in reviews stem from the USA;
- studies are typically carried out for research purposes and can tell us something about what can be achieved in ideal circumstances but not what can be achieved within the normal conditions of practice;
- individual studies report in detail on statistical significance of studies but relatively infrequently comment on the practical significance of findings;

- details of the nature of interventions, their theoretical underpinnings and the process of implementation receive limited coverage in many studies.

Systematic reviews inevitably exclude a large number of studies which do not conform to the prescribed methodological criteria. At the same time, the theory-related weakness of studies was not used as a specific criterion for exclusion in earlier health promotion systematic reviews and reviews have been criticised for this (Green, 2000). A number of reviews have, however, recorded the theory base of interventions when this was stated and this information was used to inform the conclusions drawn about particular studies. Finally, many published papers provide insufficient detail on implementation of interventions and minimum reporting requirements have been proposed to ensure that papers can be judged fully (Tilford and Delaney, 1995).

Even where there has been a readiness to use the findings from systematic reviews there is evidence that reviews have not come up to practitioner expectations because of the shortcomings noted above (Tilford et al., 1998). A further issue which has implications for practitioners drawing on reviews has recently been reported. A series of papers has examined discrepancies in the findings of systematic reviews on the same subject (Oliver et al., 1999; Peersman et al., 1999). Discrepancies between different reviews of health promotion interventions designed to change cholesterol levels and also reviews of health promotion interventions with older people were examined. The researchers noted that few effectiveness reviews in health promotion have fully reported the review methods used and that it is difficult to assess the potential bias and reliability of most reviews. They conclude that the review methods used affect the scope and recommendations of an effectiveness review. While this is not a surprising finding, it is an important point to remember when reviews evidence is being disseminated and used to inform decisions about practice.

Various responses to the limitations of health promotion systematic reviews have been made:

- health promotion is at an early stage of development and the number of evaluated studies appropriate to classic systematic review are few and use of the technique is premature;
- processes such as judicial review are to be preferred (Tones, 1997);
- there is value in the systematic review procedure but modifications appropriate to health promotion need to be made to the standard procedures – these would include extending inclusion/exclusion criteria to evidence of needs assessment in developing interventions and the use of theory to inform interventions and their implementation;
- the evidence from reviews has limitations but can usefully be used alongside evidence from other sources;
- rejection of systematic reviews based on quantitative studies and a call for systematic reviews of qualitative studies as an alternative.

Consideration has been given to modifying the data extraction forms used in Cochrane style reviews so that some of the criticisms made earlier can be addressed. At the same time other researchers have developed alternative instruments for assessing effectiveness which have given full emphasis to the nature of interventions, theory used, details of implementation and so on. For example, one instrument designed specifically for reviewing the effectiveness of health education and health promotion has been developed in the Netherlands (Veen et al., 1994; van Driel and Keijsers, 1996).

In this procedure a complete analysis of a small number of papers meeting comprehensive criteria for inclusion is provided. While the approach overcomes the shortcomings in systematic reviews in attention to theory and the processes of implementation the procedure is vulnerable to idiosyncrasies of reviewers in selecting studies for inclusion.

While it is open to reject systematic reviews it has to be acknowledged that the climate of much health promotion practice is one where evidence is expected to inform commissioning of activity and there is a demand for the type of evidence that such reviews can provide. The usefulness of systematic review evidence is well accepted in practice but, at the same time, there are concerns that other evidence should not be excluded in making decisions about interventions to implement in practice (South and Tilford, 2000). It is important to acknowledge the strengths and weaknesses of reviews, to improve them in response to some of the stated concerns and to draw careful conclusions about their usefulness in stated circumstances. It is worth noting the disadvantages of ignoring reviews evidence. While interventions might still be planned in the light of findings from research studies the studies used might be those most easily accessed rather than those which provide a sound lead on effective practice. It can be argued that it is more relevant to draw on evidence that has been derived from studies which permit generalisation. The conventional wisdom is that this comes from studies in the quantitative paradigm. Qualitative researchers are not setting out to produce generalisable findings in the sense that the term is understood in the positivist tradition although limited transferability, in a theoretical sense, can be made, as noted earlier (Mason, 1996).

## DESIGNING AND CARRYING OUT EVALUATION STUDIES

### Introduction

Any evaluation research study has to acknowledge and respond to a number of technical, political and ethical questions. We have commented in some detail on methodological considerations which underpin the whole enterprise of evaluation. In this section we will consider some aspects of carrying out evaluation and discuss *inter alia*:

- setting up an evaluation;
- obtaining resources for evaluation;
- the relationships between the sponsor of the evaluation, other stakeholders and the evaluator(s) and the setting of questions to be addressed in an evaluation study;
- the relationships between evaluator(s) and the programme;

- design and methodology adopted within the evaluation study;
- the quality of interventions being assessed;
- the generation, analysis and interpretation of data;
- the dissemination and use of evaluation findings.

Evaluation issues are being discussed mainly with reference to those situations where there is a commissioned evaluation and the evaluator comes from outside the health promotion programme to be assessed, although many aspects of the discussion would also be relevant to internal programme evaluation. In addition we will consider the skills needed by evaluators and the implications that these have for training.

### Setting up an evaluation

Evaluation is built in to many health promotion initiatives and is frequently undertaken from within the project itself. External evaluation is typically commissioned by project funders, but not necessarily from the beginning of a project. It may also be requested by a project when difficulties arise (Hawe and Stickney, 1997). Sponsors and funders of evaluations will vary in the extent to which they lay down objectives for an evaluation, prescribe the research methodology to be adopted and specify the nature of reports and subsequent dissemination. Where there is a high degree of direction the evaluator has restricted freedoms. There are two alternatives available to an evaluator when there are concerns about the degree to which an evaluation study is prescribed – to attempt to discuss the objectives and design and agree some changes or to turn down the evaluation opportunity. The latter option may not be an easy one to take unless there is alternative work available. The extent to which evaluators can argue for, and expect to maintain some independence from, sponsors has been discussed and claims for some degree of independence have been made. Simons (1989), for example, argued that when an evaluation is funded by a specific body this does not mean that the evaluation has to provide only the information that conforms to sponsors' values. The evaluator is to an extent a professional who can exercise independent judgement. Simons stated that there is a degree of consensus about the need for an initial contract between the evaluator and sponsor to secure the procedures for undertaking a study in order to prevent later misunderstandings and to provide a basis for review in the case of any disputes.

## Resources

The resources available for an evaluation can have a significant impact on what can be achieved. A proposal that 10% of the resources of any project should go to evaluation has been stated in recent WHO guidelines for policymakers (WHO, 1998a) but there are many instances where this amount is not available. To take resources from what otherwise might be used to enhance implementation can be difficult, especially if there are feelings that the impact of the project might be prejudiced. On the other hand, if the rigour of the evaluation is prejudiced the justification for continuation of the project may be less easy to make. A 10% figure may make sense in large projects but this percentage of a very small budget does not permit more than cursory evaluation. Rather than specifying a target percentage to go to evaluation it may be more relevant to use limited evaluation resources differentially. Where there is already a sound evidence base for a particular intervention a programme may simply be monitored to check that it is being implemented in ways most likely to lead to success and to pick up any unanticipated effects that may occur should programmes be tried in different circumstances from the original evaluation. Innovatory programmes can also be tried on a small scale with relatively small needs for evaluation resources. On the basis of findings a resource-rich evaluation on a wider scale may then be called for. Programmes which are likely to be costly if applied widely need more thorough-going evaluation than cheap ones. Interventions that may have negative consequences also need very thorough evaluation.

## Evaluation stakeholders

Evaluation research has to be undertaken in contexts where a wide range of people have a legiti-

mate interest in the process and outcomes of the evaluation. These stakeholders can influence the way that the evaluation can be undertaken and the subsequent use of its reports. Whatever the style of evaluation the identity and diversity of stakeholders needs to be recognised and consideration given to those whose concerns may need to be given higher priority in completing work. Where there is a commitment to interpretivist and constructivist styles of evaluation there is likely to be varying degrees of working together with some or even all key stakeholders.

## The questions to ask

The previous chapter noted that evaluation can be both formative and summative and will assess a mix of indicators in any specific programme. Evaluation questions can address the process, the impact and the outcomes of a project and, in some cases, issues of cost effectiveness. The specific questions included will relate to the needs of the sponsors of the evaluation, the views of the evaluator(s) and the number and nature of stakeholders involved in the question setting process. There will be iteration between questions asked and the methodology preferred for the evaluation. For example, evaluations adopting a participatory style and qualitative approaches will not ask the same questions as in an experimental style or a realist evaluation. We have noted the emphasis on impact and outcomes in experimental designs and the lack of emphasis on understanding of the processes of how effects are achieved. We have also noted the lack of attention in some reported evaluations to the details of interventions, their theoretical bases and full accounts of implementation. The questions asked in an evaluation need therefore to pay attention to the following:

- what was the nature of the intervention, was it informed by theory and was this theory appropriate?
- to what extent was the programme implemented according to design and what were the nature and reasons for shortcomings?
- how did programme participants receive the programme?

Evaluation questions may be stated firmly and precisely at the start of some programmes. In others new questions may emerge which need to be added in as the programme unfolds.

## Design of evaluations and methodological considerations

While an evaluator may have individual preferences the design of an evaluation may, to a significant degree, have been determined by the sponsors of an evaluation, the research questions that have been set and the situational constraints governing the evaluation. Where an evaluation is being introduced into a programme at some point after implementation has begun certain forms of evaluation design are precluded and the capacity to generate particular results will, as a consequence, be reduced. Views on the best ways to generate answers to research questions will also influence choice of design. Where an experimental or quasi-experimental design is being implemented there are technical considerations that have to be met. If these are not addressed adequately the reliability and validity of findings is compromised. Where such studies are not possible but a positivist approach is still preferred, descriptive studies based on survey design methods can be adopted. These do not claim to establish cause–effect relationships and can be of differing kinds. The most commonly used survey designs in evaluation studies are of the time series type, where a project is studied over a period of time and for variable periods after a project has ceased. There may, or may not, be comparison groups. In too many cases evaluations are planned too late to allow the acquisition of adequate baseline data or even data from the early stages of implementation. Resources may also not be available for adequate follow-up. Where the conditions for completion of an adequate baseline and follow-up survey are not in place the strength of results will, inevitably, be compromised.

When a fully qualitative evaluation study is planned this also needs to be in place for the whole history of a project and for a follow-up period to provide the richest picture. Such evaluations can be organised to some extent in advance of beginning any data collection with the intention that implementation should be broadly in accordance with agreed plans in order to deliver the required information about the project. Having said this, interpretivist designs are often more flexible and can emerge during the project history in the light of events. In many instances the requirements of the sponsor of an evaluation demand a pluralist approach combining methods which cross the methodological divide. This is increasingly the preferred and recommended approach in health promotion evaluation.

There are a variety of models for summarising the design and evaluation of health promotion programmes. A useful one has been developed and discussed fully by Nutbeam (1998). We will comment specifically on 'Action Research' designs, which have a relatively long history in health education and promotion, and on 'Realist' and 'Theory of Change' designs, which are increasingly being adopted.

### Action Research

The term Action Research has a fairly long history and was first used by Lewin in the 1940s in reviewing community projects in the USA (Lewin, 1946). As an approach it was defined earlier in Chapter 2 according to Cohen and Manion (1994). A further definition by Kemmis and McTaggart (1988 p5) is widely used:

> Action research is a form of collective self reflective enquiry undertaken by participants in social situations in order to improve the rationality and justice of their own social or educational practices as well as the understanding of these practices and the situations in which these processes are carried out. The process is only action research when it is collaborative.
>
> (p147)

In the emphasis on collaborative and participative elements Action Research is distinguishable from some other styles of evaluation. The distinctiveness of action research lies in the continuous conjunction of action and research. This is generally described as involving a spiral of self-reflective cycles of:

- planning a change;
- acting and observing the process and consequences of the change;
- reflecting on the processes and consequences;
- replanning.

An *Action Research* evaluation can consist of several rounds of problem identification, identification of possible solutions, implementation, evaluation, revision of the problem, further solutions and so on. *Action Research* projects can involve external facilitators and evaluators but may also be internally led with or without external support. Such projects differ in the extent and nature of participation between facilitators and projects and in the nature of their aims. Classifications of *Action Research* approaches typically distinguish three broad types (Box 10).

**Box 10** Characteristics of Types of *Action Research*

---

*Technical Action Research*
- Directed by persons with special expertise;
- aims to obtain more effective and efficient practice as perceived by outsiders;
- activities product centred;
- operates within existing values and constraints.

*Practical Action Research*
- Directed cooperatively between project and outsider or by project alone;
- evaluator encourages participation and self-reflection;
- aims to achieve improvement and development of practice;
- transformation of thinking.

*Emancipatory Action Research*
- Collaborative process between project and evaluator;
- responsibilities shared between participants;
- improvement and development of practice;
- involves a shared radical consciousness;
- focused on transformation of organisations.

---

In health promotion there is a predominance of projects which fit into the practical or emancipatory models and to a great extent the term *Action Research* is associated with these particular approaches. The definition above from Kemmis and McTaggart also fits these two categories The term 'participatory' *Action Research* is frequently used to describe the emancipatory model, although the fully critical theory stance is not always adopted. Projects adopting an emancipatory approach have a concern with technical and practical improvements and also the development of participants' critical consciousness through collaborative processes and, furthermore, seek changes in systems and organisations which impede desired improvements (Zuber-Skerritt, 1996). In terms of data collection action research projects have typically been eclectic and data collected can be both quantitative and qualitative as appears to be most relevant in answering research questions. The nature of the participatory and collaborative relationships will be discussed further in the following section. Participatory *Action Research* designs have been promoted, for example, in evaluating workplace health promotion (Springett and Dugdill, 1995) We will refer in some detail to an *Action Research* project to develop a health promoting school in Chapter 5 (Davis and Cooke, 1998).

### *Realist* and *Theory of Change* designs

As described earlier, *Realist* approaches address limitations in conventional experimental designs and seek to investigate and understand more adequately the ways that programmes achieve their effects in specific contexts. While a design would incorporate collection of data before and after the implementation of a project a key emphasis would be on acquiring data which relates the context of a study to mechanisms and to outcomes according to the formula:

$$outcome = mechanisms + context$$

(Pawson and Tilley, 1997)

A *Realist* evaluation might address an intervention in one specific context or might seek to understand the outcomes when the same intervention is implemented in a variety of contexts. The intention is to understand what may work for whom in what circumstances. The planning of a programme and its evaluation would need to be built around identifying a desired goals or outcomes, specifying the context variables and then the mechanisms which may or may not operate within the contextual circumstances. The programme then needs to address those elements which are likely to increase the likelihood of the desired goal being achieved. The evaluation tests the hypotheses which have been generated. Examples of realistic evaluations can be followed up in Pawson and Tilley (1997) and in evaluations of UK *Health Action Zone* developments. An example of how this model might be used is also explored with reference to smoking cessation interventions by Kaneko (1999). He provides an illustration of possible context and mechanisms for a desired outcome of persuading pregnant smokers to give up smoking where the intervention is carried out by a doctor in an antenatal clinic (see Box 11).

A closely related model for evaluation is described as a *Theories of Change* approach. This has been described by Connell and Kibisch (Wimbush and Watson, 2000) as:

> *the articulation and testing of a programme's desired outcomes and the timescale for these to be achieved, together with the processes whereby these will be arrived at, making adjustments to goals and methods on the way.*

The approach starts from the premise that social programmes entail theories of change about how a programme will work, whether these are made explicit or are implicit. Theories are expressed in the form of causal relationships. An evaluation combines both process and outcome elements and is organised around investigating the extent to which the theory holds up when a programme is implemented. As with realistic evaluation, the use of data collection methods is eclectic. A framework for the

**Box 11** *Smoking Cessation Programme*

---

*Intervention*
Visit to clinic by pregnant woman and partner where doctor explains harmful effects of smoking on unborn children and offers advice on ways of quitting.

*Outcome*
Reduction in smoking prevalence by pregnant women.

*Illustrative Context Variables*
- Amount of past experience in organising community-wide health education activities;
- existence of competing community forces, e.g. the presence of a tobacco company;
- level of environmental consciousness;
- multiple hardships such as unemployment or poverty.

An evaluation will need to examine the extent to which the social contexts enable or disable the operation of underlying mechanisms.

*Illustrative Mechanisms for Change*
- 'Medicalisation mechanism': smokers quit as a result of knowing more about the harmful effects;
- 'primary group encouragement mechanism': smokers quit in response to requests of partner;
- 'substitute mechanism': doctor advises substitute methods of stress management or weight control which are considered to be benefits of smoking.

---

evaluation of health promotion programmes which informs work undertaken by the Health Education Board in Scotland and which incorporates realistic and theory-based models has recently been published (Wimbush and Watson, 2000).

### Relationships between evaluators and programme participants

The relationship between a designated evaluator and participants in a programme is a crucial one. The main relationships are with the workers in a programme and those for whom the programme is being provided, but there can be relationships with any of the stakeholders. The questions guiding the evaluation and the methods to be used in the evaluation influence relationships. The nature of health promotion and its ideology has stimulated much discussion about research relationships. We have noted earlier the importance of relationships in interpretivist research and also in feminist research practice. A particular focus on relationships in health promotion evaluation has been with reference to the ideas of participation and collaboration in research. For example, the recent guidelines on evaluation (WHO, 1998a) had as one conclusion the proposal that those who have a direct interest in a health promotion initiative should have the opportunity to participate in all stages of its planning and evaluation and it was especially important that members of the community whose health was being addressed should be involved in evaluation. Where there is such a commitment to the adoption, at all times, of a fully participatory approach it only remains to address the practical considerations of how to do this appropriately and effectively. There are those, however, who have a broad commitment to participatory styles but do not see these as necessarily always appropriate or feasible and yet others who would argue strongly against them. It is important to examine exactly what is intended by 'participation' and collaboration in evaluation research and the arguments both for and against and assess the extent to which participation should be implemented.

In common with so many adjectives coming before the word research, participatory is not always being used in the same way. As will be discussed in the later chapter on community participation, there can be a continuum from minimal to maximal participation. In the former there can be little more than cooperation with an evaluation that has been mostly planned and implemented by outsiders, although there may be minimal consultation on some aspects. Some *Action Research* projects conforming to the technical model would provide examples of this level of participation. At the other end of the continuum there will be full collaboration on all aspects of the evaluation research process and emphasis given to establishing equality between researchers and others as set out in the model of emancipatory *Action Research*. There are reasons for adopting participatory approaches which are associated with a philosophical commitment to particular ways of working with individuals and communities and there are also practical benefits. Pollitt (1999) has summarised the main claims for collaborative research:

- collaborative evaluation is likely to possess greater validity because it will reflect the different perspectives, conceptualisations, constructions and values of all the key stakeholders in the programme/project;
- collaborative evaluation is more likely to be used because stakeholders will have participated in the evaluative process and will therefore feel a more developed sense of ownership of the final report or findings;
- collaborative evaluation is ethically superior to other forms of evaluation because it is founded on an equitable and democratic acceptance of the right of every stakeholder to have a full and equal say in the conduct of the evaluation.

In addition, in the case of health promotion, we should add the commitment to making a contribution to the emancipatory and empowering goals of health promotion through involvement of people in participatory evaluation. A majority of, but by no means all, contributors to the discussion of participatory research have a preference for interpretivist approaches. Dockery (2000), for example, in reporting on two participatory *Action Research* projects in Liverpool states that the combined use of qualitative and quantitative data collection methods, in a climate of scepticism about non-quantitative data, was seen as a powerful way of convincing key personnel of her research findings.

Achieving a fully participatory approach is challenging and a specific reflection provided by Wallerstein (1999) will be described in Chapter 9. The challenges in achieving a collaborative approach and the benefits to be gained have also been described for projects with 'out of the mainstream' young people (Harper and Carver, 1999) and with native American women (Klein *et al.*, 1999). For Harper and Carver the benefits in a project exploring HIV-related risk and prevention included the development of more appropriate research methods, recruitment of hard to reach young people, greater ease in tracking participants and increased project acceptability and credibility. The young participants reported that including them in all phases of the programme made them feel more at ease with the project and they felt that the youth perspective was truly valued and respected. The challenges included boundary issues, confidentiality, commitment and burnout. Harper and Carver concluded that collaborative research requires a strong commitment from all involved and often entails more work and effort than traditional models but can offer bountiful rewards and:

> *the synergistic knowledge and experience of university researchers, community based service providers, and out of the mainstream youth can result in the development of unique and informative research and service programmes.*

Various general reservations have been raised in the research literature about participatory approaches, particularly with reference to their adoption in evaluation research. Questions have been raised about the feasibility, in constructivist approaches, of getting all stakeholders to agree about an evaluation. Guba and Lincoln (1989) proposed the development of a contract between all stakeholders at the start of a process. Others have claimed that there are situations where the diversity is such that consensus is realistically unattainable. For example, the outcome of a research project may lead to loss for some stakeholders and gain for others, so unity on the evaluation is unlikely (Pawson and Tilley, 1997). It is also questionable, according to Pollitt (1999), how far or how often rigorous empirical investigation of effectiveness, if this is what is sought, can be combined with full stakeholder participation. Some commentators are against participatory approaches altogether in evaluation and

argue, in the interest of getting evaluation studies completed, for maintaining some distance – including contact with programme staff – in order to maintain validity and exclude sources of likely bias (Scriven, cited in Pollitt, 1999).

The size of an evaluation and preferred methodology clearly have an influence on the degree of possible participation of all stakeholders. A large-scale community-wide heart disease prevention project using a quasi-experimental design is a very different activity from a localised community project. Participation has to be easier to achieve in the latter.

While there are situations where full participation may be desirable and achievable there are others where there may be competing considerations and where prioritisation of participation over everything else would not be desirable. For example, the American Evaluation Society (Pollitt, 1999) has pointed out that evaluators have obligations that encompass the public interest and the public good and these may sometimes be in tension with the expressed interests of particular stakeholders. Pollitt has identified situations where collaborative evaluations are likely to encounter serious difficulties:

- the evaluation situation approximates to a zero sum gain between two or more of the main stakeholders;
- there are deep differences of values and world views between stakeholders;
- there is a multiplicity of stakeholders, some of which are highly dispersed, alienated and disorganised while others are concentrated, determined and highly organised;
- the sponsors of an evaluation actually want a causal type explanation of programme effectiveness.

To this we can add the difficulties of achieving a fully participatory approach when there are marked power differences between participants.

There are an increasing number of projects where efforts are made to incorporate participatory approaches and where those involved address the challenges as fully as possible. It needs to be stressed that participatory research projects do not necessarily require equal amounts of involvement from all or the same kind of involvement from all. Not all stakeholders will want or be available to participate to the same degree, but ensuring that all interests do have a voice and the less powerful are fully involved requires particular attention. Klein *et al.* (1999), for example, record the efforts needed to overcome the scepticism of native American women about involvement in research, a reflection of the negative relationships that such communities have often had with outside researchers. Boulton (1994) has also provided a thoughtful reflection on evaluating community peer education projects when there was a commitment to participatory evaluation but where this was also balanced by a commitment to the interpretation of project theory and questions of the utility of the evaluation as other integral elements of the process. In conclusion, we can suggest that while there are situations where full collaboration and participation in evaluation is desirable and potentially achievable, there are others where there are constraints which would make participation difficult.

### The quality of interventions which are under evaluation

The previous chapters have discussed what should be measured in evaluation studies and distinguished process from impact and outcome measures. In this chapter we will look in more detail at one specific issue which we have alluded to at several points in this chapter and which a number of people have addressed – measures of the quality of the interventions which are being evaluated. Speller (1998) has said that while the prime responsibility for developing quality assurance programmes lies with health promotion practitioners, researchers also need to be aware of what constitutes good quality health promotion in designing research studies. What will be defined as a quality health promotion intervention is, like everything else, open to debate. Catford (1993) offered a set of signs of quality for health promotion (Box 12).

**Box 12**   Indicators of Quality of Health Promotion

- Understanding and responding to people's needs fairly.
- Building on sound principles and understanding.
- Demonstrating a sense of direction and coherence.
- Reorienting key decision makers.
- Connecting with all sectors and settings.
- Using complementary approaches at both the individual and environmental levels.
- Encouraging participation and ownership.
- Providing technical and managerial training and support.
- Undertaking specific actions and programmes.

Some of the criteria in Box 12 are particularly relevant to judging the quality of a specific intervention; namely the correlation between the intervention and people's needs, the theoretical rationale for the intervention and provision of technical and managerial training to permit appropriate implementation of the intervention. If participation is taken as a prime criterion for any health promotion intervention this would also be added. There is now considerable attention given to needs assessment but reporting on how this has informed the designation of an intervention is commoner in evaluations of practice-based interventions than in the more narrowly research-based studies conduced by non-practitioners. Systematic reviewers have concluded that few interventions in a mental health promotion review (Tilford *et al.*, 1996) and none in a review of substance abuse interventions (White and Pitts, 1996) were based on needs assessment. The importance of the use of theory in designing interventions has been referred to earlier in the discussion of systematic reviews. Leaving aside the quality of the theory base in health promotion, the extent to which theory is drawn on and used appropriately in designing interventions can be difficult to deduce from reported research studies. In some instances theory may not be reported but can be deduced from other things that are said, but on other occasions no theory base is apparent. White and Pitts (1996) review, referred to above, concluded that none of the interventions included in their review explicitly focused on theory. In the main, interventions involved complex approaches and, if they were theory driven, were driven by a number of theoretical approaches. Boulton (1994), in describing three principles which guided her evaluation, gave as the first *the interpretation of project theory must be an integral part of evaluation.*

Theory also needs to inform the method for implementation of an intervention. An intervention designed to develop decision making skills is unlikely to succeed if the principles for achieving such changes are not appropriately incorporated. To do this may require the provision of training and other support for those involved in a project and some measures to ensure that prescribed methods are actually used. An early evaluation (Institute for the Study of Drug Dependence, 1982) reported some failure in achieving effective decision making skills in classroom situations because the theoretically based intervention for which training was actually provided was not implemented with fidelity by some teachers once isolated in their classrooms. The rationale for the methods advocated had not been fully accepted. Attention to the quality of interventions has been addressed in the various approaches to summarising effectiveness of health promotion. The IUHPE in the Netherlands gave good attention to this in its series of reviews (Veen Vereijken *et al.*, 1994) while many early systematic reviews of health promotion were less good. Those undertaken by reviewers with a knowledge of health promotion have been more sensitive to the debates and concerns within the discipline about the need to address the theory base of projects being evaluated but have been constrained by the methodology that they were expected to use as a condition of undertaking a review. Speller *et al.* (1997) proposed that existing reviews should be critically reanalysed using appropriate inclusion criteria which consider the quality of the health promotion intervention as well as that of the research.

## Carrying out data collection

This will clearly differ according to the approach adopted and the amount of control the evaluator has over the data collection. There are projects which have, basically, been set up in order to derive evidence of effectiveness and where the requirements of the evaluation research are clearly foremost. Much evaluation, however, is of programmes where the evaluation is secondary, for most stakeholders, to the planning and implementation of the programme. While the evaluator will have negotiated general access to the project it may be necessary to refine what this actually means within the day-to-day events of a project. For example, a sexual health education project within a community setting might not find it acceptable to have evaluators present in an observational capacity in sessions where particularly sensitive material was being discussed. Identifying and agreeing 'no go' areas for an evaluation from the outset can be recommended, but this is not always practicable and time will need to be found to consider these if, and when, situations arise. Where answering the research questions does not require evidence which could only be derived from specific sessions the evaluators can accept exclusion from aspects of a programme.

In evaluation research data collection instruments often have to be developed in less than ideal conditions. Many projects evolve during their life and activities cannot be fully determined at the point at which an evaluation begins. It is frequently necessary to decide at short notice how to evaluate specific activities within a project and conditions for piloting instruments may not be present. Evaluation projects also frequently incorporate a mix of methods which demands versatility of evaluators in small teams. As Boulton (1994) comments on her community-based evaluation of HIV/AIDS projects:

> we used quantitative and open ended surveys, individual and focus group interviews, participatory observation and repertory grids as well as such activities as literature reviews, attending meetings and keeping site contact sheets. ... Many of these skills had to be mastered before they were deployed. So

*much variety not only made the researcher feel that as soon as she was nearing competence in one activity she was reduced to a novice at another.*

The reactive impact of evaluators on a project, both positive and negative, cannot be ignored. The presence of an evaluator can trigger more concentrated attention to quality of implementation than may usually be the case in a project. Modifications to project activities can result in an eventual impact on achievements. The extent of impact is clearly related to the degree of participation of evaluators in the ongoing life of a project. Hawe and Stickney (1997) refer to the positive impact of evaluators in reporting on a formative evaluation of an inter-sectoral food policy coalition:

*we feel that our impact was assisted by an interview process which investigated important issues raised by previous researchers in coalition development and which indeed appeared to 'press the right buttons' for ensuing action.*

Issues of time are of particular relevance in evaluation. While non-evaluation research is not immune to considerations of deadlines, those within an evaluation can be particularly problematic. Some aspects of an evaluation may require permission from ethical committees, which can shorten the time available for data collection. Even where evaluations are commissioned prior to the start up of a project there can still be very short periods to plan the overall evaluation and to identify and discuss any possible difficulties ahead. Baseline measures may need to be developed rapidly and this can pose particular difficulties when indicators to measure complex concepts do not already exist and have to be developed. Where participatory approaches are to be adopted it is imperative to ensure that the time will be available to pursue these adequately.

### Measurement issues

These concern the measures used in evaluations used and the timing of measures. The nature of measures has been discussed in some detail in the preceding chapter. Clearly, discussion of measurement is particularly appropriate to positivist styles of evaluation but can be also be relevant to other styles of evaluation. Particular challenges at the present time are the specification of appropriate measures for use in assessing some of the newer initiatives in health promotion and the difficulties in being successful have been discussed (Hayes and Manson-Willms, 1990; Hawe, 1993). Issues around the timing of measurement were discussed earlier in relation to Type 1 and 2 errors. Evaluation resources are very often only available for a restricted period and do not support a sufficient length of follow-up time. Long-term follow-up is relatively unusual. One good example of where this was achieved was in a study of the impact of an intervention undertaken with people experiencing involuntary job loss (Vinokur *et al.*, 1991). The intervention consisted of eight group sessions over a 2 week period, based on coping resources theory and each lasting 2 hours, with recently unemployed men in the USA. The positive impact of the intervention on incidence and prevalence of severe depression symptoms among high risk individuals was maintained over the follow-up period of $2\frac{1}{2}$ years.

### Reliability and validity of methods used in evaluations

Finally we need to address issues of reliability and validity of the methods used with reference to the broad methodological approach to data collection, as well as that of specific measures. Reliability is the capacity of an evaluation to deliver similar findings if repeated by another researcher – assuming that no changes in the programme have occurred – while validity addresses questions of whether the research has adequately tapped the material needed to appropriately answer the research questions posed. The main types of validity are internal and external. The internal validity of a design is its capacity to generate definitive statements about whether or not a specific intervention produced the observed outcome. Experiments, when properly conducted, can claim the highest internal validity since they are designed to rule out extraneous causes of effects. As described earlier in the hierarchy of designs, other designs have reduced internal validity. External validity refers to the ability to permit inferences or generalisations about effects beyond the groups and contexts where interventions are tested. Experimental studies conducted with highly selected groups which may not be representative of the wider population and conducted with a degree of control which cannot be readily achieved in other situations have lowered external validity. Quasi-experimental studies, on the other hand, which lose some internal validity gain in external validity.

Research methods score differently on validity and reliability measures and decisions have to be made about what is most desired from an evaluation study. With an innovative and possibly complex intervention that would be costly to implement widely it may be important to opt for internal validity in the first instance to assess whether efficacy can be secured in the most advantageous circumstances. When it is important to know how effective something is within natural circumstances of implementation it becomes important to give greater emphasis to external validity. Where reliability is concerned those designs where the researcher has greater control over methods which can be implemented uniformly have the greater reliability. In general, methods generating quantitative data have higher reliability than those generating qualitative data.

## Interpretations of findings

These relate to the methodology adopted in the evaluation study and the constraints which govern interpretation within each approach. Within the positivist tradition there is a particular issue, noted earlier, that does not always receive the amount of attention that it should in study reports. This is the issue of the practical and policy significance of findings in comparison with their statistical significance. Systematic reviewers of health promotion have noted the small amount of consideration that is given to this issue in most published papers. In general, it can be said that while studies can generate highly significant findings in a statistical sense the findings

may be of little significance in a policy sense. Rossi *et al.* (1979) stressed that, ideally, the magnitude of change to be regarded as policy significant should be explicated as a part of the design of an evaluation. At the time they conceded that this was not often done. They also stated that it was important that all statistically significant differences should not be regarded as meaningful from a policy and planning decision making perspective. At the point at which statistical significant difference has been established between an intervention and a control group at a pre-specified level of significance a further question has to be asked. While it may be fair to say that this point is accepted in health promotion it is also clear that attention to practical significance in published literature does not appear to have increased significantly in the period since Rossi *et al.* made their comments. It may be assumed by some writers that readers can extrapolate for themselves from statistical to policy significance, but this is not necessarily the case.

In making interpretations further questions have to be asked about whether there were any aspects of the design and implementation of the evaluation study which could have biased outcomes in any way and the extent to which results are generalisable beyond the evaluation situation. Generalisability is dependent on establishing that the sample of people involved in an evaluation are representative of the population to which results are to be translated and that appropriate methods have been used in the data collection. As noted above, in the discussion of internal and external validity, experimental studies may often be undertaken with highly selected and often volunteer population groups which are not representative. Studies of the survey type using random samples of populations may be lower on internal validity but, alternatively, can score higher on external validity.

While we may have statistically significant results which it is agreed can be generalised the results may still lack policy significance. What amounts to policy significance is a matter of debate – a small difference which can be achieved across a wide population with relatively low input of resources may be adequate in some cases. On the other hand, a larger difference which would require a heavy input of resources to achieve success outside a research evaluation context may not be policy significant. The social worth of a change is also to be taken into consideration – a programme that made a small change in an aspect of health inequalities where achieving change is particularly difficult could be considered as policy significant. A further issue which is raised by Rossi *et al.* (1979) is the testing of interventions designed for wider implementation without sufficient understanding of how the policy issues are seen by decision makers who would have to implement a programme. To take the inequalities example, if an effective intervention required a redistribution of resources which would be politically risky this might not be enacted. Finally, the writers propose that to maximise the utility of evaluation findings to policy makers evaluators need to be sensitive to such considerations on two levels.

- First, the design of the evaluation should reflect policy considerations and be sensitive to relevant policy issues. Important issues need better evaluations than trivial issues. Technical decisions, such as the setting of statistical levels of significance, should be informed by policy considerations.
- Second, evaluation findings have to be assessed according to their generalisability, whether the findings are policy significant and whether the programme clearly fits with needs.

(Rossi *et al.*, 1979 p293)

In addition, it is important to recognise that even where evidence that appears to be policy significant is available this does not necessarily lead to its use. The ways that evidence is used in the policy making process has been examined more fully since the earlier lack of impact was noted in the 1960s. As noted by Whitelaw and Williams (1994), any notion of policy making being remotely 'rational' has been fundamentally challenged and 'policy making is seen as inherently chaotic and value oriented. It becomes necessary, therefore, to consider the kinds of research findings which are likely to have the most effect in

policy contexts and the ways that such findings should be made available in order to achieve their greatest effect. Whitelaw and Williams provide a valuable discussion of this issue.

The discussion above is taken very much from the perspective of an evaluator(s) making the interpretations. In those evaluations where there has been a commitment to participatory approaches or to a full-blown constructivist approach the development of interpretations will be a collaborative process. Labonte and Robertson (1996) comment on this commitment for practitioners:

> to ensure that all evaluation findings, whether quantitatively or qualitatively expressed, are interpreted by all stakeholders: practitioners, citizens, agencies, and funders. This interpretation should lead to a consensus on the best (whether that is in terms of most relevant or most appropriate) explanation for the effects of the program. This interpretation should also be subject to validity tests through hard questioning by others outside of the program process.

**Communicating findings and writing up reports**
Some evaluations may be completed and final reports written prior to communication of any findings within the project itself. This is most likely to be the style when experimental designs are used. In other styles, depending on the degree of ongoing communication between evaluators and project participants, there will be opportunities for sharing interim findings and reflections on projects. This may be held to be important in most health promotion evaluation. Early sharing of reflections ensures that the final report does not come as a 'bolt from the blue'. Where the ongoing style has been a collaborative one reports may, to varying extents, be joint productions.

Completion of evaluation reports is typically tightly time constrained and reports also need to be written up in ways that are required by the sponsors of an evaluation. This may not be in a style which is ideal for programme participants and this raises questions of the number of reports produced and their respective formats. The content of projects and the care with which material has to be written up poses particular demands in evaluation research. Evaluators can build up good relationships with project participants and it can be difficult to include material in reports which appears to fall short of full endorsement of a project. Evaluators have to remember that they have typically been employed to provide an objective and detached report of a project. The ways that information is reported can ensure that self-esteem is not damaged. As Schiroyama *et al.* (1995) point out:

> *Evaluators have a responsibility to draw constructive conclusions and project imple-mentors have a responsibility to receive even negative comments in a spirit of learning by mistakes. Achieving this level of openness, trust and positive working is a challenge to all involved in evaluation.*

A specific concern is the maintenance of confidentiality. In qualitative studies incorporation of quotations has to be done in such a way that they cannot be directly attributed unless this has been checked out. With small projects where a limited number of people are involved Finch (1986) pointed out that total anonymity can probably never be agreed. Issues of confidentiality have been particularly addressed with reference to relative power in evaluation contexts and arguments made that protection is most important with the least powerful. Finch goes on to say:

> *such considerations can be at least partially suspended in research on the powerful, who already have the means whereby they can protect themselves and in a real sense are 'fair game'.*

(Finch, 1986 p207)

### Ethical concerns

Ethical considerations run through all stages of an evaluation and have been alluded to above. It is useful to bring these together and comment separately. At the outset it can be wrong to take on an evaluation which is insufficiently resourced for questions to be answered adequately. The expec-tations of project participants that a thorough and fair appraisal will be undertaken would be inappropriate. Sponsors of an evaluation may be asking questions which cannot be met and these have to be recognised and challenged. To demand evaluation in terms of health outcomes is wrong if the project has not understood this from the start or has not been resourced in such a way that such gains could be achieved. Ethical concerns have emerged strongly in debates about methodology. For example, there is the view that it is actually wrong, in a health promotion project, to randomly assign individuals in the context of an experimental design and that the right way to proceed is through participatory approaches with full use of qualitative methods. This can be challenged where the long-term aim of achieving health gain may be better achieved with the use of methods which generate strong evidence of a type which will persuade policy makers and others. While we may have reservations about the evidence from certain types of studies, if such evidence will provide the basis for gaining further support we have to take care in rejecting such evidence. At times evaluators can gain knowledge from their contact with a project which generates concerns not directly related to the objectives of the evaluation. For example, a project which is working effectively on one area of health may, inadvertently, be impacting negatively in other areas. Evaluators have some duty to bring such matters to the attention of a project but it is debatable whether they form part of a final report in a fully explicit way. Concerns have been raised about situations where an evaluation report might impact negatively on the individuals involved or even on a whole social group. Finch (1986 p207) raised this issue following an evaluation of play groups where she felt than her findings might confirm particular stereotypes about working class parents. Kelly has examined ethical concerns about pursuing her own values – those of a feminist researcher – in conducting an *Action Research* study in schools (Kelly 1989). Finally, there are ethical considerations in witholding evidence of lack of impact of an intervention or of negative outcomes resulting from interventions.

## Dissemination of findings

As we noted at the beginning of the chapter, evaluations are undertaken for a variety of reasons and these will influence the commitment to wider dissemination and the nature of activities adopted. Experimental and quasi-experimental projects which have been initiated to assess the efficacy and effectiveness of interventions and are of appropriate quality are likely to be published in mainstream journals. Commissioned evaluations of extensive projects such as *Health Promoting Schools* which may use survey approaches or qualitative research methods also often appear as published reports. A significant proportion of health promotion evaluation activity is, however, of smaller scale projects which may be externally or internally evaluated and are written up in reports which are retained within projects or disseminated only in a limited way. Where the prime motivation of evaluation research is to seek evidence on which to develop improvements to a specific project some case can be made for restricted circulation. However, it can also be argued that any evaluation probably includes insights that would be valuable to people working in comparable projects and wider dissemination could make a contribution to improving practice. There is now a more explicit emphasis on the importance of dissemination and on dissemination which is appropriate to all potential users. There are two general, but overlapping, levels at which dissemination needs to be addressed: the dissemination of individual projects at the point of completion and the dissemination of accumulated evidence on specific areas of health promotion.

Where individual projects are concerned the nature and scale of evaluation research projects will vary considerably, but where evaluation is commissioned externally the normal procedure is the production of a final report. The audience for this report needs to be agreed. Where projects have adopted a participatory approach towards evaluation there were will be greater concerns about communicating the results of an evaluation to all stakeholders than in a strictly controlled experimental style evaluation. A decision has to be taken about the nature and forms of outputs to be generated and the nature of dissemination activities.

The dissemination of accumulated evidence on specific areas of health promotion goes on in a number of ways. The evidence from systematic reviews, for example, can be available in a full report form, through conference presentations, through workshops, via the Internet, in papers in academic journals and professional journals and through *Effectiveness Bulletins* of the type published by the Centre for Reviews and Dissemination, press releases and any further methods deemed appropriate. The limitations of paper-based dissemination are recognised, although these still predominate. This is often because resource considerations preclude the use of more varied approaches. Blackburn *et al.* (1997), in disseminating findings from an evaluation of women's smoking, included a dissemination phase to their project which would enable them to make available key findings to health practitioners and to evaluate this process. They used a user-friendly information pack which distilled research findings in ways that were relevant to practice. Positive conclusions were drawn about the method used which appeared to offer an appropriate model for disseminating research-based information. The authors emphasised the need for researchers to have a detailed understanding of the context of specific professional practice in order to achieve effective dissemination.

## Skills for evaluation

At the beginning of the chapter we asked the question about whether evaluation research differed from other types of research. We did not accept the notion of its separate nature. We can, however, in supporting the idea that there are, nonetheless, distinctive emphases to evaluation research consider whether skills for such research are in any way particular. In terms of setting research questions, selecting methodologies and designing interventions general research skills should be transferable. At the same time, there are specific elements of evaluation research which require additional skills which may not necessarily have been fully provided in earlier training. The more a project moves towards a tightly designed controlled experimental study the less some of these additional skills may be required. Most health promotion evaluation is not of this type and the additional skills are of particular importance. Skills will, in part, relate to the stage of a project. They will include the following.

- *Communication*. The capacity to communicate effectively with the range of stakeholders in a project.
- *Negotiation*. Needed at the stage of setting research questions, agreeing elements of design, gaining access to aspects of a project necessary to the answering of research questions.
- *Conflict management*. This can be called for at all stages of an evaluation study.
- *Assertiveness skills*. There can be considerable pressure not to report certain aspects of projects and it may be essential to do so if the agreed goals of an evaluation are to be met.
- *Writing skills*. Needed for all research but where there is a commitment to producing various outputs a wider range of writing styles is called upon. The capacity to ensure that a full picture of a project is provided in such a way that a project can learn from the evaluation and move forward rather than be discouraged by unnecessarily negative comment is also needed.
- Knowledge and understanding of the contexts in which dissemination is relevant and the skills to disseminate appropriately.

### Impact of evaluations

There have been many cynical observations in the literature about evaluation reports being filed away and making no impact on future practice. The more that evaluations are undertaken using a mix of methods and adopt participatory styles there is usually some impact of an evaluation at the project level during the actual evaluation process. This may not invariably be positive impact but in most cases of professionally carried out evaluation, notwithstanding instances of conflict, it can be. The evaluation report can feed into the continuing life of a project and it can influence similar practice elsewhere. The extent of influence will depend on the nature and type of evaluation study. Evidence from evaluations of health promotion activities is

increasingly being brought together and the aspiration of reviewers is that the evidence summarised will be drawn on in practice. This has been succinctly stated by Nutbeam (1996):

> *… to make continued progress in health promotion it is essential that lessons learned from research are more systematically applied to practice. Decision making should be based on the best available evidence concerning its effectiveness and it application in real life circumstances. How to improve the fit between research and practice has been a long standing dilemma in health promotion (and many other disciplines in the health and social sciences).*

Discussion of achieving evidence-based practice is beyond the scope of this chapter but this important issue is achieving active attention at the present time and an effective health care bulletin *Getting Evidence into Practice* in health care was published in 1999. This included the following conclusions.

- While individual beliefs, attitudes and knowledge influence professional behaviour, other factors including the organisational, economic and community environments of the practitioner are also important.
- A range of interventions have been shown to be effective in changing professional behaviours in some circumstances. Multi-faceted interventions targeting different barriers to change are more likely to be effective than single interventions.

The outcomes of evaluations are often expected to be influential on current and future policy making. There has frequently been the assumption that policy making is a rational process and where relevant evidence is available this will be used. As noted earlier, the way that evidence is used is now conceived of as a more complex process.

## CONCLUSIONS

This chapter has sought to examine some of the current debates about evaluation and relate these to evaluation research in health promotion. It has also dealt briefly with some of the practical challenges that relate to the different stages of an evaluation process. The chapter has, of necessity, had to be selective, but a number of the matters discussed will receive further discussion in other chapters and in the Conclusions.

The 51st World Health Assembly urged member states to:

> *adopt an evidence based approach to health promotion policy and practice, using the full range of quantitative and qualitative methodologies.*

> (WHO, 1998b)

There is a growing consolidation of views in some countries about the ways health promotion evaluation should be undertaken, which the World Health Organization is reflecting. At the same time there continues to be a healthy diversity of views about health promotion and its evaluation and this needs to be recognised. At one end of a spectrum there will be some who reject any use of positivist and post-positivist approaches to research and evaluation in health promotion and at the other end those who would argue that health promotion's development and acceptance would best be served by the building up of a strong evidence base using positivist studies designed for such a purpose. Somewhere in the middle is a consensus that evaluation research studies should be relevant to the questions being asked and in many cases a combination of quantitative and qualitative data might best meet the needs of stakeholders and generate the most comprehensive account of a project.

The discipline is relatively young and it can be argued that it is premature to be too prescriptive about what should or should not constitute health promotion evaluation. The particular nature of health promotion interventions needs to be borne in mind when considering appropriate forms of evaluation. As Nutbeam (1999) has said:

> *It is a challenge to assemble 'evidence' in ways which are relevant to the complexities of contemporary health promotion, and to*

> *avoid the possibility that this may lead action down a narrow reductionist route.*

Strong commitment to the key principles articulated in the Ottawa Charter, including the commitment to community participation in research, will privilege the choice of particular evaluation designs and practice. For example, case studies strongly informed by interpretivist approaches are favoured in some studies of healthy settings. Designs informed by critical theory are probably most in harmony with the emancipatory goals of health promotion (Vanderplaat, 1995; Poland, 1996). At the same time it is clear that *Realist* evaluation and *Theory of Change* models are increasingly being seen as relevant to evaluation of complex interventions which typify much health promotion.

Despite strong reservations about some evaluation methods in working to achieve the ultimate goals of health promotion the best strategy may sometimes be to draw on a variety of evidence, including that from pure and quasi-experimental studies. For example Fraser *et al.* (1995), in reviewing quantitative evaluations of health promotion, remind us that:

> *carefully used, they can lead to greater understanding of important issues and provide evidence on which to base future policy and practice.*

Given the purpose of the book and the wide variety of activities that are contained within the concept of health promotion we will draw on evidence from all types of study as we examine the effectiveness of interventions in selected settings in the remaining chapters.

## REFERENCES

Armstrong, D. (1983) *Political Anatomy of the Body: Medical Knowledge in Britain in the 20th Century.* Cambridge University Press, Cambridge.

Basler, H. D., Brinkmeier, U., Buser, K. and Gluth, G. (1991) *Nicotine gum assisted group therapy in smokers with an increased risk of coronary disease – evaluation in a primary care setting. Health Education Research*, 7 (1), 87–96.

Benson, K. and Hartz, J. A. (2000) *A comparison of observational studies and randomised controlled trials. The New England Journal of Medicine*, 342 (25), 1878–1886.

Bhaskar, R. (1975) *A Realist Theory of Science.* Harvester, Brighton.

Blackburn, C., Graham, H. and Scullion, P. (1997) *Disseminating research findings on women's smoking to health practitioners: findings from an evaluation study. Health Education Journal*, 56, 113–124.

Blaikie, N. W. H. (1991) *A critique of the use of triangulation in research. Quality and Quantity*, 25, 115–136.

Boulton, M. (1994) *The methodological imagination.* In M. Boulton (Ed.) *Challenge and Innovation, Methodological Advances in Social Research on HIV/AIDS.* Taylor and Francis, London.

Broughton, W. (1991) *Qualitative methods in program evaluation. American Journal of Health Promotion*, 5 (6), 461–464.

Bulmer, M. (1982) *The Use of Social Research: Social Investigations in Public Policy Making.* Allen and Unwin, London.

Campbell, D. T. and Stanley, J. C. (1963) *Experimental and Quasi-Experimental Designs for Research.* Rand-McNally, Chicago, IL.

Catford, J. (1993) *Editorial. Auditing health promotion: what are the vital signs of quality? Health Promotion International*, 8(2), 67–68.

Chalmers, A. F. (1982) *What is This Thing Called Science?, 2nd edn.* Open University Press, Milton Keynes.

Cochrane, A. (1972) *Effectiveness and Efficiency: Random Reflections on Health Services.* Nuffield Provincial Hospitals Trust, London.

Cochrane Collaboration (1993) *Introductory Brochure.* UK Cochrane Centre, Oxford.

Cohen, L. and Manion, L. (1994) *Research Methods in Education, 4th edn.* Routledge, London.

Davies, J. and Cooke, S. (1998) *Parents as partners for educational change.* In B. Atweh, S. Kemmis and P. Weeks (Eds) *Action Research in Practice.* Routledge, London.

Denzin, N. (1970) *The Research Act in Sociology.* Butterworths, London.

Dickerson, K., Scherer, R. and Lefebvre, C. (1994) *Identification of relevant studies for systematic reviews. British Medical Journal*, 309, 1286–1291.

Dockery, G. (2000) *Participatory research: whose roles, whose responsibilities?* In C. Truman, D. M. Mertens and B. Humphries (Eds) *Research and Inequality.* UCL Press, London,.

Eisner, E. W. (1985) *The Art of Educational Evaluation.* Falmer Press, London.

Everitt, A. and Hardiker, P. (1996) *Towards a Critical Approach to Evaluation.* Macmillan, London.

Finch, J. (1984) *"It's great to have someone to talk to". The ethics and politics of interviewing women.* In C. Bell and H. Roberts (Eds) *Social Researching: Politics, Problems and Practice.* Routledge and Kegan Paul, London.

Finch, J. (1986) *Research and Policy: The Uses of Qualitative Methods in Social and Educational Research.* Falmer Press, London.

Fraser, E., Bryce, C., Crosswaite, C., McCann, K. and Platt, S. (1995) *Evaluating health promotion: doing it by numbers. Health Education Journal*, 54, 214–225.

Freire, P. (1972) *Pedagogy of the Oppressed.* Penguin, Harmondsworth.

Green, J. (2000) *The role of theory in evidence based health promotion practice. Health Education Research*, 15 (1), 125–129.

Green, L. W. and Lewis, F. M. (1986) *Measurement and Evaluation in Health Education and Health Promotion.* Mayfield, Palo Alto, CA.

Guba, E. G. and Lincoln, Y. (1989) *Fourth Generation Evaluation.* Sage, Newbury Park, CA.

Guba, E. G. and Lincoln, Y. S. (1998) *Competing paradigms in qualitative research.* In N. K. Denzin and Y. S. Lincoln (Eds) *The Landscape of Qualitative Research: Theories and Issues.* Sage, London.

Habermas, J. (1972) *Knowledge and Human Interests.* Heinemann, London.

Harper, G. W. and Carver, L. J. (1999) *'Out of the mainstream' youth as partners for collaborative resarch: exploring the benefits and challenges. Health Education and Behaviour*, 26 (2), 250–265.

Harre, R. (1972) *The Philosophies of Science.* Blackwell, Oxford.

Harvey, L. (1990) *Critical Social Research.* Unwin-Hyman, London.

Hawe, P. (1993) *Capturing the meaning of 'community' in community intervention evaluation: some contributions from community psychology. Health Promotion International*, 9 (3), 199–210.

Hawe, P. and Stickney, E. K. (1997) *Developing the effectiveness of an intersectoral food policy coalition through formative evaluation. Health Education Research*, 12 (2), 213–226.

Hayes, M. V. and Manson-Willms, S. (1990) *Healthy community indicators: the perils of the search and the paucity of the find. Health Promotion International*, 5 (2), 161–166.

Hodgson, R. and Abbasi, T. (1995) *Effective Mental Health Promotion: Literature Review*, Technical Report 13. Health Promotion Wales.

Hosman, C. M. H. and Veltman, N. E. (1994) *Prevention in Mental Health: A Review of Effectiveness of Health Education and Health Promotion*. Landelijk Centrum GVO, Utrecht.

House, E. R. (1993) *Professional Evaluation*. Sage, Newbury Park, CA.

Institute for the Study of Drug Dependence (1982) *Facts and Feelings About Drugs But Decisions About Situations*. ISDD, London.

Kaneko, M. (1999) *A methodological inquiry into the evaluation of smoking cessation programmes. Health Education Research*, 14 (3), 433–441.

Keat, R. and Urry, J. (1975) *Social Theory as Science*. Routledge, London.

Kelly, A. (1989) *Education or indoctrination? The ethics of school based action research*. In R. G. Burgess (Ed.) *The Ethics of Educational Research*. Falmer Press, London.

Kemmis, S. and McTaggart, R. (1988) *The Action Research Planner, 3rd edn*. Deakin University Press, Geelong.

Kippax, S. and Van den Ven, P. (1998) *An epidemic of orthodoxy? Design and methodology in the evaluation of the effectiveness of HIV health promotion. Critical Public Health*, 8 (4), 371–386.

Klein, D., Williams, D. and Witbrodt, J. (1999) *The collaboration process in HIV prevention and evaluation in an urban American Indian clinic for women. Health Education and Behaviour*, 26 (2), 239–249.

Kuhn, T. (1970) *The Structure of Scientific Revolutions*. University of Chicago Press, Chicago, IL.

Labonte, R. and Robertson, A. (1996) *Delivering the goods, showing our stuff: the case for a constructivist paradigm for health promotion research and practice. Health Education Quarterly*, 23 (4), 431–447.

Lawton, D. (1980) *The Politics of the School Curriculum*. Routledge and Kegan Paul, London.

Lewin, K. (1946) *Action research and minority problems. Journal of Social Issues*, 2 (4), 34–46.

Lyotard, J. (1984) *The Postmodern Condition: A Report on Knowledge*. Manchester University Press, Manchester.

Mason, J. (1996) *Qualitative Researching*. Sage, London.

Mays, N. and Pope, C. (1995) *Rigour and qualitatitve research. British Medical Journal*, 311, 109–112.

McQueen, D. (1986) *Health education research: the problem of linkages. Health Education Research*, 1 (4), 289–294.

Milburn, K., Fraser, E., Secker, J. and Pavis, S. (1995) *Combining methods in health promotion research: some considerations about appropriate use. Health Education Journal*, 54, 347–356.

Muir Gray, J. A. (1997) *Evidence Based Health Care*. Churchill Livingstone, Edinburgh.

NHS Centre for Reviews and Dissemination (1996) *Undertaking Systematic Reviews on Research and Effectiveness: CRD Guidelines for Those Carrying Out and Commissioning Reviews*. NHS CRD, University of York, York.

NHS Centre for Reviews and Dissemination (1999) *Preventing the Uptake of Smoking in Young People*, vol. 5. University of York, York.

Nutbeam, D. (1996) *Achieving 'best practice' in health promotion: improving the fit between research and practice. Health Education Research*, 11, 317–326.

Nutbeam, D. (1998) *Evaluating health promotion – progress, problems and solutions. Health Promotion International*, 13 (1), 27–44.

Nutbeam, D. (1999) *The challenge to provide 'evidence' in health promotion. Health Promotion International*, 14 (2), 99–101.

Nutbeam, D., Smith, S., Murphy, S. and Catford, J. (1993) *Maintaining evaluation designs in long term community based health promotion programmes: Heartbeat Wales case study. Epidemiology and Community Health*, 47, 127–133.

Oakley, A. (1981) *Interviewing women: a contradiction in terms*. In H. Roberts (Ed.) *Doing Feminist Research*. Routledge, London.

Oakley, A. (1990) *Who's afraid of the randomised controlled trial? Some dilemmas of the scientific method and good research practice*. In H. Roberts (Ed.) *Women's Health Counts*. Routledge, London.

Oakley, A. (1998) *Experimentation in social science: the case of health promotion. Social Sciences in Health*, 4 (2), 73–89.

Oakley, A. and Fullerton, D. (1996) *The lamp post of research: support or illumination? The case for and against randomised control trials*. In A. Oakley and

H. Roberts (Eds) *Evaluating Social Interventions*. Barnados, Ilford.

Oliver, S., Peersman, G., Harden, A. and Oakley, A. (1999) *Discrepancies in findings from effectiveness reviews: the case of health promotion for older people in accident and injury prevention. Health Education Journal*, 58, 66–77.

Oxman, A. D. (1994) *Section VI: Preparing and maintaining systematic reviews. In The Cochrane Collaboration Handbook*. Cochrane Collaboration, Oxford.

Parlett, M. and Hamilton, D. (1972) *Evaluation as illumination: a new approach to the study of innovatory programmes*, Occasional Paper 9. Centre for Research in Educational Sciences, University of Edinburgh.

Pawson, R. and Tilley, N. (1997) *Realistic Evaluation*. Sage.

Peersman, G., Harden, A., Oliver, S. and Oakley, A. (1999) *Discrepancies in findings from effectiveness reviews: the case of health promotion to change cholesterol levels. Health Education Journal*, 58, 192–202.

Perry, C. I., Kelder, S. H. and Klepp, K. (1994) *Community wide cardiovascular prevention in young people: long term outcomes of the Class of 89 study. European Journal of Public Health*, 4, 188–194.

Poland, B. (1992) *Learning to 'walk our talk' the implications of sociological theory for research methodologies in health promotion. Canadian Journal of Public Health*, Suppl. 1, S31–S46.

Poland, B. D. (1996) *Knowledge development and evaluationin, of and for Healthy Community iniatives. Part 1: guiding principles. Health Promotion International*, 11 (3), 237–247.

Pollitt, C. (1999) *Stunted by stakeholders? Limits to collaborative evaluation. Public Policy and Administration*, 14 (2), 77–90.

Popay, J., Rogers, A. and Williams, G. (1998) *Rationale and standards for the systematic review of qualitative literature in health services research. Qualitative Health Research*, 8 (3), 341–351.

Popper, C. (1959) *The Logic of Scientific Discovery*. Hutchinson, London.

Rabinow, P. (Ed.) (1984) *The Foucault Reader*. Penguin Books, Harmondsworth.

Rawson, D. (1992) *The growth of health promotion theory and its rational reconstruction: lessons from the philosophy of science*. In R. Bunton and G.

Macdonald (Eds) *Health Promotion Disciplines and Diversity*. Routledge, London.

Rossi, P. H., Freeman, H. E. and Wright, S. R. (1979) *Evaluation: A Systematic Approach*. Sage, London.

Sackett, D. Rosenberg, W., Muir Gray, J. A., Haynes, B. and Richardson, S. (1996) *Evidence-based medicine: what it is and what it isn't. British Medical Journal*, 312, 71–72.

Schiroyama, C., McKee, L. and McKie, L. (1995) *Evaluating health promotion projects in primary care: recent experiences in Scotland. Health Education Journal*, 54, 226–240.

Schwandt, T. A. (1998) *Constructivist, interpretivist approaches to human inquiry*. In N. K. Denzin and Y. S. Lincoln (Eds) *The Landscape of Qualitative Research, Theories and Issues*. Sage, London.

Scott, D. (1998) In D. Scott and R. Weston (Eds) *Evaluating Health Promotion*. Stanley Thornes, Cheltenham.

Secker, J., Wimbush, E., Watson, J. and Milburn, K. (1995) *Qualitative methods in health promotion research: some criteria for quality. Health Education Journal*, 54, 74–87.

Silverman, D. (1985) *Qualitative Methodology and Sociology*. Gower, Aldershot.

Simons, H. (1989) *Ethics of case study in educational research and evaluation*. In R. G. Burgess (Ed.) *The Ethics of Educational Research*. Falmer Press, New York, NY.

South, J. and Tilford, S. (2000) *Perceptions of research and evaluation in health pormotion practice and influences on activity. Health Education Research*, 15 (6), 729–741.

Speller, V. (1998) *Quality assurance programmes: their development and contribution to improving effectiveness in health promotion*. In D. Scott and R. Weston (Eds) *Evaluating Health Promotion*. Stanley Thornes, Cheltenham.

Speller, V., Learmonth, A. and Harrison, D. (1997) *The search for evidence of effective health promotion. British Medical Journal*, 315, 361–363.

Springett, J. and Dugdill, L. (1995) *Workplace health promotion programmes: towards a framework for evaluation. Health Education Journal*, 54, 88–98.

Thompson, J. C. (1992) *Program evaluation within a health promotion framework. Canadian Journal of Public Health*, Suppl. 1, S67–S71.

Tilford, S. (1982) *Implementation of SHEP 13-18 in Leeds schools*, unpublished report. Leeds Polytechnic, Leeds.

Tilford, S. and Delaney, F. (1992) *Editorial: Qualitative research in health education. Health Education Research*, 7 (4), 451–455.

Tilford, S. and Delaney, F. (1995) *Assessing the effects of mental health promotion interventions; methodological and substantive concerns*, paper presented at the IUHE Conference on Quality and Effectiveness, Turin.

Tilford, S., Delaney, F. and Vogels, M. (1997) *Effectiveness of Mental Health Promotion Interventions: A Review*. Health Education Authority, London.

Tilford, S., Godfrey, C., White, M., Nicholson, F. and South, J. (1998) *Evidence based health promotion: commissioning interventions for the prevention of smoking in young people*, unpublished report.

Tilford, S., Errington, R. and Nicholds, A. (2000) *Evaluation of Leeds Occupational Health Project*. Centre for Health Promotion Research, Leeds Metropolitan University, Leeds.

Tones, B. K. (1997) *Editorial: Beyond the randomised controlled trial: a case for judicial review. Health Education Research*, 12 (2), i–iii.

Tones, B. K. (2000) *Evaluating health promotion: a tale of three errors. Patient Education and Counseling*, 39, 227–236.

Vanderplaat, M. (1995) *Beyond technique: issues in evaluating for empowerment. Evaluation*, 1 (1), 81–96.

Van de Ven, P. and Aggleton, P. (1999) *What constitutes evidence in HIV/AIDS education. Health Education Research*, 14 (4), 46–472.

van Driel, W. G. and Keijsers, J. F. E. M. (1997) *An instrument for reviewing the effectiveness of health education and health promotion. Patient Education and Counseling*, 30, 7–17.

Veen, C. A., Vereijken, I., van Driel, W. G. and Belien, M. A. (1994) *An Instrument for Analysing Effectiveness Studies on Health Education and Health Promotion*. Dutch Centre for Health Promotion and Health Education and IUHPE/EURO, Utrecht.

Vinokur, A. D., van Ryn, M., Gramlich, E. M. and Price, R. H. (1991) *Long term follow up and benefit-cost analysis of the jobs program: a preventive intervention for the unemployed. Journal of Applied Psychology*, 76 (2), 213–219.

Wallenstein, N. (1999) *Power between evaluator and community: research relationships within New Mexico's healthier communities. Social Science and Medicine*, 49, 39–53.

White, D. and Pitts, M. (1997) *Health Promotion with Young People for the Prevention of Substance Abuse*. HEA, London.

Whitelaw, A. and Williams, J. (1994) *Relating health education research to health policy. Health Education Research*, 9 (4), 519–526.

Wiggers, J. and Sanson-Fisher, R. (1998) Evidence based health promotion. In D. Scott and R. Weston (Eds) *Evaluating Health Promotion*. Stanley Thornes, Cheltenham.

Wimbush, E. and Watson, J. (2000) *An evaluation framework for health promotion: theory, quality and effectiveness. Evaluation*, 6 (3), 301–321.

WHO (1998a) *Health Promotion Evaluation: Recommendations to Policymakers*. WHO, Geneva.

WHO (1998b) *Fifty First World Health Assembly: Health Promotion*. WHO, Geneva.

Zuber-Skerritt, O. (1996) *Emancipatory action research for organisational change and management development*. In O. Zuber-Skerritt (Ed.) *New Directions in Action Research*. Falmer Press, London.

# PART TWO

# 4 SETTINGS AND STRATEGIES

This second part of the book will consider questions of effectiveness, efficiency and equity from the perspective of settings and strategies for health promotion. The term 'setting' refers to the context in which health promotion takes place. It may be a particular location, agency or organisation, such as family or workplace. On the other hand, it may be more informal and less tangible, such as the 'community'. The contemporary guiding principle for reviewing health promotion in settings is now termed a 'settings approach' and, as we will note below, this particular orientation is more than merely identifying a convenient location for accessing different population groups. A detailed review of the whole range of settings is beyond the scope of this book and we will content ourselves with illustrating the implications of a settings approach for reviewing effectiveness by considering the school, the health care context and the workplace.

The notion of strategy is somewhat vague. As used here it refers to the development of a plan designed to achieve certain valued goals or outcomes. It is considered to operate at a higher 'macro' level by comparison with 'methods' which are viewed as more specific. Methods are used as part of a strategic plan. For instance, methods such as face-to-face counselling or simulation and gaming would be used as part of a broader strategy to promote the personal and social development of young people. Practising effective non-verbal communication, by repetition and video feedback, would be used as part of a number of methods designed to provide health workers with 'reticulist' (networking!) skills that might be used as part of a strategy to develop inter-sectoral collaboration between different agencies in a health promoting coalition. For further discussion of the relationship between strategy and methods see Tones (1993) and comments in the *Introduction* to the 2nd Edition of this text.

In this book we view the employment of mass media as a strategic exercise rather than a setting – largely because of recommendations that mass media should be used in support of other, settings-based, approaches. Again, we could reasonably identify the process of inter-sectoral working and the establishment of coalitions as strategic operations which are not settings *per se* but have their own theoretical base and even ideological underpinning.

We will, in this chapter, explore further the nature and meaning of a 'settings approach'. However, before doing so some consideration will be given to an especially useful concept that has practical and theoretical significance for the identification and specification of particular settings for health promotion initiatives. The concept is generally known as a 'health career'.

## THE CONCEPT OF HEALTH CAREER

In brief, a health career analysis charts individuals' progress throughout their lifespan and notes the ways in which various factors over time cumulatively influence their health. The insights gained from this examination can help with the needs assessment stage of programme planning by providing insight into the nature and strength of earlier events, both acute and chronic, that have a bearing on the current state of 'readiness' for health promotion interventions. Secondly, by being able to anticipate future health damaging influences, anticipatory guidance can be provided and perhaps some degree of 'inoculation' against these negative influences. Thirdly, by identifying the sources of these various contributions to health – for good or ill – agencies and organisations might be enlisted as 'settings' for the provision of health promotion.

Perhaps the earliest use of a career line analysis for health promotion – certainly in the UK – is due to Baric, who applied a functionalist, sociological approach to the definition of health career and applied this *inter alia* to smoking (Baric, 1974). The theoretical underpinning of the approach centred on the construct of socialisation and the progress made by individuals in given cultures from one role to another over the lifespan. Figure 4.1 (Baric, 1996 p261) illustrates this progress schematically.

Figure 4.1 illustrates the progress of an individual in a Western culture as (s)he negotiates a series of transitions through childhood, via school entrance, through the process of higher education and/or work (or extended unemployment) through to retirement and, ultimately, death. At each stage 'socialisation agencies', such as the family, school and the workplace, exert a normative effect on individuals. As they proceed on their 'career' the nature and strength of these effects will vary and as the child grows older (s)he will be exposed to an ever-widening number of influences.

## Socialisation and the health career

The influences on a health career are best explained in terms of socialisation, i.e. the direct or indirect effects of social norms on individuals'

health-related behaviours and practices – and, importantly, their construction of the reality they experience in terms of knowledge and beliefs together with values and attitudes. As Mussen *et al.* (1974) put it, *Socialisation is the process by which the individual acquires those behaviour patterns, beliefs, standards and motives that are valued by, and appropriate in his own cultural group and family.*

Primary socialisation is the term applied to the early influence of the home, parents and close kith and kin. It is usually a relatively informal set of procedures – often characterised by Skinnerian conditioning in that parents reward or punish their children for developing desirable or undesirable attitudes and practices; they also offer models of behaviours which may or may not be health promoting! Children internalise parental values – which traditionally also reflect local/sub-cultural norms. According to many decades of developmental psychology, the process of primary socialisation can be dramatically powerful and, according to the so-called *Law of Primacy*, influences occurring during these early years are both deep-seated and enduring.

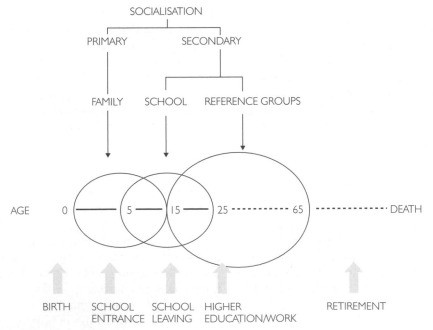

**Figure 4.1** Socialisation and the Health Career

**Box 1**  *A Law of Primacy*

> *Give me the child and I will give you the man*
> – Jesuit maxim relating to the first seven
> years of life and cited in the first publication
> of the influential cohort study directed by the
> National Children's Bureau (Davie *et al.*,
> 1972).

It is at this early stage that the foundations of
personality may be dramatically shaped and the
'starting position' established for individuals'
future health-related behaviour – for instance, not
only early influences on future respiratory capability but perceptions of the normality of smoking; not only taste preferences for sugar and salt,
for example, but also attitudes to food.

Secondary socialisation, on the other hand,
refers to the concerns of more formal agencies to
instil values and interpretations of what is or is
not important to the life of a particular culture or
community. It is wrong to think of the school, for
instance, as a neutral purveyor of knowledge: the
very act of developing and teaching a particular
curriculum involves a selection from culture. The
curriculum is socially constructed. In addition to
greater formality, secondary socialisation agents
are (usually) less emotionally involved in the
process and outcomes.

The term 'anticipatory socialisation' is used by
Baric and others to refer to the commonly
observed process whereby individuals adopt
norms in anticipation of some future status (one
of the oft-cited motivations for the adoption of
smoking by adolescents 'precocity' or 'early anticipation of adulthood', provides an illustration of
this phenomenon). Again, the adoption of behaviours, values and attitudes attributed to members
of certain 'reference groups' is due to anticipatory
socialisation. It is not at all uncommon for young
people to ape the behaviours of groups to which
they aspire but to which they do not belong.

Finally, the notion of 're-socialisation' merely
describes attempts to reverse or change existing
normative behaviours; the often desperate
attempts of health promoters to persuade people

to change lifestyles rooted in earlier socialisation
offers a prime example of the phenomenon!

**Box 2**  Socialisation and Social Control

> *Socialisation thus represents an important
> instrument of social control, by means of which
> societies ensure that the newly integrated
> individuals conform to social norms inherent
> in the institutions of the relevant society.*
> (Baric, 1996 p259)

## The power of social norms

A belief in the power of social norms is central to
Baric's earlier discussions of health career (see for
example Baric, 1975; Baric *et al.*, 1976). In short,
it is assumed that individuals will not merely be
governed by internalised normative pressures but
may also be controlled by external pressures. This
view, of course, reflects assertions made in Chapter
2 about the contribution of the *normative system*
on individuals' intentions to act. However, Baric's
view of individuals progressing throughout life
from one status to another provided quite an interesting slant on normative pressure. The rationale is
as follows: when someone enters a given status –
e.g. pregnancy – they assume a role embodying a
number of expectations about what are appropriate or inappropriate behaviours and, indeed, the
kinds of value that are expected in respect of the
role. If individuals deviate to a greater or lesser
extent from the expectations associated with that
role, they will be subjected to normative 'sanctions'. These expectations, of course, may or may
not be judged appropriate by professionals – for
instance a cultural expectation that women should
eat for two would be judged as inappropriate by
paediatricians – on the premise that such a norm
may be virtually synonymous with maternal convictions that bonny babies bounce with obesity! On
the other hand, if it were possible to influence normative expectations to the extent that smoking and
alcohol consumption were a contradiction in terms
for pregnant women, the full force of sanctions
might dissuade women from smoking and drinking
while they were pregnant. Indeed, having inter-

nalised those norms, they would presumably not even contemplate the possibility. A similar point was made in Chapter 2 about the normative pressures on choice of infant feeding in a culture virtually totally dominated by breast feeding.

In terms of the dynamics of the *Health Action Model* we might on occasions witness an agonising conflict between addiction and normative pressure! Baric proceeds to take the discussion beyond the specific roles such as pregnancy and argues that if health education could create a generic 'at-risk' role it would only be necessary to ensure that people understood that they were indeed at risk (cf. the *Health Belief Model* notion of susceptibility) for normative pressures to 'kick in' (Baric, 1969).

## Health career and choice of settings

While retaining the valuable notion of socialisation, later applications of the health career tended to provide a more psychological and pedagogical perspective (see for example Tones, 1979, 1981). A major focus of this somewhat different formulation is twofold: (1) to argue that appropriate health education be made available to young people at the appropriate point on their health career; (2) to identify the range of possible settings for providing appropriate quality education. The first of these two imperatives was, of course, by no means new and educationists had long recognised the importance of devising a 'spiral curriculum'. In short, teaching should be provided on a given topic or in relation to a particular issue at an appropriately early point in the child's development and then subsequently re-visited on future occasions. During these later visits the subject matter might be presented in greater breadth or depth and, importantly, in a way appropriate to the child's developmental stage. The situation is particularly well illustrated by recommendations about the most appropriate means of teaching about sexuality: first (pre-school) answer honestly questions asked by children but at the appropriate level; secondly, focus on biological dimensions associated with reproduction but with some introduction to issues such as caring and responsibility; thirdly, focus on gender relationships; finally, discuss issues around contraception and different sexual orientations.

Of course, it is now a routine part of health promotion practice that the potential and actual role of settings should be integrated and coordinated in an effort to gain an accumulating critical mass of influence that will be difficult to resist. Figure 4.2, which has been used in the context of promoting sexual health (Green and Tones, 2000), describes the psychological–pedagogical dimensions of health career.

It will be noted that the career line is represented as a kind of multiple co-axial cable. This is intended to demonstrate the concentric series of influences on an individual that were described in Chapter 2 (indeed, the *Health Action Model* could be conceptualised as a cross-sectional analysis of a moment in time of an individual's health career). The central core represents a person's socialised values, attitudes, beliefs, etc.; peripheral layers relate to current normative effects from significant others and the internalisation of the normative effects of mass media and, of course, the material circumstances of a given culture or sub-culture that may channel an individual along a healthy or unhealthy career.

One final thought might be introduced at this point: if primary socialisation is so powerful, what hope is there for re-socialising people and directing them into a healthy life career? For those who feel despondent at the prospect implied by this query, we should make three observations: (1) there is increasing evidence that there is a two-way interaction between parent and child and it is not always clear who is manipulating whom!; (2) socialisation systems – even in totalitarian states – are frequently inefficient and there is, therefore, potential for change; (3) primary socialisation (like any socialisation) can be controlling or emancipatory. Indeed, it is possible to specify the kind of child rearing experience that would be empowering and salutogenic. On the other hand, consideration of the effects of really depowering and alienating environments should caution against false optimism. It is for these reasons that we argue for major policy initiatives to combat the effects of disadvantage and the importance of seeking to maximise the effects of health promotion by adopting a developmental perspective that utilises to the full the potential of a settings approach.

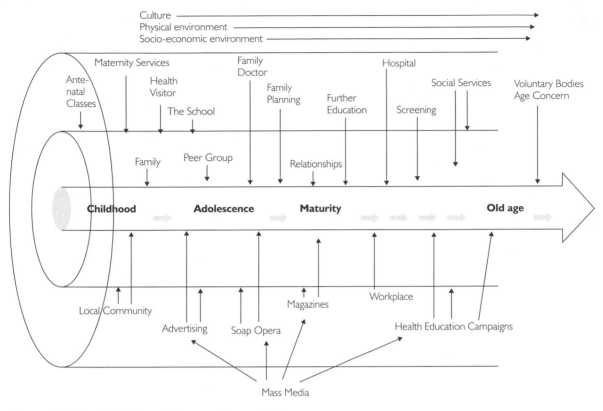

*Figure 4.2* The Health Career (Green and Tones, 2000)

---

**Box 3** Socialisation for Emancipation?

In addition to offering a geographical structure in which health promoters may operate, settings are socially constructed entities having a socialisation function. The curriculum of schools is a social construction rather than an objective list of all existing knowledge and unanimously agreed values. A setting may seek to shape the behaviour of its constituent individuals and agencies. The shaping process may be restrictive and conservative; alternatively, it may be radical, creative and emancipatory. The prime concern of health promotion within or without settings should also be radical and emancipatory.

## THE *SETTINGS APPROACH*

As indicated in our earlier reference to the applicability of the health career as a programme planning aid, health educators have always looked enviously at a number of settings and the opportunities they provide for accessing an at-risk group or target population. It was of course important to identify the peculiar characteristics of each setting before negotiating entry! Whitehead and Tones (1990), for example, identified five fundamental questions that should be borne in mind when considering how best to develop settings-based programmes (Box 4).

**Box 4**  Five Questions to be Addressed When Working in Settings

- *The question of access*
  What kind of target group is accessible through this setting ? How many people will be reached? How easy will it be to reach them?
- *The question of philosophy and purpose*
  Has the institution with which the strategy is associated a particular philosophy or goal?
- *The question of commitment*
  How committed are the institution and its members to the preventive philosophy underpinning the aims (of health education)?
- *The question of credibility*
  How credible are the institution and the people in it who will act as health educators? How will the public respond to them?
- *The question of competence*
  Irrespective of commitment, do the potential health educators have the necessary knowledge and communication/education/training skills needed to promote efficient learning?

  (after Whitehead and Tones, 1990 p19–20)

## Emergence of the *Settings Approach*

Although the five questions listed in Box 4 have practical value, the *Settings Approach* involves much more than merely delivering health education in, for example, school, workplace, hospital or (*a fortiori*) in the community. Its origins are generally considered to have emerged from the Lalonde Report – to which reference was made in Chapter 1. At a simple level a *Settings Approach* can be compared, in terms of strategic guidelines, with a focus on health issues or problems – or on particular population or 'target' groups. More significant, however, is the emphasis placed by the Ottawa Charter on '*creating supportive environments*' for developing a settings-based activity. The statement *Health is created and lived by people within the settings of their everyday life; where they learn, work, play*

*and love* … further legitimised, as it were, the discourse of the *Settings Approach* as something more than delivery in specific and convenient contexts and geographical locations (WHO, 1986 p2). The Ottawa Charter also suggests what is perhaps the easiest way of describing the key elements of a *Settings Approach* in its celebration of the centrality of 'healthy public policy'. This relates to the 'formula' mentioned in Chapter 1 that asserts that health promotion is essentially grounded in the multiplicative relationship between health education and healthy public policy. This relatively basic formulation is seen in Figure 4.3 (Tones, 1992), which provides a schematic representation of the curriculum of a health promoting school that emphasises the role of policy and education (teaching) in achieving empowering outcomes. Empowerment is mediated by the curricular domains of '*Lifeskills Teaching*' and '*Social Education*', which are considered necessary supplements to the traditional provision of '*Health Knowledge*'. '*Health Issues*' and '*Health Skills*' are at the interface between social education and 'lifeskills teaching', respectively and 'health knowledge'. Health knowledge is viewed as the provision of knowledge and understanding about factors relating directly to preventive outcomes.

Following Ottawa, the development of health promotion theory and strategy was paralleled by a continuing commitment by WHO to the *Settings Approach* and its progress into the 21st century was re-affirmed at the Jakarta Conference (WHO, 1998) together with its roots in the *Healthy Cities* movement.

It is reasonable to ask what differentiates a *Settings Approach* from other 'ideologically sound' and technically sophisticated health promotion projects. Apart from the inefficient strategy of using mass media without inter-personal support, such projects must clearly operate within some setting or other – or transcend the boundaries of settings. Is it a matter of focusing in on separate settings within an overall scheme to identify and specify their particular contribution to the whole? Is it mere convenience to simplify complexity by having circumscribed boundaries – either geographical or socio-cultural? Is it easier, as noted elsewhere, to use a location such as

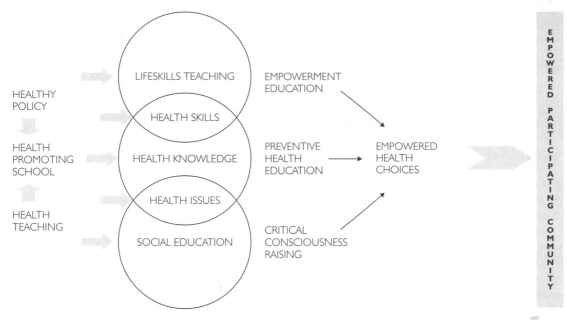

**Figure 4.3** PSHE and Citizen Empowerment

a city as a test-bed for key principles such as those embodied in the Ottawa Charter? What is the influence of relative size? For instance, a health promoting market would exist within a health promoting village or community which, in turn, might exist within a health promoting city.

Again, in principle, a number of cities could exist within a health promoting island – and, of course, some large countries (or even continents) are islands. Observations in the Report of the Jakarta Conference (WHO, 1998) help clarify these matters (see Box 5).

**Box 5** Healthy Cities/Villages/Islands/Communities

*Being started as a health promotion demonstration project in the European Region of WHO in 1986, the Healthy Cities initiative is now an established global movement. One of the very first agreements the participants established was that 'Healthy City' is the catch phrase for a wide variety of health promotion programmes related to larger scale contained living arrangements. Therefore, healthy islands, communities, and villages – in spite of their unique social and geographic set-ups – would all fall under the one slogan. The approach has become an umbrella for many other setting approaches, e.g. in schools, hospitals and market places. It contributes to the establishment of high quality physical infra-structures, psychosocial environment, and sustainability of health action. It effectively combines the 'art' and 'science' dimensions of public health, linking ideas, visions, political commitment and social entrepreneurship to the management of resources, methods for infrastructure development, and the establishment of procedures to respond to community needs. Intersectoral work is an integral part of the movement, with many partnerships already in place. Whatever the size of the target population (be they inhabitants of mega-cities or of small islands), the importance of action at the local level is identified as essential.*

(WHO, 1998 p4)

Galea *et al.*'s (2000) discussion of *Healthy Islands* in the Western Pacific provides further enlightenment. They refer to '*elemental*' settings by which they mean

> ... *one which is indivisible for the purpose of organizing meaningful health promotion and health protection programmes. This elemental setting can be described as having three characteristics:*

> - *it is small enough for its members to self identify as belonging to that setting and to engender a sense of one entity;*
> - *it has distinguishing social, cultural, economic and psychological peculiarities; and*
> - *it has a recognizable formal or informal administrative structure to which health promotion or health protection activities can link.*

Clearly the island setting is viewed as *relatively* small. It has the potential for the development of a sense of community. Health promotion within the setting will take account of and address the peculiar socio-economic, cultural and health needs of that community. Key features of the *Health Promoting Island* were identified in the Yanuca Island Declaration (WHO, 1995) and these are listed in Box 6.

**Box 6**  Healthy Islands

---

*Healthy islands should be places where:*

- *children are nurtured in body and mind;*
- *environments invite learning and leisure;*
- *people work and age with dignity;*
- *ecological balance is a source of pride.*

(Galea *et al.*, 2000)

---

A meeting of ministers at Rarotonga (WHO, 1997) identified a list of major goals to be addressed by *Healthy Islands*. These goals comprise an eclectic mix of different health outcomes that doubtless reveal their pedigree in developing countries' concerns within a context of primary health care. They look somewhat different from the typical 'process

goals' of *Healthy Cities* initiatives – although, of course, due acknowledgement is made of the Ottawa Principles. They are:

- adequate water supply and sanitation facilities;
- nutrition, food safety and food security;
- waste management;
- housing;
- human resources development;
- communicable and non-communicable disease prevention and control;
- lifestyle and quality of life issues;
- reproductive and family health;
- promotion of primary health care;
- social and emotional well-being;
- population issues;
- ecological sustainability; information management;
- tobacco or health;
- alcohol and substance abuse;
- environmental and occupational health.

(WHO, 1997 pp170–171)

## A perspective from Sundsvall

Sundsvall was the location for one of the major conferences following up Ottawa themes. Its central concern was the provision of 'supportive environments for health' – and, of course, a major purpose of the *Settings Approach* is just that – to provide environmental support for healthy actions. The Sundsvall statement (Pettersson *et al.*, 1992) notes that a supportive environment refers to both physical and social aspects of people's surroundings:

> *It encompasses where people live, their local community, their home, where they work and play. It also embraces the framework which determines access to resources for living, and opportunities for empowerment. Thus action to create supportive environments has many dimensions: physical, social, spiritual, economic and political. Each of these dimensions is inextricably linked to the others in a dynamic interaction.*

(p45)

In terms of the importance of research providing 'illumination', Sundsvall assembled some 171 'stories' illustrating the various conference themes. Three examples from the workplace, the hospital sector and an educational setting will be provided here in advance of more complete discussion in chapters to come. The first describes the first WHO 'healthy hospital' established in Vienna. Box 7 exemplifies the format of the Sundsvall stories in its categorisation system: Problem; Solution; Strategies; Outcomes.

**Box 7** A Healthy Hospital in Vienna

> *Problem*
> Stress among staff, unsatisfactory working conditions and occupational safety practices. Inadequate quality of services, shortage of space, inefficiency, dissatisfied patients, relatives and politicians.
>
> *Solution*
> Establishing a WHO model project *'Health and Hospitals'* to develop the concept of the *'Health Promoting Hospital'* and implement appropriate strategies, structures and procedures according to the Ottawa Charter of Health Promotion.
>
> *Strategies*
> Re-orienting the organisation, providing appropriate and essential services, empowering and enabling, mediating, mobilising resources, developing policy, and applying innovative approaches.
>
> *Outcomes*
> Higher quality of medical, nursing and social services, higher job satisfaction among staff, higher status and reputation of hospital, beginning of integration of the hospital into its regional environment, addressing more consciously the well-being of patients and relatives, and reorganising services, working practices, functions, space, etc.
>
> (after Haglund *et al.*, 1991 story 121)

A story from Indonesia makes reference to one of the key features of the *'Health Promoting*

*School'* – as we will see later. Two recognised settings are involved – the home and the school. It emphasises the importance of school and community links. In this case the school children act as 'outreach workers' – a notion that will be familiar to those who know the *Child-to-Child Project*. The 'strategies' listed in Box 8 encompass key principles of health promotion – and of the *Settings Approach*.

**Box 8** Children Teach Parents About Diarrhoea in Indonesia

> *Problem*
> Parents who were hard to reach through formal means needed information on how to prevent dehydration.
>
> *Solution*
> Children were prompted to teach parents the information about dehydration that they learned in school.
>
> *Strategies*
> * Building alliances (between school and families).
> * Empowerment (of children and their parents).
> * Mobilising resources (the children).
> * Re-orienting organisations (locally relevant information was added to the school's curriculum; children were prompted to be the 'teachers' instead of the learners).
>
> (after Haglund *et al.*, 1991 story 31)

The final example of a Sundsvall story is set in the workplace. It illustrates an important principle of health promotion – the use of research to stimulate social action together with advocacy, participation and community mobilisation. The Karolinska Institute in Stockholm collaborated with the University of Nicaragua to address the health problems of workers in a gold mine. As we will note in a later chapter, examples of radical health promotion programmes in the workplace are relatively rare – and this particular project is therefore of particular value.

**203**

**Box 9** A Swedish–Nicaraguan Project to Improve Miners' Health

---

*Problem*

Health problems among miners and their families in the mining community of El Limon, Nicaragua.

*Solutions*

Joint Swedish–Nicaraguan research project, community involvement in defining problems and solutions.

*Strategies*

Community involvement and mobilisation. By involving the community members, it was possible to rapidly design and implement several programmes to change the situation, e.g. focused intervention measures directed against hearing problems and lung disorders.

*Outcomes*

Results from the assessment of the health conditions of the miners and their families was the basis for formulating long-term health programmes. A local literacy campaign was started and the construction of houses, latrines and potable water projects was speeded up. Garbage disposal improved.

(after Haglund *et al.*, 1991 story 134)

---

## The *Healthy Cities* movement

In many ways the *Healthy Cities* initiative is the archetypal setting – both conceptually and chronologically. It paved the way for WHO's expansion into other settings such as school, hospital and workplace. A full discussion is beyond the scope of this chapter, but the venture has been fully examined elsewhere (see for example Hancock and Duhl, 1988; Kickbusch, 1989a, b; Tsouros, 1995; Duhl 1996; Flynn, 1996) As Mittelmark (1999) has observed in a lucid account, the period 1984–1986 was pivotal for the development of the project, which was conceived at a Canadian workshop concerned to improve the health of Toronto (Draper *et*

*al.*, 1993). Mittelmark reports how Duhl (1985) made one of the first formal presentations of the concept of a healthy city at a conference organised by the Canadian Public Health Association. The *Healthy Cities* initiative developed at sufficient pace to be ready to incorporate WHO's 38 European targets for health and to act as a test bed for applying the principles of the Ottawa Charter that were promulgated in 1986. Although now modified, the 38 targets are worth consideration – especially in the context of the emergent *Settings Approach*. They therefore appear in Appendix 5. At a Conference in Lisbon in 1986 representatives from 21 European cities discussed the development of the project and, according to Baric (1996) accepted a definition of health as

> *… a social rather than a narrowly medical concept, which meant that the improvements can only occur from a partnership of all the institutions and organisations, as well as the inhabitants, in a city.*

This focus on inter-sectoral working reflected the Ottawa conclusions and would become part of the principles incorporated in the settings approach generally.

The *Healthy Cities* project was formally established at the start of 1987 and 11 European cities became founding members of the 'WHO approved' network. By 1992 this had grown to over 500 cities in Europe and 300 cities in other parts of the world. Mittelmark assesses current (i.e. 1999) numbers as more than 1000 cities (see http://www.who.ch/peh/hlthcit/index.htm). A limited number of cities initially received WHO approval and 'entry to the club' depended on would-be members demonstrating a strong commitment towards the Ottawa Charter and *Health for All* principles together with a clear political commitment to develop and implement the *Healthy City* strategy. Cities must also show they were prepared to make available the necessary resources – financial and personnel – and would both support national developments and collaborate with the *Healthy City Network* internationally.

Tsouros (1990) emphasised the empowerment mission of the movement, as ... *a means of legitimizing, nurturing and supporting the process of community empowerment.*

Hancock (1993) asserted that the

*... three key elements relating to health are a positive model of health, an ecological model of health and a concern with health inequalities. The major elements concerned with strategies focus on process, public policy and community empowerment.*

(p14)

Hancock also notes that

*The most fundamental salutogens are of course such basic human needs as food, shelter, clean water, a safe environment and peace...*

He also observes that this

*... set of factors that are met almost entirely for the citizens of the Western industrialized cities, ... are still lacking for many who live in the cities of the less developed nations.*

He also refers to other desirable salutogenic factors such as, social networks, a sense of self-esteem, power and control over the events and conditions of one's life, income, a sustainable ecosystem. The relevance of these observations to

**Box 10**   Ten Criteria for a *Healthy City*

1 A clean, safe, high quality physical environment (including housing quality).
2 An ecosystem which is stable now and sustainable in the long term.
3 A strong and mutually supporting community with a high degree of participation and community control.
4 The meeting of basic human needs (for food, water, shelter, income, safety) for all the city's people.
5 Access to a wide variety of experiences and resources with the possibility of multiple contacts, interaction and communication.
6 A diverse city economy which is innovative, import-replacing and both self-reliant and actively trading with other cities and its own hinterland.
7 The encouragement of citizens to relate to the past, with their cultural and biological heritage and with other groups and individuals.
8 A city form that is compatible with and enhances the above parameters and behaviours.
9 An optimum level of appropriate health care services accessible to all.
10 High health status.

(after Baric, 1996 p323)

our discussion of social capital and empowerment in Chapter 1 will doubtless be apparent.

Other agreed criteria for a successful *Healthy City* are given in Box 10.

We might at this juncture reiterate the point that, in respect of philosophy and principles, what obtains for *Healthy Cities* also obtains for settings generally. We will comment later about implications for research and criteria for judging success. In the meantime, we will give some further thought to the definition of the *Settings Approach*.

## THE *SETTINGS APPROACH*: A SOMEWHAT CONTESTED CONCEPT?

Although it seems clear enough that the *Settings Approach* should encapsulate the principles of Ottawa and Jakarta, in practice it is probable that settings may be viewed as merely a location not only for delivering health education but for delivering a *Medical Model* of health education!

**Box 11** The *Settings Approach*

> *The setting, as a system, can be considered to have an 'input' (clients), a production process (care and treatment) and an output (health gain of clients). The main variable in this equation is the difference in clients according to their readiness and competence related to coping and the management of their health problems (input), resulting in a difference in the health gain (output) provided the process is standardised and optimised (i.e. the best available).*
>
> (Baric, 1994)

Baric's (1996) definition of setting appears in Box 11. He also observes (1996) that there is

> *... a qualitative difference between health promotion in a setting and a health promoting setting ... . The main characteristics of a health promoting setting are a recognised status, an approved monitored programme, total involvement of the staff and participation in a network of similar settings.*

He illustrates this observation by identifying three 'general aims' for health promoting settings together with some 39 objectives. A selection of these is reproduced in Table 4.1.

Green *et al.* (2000) aspire to adopt a 'critical social science perspective' on the notion of 'setting' that aims to challenge and re-assess the way in which it is conceptualised. This involves arguing against the conventional instrumental view mentioned earlier in this chapter with its underpinning notion of a 'captive audience' to be persuaded and manipulated. They remind us that settings are not necessarily homogeneous or politically neutral. They argue that their viewpoint leads inevitably to a point where they must ... *view the boundaries between settings as permeable* ... (a relevant observation for the imperative of inter-sectoral working!) and acknowledge the existence of

> *... pre-existing social relations in the setting (e.g. management–labor relations) that can*

influence how health promotion initiatives are framed and perceived by different players in the setting, how well they are supported (and by whom), and what their impact will be in the short and long term.

They, therefore, argue strongly for an ecological approach to defining a settings approach:

> *Settings can be conceptualized as both (a) physically bounded space-times in which people come together to perform specific tasks (usually oriented to goals other than health) and (b) arenas of sustained interaction, with preexisting structures, policies, characteristics, institutional values, and both formal and informal social sanctions on behavior.*
>
> (p23)

Wenzel (1997) also feels a critical, ecological approach is central to the definition of setting and he takes issue with Baric's (1994) definition (Box 11). He notes that a foreword to Baric's monograph by a staff member of the WHO Regional Office for Europe lends an air of authority to this definition – a not unreasonable though possibly inaccurate assumption! He considers that conceptualisation is mechanistic and over-simplistic; it also tends to focus on a *Medical Model* with its references to 'care and treatment' and implicitly encourages manipulation and even 'victim blaming'. Wenzel feels that the 'true' *Settings Approach* must incorporate physical, mental and social well-being. He is moved to cite Lowell Levin's classic (1984) caution that *health may be the ultimate disease* (if a 'healthist' manipulative stance is adopted).

In contrast, Wenzel describes a setting as:

- *a socially and culturally defined geographical and physical area of factual social interaction, and*
- *a socially and culturally defined set of patterns of interaction to be performed while in the setting.*

It is certainly important to adopt a rather more detached view of setting than is usually the

***Table 4.1***    Baric's Objectives

General Aim 1: Creating a healthy environment for staff and clients

Specific Aim 1.1
| | |
|---|---|
| Objective 1.1.1 | Securing a healthy working environment |
| (Indicator: | Level of safety at workplace) |
| Objective 1.1.2 | Ensuring job satisfaction of staff. |
| (Indicator: | Level of motivation and turnover of staff) |

Specific Aim 1.2    Proper accommodation for staff and clients
| | |
|---|---|
| Objective 1.2.2 | Ensuring proper accommodation for clients |
| (Indicator: | Level of complaints by clients) |
| Objective 1.2.3 | Ensuring appropriate commuting facilities |
| (Indicator: | Level of complaints) |

Specific Aim 1.3.    Availability of healthy nutrition for staff and clients
| | |
|---|---|
| Objective 1.3.1 | Assessment of existing nutritional values |
| (Indicator: | Meeting standards for healthy nutrition) |
| Objective 1.3.2 | Provision of a healthy diet |
| (Indicator: | Selection of food on offer) |

Specific Aim 1.4.    Prevention and treatment
| | |
|---|---|
| Objective 1.4.1 | Prevention of health threats for staff |
| (Indicator: | Changes in staff health behaviour) |
| Objective 1.4.2 | Prevention of health threats for clients |
| (Indicator: | Changes in client health behaviour) |

Specific Aim 1.5.    Care and relationships
| | |
|---|---|
| Objective 1.5.2 | Improvement in staff–client relationships |
| (Indicator: | Level of conflict and complaints) |
| Objective 1.5.4 | Improvement in client satisfaction |
| (Indicator: | Level of satisfaction of client needs) |

General Aim 2: Integrating health promotion into the daily activities of the setting

Specific Aim 2.1    Consideration and satisfaction of the health needs of the staff
| | |
|---|---|
| Objective 2.1.3 | Ensure that the staff working conditions are compliant with reduction of risk at work |
| (Indicator: | Level of stress, accidents, conflicts, etc.) |
| Objective 2.1.4 | Ensure general health of the staff |
| (Indicator: | Level of utilisation and timing of curative health services) |

Specific Aim 2.3    Assessing and meeting the needs of the immediate social environment
| | |
|---|---|
| Objective 2.3.1. | Ensuring the social support from the client's immediate family and relatives |
| (Indicator: | Level of support, type of conjugal roles, type of family cycle of development) |

General Aim 3: Initiating and participating in community developments

Specific Aim 3.1    Initiating and promoting the *Health Promoting Setting* movement in the community
| | |
|---|---|
| Objective 3.1.2 | Public meetings for representatives of other settings to learn about the concept of 'health promoting settings' |
| (Indicator: | Attendance rate, comments and commitments of the attending representatives of other settings) |

Specific Aim 3.2    Networking with other similar health promoting settings
| | |
|---|---|
| Objective 3.2.2 | Creating and/or joining the national network of similar health promoting settings |

Specific Aim 3.3    Creating healthy alliances with other health promoting settings on the local, national and international levels
| | |
|---|---|
| Objective 3.3.1 | Establishing mechanisms for cooperation with other health promoting settings on a local level (e.g. hospitals, schools, services, enterprises, prisons, etc.) |

*Adapted from Baric (1996, pp. 308–313). The original list contains 39 objectives derived from the Specific Aims.*

case. Not unreasonably, we tend to consider the 'geographical' aspect of setting – the school buildings, the office block, the clinic and the physical features of the neighbourhood – as mere bricks and mortar or other materials in which the drama of human interaction occurs. The reference to drama is itself suggestive and helps draw our attention to the symbolic nature of scenery. Indeed, in their examination of the meaning of landscape, semiologists have jolted our view of the taken-for-granted features of physical circumstances. For instance, Duncan and Duncan (1992) have discussed the importance of deciphering the ... *complexity and instability beneath the apparent simplicity of the everyday cultural landscape.* Landscape should be interpreted as a *'signifying system'* steeped in ideology. The authors draw attention to the intriguing case of Hachette's *Blue Guides* for tourists which they argue are 'agents of blindness' focusing travellers' attention on a limited range of landscape features and which thus *'overpower' or 'mask' the 'real' spectacle of human life and history* (or, more accurately, an alternative real spectacle). The picturesque scenario portrayed by Hachette – according to Duncan and Duncan – relates to a bourgeois ideology. More particularly, Hachette's (doubtless entirely unconscious) social construction of landscape can be characterised as ... *a 19th century 'Helvetico-Protestant morality' in a hybrid compound of the culture of nature and Puritanism* involving ... *regeneration through clean air, moral ideas at the sight of mountain tops, summit climbing as civic virtue... an individualistic ideology – morality equated with effort and solitude.* According to the authors, the *Blue Guides* provide *'uplift without effort'.* The formulation of a health promotion strategy leading to the physical and social construction settings that provided 'health without effort' would indubitably be greeted with considerable enthusiasm!

Wenzel (1997) also questions the WHO's (1993) observations in the context of specifying 'Health for All' targets (Box 12).

**Box 12**   Creating Health Promoting Settings

*The challenge is to offer incentives and support for the creation of settings where physical characteristics and social processes interact to enhance healthy living. Housing and neighbourhood can be designed to strengthen the supporting and caring functions of families and friends. Schools and recreation areas can encourage social experiences that shape and maintain healthy behaviour among children. Workplaces can be safe and offer opportunities to be productive in an environment that encourages healthy lifestyles.*

(WHO, 1993 p67)

While this exhortation undoubtedly emphasises the importance of an ecological approach and argues for the provision of supportive environments for health choices, Wenzel rightly draws attention to the omission of emphasis on community participation – of the creation of active participating communities within each setting. It would, however, be churlish to accuse WHO of lacking commitment to participative approaches given its increasing tendency to define health promotion as essentially a strategy for helping people gain control over their lives and their health!

On the other hand, Wenzel approves of Moos' analysis of setting (Box 13).

**Box 13**   Characteristics of Settings According to Moos

1  Behaviour settings have one or more *standing patterns* of behaviour. These patterns of behaviour are not the behaviour of individuals, but of people *en masse*.
2  Behaviour settings involve not just behaviour but also a *milieu* that is physical and may include man-made objects such as buildings, streets, or chairs.
3  The *physical milieu surrounds or encloses* the behaviour.

4 The standing patterns of behaviour in the setting are <u>*similar in structure*</u> to the milieu. That is, the physical and temporal aspects of the setting, and the standing patterns of behaviour in the setting are interdependent.

(Moos, 1976 pp215–216; cited in Wenzel, 1997)

Wenzel also draws our attention to Bronfenbrenner's (1979) well-known ecological perspective on developmental psychology (Box 14). It will doubtless be apparent that this perspective is consonant with the *Health Career Model* discussed at the beginning of this chapter. It is also consistent with our review, in Chapter 1, of the different levels of social influence on health – and with our assertions in Chapter 2 about the importance of *Social Learning Theory*'s notion of 'reciprocal determinism'.

**Box 14**   Reciprocal Determinism and Human Development

*The ecology of human development involves the scientific study of the progressive, mutual accommodation between an active growing human being and the changing properties of the immediate settings in which the developing person lives, as this process is affected by relations between these settings, and by the larger contexts in which the settings are embedded.*

(Bronfenbrenner, 1979 p21)

We commented in Chapters 1 and 2 on the different 'layers' of influence on individual health and health choices and utilised the standard terms, macro, meso and micro. Bronfenbrenner uses four layers or systems: 'macro', 'exo', 'meso' and 'micro'. In the author's words:

*The ecological environment is conceived topologically as a nested arrangement of concentric structures. ... A micro-system is a pattern of activities, roles, and interpersonal relations experienced by the developing per-son in a given setting with particular physical and material characteristics.*

*A meso-system comprises the interrelations among two or more settings in which the developing person actively participates (such as, for a child, the relations among home, school, and neighbourhood peer group; for an adult, among family, work, and social life).*

*An exo-system refers to one or more settings that do not involve the developing person as an active participant, but in which events occur that affect, or are affected by, what happens in the setting containing the developing person.*

*A macro-system refers to consistencies, in the form and content of lower-order systems (micro-, meso- and exo-) that exist, or could exist, at the level of the subculture or the culture as a whole, along with any belief systems or ideology underlying such consistencies ... the system's blueprints differ from various socioeconomic, ethnic, religious, and other subcultural groups, reflecting contrasting belief systems and lifestyles, which in turn help to perpetuate the ecological environments specific to each group.*

(Bronfenbrenner, 1979, pp25–26; cited in Wenzel, 1997)

The *Health Career* described in Figure 4.2 should be regarded as demonstrating individuals' progress though their lifespan while subjected to the influence of different 'layers' as described by Bronfenbrenner.

## PROBLEMS FOR A *SETTINGS APPROACH*

In the light of increasing enthusiasm for the *Settings Approach*, Green *et al.* (2000) suggest that it would be unwise to ignore certain problems and difficulties.

### Stakeholder conflict

As will be apparent in later chapters, there is almost inevitably a number of different 'stakeholders' in any given setting (for instance in the workplace these include workers (and their families), trade unions and different levels of management). Apart from the necessity to work with and reconcile these different interests, there is a danger that health promoters might find themselves seeking alliances with the most powerful 'gatekeepers' in order to gain entry to the target group and thus acquiring ambivalent or even hostile status in the eyes of the major client group.

### Losing sight of marginal groups

As Green *et al.* observe, the strength of a *Settings Approach* for accessing large client groups may also be its weakness,

> ... *for the settings in which one is to find the unemployed, the homeless, the disenfranchised youth, the illegal immigrants, and so forth are not as well defined. Indeed there is considerable selectivity in what settings are addressed ... health promotion has chosen to privilege some settings ... as being more 'legitimate' sites of practice than others (e.g. bingo halls, nightclubs, street corners, public washrooms, and other 'sites of resistance'). Kickbusch (1995) argues that we need to move toward considering these 'less obvious' settings, beyond hospitals, corporations, prisons, or other 'total institutions'. The unconventional settings for health promotion are in many cases those (a) in which the health-adverse behaviors that have traditionally been of concern to health professionals are perhaps most common; (b) that are the least 'formal' in terms of the social organization of interaction (and therefore the least amenable to bureaucratic intervention and control, possessing few of the formal channels of power of formalized institutions); i.e. they are more fluid in structure and therefore less amenable to formal regulation ... and (c) that are most likely to challenge the historically middle-class, rational actor, deferred gratification, health-as-superordinate-goal, professional, expertise-oriented bias characteristic of much ... health promotion.*

> (p25)

While not seeking directly to address those settings and situations in which the 'standard' *Settings Approach* is not directly relevant, in later chapters we have considered it appropriate to give some detailed thought to the contribution of mass media to health promotion: and mass media, quite clearly, do not constitute a setting. Moreover, we separately consider the notion of community development – which would typically be concerned with the kinds of marginal circumstances mentioned above – and 'community organisation' or, more accurately, community-wide programmes that usually focus on a specific preventive goal and which tend to have a 'top-down' approach – with or without some degree of community participation.

### Complexity of a settings analysis

A third problem with ecological versions of the *Settings Approach*, is the fact that there are so many interacting and interlocking variables that health promoters might well be forgiven for preferring simpler options! In the words of Green *et al.*, *Ecological Complexity Breeds Despair!*

**Box 15**  Does Ecological Complexity Breed Despair?

> Since the sophisticated pursuit of wide ranging health promotion goals within the context of complex social and economic systems is a *sine qua non* for efficient programme design, health promoters, like their clients, may well benefit from aspiring to the empowered state! Following Antonovsky's 'negentropic' imperative, they should ideally feel that their professional life is both manageable and meaningful. Accordingly, adoption of a post-modern perspective may not be too helpful!

### The challenge of new paradigm research

The ecological dimension of a settings approach, together with its concern with salutogenic goals, pose problems for traditional researchers. A new gold standard is needed and its pursuit may involve a degree of conflict and power play among different stakeholders in the research community.

# RESEARCHING HEALTH PROMOTING SETTINGS

The *Healthy Cities* initiative has been in existence longer than any of the other settings approaches promoted by WHO. It has also been subjected to considerable debate and a good deal of research. For these reasons, we can identify a number of issues that have relevance for researching settings in general. More particularly, it is important to consider the research philosophy as revealed by the kinds of indicator of effectiveness that have been typically used and the research methodology espoused. There is also some evidence of the actual level of success achieved by *Healthy Cities* programmes.

## Philosophy and indicators of success

The philosophical perspective of *Healthy Cities* is both implicit and explicit. In short, the model of health mirrors WHO's original holistic definition while acknowledging that health is also, importantly, a 'resource for achieving a socially and economically productive life'. It adopts an ecological approach to health promotion and, according to Davies and Kelly (1993), it has a strong post-modern theme in its ... *fundamental epistemological shift in the conceptualization of health itself* and its acceptance of multiple realities. It is also ... *a political programme which is about a change in power relations in respect of health and illness* ... .

The six research priorities identified by Tsouros and Draper (1993) also reveal its philosophical foundation (Box 16).

***Box 16*** Research Priorities for *Healthy Cities* Programmes

- *Equity*. Reducing inequalities in health is a universal *Healthy Cities* priority.
- *Prerequisites for Health*. Poor housing, inadequate food, limited education, prolonged unemployment, poor access to primary care and few opportunities for leisure and recreation.
- *Policy and Programme Impact*. Urban planning and housing policy, traffic and pollution control, development of recreational

facilties and improvement of public transport on health.
- *Inter-sectoral Action*. Challenges to traditional patterns of organisations and management in the public sector.
- *Community Participation*.
- *Strategic Planning*. Development of urban environments that are supportable and sustainable. Health is linked with well-being and to social and cultural development. The concept is ecological.

*(after Tsouros and Draper, 1993 pp31–33)*

As observed in Chapter 2, what are classed as 'intermediate' and even 'indirect' indicators of effectiveness for certain programmes may well be deemed indicators of effective outcomes for others. Improving the health status of disadvantaged groups and creating a more equitable distribution of resources are manifestly desirable outcomes – as is the achievement of community empowerment. It also seems to be the case that for many working in the *Healthy Cities* movement, inter-sectoral working and a 'sense of community' may also be regarded as end-points rather than operating instrumentally to achieve ultimate outcomes. For whatever reason, it might be argued that virtually all of the recorded effects of programmes describe process rather than outcome.

## Importance of clear identification of indicators

The revised aims of the Noarlunga project in Australia make interesting reading. Although they are aims, the implications for identifying different categories of indicator are quite evident.

1  *To involve government agencies, non-government organizations and other sectors in the development of local health policies and actions which seek to establish a social, economic and physical environment conducive to health.*

2  *To implement the Healthy Cities project in a way that defines and promotes*

*equity of access to the resources neces-sary to maintain good health and improve poor health.*

3 *To increase community awareness of social perspectives on health, in particu-lar the social determinants of illness.*

4 *To encourage local health services' reorientation towards health promo-tion.*

5 *To implement and evaluate demonstra-tion projects focusing on intersectoral cooperation and community involve-ment.*

6. *To evaluate the process and the outcome of the Healthy Cities project at the local level, using a common national frame-work.*

(Baum, 1993 p92)

In the terminology used in Chapter 2, five of the aims are indirect indicators relating to the development of 'healthy public policy'. For exam-ple, Aim 1 involves inter-sectoral working – in order to develop policy – in order to achieve the outcome of environmental change – in order to achieve the end-point outcome of reducing disad-vantage.

Aim 2 is concerned to achieve policy in order to improve access to health enhancing 'resources' – presumably in order to achieve the end-point of health (apparently including disease prevention and treatment). Indicators of the successful attain-ment of Aim 5 would demonstrate inter-sectoral working and community participation – presum-ably on the assumption that other more distal out-comes would result from the successful attainment of this goal. Aim 3, on the other hand, might well generate indicators of an 'intermedi-ate' nature – resulting from health education – and might include the kinds of measure to which reference is made later in the context of social marketing approaches and, more particularly, appropriate interpretation and accurate recall of the message. Hopefully, the evaluation would also demonstrate a high level of public acceptance of the message together with a positive attitude to its substance.

To reiterate our earlier argument: precise spec-ification of indicators in the context of a web of influences operating over time and across agen-cies will enhance the effectiveness of both evalua-tion and programme design. The specification of indicators, of course, must be based on a respectable theoretical framework (notwithstand-ing post-modern objections!).

## Formative evaluation and the primacy of process

It is self-evident that the vast majority of evalua-tion efforts within the *Healthy Cities* movement centres on process. For instance, an evaluation of the *Healthy City* project in Glasgow (McGhee and McEwen, 1993) reported on the process of recruiting lay 'volunteers' (a strategy reminiscent of the *North Karelia Heart Disease Prevention Project* – discussed in a later chapter). Semi-struc-tured interviews were carried out with two groups of 10 volunteers. Indicators included: types of activity undertaken; levels of confidence in work-ing with different client groups; problems experi-enced in performing their volunteer roles (mainly organisational – lack of identified space, lack of time, lack of status and knowledge, lack of confi-dence and lack of a creche); perceptions about collaboration with other volunteer workers, working group members and project executive group members. Rather intriguingly, health out-come indicators were recorded for the volunteers! Reported perceptions of improvements in own health improved over time in all cases and seven of nine volunteers claimed to have made lifestyle changes!

The project also employed *intermediate* indica-tors to assess levels of popular awareness about the project.

The Glasgow project had used process data to gain insight into the nature of the processes involved. However, 'milestone' process data are also quite common and Hancock (1993) lists 11 kinds of information describing the features of successful *Healthy Cities* projects and which can be used as 'milestone' targets along the road to success (see Box 17).

**Box 17** Characteristics of a Successful *Healthy Cities* Project

- Strong political support
- Effective leadership
- Broad community ownership
- High visibility
- Strategic orientation
- Adequate and appropriate resources
- Sound project administration
- Effective committees
- Strong community participation
- Inter-sectoral collaboration
- Political and managerial accountability

(after Hancock, 1993 p21)

## Formative and illuminative evaluation

Whereas process measures feature most frequently in *Healthy Cities* evaluations, there is occasionally evidence of formative evaluation at work. For instance, Baum (1993) describes the way in which information generated in the pilot period of the initiative raised awareness about the poor quality of water in a local estuary. As a result of media publicity, public meetings and advocacy work, a number of groups and working parties were formed to address the problem. Respondents from the community judged that the *Healthy City* project had been valuable in opening pathways to ministers and generally acting as an advocate.

Curtice (1993) demonstrates the value of using process information for illumination in the form of an illustrative, albeit fictitious, 'mid-term report' from a project coordinator.

A flavour of this exemplar of illuminative evaluation (or the use of 'stories') is in Box 18. For a more complete (and factual) exemplar, see Labonte's report in Appendix 2.1.

**Box 18** A Project Co-ordinator's Mid-term Report

*We have spent a lot of energy in the two years establishing the intersectoral group … . When we got involved in the pilot project to reduce accidents on a local estate we began to feel that we really had established the personal and organizational links which might make a difference … . At times the project structures seem far more fragile. City politics are dominated by the issue of financial cutbacks and the project seems to be marginalized. A few key individuals switch their attention elsewhere and some of the links between different groups break down. … Nonetheless, some activities are flourishing. When we started, there were a number of groups around who were already working on health issues and who shared quite a lot of our basic concerns, so we got involved with them and now we have a couple of local pilot projects … . We have drawn up a strategy for community development in health which is going to the health authority, and the elements of a comprehensive health policy for the elderly have emerged from the elderly forum set up by the project which has a membership drawn from health care and social work agencies and carers/groups.*

(Curtice, 1993 p41–42)

## Research methodology

It will by now be clear that the preferred (almost the only) research paradigm typically adopted in *Healthy Cities* research is ethnographic and qualitative – both epistemologically and practically. One particular point of significance – in the context of the re-iterated emphasis in this book on empowerment – is the point of principle that health promotion should adopt empowering research strategies, i.e. it should not only ensure that the research results are fed into health improvements for the client group but that clients should be actively involved in the research process itself.

A valuable discussion of this principle is provided by Smithies and Adams (1993). They remind us of the contribution of Feuerstein (1986) in identifying the key features of client involvement in research and provide a schematic representation of this process – and this is reproduced in Figure 4.4.

A final, but highly important, point about methodology will be made. We mentioned above the importance of *formative evaluation*. However, if health promotion is the militant wing of the public health, we would hope to develop participatory evaluation to the point where it becomes action research and results in significant political and social change. A modified model of the Freirean approach to empowerment and action was discussed in Chapter 1 and serves as a basis for radical, action research. Hunt provides one of the most important examples of such radical action in recent years and her experience has been located within the ambit of a *Healthy Cities*

approach (Hunt, 1993).

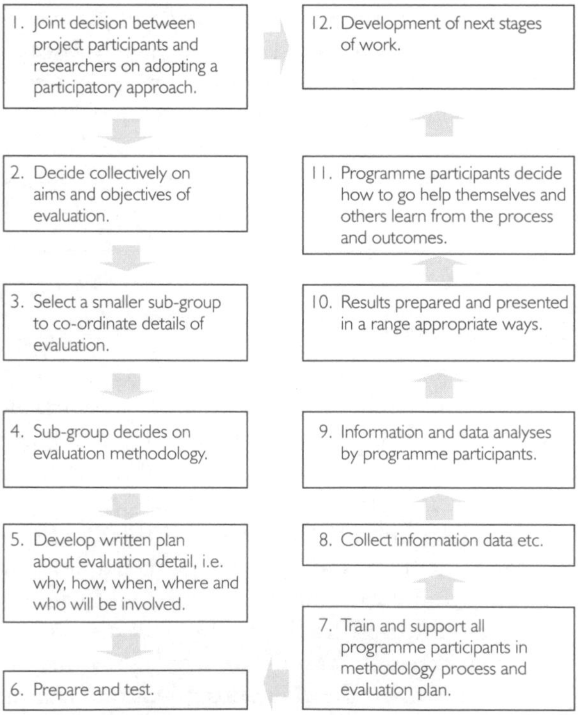

In brief, Hunt provides two illuminating and related case studies of the ways in which research into housing and health resulted in tangible action to reduce the negative effects of damp housing: in a very real sense, case studies into praxis in the city. The first study involved the community in a coalition of professional workers researching problems associated with housing and health. The research method included a double-blind study of 300 council houses and those living in them. Individuals' health status was related to housing conditions – and particularly evidence of damp and visible mould. The results demonstrated quite categorically that there were statistically significant and strong links between the presence of damp and health problems in women and children. This association could not be attributed to individual behaviours or lifestyle.

Although the study received publicity, little of practical moment happened. Accordingly, a second study was initiated – again involving the commitment and cooperation of the client group together with inter-sectoral collaboration between a number of disciplines and professions. This second research project established a dose–response relationship between the levels of mould in the air and on the walls of the houses and the extent and nature of symptoms in children. The relationship was independent of smoking in the household, unemployment, income, household composition, the presence of pets and type of cooking facilities.

The research report was discussed with the community and widely publicised. Tenants set up press conferences, a paper was published in the *British Medical Journal*, questions were asked in Parliament. There was widespread media reporting.

A raft of changes resulted from the publicity derived from the report. Amongst other results, the report was used ... *to change housing priorities in Glasgow and pressurise government to allow more revenue to be raised for housing. For the first time, the council publicly embraced the responsibility for ill health caused by its own housing ... the Institute of Environmental Offi-*

**Figure 4.4** Participatory Approach to Evaluation

cers recommended a change in the 'tolerable standard' of dampness in housing regulations and the report ... also influenced the obtaining of a grant by the tenants' group in Glasgow from the European Community for a £1.3 million Solar Energy Demonstration Project in Glasgow.

In short, real policy changes resulted from this research. Not surprisingly perhaps, Hunt reported that there were several negative consequences of the political nature of the research and its 'critical consciousness raising' (Box 19).

**Box 19** Political Repercussions of Research on Damp Housing

> Officials at the Scottish Office indicated their displeasure that the research had been done at all, that they had not been made aware of it and the political implications. Warnings about career consequences, veiled and not so veiled, were received by members of the research team. A few members of more traditional Community Medicine Public Health departments showed signs of resentment that their territory was being poached upon by people who were not even medically qualified. Jealousy and friction was also evident between tenants groups as some appeared to get more publicity and more attention than others, and there was a feeling that some areas which were more visible in the media would get a disproportionate amount of housing money. The researchers were also treated with resentment by some community workers for pre-empting their role with tenants and for 'hogging' the publicity. There were also unforeseen medicolegal consequences. The research led to an increase in the number of tenants who brought legal action against Glasgow district council and the council found itself in the position of being sued on the basis of work it had itself commissioned.
>
> (Hunt, 1993 p79)

Not only is health promotion inherently political – so is health promotion research!

## Effectiveness of *Healthy Cities*: general results

The degree of success greeting Hunt's research is unusual. General evaluations of the *Healthy Cities* programmes have been much less conclusive. For instance, the WHO Project Office reported on the first two to three years of the project. It examined both process and outcome effects (the process measures were concerned with factors leading to political commitment and the kinds of organisational and managerial structures that were developed to achieve project goals). As Tsouros and Draper (1993) report, the kinds of outcome addressed had to do with progress in ... *promoting equity and in dealing with particular lifestyle, environmental and health service problems*. As regards the effectiveness of the programme at that relatively early stage in its history, *in general, cities have made more progress in developing structures and processes than in introducing innovative policies and programmes*. The evaluation contains a particularly important lesson for those seeking to achieve broad 'social' goals within the context of inter-sectoral working: it will probably take a lot longer than anticipated! As Tsouros and Draper observe, *In many cities, the length of time between political acceptance of the project idea and the achievement of the real changes in policies and programmes has been longer than expected by both WHO and local practitioners.*

Mittelmark (1999) comments on the expanded review of 35 project cities five years into the programme (Draper *et al.*,1993), noting that ... *some cities had done a great deal and others had done very little*(!). He also pointed out that in many cases the establishment of a *Healthy Cities* programme was the main project activity. It appears that

> ... *only 15 of the 35 cities had begun or completed the preparation of comprehensive city health plans, which in an important sense is the main objective of the Healthy Cities approach to health promotion.*

The degree of political commitment and level of resources were important factors in determining progress, together with the existence of steering committees representing key agencies, political links and community participation. Successful cities also had

> ... specialized groups for management and technical support, the roles and responsibilities of committees and working groups were defined clearly, and projects were staffed at the level of a full-time coordinator or more.

A more intensive and more recent review of the effectiveness of *Healthy Cities* is reported by Goumans and Springett (1997). Five key issues were identified as a basis for interviewing informants in 10 cities in UK and the Netherlands. They were:

- *extent of supportive national strategies;*
- *development of formal structures that see health as part of mainstream activity of all key organizations and departments;*
- *existence of shared ownership and commitment by all organizations and communities involved;*
- *development of core activities within the organizations involved which create the capacity needed for healthy public policy development and implementation;*
- *agenda-building.*

(pp313–314)

The findings revealed that most respondents felt that 'Healthy Cities' had made a difference – certainly in the awareness-raising and agenda-setting domain. There seemed to be a feeling that projects had succeeded in influencing public policy to some degree but it was clearly difficult to attribute policy changes to the project nor were people able to identify what the policy benefits had been. Long-term policy making had been lacking and ... *had been discussed largely in terms of developing a health plan.*

Part of Goumans and Springett's conclusion is worth citing since it acknowledges the difficulties facing any complex, wide-ranging and ecologically diverse settings approach.

*Building healthy public policy is a time-consuming process, because it involves developing a new infrastructure supportive to health promotion and it requires a critical mass of people to hold in their consciousness the vision involved. 'Healthy Cities' is asking for a radical change and this change is only beginning to happen in a few places. Health, as opposed to health care, still does not have solid place on the political agenda. It is hardly discussed, it is not problematic, and it is not politically interesting. Strategies need to be developed to change this or 'Healthy Cities' will continue to be largely professionally driven and will remain vulnerable to political whim.*

(p321)

So what should we look for in considering *Settings for Health Promotion*?

- We should distinguish settings from strategies and note their interdependence.
- We should consider the extent to which health promotion in different settings makes appropriate use of insights that can be gained from a health career perspective.
- We should ask whether a given setting is being used merely as a locus for delivering health education or whether it, at least, incorporates the support of healthy public policy.
- We should ask to what extent its focus is relatively narrow and fixated on the prevention of disease or whether it has a relatively broad, ecological perspective on health.
- We should ask to what extent it incorporates the principles of Ottawa and Jakarta and seeks to empower and provide a radical challenge to the status quo ante in pursuit of equity.

From what has been written in this chapter the reader might expect that we would evaluate the contexts selected for further discussion in subsequent chapters solely from a healthy settings perspective – drawing on evidence of research deemed most appropriate to evaluating these holistic developments with their particular ideology. We will, indeed, seek to include such evaluations where these are available. However, a considerable body of current health development work in workplaces, schools and health care is best described as health education. Some of this does take place within the context of the kind of settings approach discussed earlier, i.e. holistic health promotion which incorporates supportive policy. On the other hand, a great deal of activity does not occur in this way. While the adoption of the settings approach is proceeding very rapidly, developments in many countries are still at a very early stage. As we have emphasised in previous chapters, health education is a component of health promotion, whether or not it is occurring within a healthy settings approach. It is, therefore, still important to know to what extent health education activities are effective. Globally there are major health concerns where health education has a continuing role to play in addressing the problems. For example, while a number of social and economic changes are necessary in response to the HIV AIDS problem and it can be argued persuasively that these ought to be prioritised, it is generally acknowledged that this is not yet happening. Accordingly, education is, and will remain for some time, of major importance. We will therefore continue to review health education activities as well as achievements in developing health promoting settings. While accepting that the ideology of health promotion would suggest that certain evaluation methodologies are more appropriate, we will draw on literature which has used the full range of research approaches for reasons discussed in the previous chapter. It will be apparent to readers that the balance between the types of research studies which have been carried out to examine effectiveness varies from one setting to another.

## REFERENCES

Baric, L. (1969) *Recognition of the "at-risk" role*. International Journal of Health Education, XII (1), 2–12.

Baric, L. (1974) *Acquisition of the smoking habit and the model of "smoker's careers"*. Journal of the Institute of Health Education, 12 (1), 9–18.

Baric, L. (1975) *Conformity and deviance in health and illness. International Journal of Health Education*, XVIII (1), 1–12.

Baric, L. (1994) *Health Promotion and Health Education in Practice*. Module 2: *The Organisational Model*. Barns Publications, Hale Barns.

Baric, L. (1996) *Handbook for Students and Practitioners*. Barns Publications, Hale Barns.

Baric, L., MacArthur, C. and Sherwood, M. (1976) *A study of health education aspects of smoking in pregnancy. International Journal of Health Education*, XIX (2), 1–17.

Baum, F. (1993) *Noarlunga Healthy Cities Pilot Project:* I. *The contribution of research and evaluation*. In J. K. Davies and M. P. Kelly (Eds) *Healthy Cities: Research and Practice* Routledge, London.

Bronfenbrenner, U. (1979) *The Ecology of Human Development. Experiments by Nature and Design*. Harvard University Press, Cambridge, MA.

Curtice, L. (1993) *Strategies and values: research and the WHO Healthy Cities project in Europe*. In J. K. Davies and M. P. Kelly (Eds) *Healthy Cities: Research and Practice* Routledge, London.

Davie, R., Butler, N. and Goldstein, H. (1972) *From Birth to Seven*. Longman, London.

Davies, J. K. and Kelly, M. P. (Eds) (1993) *Healthy Cities: Research and Practice*. Routledge, London.

Draper, R., Curtice, L., Hooper, J. and Goumans, M. (1993) *WHO Healthy Cities Project: Review of the First Five Years (1987–1992)*. WHO, Copenhagen.

Duhl, L. (1985) *Healthy cities. Health Promotion*, 1, 55–60.

Duhl, L. J. (1996) *An ecohistory of health: the role of "Healthy Cities". American Journal of Health Promotion*, 10 (4), 258–261.

Duncan, J. S. and Duncan, N. G. (1992) *Ideology and bliss: Roland Barthes and the secret history of landscape*. In T. J. Barnes and J. S. Duncan (Eds) *Writing Worlds: Discourse Text and Metaphor in the Representation of Landscape*. Routledge, London.

Feuerstein, M. T. (1986) *Partners in Evaluation: Evaluating Development and Community Programmes with Participants*. Macmillan, London.

Flynn, B. C. (1996) *Healthy Cities: towards worldwide health promotion. Annual Review of Public Health*, 17, 229–309.

Galea, G., Powis, B. and Tamplin, S. A. (2000) *Healthy islands in the Western Pacific – international settings development. Health Promotion International*, 15 (2), 169–178.

Goumans, M. and Springett, J. (1997) *From projects to policy: "Healthy Cities" as a mechanism for policy change for health? Health Promotion International*, 12 (4), 311–322.

Green, J. and Tones, B. K. (2000) *Sex and the world*. In H. Wilson and S. McAndrew (Eds) *Sexual Health: Foundations for Practice*. Bailliere-Tindall, London.

Green, L. W., Poland, B. D. and Rootman, I. (2000) *The settings approach to health promotion*. In L. W. Green, B. D. Poland and I. Rootman (Eds) *Settings for Health Promotion: Linking Theory and Practice*. Sage, Thousand Oaks, CA.

Haglund, B. J. A., Pettersson, B., Finer, D. and Tillgren, P. (1991) *The Sundsvall Handbook: "We Can Do It"*. Karolinska Institute, Stockholm, Sweden.

Hancock, T. (1993) *The Healthy City from concept to application: implications for research*. In J. K. Davies and M. P. Kelly (Eds) *Healthy Cities: Research and Practice* Routledge, London.

Hancock, T. and Duhl, L. (1988) *Promoting Health in the Urban Context*, WHO Healthy Cities Papers no. 1. WHO, Copenhagen.

Hunt, S. M. (1993) *The relationship between research and policy: translating knowledge into action*. In J. K. Davies and M. P. Kelly (Eds) *Healthy Cities: Research and Practice* Routledge, London.

Kickbusch, I. (1989a) *Good Planets are Hard to Find*, WHO Healthy Cities Papers no. 5. WHO, Copenhagen.

Kickbusch, I. (1989b) *Healthy Cities a working project and growing movement. Health Promotion*, 4 (2), 77–82.

Kickbusch, I. (1995) *An overview to the settings based approach to health promotion*. In T. Theaker and J. Thompson (Eds) *The Settings-Based Approach to Health Promotion; Report of an International Working Conference*. Hertfordshire Health Promotion, Hertfordshire.

Levin, L. S. (1984) *Health – the ultimate disease*. In WHO Regional Office for Europe (Ed) *Health Promotion: Concepts and Principle*. WHO Regional Office for Europe, Copenhagen, pp. 18–19.

McGhee, S. and McEwen, J. (1993) *Evaluating the Healthy Cities Project in Drumchapel, Glasgow*. In J. K. Davies and M. P. Kelly (Eds) *Healthy Cities: Research and Practice* Routledge, London.

Mittelmark, M. B. (1999) *Health promotion at the community wide level: lessons from diverse*

perspectives. In N. Bracht (Ed.) *Health Promotion at the Community Level: New Advances*. Sage, Thousand Oaks, CA.

Moos, R. H. (1976) *The Human Context. Environmental Determinants of Behavior*. Wiley, New York, NY.

Mussen, P. H. and Conger, J. (1956) *Child Development and Personality*. Harper and Brothers, New York, NY.

Pettersson, B., Tillgren, P., Finer, D., Haglund, B. and Macdonald, H. (1992) *Playing for Time … Creating Supportive Environments for Health*, Report from the 3rd International Conference on Health Promotion, Sundsvall, Sweden, 9–15 June, 1991. People's Health Vasternorrland, Sundsvall.

Smithies, J. and Adams, L. (1993) *Walking the tightrope: issues in evaluation and community participation for Health for All*. In J. K. Davies and M. P. Kelly (Eds) *Healthy Cities: Research and Practice* Routledge, London.

Tones, B. K. (1979) *Socialisation, health career and the health education of the schoolchild. Journal Institute of Health Education*, 17 (1), 23–28.

Tones, B. K. (1981) Affective education. In J. Cowley and T. Williams (Eds) *Health Education in Schools*. Harper and Row, London.

Tones, B. K. (1992) *Empowerment and the promotion of health. Journal of the Institute of Health Education*, 30 (4), 133–137.

Tones, B. K. (1993) *Methods, strategies and settings in health education: emergent ideologies and the ascendancy of theory. Health Education Journal*, 52 (3), 125–139.

Tsouros, A. (1990) *Healthy cities means community action. Health Promotion International*, 5, 177–178.

Tsouros, A. D. (1995) *The WHO Healthy Cities Project: State-of-the-art and future plans. Health Promotion International*, 10, 133–141.

Tsouros, A. and Draper, R. A. (1993) *The Healthy Cities Project: new developments and research needs*. In J. K. Davies and M. P. Kelly (Eds) *Healthy Cities: Research and Practice* Routledge, London.

Wenzel, E. (1997) *A comment on settings in health promotion. Internet Journal of Health Promotion*, 1, 1–9. (http://www.monash.edu.au/health/IJHP/1997/1)

Whitehead, M. and Tones, K. (1990) *Avoiding the Pitfalls: Notes on the Planning and Implementation of health Education Strategies and the Special Role of the H.E.A.* Health Education Authority, London.

World Health Organization (1986) *Ottawa Charter for Health Promotion. Health Promotion*, 1 (4), i–v.

World Health Organization (1993) *Health for All Targets. The Health Policy for Europe*. WHO, Copenhagen.

World Health Organization (1995) *Yanuca Island Declaration*. Regional Office for the Western Pacific, Manila.

World Health Organization (1997) *The Rarotonga Agreement: Towards Healthy Islands*. Regional Office for the Western Pacific, Manila.

World Health Organization (1998) *The Jakarta Declaration on Leading Health Promotion into the 21st Century*. WHO, Geneva.

# 5 HEALTH PROMOTION IN SCHOOLS

## INTRODUCTION

Societies have long recognised the potential offered by schools for influencing young people in their formative period. It has been estimated that in those countries where children have the opportunity to attend school from the ages of 5 to 16 years something like 15,000 hours are spent there (Rutter *et al.*, 1979). Not surprisingly, therefore, schools have been identified as one of the main settings for health promotion. Their stated advantages have included the potential:

- to reach a significant proportion of those of school age;
- to reach people at a particularly significant stage of life in the development of health knowledge, attitudes and behaviours and the capacity, therefore, to influence current and future health;
- to build links with communities and develop two-way actions that can influence health;
- to reach children with preventive health services.

As summarised by the American Public Health Association (Allensworth and Wolford, 1988):

*The school, as a social structure, provides an educational setting in which the total health of the child during the impressionable years is a priority concern. No other community setting even approximates the magnitude of the school education enterprise – thus it seems that the school should be regarded as a social unit providing a focal point to which health planning for all other community settings should relate.*

At the same time it is important not to place unrealistic demands on the school.

*School definitely cannot counteract all the stressors and tensions originating in other life spheres such as unfavourable economic conditions, dysfunctional families or lack of supportive friends. Above and beyond that, school in and of itself bears a considerable risk potential for the healthy development of the young.*

(Hurrelman *et al.*, 1995)

## SCHOOLS AND HEALTH

While we are particularly concerned to assess the activities in schools which are designated either as health education or health promotion it needs to be emphasised that there is a clear relationship between access to education in general and health. A recent UK document *Saving Lives* (Department of Health, 1999) had this to say:

*People with low levels of educational achievement are more likely to have poor health as adults. By improving education for all we can tackle one of the main causes of inequality in health … . Education can also contribute to general improvements in health by enhancing people's ability to secure opportunities for work.*

Overcoming inequalities in health within and between countries and between the 'North' and 'South' is a key development goal and formal educational structures have important contributions to make to the achievement of such a goal (for North and South see footnote in Chapter 9).

Education can influence health, both directly and indirectly. Directly, the school environment, activities in the curriculum and school health services can influence current health. Health education in schools can also contribute to future health. Indirectly, educational achievement influences occupational opportunity and material circumstances and, ultimately, health. It is in the light of the recognition of the importance of education to achievement of health and other valued social goals that efforts to secure access to education for all children has been a global objective. During the last century goals for universal access to education were set although not achieved. In 1985 UNESCO estimated that 105,000,000 children between 6 and 11 years did not receive any formal education, of which 70% were in the least developed countries and 60% were girls. By 1990 the estimate had risen to 130,000,000 following the structural adjustment programmes in the late 1980s. The end of century goals following the 1990 World Summit for Children were that all children would receive basic education and 80% of boys and girls would complete primary education. By 1995 UNICEF reported that just under 50% of countries were on target to reach the 80% goal. It is difficult to document progress since accurate information from many countries is not yet available (Grant, 1995).

The contribution of schools to the achievement of health has been clearly identified in a number of WHO documents (WHO, 1978, 1996, 1997). The Alma Ata Document (WHO, 1978) stated:

*Schools could provide the efficient means to attain all of the eight components of primary health care and could ensure that young people can be educated to have a good understanding of what health means, how to achieve it, and how it contributes to social and economic development.*

Twenty years later The WHO said:

*School health programmes that co-ordinate the delivery of education and health services and promote a healthy environment could become one of the most efficient means available for almost every nation in the world to improve significantly the well being of its people. Consequently such programmes could become a critical means of improving the condition of humankind globally.*

(WHO, 1997)

The particular importance of education for girls is shown by evidence that a 10% increase in female literacy reduces child mortality by 10% while increased male literacy has little effect (World Bank, 2000). It must be emphasised that unrealistic goals should not be set for schools in relation to the current and future health of young people. The education sector can only go so far in impacting on the factors that seriously damage the health of children of school age and subsequently. Poverty, for example, is a main, if not the major, determinant of health and education can make only so much contribution to redressing poverty. Conflict within and between countries also has a major impact on the health of children and again education can only make limited contribution to amelioration of such effects. A UK document concerned with inequalities and health (Acheson, 1998) recommended:

*the provision of additional resources for schools serving children from less well off groups to enhance their educational achievement ... . Funding mechanisms should be more strongly weighted to reflect need and socioeconomic disadvantage.*

## HISTORICAL BACKGROUND AND THE EMERGENCE OF THE HEALTH PROMOTING SCHOOL

Efforts to secure the provision of both health education in schools and specialist school health services have a relatively long history. More recently the holistic development of schools as health promoting settings has become a focus for activity. The stimuli for the development of health education and related activities in schools have varied over time and between countries but it has to be acknowledged that at a global level the WHO has made a singular contribution to setting an agenda for thinking and practice. The 1950s provide a useful starting point for noting some key points of the development.

The Expert Committee on School Health Services (WHO, 1951) emphasised the importance of developing satisfactory health education programmes, supportive teacher training and innovative teaching methods. Endorsement of the emphasis on health education in schools was provided by a subsequent Expert Committee (WHO, 1954). Although this document did not use the current language of 'health promoting schools' many of the criteria specified for such schools are mentioned in this early document. It also recommended that as part of teacher training students should experience cooperative relationships between school- and community-based public health workers and collaborative working with them. This committee recommended that the WHO, in collaboration with UNESCO, should convene a conference or study group to explore the fostering of teacher training for health education and *Planning for Health Education in Schools* was published (WHO, 1966).

Throughout the 1970s and 1980s WHO produced a number of reports and technical discussions addressing features of the health of children and young people, including observations on school health education (WHO, 1977, 1979, 1986 1989). A number of similar principles and recommendations can be identified in the documents:

- the need to recognise the two-way relationship between health and education;
- the matching of health education programmes to local needs and problems;
- enhancement of the role of schools in local communities by establishing closer relationships between children, teachers, parents and community members;
- greater cooperation between health, education and social authorities;
- increase in appropriate interdisciplinary collaborative research;
- the use of innovative teaching methods, including the participation of children in community health projects.

When discussing the health of young people, which it describes variously as 'adolescents' or 'youth', the WHO has placed emphasis on the participation of young people themselves in the assessment of their needs and in the planning, implementation and evaluation of programmes. For example, it proposed (WHO, 1993a, b) that young people should have a role in the decision making procedures in all matters relating to health. A global review of the status of school health education was prepared in 1990 for presentation at the World Conference on Education For All in Thailand. It documented the nature and range of successful initiatives, stressed the importance of health education for all children irrespective of whether they are able to attend schools and set out challenges and issues for action, including:

1 Linkage of health education with the Education For All initiative.
2 The need for policies on school health education and for joint education and health sector implementation strategies.
3 Curriculum development based on the health needs of different age groups and taking the sociocultural context into account. Inclusion of parents and community leaders on curriculum development committees.
4 The need to give due weight in schools to personal and social development.
5 Teacher training and other curricula support for health education.
6 High priority to the pivotal role of teachers in the promotion of health in schools and communities.
7 Schools must be health promoting institutions.
8 School health education must be planned and implemented in the context of the pupils/families and the wider community.

(WHO, 1990)

From the 1990s there has been wide adoption of the language of 'health promoting schools'. defined as follows:

> *The health promoting school aims at achieving healthy lifestyles for the total school population by developing supporting environments conducive to the promotion of health. It offers opportunities for, and requires commitments to, the provision of a safe and health enhancing environment.*

(WHO, 1995)

The origins lie in the recognition that all aspects of the school and influences in the wider community make their separate and interacting influences on health in schools. The UK can be given some credit for getting the idea going in a practical way. In-service training in 1979 for teachers to deliver the *Schools Council Health Education Project* (Schools Council/HEC, 1982) included identification of the elements of the health promoting school and support for teachers in generating targets for developing individual schools in a health promoting direction. The take-up of such ideas developed slowly through the 1980s.

A European Network of Health Promoting Schools was set up in 1992 as a joint initiative between the Council of Europe, the World Health Organisation European Office (WHO/EURO) and the Commission of the European Communities. In 1993 the European Parliament called on the Commission for European Communities and its member states to:

> ... *encourage the establishment throughout the community of pilot projects which adopt a comprehensive approach to health education by involving not only schools but also families, local communities, sports clubs, voluntary services etc. These measures should be pursued as an integral part of the European Network of Health Promoting Schools Projects.*
>
> (European Parliament, cited in St Leger, 1998)

The initiative has been taken forward in a number of ways. In some countries and regions the promotion of healthy school awards has been the organising format for furthering the health promoting schools idea (Moon *et al.*, 1999). National policy documents have also endorsed the health promoting school concept. The major publication on redressing inequalities in health, the *Acheson Report*, referred to earlier, included as one of its recommendations the further development of 'health promoting schools' initially focused on, but not limited to, disadvantaged communities.

## MODELS OF THE HEALTH PROMOTING SCHOOL

The health promoting school goes significantly beyond the provision of health education in the classroom. The concept of such schools includes a number of elements:

- the school as an environment;
- the formal and informal curricula;
- the hidden curriculum and ethos of the school;
- the links with families and other aspects of the community;
- health and social services.

Different writers have identified and grouped the elements in slightly different ways (Box 1).

**Box 1** Elements of Health Promoting Schools

> 1 *Health education in the formal curriculum and through pastoral care.*
> 2 *The hidden curriculum – including the caring relationships, the examples set by teachers, the relationships developed between home and school, and the physical environment and facilities of the school.*
> 3 *The health and caring services providing health screening, immunisation, first aid, and psychological services.*
>
> (Young, 1992)
>
> 1 *Enhanced education for health through the formal curriculum.*
> 2 *Improvements in the physical and social environment for pupils and staff to work in, including attention to how the organisation of the school encourages or inhibits healthy living.*
> 3 *Expansion of school/wider community links.*
>
> (Tones, 1999)

Within the European Network of Health Promoting Schools the three broad areas are broken down into 12 criteria which schools are expected to address.

### Twelve criteria for health promoting schools

1 Active promotion of the self-esteem of all pupils by demonstrating that everyone can

make a contribution to the life of the school.

2  The development of good relations between staff and pupils and between pupils in the daily life of the schools.

3  The clarification for staff and pupils of the social aims of the school.

4  The provision of stimulating challenges for all pupils through a wide range of activities.

5  Using every opportunity to improve the physical environment of the school.

6  The development of good links between the school, the home and the community.

7  The development of good links between associated primary and secondary schools to plan a coherent health education curriculum.

8  The consideration of the role of staff exemplars in health-related issues.

9  The active promotion of the health and well-being of school staff.

10  The complementary role of school meals (if provided) to the health education curriculum.

11  The realisation of specialist services in the community for advice and support in health education.

12  The development of the education potential of the school health services beyond routine screening towards active support for the curriculum.

(Parsons *et al.*, 1977)

These criteria can, of course, be used to generate indicators for evaluation.

## IDEOLOGIES OF HEALTH EDUCATION AND HEALTH PROMOTION IN SCHOOLS

Chapter 1 provided a full discussion of models of health promotion. Schools may use, explicitly or implicitly, all of the models discussed. For example, various external agencies have expectations that children in schools will be encouraged to adopt health promoting behaviours and evaluation will assess the extent to which they are successful in achieving such a goal. Schools, in seeking to respond to these expectations, have implemented interventions informed by the various elements of a preventive approach. At the same time schools are in the business of developing knowledge and the cognitive skills of problem solving and decision making and the educational approach fits this central purpose. Schools, it can be suggested, have a more ambivalent relationship with health promotion models centring on concepts of empowerment and social change. Developing individual empowerment, within limits, might fit with the simple educational model but pursuit of empowerment as collective action to bring about social change could be seen as problematical. Given the ages during which children are at school and the agreed, as well as contested, expectations of what schools are for, we would expect to find all models being drawn on according to time, place and age of children. For example, even where there are reservations about drawing on the elements of the *Preventive Model* its use would be justified in some circumstances. For example, use of a preventive approach would be endorsed in work with young children in the context of acting *in loco parentis* and in recognition of their underdeveloped capacity to make informed choices.

The division between an *Educational Model* and an *Empowerment Model* is not always clear cut as far as the content of activities is concerned. One way to make the distinction can be through locating the source of the impetus for activities and the end goals which are sought. For example, schools may build in activities designed to develop self-efficacy in order to enable young people to benefit from educational opportunity and to support employment seeking at a later stage. Alternatively, such work can be in response to young people's identification that they need to be self-efficacious in order to be able to bring about changes in their lives. Ideas associated with empowerment have predominantly been associated with progressive ideologies of education and more closely associated with individual empowerment than with developing community empowerment. As the writings of Freire and other critical theorists and, more recently, the ideas associated with the health promotion movement began to have an influence in schools we have seen some broadening of the conceptions of empowerment

(Kalnins *et al.*, 1992). In describing the *Empowerment Model* in schools Hagquist and Starrin (1997) have suggested that this presupposes a mobilisation of persons and is characterised by:

- joint action by pupils;
- development work must be directed by participants;
- participants must be enabled actively to participate in the production of the necessary knowledge in order to enable changes to be introduced efficiently;
- development of individual capabilities.

They summarise the model as:

> *all those involved in the school should actively participate in all stages of the local work for change, constantly maintaining a democratic dialogue with each other. Teachers and other staff can play the role of facilitators of the empowerment process among the pupils. The starting point is pupils participation in identifying problems and needs. Subsequent steps are aimed at investigation and analysis, preparing a proposal for change, formulating an action programme and implementing changes. Pupils, teachers and others should jointly monitor what has resulted.*

Addressing the social and environmental determinants of health is central to health promotion. While the raising of awareness about such causes has not been ignored, it has not appeared to rank highly in importance as an aim with teachers in practice, or in training. In a survey by Nutbeam *et al.* (1987) teachers rated topics in order of perceived importance. The environment and health were rated as very important by only 28% of respondents. From a national survey of preparation for health promotion in initial teacher training in England and Wales Walsh and Tilford (1998) reported that only one third of courses covered environmental aspects of health or addressed health inequalities. Relatively few early health education curriculum support materials were strongly informed by broad empowerment/social change approaches, although there

were some notable exceptions (Dorn and Nortoft, 1982; Anderson, 1986). The health promoting school concept might be expected to stimulate adoption of more radical approaches and we will consider the extent to which it appears to have done so later in the chapter.

## EVALUATING HEALTH PROMOTION IN SCHOOLS

Given the growing importance of the whole-school approach to health promotion the major emphasis of our attention to evaluation could arguably be given to discussing the measures of success in achieving health promoting schools and identifying achievements. However, despite support for the idea of health promoting schools the full dissemination of the idea is not yet complete and schools in very many countries continue to focus predominantly on health education initiatives carried out within the formal and informal curricula. Early evaluations largely focused on success in achieving classroom-based health education goals. Gradually evaluations were undertaken, especially in the USA, of classroom interventions in the context of community-wide programmes. These comprehensive programmes often included activities covering the main elements specified for health promoting schools, although not designated as such. Most recently, published evaluations of the 'health promoting schools' approach have emerged, predominantly, but not solely, from Europe and Australia. In reviewing evidence we will be examining the effectiveness of health education interventions – which may, or may not be, in the context of health promoting schools initiatives – together with evidence of success in achieving the broader goal of health promoting schools. We will comment on approaches to evaluating health education interventions followed by approaches to evaluating health promoting schools

### Evaluation of health education interventions

Methodological approaches to the evaluation of school health education initiatives have broadly paralleled those in health education more generally, as discussed in Chapter 3. There has been widespread use of true and quasi-experimental design approaches, although these have been used rather more extensively and thoroughly in the USA than elsewhere. A large number of before–after studies, with or without a comparison group, have also been published. While most content areas of health education have been evaluated, certain topic areas have been subjected to more activity than others – substance use and misuse, nutrition and sexual health education, including HIV/AIDS prevention, stand out as examples. A large number of reviews have been reported and we will draw on the conclusions of such studies. Throughout this book we have noted the ambivalence about systematic review evidence in health promotion. We will draw on systematic reviews in this chapter since they bring together a large part of the literature, but confining discussion to this evidence alone would fail to meet many readers' needs and we will also draw on additional studies as appropriate to discussion. There are many school-based evaluation studies which do not meet the methodological criteria for inclusion in systematic reviews as they are typically applied. Such studies can generate either quantitative or qualitative data or a combinations of both. For example, case studies from schools evaluating the development of comprehensive health education curricula or the adoption and implementation of specific curriculum projects have adopted action research approaches and generated quantitative and qualitative data. These studies can provide us with some of the richest insights into health promotion in schools.

## Evaluating health promoting schools initiatives

The development of the holistic health promoting schools concept has stimulated active consideration of evaluation issues. Evaluations may seek to generate evidence of the extent to which the development of health promoting schools has progressed overall, in countries or in regions, and also of evidence of success within individual schools. It has been necessary to consider the development of indicators for measuring the suc-

cess of such complex initiatives. To the extent that health promoting schools initiatives are informed by the Ottawa Charter principles it becomes central to consider to what extent a participatory approach to evaluation will be adopted. To what extent, for example, are young people themselves involved in developing indicators for health promoting schools, in deciding on the nature of evaluations and participating in the process of completing and writing up evaluations? There have been some reflections on evaluation of the health promoting school developments. Parsons *et al.* (1996) referred to the WHO definition for health promoting schools and the 12 criteria listed above and pointed to their emphases on provision rather than on specific behaviour change goals. They commented:

> *The significance of this is not to indicate error or oversight but that different audiences may have different, even competing expectations of the health promoting school and different preferred foci for evaluation.*

We can expect, therefore, to see differences in the weighting given to process, impact and outcome indicators. Where there is a strong emphasis on empowerment and participation there will, inevitably, be a reduced emphasis on following up specific individually focused health behaviour goals, although behaviours associated with achieving health-related social and environmental change might be addressed. There is clearly a tension between the settings-based ideology of this development and pressures for accountability through evidence on narrowly focused health and behaviour indicators. This has been emphasised by Rowling and Jeffries (2000):

> *the simplified perspective represented in the accountability perspective brushes aside the complexity represented in the interplay of the structural and organisational milieu with the process and personal elements, that operate in the development of the Health Promoting School.*

Individual countries within the wider networks such as the *European Health Promoting School* may put individual interpretations on the health promoting school model and seek to prioritise particular processes and outcomes in evaluations. In communicating the idea of evaluation of the health promoting school beyond the selected small number of schools taking part in pilot programmes a strong emphasis on process goals may be more difficult to transmit than one which emphasises what are clearly recognised to be health related outcomes. The more general and wide ranging the process goals the more difficult it may become to distinguish the idea of the health promoting school from an idea of what education should offer in its entirety.

A recent systematic review of health promotion in schools (Lister-Sharp *et al.*, 1999) was divided into two components – one an assessment of the effectiveness of health promoting schools and the other of health promotion interventions (strictly speaking health education) in schools. Reflecting on the first of the reviews the researchers said that because of the philosophical approach to health promoting schools and their emphasis on process they saw the inclusion of only the particular types of study normally incorporated in systematic reviews as problematical:

> *There are difficulties with the application of the experimental model to health promoting interventions which arise from the need for active participation in health promotion programmes and this is well acknowledged.*

The evaluation challenges in assessing the effectiveness of the health promoting school were discussed by Lister-Sharp *et al.*, including the lack of agreement on appropriate methods and they also commented on the particular focus of evaluations which had been published:

> *The health promoting school concept sits uncomfortably within a framework for evaluation that requires the demonstration of physical and health related behaviour outcomes. Yet these outcomes were those most commonly employed in the studies we identified and only a minority of studies evaluated the impact of the interventions on mental well being.*

## Health promotion in schools: indicators of success

### Health promoting schools

While schools are unlikely to deny that they are concerned to do anything other than promote the health of their members not all will have adopted the holistic notion of the health promoting school as described above. In some cases, therefore, indicators of success may largely focus on knowledge, attitudes, values and health promoting behaviours at the individual and group levels. As schools implement the full health promoting school idea indicators of achievements in all the areas identified as part of the health promoting school will need to be addressed. The number of stakeholders with an interest in the health promoting school developments may have competing views on appropriate indicators for assessing successes and different degrees of influence in determining the indicators which are used. Where there is particular concern to assess the combined success of a health promoting school initiative at regional, national or international levels there are likely to be pressures to measure success against some agreed common indicators. While such indicators can include process ones there may be pressures to obtain, or even give priority to, outcomes evidence. For a project informed by health promotion ideology which prioritises process and especially the active participation of young people themselves in the achievement of health promoting schools there will be a reluctance to have these values compromised by pressures to achieve on behavioural goals. Illustrative goals and examples of the content of indicators for the various elements of the health promoting school, from policy through to individual level, are described in Box 2. Within each element of the health promoting school there will be discussions about what might be appropriate goals and indicators. Indicators need to be fully specified in order to derive appropriate measures. Such measures might be in percentage terms or, alternatively, the existence of qualitative evidence would be used. In many cases indicators might be staged such that progress towards stated goals can be fully documented.

There is an ongoing project to develop indicators for health promoting schools at the European level and publication is planned for 2001. This project will be developing objectives, indicators and criteria for success for the health promoting school at international, national, school and community level, together with general recommendations on evaluation of this programme.

**Box 2** Examples of Indicators for Assessing Health Promoting Schools

---

*National*

*Policy*
Goal: health promotion should have a place in school national curricula and should have parity with other subjects.
Indicators: national curriculum documents.

*Educational training to support health promotion initiatives*
Goal: all people completing teacher training should have participated in a course of health promotion in order to prepare them to contribute to the development of health promoting primary and secondary schools.
   Indicators: specified curricula in teacher training courses with evidence from assessed work and school practice of knowledge of health promoting schools.

*School*

*Policy*
Goal: schools will have a general health promotion policy and specific policies for aspects of health as required.
Indicators: existence and content of policies.

*Curriculum*
Goal: all young people should have access to a comprehensive programmes of health education throughout the years of formal education which conforms to national curriculum requirements.

Indicator: timetabled as stated subject or identified contextually.

*Individual*
Goal: all children and young people should be enabled to make health promoting behavioural choices.
Indicators: choices in school meals; assessed competence in decision making.

*Hidden curriculum*
Goal: that young people should receive messages that they are valued and have a participatory role in school activities.
Indicators: participation in policy making activities in schools; pupil reports.

*Environment*
Goal: all aspects of the school environment should be supportive of health.
Indicators: shady as well as sunny outside play and recreation areas; water and sanitation; school gardens; design, lay out and decoration of buildings.

*Community links*
Goal: to develop a range of linkages and activities with families communities and other institutions.
Indicators: degree of involvement and nature of linkages with health service staff; joint school–community actions; parental involvement in development of health promotion policies.

---

### Health education in schools

As we have noted, the major proportion of reported evaluations of school programmes are of health education initiatives undertaken at classroom level. Studies address either single indicators or various combinations of intermediate and outcome indicators. Early evaluations tended to focus heavily on knowledge and beliefs, attitudes and relatively simple behaviours, but more complex competencies such as coping strategies and decision making were also addressed. While a large number of studies have measured successes with reference to specific health behaviours and their associated variables, others have assessed the achievements of general personal attributes and transferable skills. Indicators of success can include knowledge and beliefs, attitudes, self-esteem, self-efficacy, empowerment, a variety of communication and social interaction skills, specific health behaviours, decision making, advocacy and so on.

### Efficiency and equity

In addition to addressing questions of effectiveness we have also to consider efficiency and equity. Efficiency concerns will be addressed in assessing alternative methods and the most appropriate timing of interventions in reaching goals. Measures of equity can include policies to redress inequalities, equal opportunities to access national (or local) resources to support health promoting school initiatives and the identification and appropriate responses to the health education needs of all young people.

Before examining evidence of success we will comment briefly on schools as contexts for evaluation research and on methods of data collection.

## SCHOOLS AS A CONTEXT FOR EVALUATION RESEARCH

While teachers routinely assess many aspects of pupil performance they have not typically been required to undertake research-based evaluations of curriculum provision and they have not routinely been trained as researchers. The action research movement triggered, in some countries, a growth in classroom-based evaluation in schools in a number of countries (Elliott, 1991), although it is hard to estimate how often health education developments were the subject of action research projects. A considerable proportion of published health education interventions, particularly in the USA, have been carried out by researchers external to schools. There are a number of reasons which can be suggested for the relatively low amount of school initiated evaluations of health education:

- failure to acknowledge the importance of evaluating a subject area which has traditionally had lower status within the curriculum;

- lack of skills for evaluating some of the key components of health promotion, e.g. attitudes and values, decision making skills, empowerment, school community links and alliances;
- a shortage of time and other resources to support evaluation, especially in the context of escalating demands on teachers;
- limited preparation in initial teacher training for evaluation of health promotion;
- the continued existence of competing ideas of health promotion and debates about the aims of school health promotion can generate conflict about evaluations and resulting inaction.

There are probably no aspects of evaluation which are unique to schools, although there are some which are more of an issue in this context than in some others. They include the following.

1 Delineating what should be included in evaluation of health promotion. The more broadly the goals of health promotion are defined the more difficult it becomes to differentiate these from the general goals of education.
2 Where the total health education programme in the school is to be evaluated identifying exactly where it is occurring within the school curriculum can be challenging. In the secondary sector, for example, it can be provided through: coordinated inputs across a number of curriculum areas such as biology, physical education, language and so on; as a component of personal, social and health education (PSHE); in the context of tutorial time; or a combinations of all of these. When the contributions from other aspects of the school are to be added in the evaluation task becomes complex.
3 Where health behaviours are the focus for evaluation there are two particular issues. First, many behaviours which are to be addressed typically occur outside the school context and evaluators must rely on reported measures. Second, some activities will be oriented towards behaviours that do not occur until differing periods after young people leave school. Because of the difficulties in carrying out long-term evaluations there will need to be a reliance on intermediate indicators.

4 Where there is a commitment to empowerment approaches it will be necessary to engage with and resolve the difficulties of operationalising and measuring some of their component concepts. Enabling young people themselves to play a full role in the evaluations is also a challenge and there may be a reluctance to facilitate this involvement.

5 Given the ages of children and young people in formal education there are issues about appropriate forms of data collection and around consent to involvement in evaluations.

## Data collection techniques in school evaluations

Above a certain age most methods used with adults can, theoretically, be used with young people. The use of true experimental designs, even where deemed appropriate, can be practically difficult where interventions normally take place in school classes which cannot be rearranged for research purposes. Randomisation of pupils to new groups as required by an experiment is, therefore, not practically feasible. All the issues raised earlier about experimentation also apply to interventions with young people. Where experimental approaches have been undertaken quasi-experimental designs using existing groups have often been preferred.

With young children there are methods which are not appropriate. The use of written questionnaires before literacy is fully established are a case in point. The complexity of language and the concepts used in surveys need to be judged according to cognitive and social development. Questionnaires, if used, need to be interesting and fun to answer.

Ethical issues should be foremost in undertaking research with children. These include attention to the procedures for gaining access to children, their consent to participation and confidentiality at all stages of a research process. While such issues are important in research with any group of people they are arguably even more so with children but have not always been adequately recognised (Morrow and Richards, 1996). They remind us of the following:

- in terms of methodology researchers need to think carefully about the standpoint from which they are studying children and the ethical implications of that standpoint;
- researchers need to be aware that their responsibilities as adults towards children must be fulfilled and ensure that children do not suffer harm at any stage of the research process;
- researchers must be wary of assuming that children are a homogenous group; the accounts children give of themselves will be affected by a number of variables related to the individual child, where and how data are collected and the personal style of the researcher.

They make a useful point in support of the use of multiple methods in research with children:

*In practical terms, over reliance on one type of data collection can lead to biases, and given children's relatively powerless position in society, it might be that drawing on a range of creative methods, and using multiple research strategies might be a useful way forward.*

Some specific techniques have been developed for use with children. With young children there has been increasing application of the 'draw and write' technique where children are invited to draw their answer to questions posed and then to write about what they have drawn. The technique can be used as both a quantitative and qualitative tool and singly or in combination with other methods (Porcellato *et al.*, 1999). Examples of studies in which it has been used include those of Barnett *et al.* (1995), Pridmore and Bendelow (1995), McGregor *et al.* (1998) and McWhirter *et al.* (2000). 'Draw and write' has recently been subjected to critical appraisal (Backet-Milburn and McKie, 1999). They argued that although the technique has made an important contribution to health education research a number of methodological, analytical and ethical issues can be raised about it. They ask whether children give back to researchers what they feel they want to hear. The evidence reported from requests to children to draw 'what makes or keeps you healthy' has tended to elicit from children a more conventional and limited picture of health than can be discovered in the use of other methods. Questions are also raised about the quantitative analysis of what is essentially a qualitative method. Where ethical issues are concerned they note that, given the importance of access and consent, it is important to reflect on whether particular methods, including drawing, lead children to reveal more than they might otherwise choose to do so. They concluded:

*...health education research with children must involve taking children seriously as social actors and query the assumption that drawing enables children to communicate their thoughts any more than does conversational language.*

Some of the techniques used in participatory appraisal, which will be considered in Chapter 9, can also be used in research with children, a point made by Morrow and Richards (1996):

*Using interactive and participatory research methods may be a useful way of researching children – and it is interesting to note that much of the impetus for participatory methods is coming from developing countries, where children are participants in society (at least at the level of production) to a much greater extent than in the UK.*

For the remainder of the chapter we will review the evidence of effectiveness of school health promotion under the following headings:

- policy;
- the overall impact nationally and internationally of health promotion in schools with reference to health education and to health promoting school developments;
- specific health promoting school evaluations;
- health education interventions.

## POLICY – INTERNATIONAL AND NATIONAL

Developments at the policy level provide a context which can support or inhibit the development of health promotion at the school level. It is important to assess the extent and nature of policy developments. Such policies can include general education policies, policies on health promotion as a totality or policies on specific elements. In addition, there are policies in other sectors which have a direct or indirect bearing on children's health. While the existence of policy can be necessary to achieve action it is rarely sufficient. There are numerous examples of policies which have never sufficiently influenced practice. Reviewing all the policy areas which can have an impact on the health of children and young people is beyond the scope of this chapter. Policy areas of significance will also vary from country to country. We will comment specifically on designated policy on health promotion in schools.

The World Health Organization is the lead player in generating policy at regional and global levels. While their policies are not binding on nations they do provide a background context which influences national level policies. The invitation from the central office of the WHO in Geneva to take up the health promoting schools concept has been responded to in all WHO regions with the subsequent developments having their own particular flavour. In the European Region 37 countries were reported to be in the network by 1997 (St Leger, 1999). In the Western Pacific Region the health promoting schools concept was articulated in *New Horizons in Health* and by 1995 had been adopted by the 32 member nations (St Leger, 1999).

At the national level countries have policies on health and on education both of which may incorporate policy statements on school health promotion. These statements may directly recognise the role of the health promoting schools movement but can also omit to do so even where there is participation in the development. Policies can be directed towards school health promotion as a whole or to specific health areas, with drugs education (including tobacco and alcohol) and sexual health education (family life in some countries) being very common examples. In commenting on policy on health promotion we will illustrate the discussion with references to the UK and, briefly, to Australia.

National policies on education and health in the constituent countries of the UK have included statements on school health education. In the English *Health of the Nation* policy document (Department of Health, 1992) schools were given a clear role as a setting for the provision of health education. When the Education Reform Act in 1988 (Her Majesty's Government, 1988) initiated a National Curriculum for education there was limited attention to health promotion, although pupils were given an entitlement to personal, social and health education. Curriculum guidelines were issued to guide health education provision. Education legislation (Department of Education, 1994) made sex education compulsory in schools and the national orders for science included elements of sex and drugs education. The current government has addressed health in schools through health and education policy documents. A White Paper *Excellence in Schools* stated a commitment to early years education and to helping all schools become healthy schools (Department for Education and Employment, 1997). The most recent major policy document *Saving Lives: Our Healthier Nation* has promoted the *Healthy Schools Programme*, defining a healthy school as one where good health and social behaviour underpin effective learning and academic achievement (Department of Health, 1999). A national *Healthy Schools Scheme* will build links between education and health authorities to provide the context and support for school communities. The scheme encourages schools to become healthy schools by establishing and consolidating partnerships in order to improve the health of pupils and staff and the wider community (Aggleton *et al.*, 2000).

Australia's goals and targets for health for the year 2000 and beyond involve the school curriculum, school environment and the interface between schools and community and links with health and welfare services. A national network of healthy school communities and the Australian Education's *Nation Goals for Schooling* provided guidelines for the development of health promoting schools (Colquhoun, 1997, Lynagh *et al.*, 1997).

Policy in relation to specific health topic areas

has also been generated either with reference to health promotion as a whole or for specific named areas. For example, we can comment on drugs policy in the UK. Requirements for drug education in schools were included within the statutory orders for science in the national curricula in the UK. These required particular areas of content for drug education. In addition, the curriculum guidelines for health education advised on the extension of drug education beyond the statutory requirements by examining drugs, society and behaviour. The recommendations contained within the publications have been summarised (Allott *et al.*, 1999) (Box 3).

*Box 3* Drug Education Recommendations

---

*Providers*
Education should be led by teachers
There should be multi-agency support

*Methods*
Needs based
Providing information
Teaching decision making skills
Interactive teaching methods
Integrated into the curriculum
Maintained across the life span

*Research and Evaluation*
Drug education should be evidence based
Programme effectiveness should be evaluated

---

The nature and extent of school level policies in Wales and England has been reported from a study by Thomas *et al.* (1998) All secondary schools in Wales together with a representative random sample of 546 secondary schools from England were involved in a questionnaire-based survey. The survey investigated:

- the breadth and implementation of health-related policies;
- the involvement of outside agencies in the development of health-related policies;
- the frequency of reviewing health-related policies;

- the time incentives given to teachers for health education responsibility and the frequency of in-service training undertaken by teachers;
- the degree of awareness of the term 'health promoting school'.

Response rates of 53% in Wales and 44% in England were achieved. Selected results included: in Wales 76.9% of schools and in England 58.5% had a defined health education policy. Where policies for specific areas of health were concerned the figures for Wales and England are shown in Table 5.1.

Significant differences between the two countries for all specific health policies were found. In both countries only small percentages adopted policies written by their local education authorities (23.4% in Wales and 12.4% in England) while the majority developed their own (76.6% in Wales and 87.6% in England). Implementation of policies was largely the responsibility of several people but no school reported the involvement of parents or pupils. Over three-quarters of schools in both countries involved a wide variety of outside agencies and other professionals – in developing health-related policies the three most commonly cited in both countries were school nurses, district health promotion units and local authority advisory teachers. Figures for in-service training to support health education again differed between the two countries – 81.4% in Wales and 68% in England.

The impact of having policies in place needs to be examined. In a recent review St Leger (1999),

with reference to Australia, notes that despite the range of topics for which school level policies have been generated few studies have documented health outcomes with reference to the existence of policies. Some Australian evidence suggested that health gains were achieved when policies were adopted but the studies available did not include control schools. St Leger concludes:

> *The policy component in most of the international and national document frameworks of health promoting schools is not supported by evidence which indicates tangible health benefits can be achieved because policies are in place.*

Such a conclusion is a pointer to the need for further evaluation of the impact of policy.

In the next section we will consider the overall impact of health promotion in schools, beginning with health education interventions and then the health promoting schools.

## The overall impact of health promotion in schools – nationally and internationally

### Health education

There have been efforts to draw some summary conclusions about the overall effectiveness of health education drawing on interventions across countries. Many of these efforts preceded any widespread adoption of the health promoting school idea although multi-component interventions in more than one sector were included. In addition to summarising the effectiveness of health education as a whole there have also been

***Table 5.1*** A Summary of the Frequency of Health Education Policies

| Policy relating to | Wales | | | England | | |
|---|---|---|---|---|---|---|
| | % | *n* | rank | % | *n* | rank |
| Smoking | 82.8 | (77) | 1 | 59.5 | (119) | 2 |
| Alcohol | 80.6 | (75) | 2 | 58.5 | (117) | 3 |
| Illegal drugs | 80.6 | (75) | 2 | 59.5 | (119) | 2 |
| Nutrition and healthy eating | 79.6 | (74) | 3 | 56.5 | (113) | 4 |
| Physical exercise | 76.3 | (71) | 4 | 54.0 | (108) | 5 |
| HIV/AIDS | 75.5 | (71) | 5 | 61.3 | (122) | 1 |
| Pupils | 46.2 | (43) | 6 | 41.8 | (84) | 6 |
| Pupils and teachers | 43.5 | (40) | 7 | 31.9 | (65) | 7 |

many examples of attempts to generalise about overall effectiveness in specific topic areas. The difficulties in providing evidence for the success of health education across a nation has long been recognised. In 1985 Newman commented that schools are organised to facilitate learning, not to conduct evaluative research (Newman, 1985). In the interim period the growing pressures on schools in many countries to be more accountable has led to a change in attitudes to evaluation. While there are growing expectations and requirements that evaluation will happen these do not necessarily apply equally to all subjects and lower status subjects such as health education are less open to pressures. It should also be noted that much of the increase in evaluation is top down and imposed and not necessarily linked with professional development for evaluation.

Over the years pessimistic comments have been made about the general successes of what was then described as school health education. In 1992 The US contributor to the Geneva Conference on comprehensive school health education (WHO/UNESCO/UNICEF, 1992) reported progress during the previous 10 years but claimed that there was evidence that the gap between the state of the art and actual practice was larger than in any other area of the curriculum.

Some of the better early evidence came from national level surveys in the USA in the 1980s. The School Health Education Evaluation (SHEE) (Gunn *et al.*, 1985) was a study of four different health education programmes in 20 states and involved 30,000 children. As an evaluation it addressed the perceived need for experimental studies carried out in exemplary fashion and also the need for representative studies of the health education curriculum in natural surroundings. The full evaluation included studies of the four curricula in normal classroom situations and an experimental study of one project, the *School Health Curriculum Project* (Gunn *et al.*, 1985). Reviewing the SHEE evaluation Cooke and Walberg (1985) described it as of the highest quality with respect to inferences about causal connections and the generalisations that it promoted. Health educators now had, they said, a large scale

credible study to support their advocacy for school provision.

The evaluation was undertaken using a pre-test–post-test questionnaire and addressed the learning objectives that experts and parents stated as the most important for children of 8–11 years. These included ten knowledge, four attitude and three practice areas. Significant increases in knowledge were achieved in study classrooms when compared with controls. Smaller, but still significant, increases were also found for attitudes and self-reported practices. The effectiveness of programmes was linked, not surprisingly, to the extent to which the projects in question were fully implemented, although it was noted that incomplete implementation had less impact on knowledge than on attitudes and practice areas. The amount of in-service training received by teachers was also related to programme implementation measures: the fully trained completed a greater percentage of the programmes with greater fidelity than the partly trained, who were, in turn, better than the untrained. The overall results of the study were summarised:

> *the study shows, in general, that health education does make a difference, that it works better when there is more of it, and that it works best when it is implemented with broad scale administrative support for teacher training, integrated material and continuity across school years.*
>
> (Greenberg, 1985)

Although received with some enthusiasm, the SHEE did have its limitations. On its own admission the study sample was mainly white and middle class, although the reasons for this were not made clear. The follow-up period was not as long as had been wished for and the study was confined to younger children. Although it did focus on some outcomes related to an empowerment approach, no comprehensive assessment of these outcomes was offered. Most importantly, it needs to be stressed that the gains identified in this evaluation were recorded when the programmes concerned were in the early active stages of implementation. Maintenance of long-term implementation is difficult.

There have now been a large number of systematic reviews of the successes of schools health education in particular health areas and a recent 'review of reviews' has been completed by Lister-Sharp *et al.* (1999). Their conclusion was that:

> *school health promotion (i.e. education) initiatives can have a positive impact on children's health and behaviour but do not do so consistently. It would appear that most interventions are able to increase children's knowledge but that changing other factors which influence health, such as attitudes and behaviour, is much harder to achieve, even in the short term. Overall, a multifaceted approach is likely to be the most effective combining a classroom programme with changes in the school ethos and/or environment and/or with family/community involvement. This is consistent with the health promoting schools approach.*

This conclusion is an indicator of what can be achieved by health education taken as a whole but it is also a clear reminder of the difficult challenge in achieving success. Within this summary verdict there is evidence of some successes. Lister-Sharp *et al.*'s summary of achievements is provided in Box 4.

Readers should be reminded that this review of reviews could only include topics in health education where previous systematic reviews had been undertaken. The strengths and limitations of systematic review evidence were discussed in Chapter 3. As noted earlier, systematic reviews have tended to draw on studies from a limited number of countries since those countries are more likely to have carried out and reported studies which fit the methodological criteria applied in reviews. General commentary reviews, as distinct from systematic reviews, have also tended to be biased in a similar direction for the simple reason that resources are more likely to have been available in some countries to support research. Even where studies have been carried out, dissemination of findings is not equally easy. A valuable document (Hubley, 1998) has brought together and discussed a full range of school health education interventions in developing countries. He concluded that evaluation was not

**Box 4** Positive Outcomes in School Health Education Programmes

---

*Usually Achievable*
Improvement in health-related knowledge.
Reduction in intention to smoke, drink and take drugs.
Development of health protecting skills: resistance/refusal; abuse prevention skills.
Improvement in health promoting behaviour: wearing of cycle helmets and seat belts.
Improvement in physical fitness.
Environment improvement: school meals; safer roads.

*Sometimes Achievable*
Improvement in psychological health:

- self-concept;
- self-efficacy;
- coping skills;
- interpersonal communication skills.

Development of specific skills: road crossing; tooth brushing; sun protection.
Improvement in dietary intake.
Improvements in cholesterol levels.
Postponement of initiation of smoking.

*Rarely or Not Achievable*
Reductions in specific behaviours: alcohol consumption; drug misuse; high risk sexual behaviour; long term smoking rates.
Reduction in weight.
Improvements in self esteem.
Improvements in attitudes towards drinking, smoking, drug taking.

---

always done very well and results were poorly documented. The difficulties in generalising from the wide range of programmes in his review was pointed out but Hubley drew what he described as tentative conclusions.

1 There is a rich collection of relevant experience within the published literature on school health

promotion and more specifically school health education in developing countries.

2 There is evidence that school-based health education activities can bring about changes in knowledge and sometimes behaviour in the short term.

3 There are very few studies that investigate the scaling up from the small to large scale interventions.

4 There are very few published studies that follow up programmes over time or report a process of monitoring or formative evaluation.

5 There are published accounts of school-based activities in developing countries for specific health topics such as nutrition, smoking, sex education, AIDS, dental health, etc. However there are very few studies that look into the implementation of broad-based health education curricula.

6 With the exception of dental health there are few studies that combine biomedical interventions with the development of curricula.

7 It is difficult to generalise from published studies of health education in developing countries on the ingredients that contributed to success or failure as they do not always contain sufficient data – especially qualitative data. However, the following would appear to be important: an initial needs assessment which takes into account and involves teachers, parents and children, training of teachers, follow-up support of teachers and community-based activities.

8 Although needs, context and resources differ greatly there is considerable value in sharing experience in school health promotion between developed and developing countries on educational methods, research and evaluation.

Before leaving this section we should also refer to a valuable review of current policy and practice related to health and AIDS education in primary and secondary schools in Africa and Asia (Barnett *et al.*, 1995). Their report draws on published and unpublished literature and on empirical work in Pakistan, India, Uganda and Ghana. The study methods used key informant interviews and documentary analyses of policy and practice. Space precludes a full discussion of this report but a summary of case studies for one of the study countries is provided in Box 5.

**Box 5** Uganda

Uganda has many exciting developments of innovation and development within school health education generally and HIV/AIDS education particularly. There is a well established School Health Education programme, which is supported by policy, by established coordinating mechanisms at central level, and is relatively well researched both from the angle of needs assessment and evaluation. HIV/AIDS education is integrated into this work and is well resourced with innovative materials and a specially trained teams of trainers. Programme implementation is reasonably effective although a number of problems have inevitably arisen – including the need to establish a much better local coordination and strengthening of planned but so far insufficiently implemented monitoring and evaluation systems.

Evidence from the young people themselves shows insight into a variety of health issues – including a detailed understanding of AIDS prevention. There are a number of concerns which stand out – including observations on environmental health and sanitation, on different aspects of nutrition, drugs, a variety of diseases, and more personal concerns focused on family life (especially mistreatment at home) and success and failure at school. AIDS was the most frequently mentioned illness (at a stage in data collection when the young people were not aware of our interest in AIDS). This contrasted with the other three counties, where there was little or no general indication of a concern about AIDS amongst young people. In terms of moving forward on AIDS education there is much to commend in terms of current practice, and obvious areas which now need to be developed including more emphasis on the development of life skills counselling options in schools training teachers in the use of interactive teaching methods.

## OVERALL SUCCESS OF HEALTH PROMOTING SCHOOLS

In this section we will comment on the overall success in achieving health promoting schools drawing on cross-national reviews and studies of individual country developments. For the health promoting school approach Lister-Sharp *et al.* (1999) concluded:

> *the health promoting school initiative is a new, complex developing initiative and the optimum method of evaluation is currently under debate. There are indications that this approach is promising The development of programmes to promote mental and social well being would be likely to improve overall effectiveness and the impact of staff health and well being needs more consideration, The development of measures for mental and social well being is important for future evaluation. Continued investment, and ongoing evaluation are necessary to provide evidence about the effectiveness of this approach.*

These conclusions may seem limited given the extent of recent efforts to develop this idea. They might also be challenged because the systematic review procedure excluded some studies. It should be noted, however, that the reviewers set methodological criteria which were not confined to controlled trials. It can be argued that the before–after studies which were asked for would be necessary if evidence was being sought to demonstrate that major investment in the health promoting schools approach was justified. This is not to say that quite different evaluation studies are not also relevant and important. Detailed case studies of individual school developments or developments within a district using qualitative methods of inquiry are vital if we are to acquire an in-depth understanding of the factors which support and detract from the health promoting school development. They are also useful in gaining a sense of the aspects of health promotion that are readily taken up in schools and those which tend to be given lesser attention and the reasons for these variations.

A study which has attempted to draw some general conclusions about the combined success of health promoting schools was undertaken in six European countries. Parsons *et al.* (1996) based their research on interviews, analysis of documentation and some classroom observation and reported:

1  The *European Network of Health Promoting Schools* (ENHPS) is seen by member states as an internationally credible vehicle for developing public health policy, forging healthy alliances and stimulating community action.
2  The Network has become a major influence on the development and enhancement of health education and health promotion in schools across Europe.
3  ENHPS has the potential to foster internationalism and equality of opportunity in the field of health promotion on a scale which has yet to be realised in other settings for health promotion.
4  The Network has evoked a high degree of enthusiasm amongst personnel at macro, meso and micro levels of operation, management and control of school-based health promotion.
5  ENHPS has operationalised in the school setting a philosophy of health promotion which reflects an eco-holistic approach. As a project with a short life to date it has stimulated and tested ideas and practices and laid a foundation for deeper and wider developments.

They also offered a wide ranging set of recommendations to guide continuing developments.

Early studies of the impact of the health promoting school development within a specific country were reported from Wales (Nubeam *et al.*, 1987; Smith *et al.*, 1992). Their evaluations were designed to assess the key components of health promoting schools:

- the content and development of the health education curriculum;
- the implementation of health-related policies;
- the involvement of outside agencies and other professionals;

- teacher understanding of the health promotion concept.

The earlier study in 1987 had highlighted, according to Nutbeam (1992), the gap between the concept of the health promoting school and current practice in UK schools.

The later study, a survey based on a random sample of 87 Welsh schools, used a structured interview schedule to collect data (Smith *et al.*, 1992). Shortcomings in the range of indicators used were noted particularly in relation to links between the schools and the wider community. There were positive findings from the study.

- all schools taught health education and 60% taught it to all pupils in all five years of secondary school;
- sixty-eight (78%) of the schools had a designated health education coordinator;
- almost all schools provided teaching in the school career about substance misuse, healthy sexuality, personal hygiene, nutrition, exercise and dental health;
- three-fifths of schools had written policies or rules about smoking but less than a third mentioned policies about alcohol and illegal drugs;
- only one in seven schools had policies which restricted the smoking by teachers;
- most health education coordinators were unfamiliar with the health promoting school concept.

As Smith *et al.* comment:

*Many of those who thought their school was a health promoting one or close to becoming one were incorrect in their belief, judged by criteria concerning curriculum organisation, supportive policy developments and community involvement.*

Commenting in an editorial, Nutbeam (1992) said:

*progress in Europe and elsewhere will be dependent on finding ways of improving understanding of the concept of the health promoting school and closing the gap between concept and practice. This will require among other things continued leadership from international and national agencies for better health, continued research which provides evidence of effect and the development of relevant policy and supportive teacher training to ensure implementation.*

In a later study referred to earlier (Thomas *et al.*, 1998) in which schools in Wales and England were compared it was reported that about the same proportion in both countries rated themselves as health promoting schools (60.7% in Wales and 63.5% in England). There was greater awareness of the term 'health promoting school' in Wales than England (79.7 and 58.2%) and significantly more schools in Wales were able to define the term (90.0 against 74.4%). Schools were assessed on their health promoting nature against seven criteria:

1 a defined policy on health education;
2 policy aimed at both pupils and teachers;
3 policy related to smoking, alcohol, physical exercise, nutrition and healthy eating, illegal drugs and HIV/AIDS;
4 a health education coordinator appointed;
5 time allowance to develop a health education curriculum;
6 the coordinator had undergone in-service training
7 involvement of outside agencies in development of health related policies.

Using all seven factors only tiny proportions of schools were health promoting (Wales 2.9%, England 5.5%). The writers concluded that schools did not appear to be familiar with the health promoting school concept, especially in England. This reinforced the findings from earlier studies. While welcoming the apparent increase in other agencies and professionals in policy development the lack of pupil involvement contradicted the health promotion philosophy of developing self-efficacy, empowerment, decision making and advocacy. This evaluation did not address one key element of the health promoting school concept – that of links with families and communities.

## Effectiveness of specific health promoting school interventions

Lister-Sharp *et al.*'s (1999) review brought together evaluations of the health promoting school and other programmes not specifically designated as health promoting school but which, nonetheless, contained actions directed towards the key elements of health promoting schools as listed below. One hundred and eleven studies providing background material or evaluations of projects were identified and 12 were included in the final review (see Box 6). Studies were included which met three criteria (revised from earlier more stringent ones).

1 Explicit health promoting schools developments or interventions utilising the health promoting schools approach with children and young people aged from 5 to 16 years. There should be evidence of active participation by the school and studies should provide details of the components and delivery of the intervention. Programmes should include health promotion activity in the areas of:

1.1. ethos and/or environment of the school;

1.2. the curriculum;

1.3. family and/or community.

2 Controlled studies with a comparison group or a before–after design with no comparison group.

3 Studies should include and report health-related outcomes (including health -related behaviours).

The criteria used are open to challenge and many might claim that the second and third were not fully appropriate to the philosophy underpinning the health promoting school development. The studies which met the criteria are listed in Box 6.

**Box 6** Studies of Health Promoting Schools Approaches in Systematic Reviews

| Study | Focus |
|---|---|
| 1 HEA/ENHPS (1997) UK (Jamison *et al.*, 1998) | Health promoting schools |
| 2 Wessex Healthy Schools UK (Moon *et al.*, 1999) | Healthy schools award scheme |
| 3 Health Promotion Schools of Excellence USA (Sobczyk *et al.*, 1995) | Health Promotion Schools of Excellence Programme |
| 4 Healthy eating policy UK (Young 1993) | Healthy eating as part of whole schools approach |
| 5 Great sensations (USA) (Coates *et al.*, 1985) | Cardiovascular health |
| 6 CATCH USA (Luepker *et al.*, 1996) | Cardiovascular health |
| 7 Heart Smart (USA) (Arbeit *et al.*, 1992) | Cardiovascular health |
| 8 Projects SHARP, CHEK and PGHCP/SHCP USA (Dushaw, 1984) | Multiple topics |
| 9 Anti-bullying programme (UK) (Arora, 1994) | Mental health, safety |
| 10 Sunshine and skin health (Buller *et al.*, 1994) | Skin cancer |
| 11 Dental hygiene programme (Agerbaek *et al.*, 1979) | Dental hygiene |
| 12 Denmark school and community pregnancy prevention programme (Vincent *et al.*, 1987; Koo *et al.*, 1994) | Sexual health and pregnancy preparation |

Of these studies only four were fully designated as health promoting schools evaluations – three of these were general developments and one was of a healthy eating policy – while the remaining eight employed a health promoting schools approach according to the criteria specified. We will comment on the findings of two of the general projects and that on healthy eating policy. The single topic route typifies a way that some schools may begin to address the health promoting schools development. The three programmes were the *HEA European Network of Health Promoting Schools* evaluation, the *Wessex Healthy Schools Award* and the healthy eating policy. The design of the three studies is described in Box 7.

**Box 7** Health Promoting Schools Evaluations

*HEA European Network of Health Promoting Schools*

Forty-eight English schools allocated to 16 matched triads. In each triad random allocation to intervention (described as pilot) and comparison schools – reference 1 and reference 2. Eighteen primary (5–11), 21 secondary (11–16/18) and nine special schools.

Qualitative and quantitative data through cross-sectional and longitudinal surveys carried out in 1994–1996.

Measures: knowledge, attitudes, self-esteem and self-reported behaviours through the use of a longitudinal survey. Qualitative data also obtained from a cross-sectional survey. Data on contextual factors and perceptions of programmes from school staff.

*Wessex Healthy Schools Award*

Eleven secondary schools participated in the award plus five matched control schools.

Qualitative and quantitative data using audit, curriculum and policy review, semi-structured interviews, focus groups and self-completed questionnaires.

Baseline data in 1995 and follow-up in 1997.

*Healthy Eating Policy*

Three schools – one intervention and two controls in which data was collected only after the evaluation.

Used pupil questionnaires and structured staff interviews.

Results reported included:

- improvements in schools in health knowledge but little difference between pilot and reference schools;
- pupils in pilot secondary schools were less likely to report smoking and drinking alcohol at the beginning and the end of the project;
- most people interviewed were aware of and supported the health promoting school initiative;
- teachers were cautious about the learning gains in less quantifiable areas;
- levels of self-esteem in most schools in the study rose, more in primary than secondary schools, with some pilot schools showing greater rates of improvement than reference schools;
- pilot school pupils were less likely to be bullied;
- many schools broadened their concepts of health promotion; only a minority developed broad health promotion policy documents, with most developing policies for specific topics;
- simple environmental changes in the schools where pupils were involved in planning and development had a significant impact on pupil behaviour and self-esteem;
- by the end of the project many pilot schools were attempting to increase curriculum time for health topics;
- there was a marked increase in the number of whole staff development activities on health in the pilot schools.

In this evaluation detailed qualitative case studies are also provided.

The *Wessex Schools Award* is illustrative of a way that the health promotion concept has been taken forward in England, with this particular award offering a model for others. The programme was developed through an alliance between education and health authorities and local schools. Schools agreed objectives and targets with a health promotion officer (a specialist practitioner in England usually employed by a health authority) or a teacher advisor and within the constraints of resources and priorities. The Award aims to enable schools to become 'health promoting' schools as defined by the WHO. No additional theory base for the Award is described. The content of the pro-

In the HEA study schools provided their health education plans identifying the activities they would undertake in order to develop as health promoting schools. The contents of the programmes in the schools varied but all were expected to address the three domains of the *European Network* as noted above. Funding for participating schools was provided – up to £18,000 a year for the three years – plus various types of professional support.

grammes varied between participating schools The evaluation was a quasi-experimental study in which random assignment was not used since this was not acceptable to the schools wishing to participate in the award. There were difficulties in securing an equivalent number of matched schools to act as controls and this was reported as having an impact on the power to detect statistically significant results. The evaluation involved pupils, teachers, support staff and parents, school governors and health promotion officers and used both quantitative and qualitative data. Nine key areas are included in the 15 month Award scheme:

- the curriculum;
- links with the wider community;
- a smoke-free school; healthy food choices;
- physical activity;
- responsibility for health;
- health promoting workplace;
- environment;
- equal opportunities;
- access to health.

(Rogers, cited in Moon et al., 1999)

Schools were expected to act on the curriculum as a whole and on a minimum of two targets within the other eight areas. The amount and type of resources to schools varied but in all cases these were small by comparison with those received in the European study. Results included the following.

- Intervention schools made progress in all key areas except in taking responsibility for health and physical activity. Intervention schools performed better but differences between intervention and control schools did not reach statistical significance.
- Surveys of parents, governors and teachers at baseline and follow up identified that many did not feel well informed about the scheme and level of consultation and availability of training was variable. The scheme was positively viewed at follow up.
- Pupils were not always aware of schools participation.
- Health-related knowledge was high at baseline and there was little change.

- Schools found it difficult to work towards smoke-free environments and healthy eating, although supportive local authority policies were in place. At the same time the Award was associated with impact on pupils smoking. Self-reported smoking rose in 12/13 year olds but less in intervention schools and positive but non-significant impacts were made on drug use with 16 year olds – but not 12/13 year olds. Inconclusive results were reported for alcohol and healthy eating and there were no significant impacts on exercise.
- Older girls made greater progress in all target areas.
- Participation in the scheme had a positive impact on curriculum-based health education and pupils benefited from more use of participatory approaches to teaching.
- No information was provided on the social and psychological impacts of the Award scheme.
- Barriers to change included time and resources, poor facilities and catering services.
- The award appeared to have a positive impact on school management structures and processes.

Limitations in the study were noted: the lack of a specific focus on the achievement of whole-schools approaches and shortcomings in its assessment of the impact of the Award on the school environment. With reference to the former there were suggestions from the data that it was unlikely that whole-school approaches had been achieved and for the latter the need for an appropriate evaluation methodology to assess the achievement of healthy environments was identified.

The third study by Young (1993) was of a healthy eating policy intervention developed in the context of a whole-school approach to health promotion. Pupils in the 13–14 year age group were involved. The programme was developed through discussions with pupils, parents, teachers, school meals staff and health education staff from the health authority. The content was based on the Scottish Health Education Group document Promoting Good Health – Proposals for Action in Schools (1990) and included the following components:

## Environment:

- changes to food and drinks available in schools;
- healthier ingredients and cooking methods used in school catering;
- school kitchen available in breaks for the preparation of healthy snacks;
- no tuck shops allowed;
- dining room displays on healthy eating;
- headteachers highlighted theme in school assemblies.

## Curriculum:

- relevant topics incorporated into several subject areas.

## Family/community:

- parents involved in programme development and ongoing cooperation was sought; school handbook described changes made.

## Results from the study included:

- higher percentage of pupils choosing the school meals in the intervention school;
- intervention school pupils had significantly fewer snacks and these were also healthier ones;
- self-reported breakfast consumption was comparable in intervention and control schools;
- no differences were found in consumption of confectionery and fizzy drinks outside school.

The intervention was theory based and did involve a range of stakeholders.

Gains were reported, although some indicators of health promoting schools were addressed more directly than others. This is perhaps as it should be if schools are developing their own ways forward towards the health promoting schools idea. The healthy eating policy approach may demonstrate that the whole ethos of a health promoting school can be better communicated and the idea adopted if built initially around one aspect of the school. Drawing on *Communication of Innovations Theory* it can be suggested that a holistic approach to healthy eating is easier to communicate as an innovation than the achievement of the whole school as a health promoting one.

While evaluations of the health promoting school concept are seeking to assess the success in achieving all key indicators we can comment briefly on studies which have looked specifically at one of the more challenging dimensions of the health promoting schools developments – that of establishing school–community links.

### School–community links

Links with the community are a key element of the model of the health promoting school. Back in 1980 one of the early health education projects in the UK (Schools Council/HEC, 1982), which was also built around the concept of health education in the context of the health promoting school, emphasised the building of community links and activities. There was no strong evidence that such developments happened at the time. According to St Leger (1998) there are few studies which show how these partnerships may be established and how they might better contribute to better health outcomes for students. As far as the published literature is concerned this is an element of the health promoting schools development that does appear to have been addressed in a rather more limited way than some other aspects. There are, however, initiatives which do illustrate school–community partnerships, although they have not all been subjected to equally rigorous evaluation. The first to be discussed, because it has been implemented worldwide and has had considerable influence, is the *Child to Child Initiative*. It pre-dates the European initiated health promoting school idea and was originally developed to enable young children with caring responsibilities for their siblings to do this in health protective and promoting ways. The programme has developed further and its principles were articulated in 1990 by Hawes (cited in Hubley 1998).

1 The concept of primary health care: developing the power of individuals and communities to take responsibility for the betterment of their own health.
2 Faith in the power of children to spread health messages and health practices to younger children, peers, families and communities but at the same time the conviction that they would embody and profit from it.

3 Belief that health education at every level of health learning must be accompanied by health action.
4 Conviction of the need for joint action between education and health workers at all levels.

The emphasis is quite strongly on children as educators in their communities with a role in primary health care and the links emphasised are between education and health workers.

The programme has been introduced in more than 80 countries. Activity sheets and teachers guides have been produced in around 20 languages and in some countries attractively produced readers incorporate good story lines and health themes and offer an excellent means of combining literacy and health in the curriculum. A large number of case studies and other small evaluations of initiatives have been generated but not widely disseminated, leading to the project being less well known than is deserved. A literature review by Lansdown (1995) concluded:

> *There is a plethora of papers describing the developments of Child to Child and a handful of evaluations. Since an earlier 1991 review there have still been no ethnographically based accounts … . There is a dearth of well controlled studies of the impact of Child to Child on health behaviours or status using a rigorous design. There is, however, a growing interest in research, with what is hoped will be a productive tension between advocates of qualitative and quantitative methods … .*

> (in Hubley, 1998)

The *Child to Child Initiative* has introduced active learning methods to many countries where they were not widely used in schools. Overall conclusions about its overall impact and effectiveness have yet to be developed.

A good example of a project which describes partnerships between schools and the community – in this case parents – and is oriented towards the school environment is described by Davis and Cooke (1998). This is an ongoing action research project. Initiated by parents who wanted their children's intellectual, physical and social development to be developed in school the parents were equally motivated by the wish that education be empowering. They recognised the potential to address concerns about the school through a health promoting schools approach which would make positive changes for children, address teacher's concerns and involve parents. The originators were committed to participatory action research approaches to implementing the health promoting school concept and stated:

> *The participatory action research approach reinforces the health promoting school's capacity to empower individuals and communities to take action for healthier lives and healthier environments.*

The project took place in Brisbane, Australia, in a primary school for 500 children where in 1992 there was general dissatisfaction with aspects of the school environment. As in any action project the identification of a starting point was a shared decision and the project aim was to improve the physical and social environment through empowering children and adults to actively create the type of school environment they wanted. The Ashgrove project was described as shaped by its own unique combination of personal and contextual influences (Box 8).

The project followed the typical stages of the first spiral of an action research process.

Step 1. Create a shared vision of a healthy school.
Step 2. Select the priority issues.
Step 3. Develop an action plan.
Step 4. Put the plan into action.
Step 5. Evaluate progress and plan for the future.

In reflecting on the project after 4 years the writers had a number of observations.

- That the Participatory Action Research (PAR) process was re-aligning relationships – with parents, children and school staff working together, solving common problems and sharing in the solutions.
- Positive observations were made by teachers and parents of the process although sustaining participatory approaches had not been easy.

*Box 8* Characteristics of the *Ashgrove Project*

- It was initiated by parents rather than teachers in contrast to many other projects.
- It has a strong community development orientation.
- It is holistic, dealing not only with human interactions but also with the relationships between people and environments.
- It has developed a different way for parents to relate to the schools and for teachers and parents to relate to each other.
- It overtly links social justice, health promotion and environmental education.
- It has widened and strengthened links for the school with community groups and local and state government.
- It is both responding to and part of recent initiatives at local, state and federal government levels for greater pro-active community input and participation.

- A goal of the project had always been the active participation of the children in creating positive change. There was initial disappointment at the level of children's involvement with teachers and some parents seeing children as users of the improved environment rather than as decision makers and actors in creating the process. There was a reluctance to involve all children in contrast to a small group of them.

Comment about the process was offered:

*I think that until adults feel totally comfortable with the process themselves, it's very difficult to introduce children into the situation. Possibly you know, if you used this process with children, they might operate it much better than adults do.*

(School Principal)

Finding more effective ways to ensure children's participation became an important priority for the project team. Different ways of seeing the school grounds emerged, based on new understandings of the environment:

*It's not about putting an extra fort in the playground, this is a plan for the next 20 years. It's a compete revision of the way in which we have looked at everything to do with playgrounds.*

(Parent)

*… in the playground, that's where a lot of skills to relate to people are learned. Or not learned.*

(Parent)

Using a partnership model for decision making with people used to working hierarchically had been challenging and there had been negativism and loss of momentum. A number of principles, practices and observations were drawn from the project (Box 9).

To date there is a relatively small number of studies to support strong conclusions on the whole health promoting school approach to health promotion, although there is an increasing amount of positive comment on developments. Although specific health topic areas are addressed in studies the holistic conception of the health promoting school has still to be effectively communicated on a wide scale. For the idea to really take off teachers need to have a good understanding from their initial training which could be built on subsequently through in-service training. The survey in England and Wales of teacher training provision referred to earlier (Walsh and Tilford, 1998) revealed that only about a half of the 69 courses for which there was evidence included work on the health promoting school. The curricula of courses were largely oriented towards the specific health topics required within the national curriculum, namely substance use and misuse, sex education, HIV/AIDS and inter-personal relationships. Only a third of courses included environmental aspects of health and inequalities. Data collection took place in 1995 and there may now have been some changes.

**Box 9**

- Effective communication is fundamental
- Creating a shared vision is an essential component
- Change can come from any part of an organisation
- Adults need 'empowering' too. Children may more readily demonstrate such processes and may be effective models and teachers for adults
- Criticism and conflict are to be expected and can be seen as an indicator that paradigm shift is under way as new ideas and new ways of operating confront the usual way of doing things
- Changes do not come quickly
- With the increasing demands on teachers achieving curriculum change and children's involvement may take longer to evolve for a parent-initiated project
- The commitment of key facilitators is essential
- There is a danger of volunteer burn-out
- Measuring outcomes for projects that make long-term investments in building futures which are healthy, just and sustainable can be difficult

The lack of knowledge of the health promoting school concept in those countries discussed so far may be partly a result of lack of communication about the idea beyond the network of schools involved in the pilot *European Schools Network*. The development of healthy schools schemes ought to change this, although there is a danger that emphasis on certain specific aspects of health may obscure a full adoption of the holistic concept.

Finally, we can comment on two summaries of what are key factors in taking the health promoting school initiative forward, the first identifying three main principles and the second a more general set of recommendations. Rowling and Jeffreys (2000) offer as guiding principles:

- capacity building – involving initiatives at national, state and local level;
- inter-sectoral collaboration and mediation – involving collaboration, community ownership and consultation;
- equity – realised through the allocation of resources according to local needs.

Denman (1999) has drawn from a number of evaluations the common issues in developing the health promoting school and points to the importance of the following:

- a school-based review as the first step to facilitate the change process;
- a designated coordinator, with time, status, vision and skills to plan and lead staff in health promotion;
- a health promoting school policy and detailed development plan for health promotion;
- a budget and adequate resources for health promotion;
- strong management support and involvement;
- good management and communication structures in school; consultation and involvement of teaching and non-teaching staff, parents and pupils through, for example, a health promoting school working group;
- a clear contract with outside agencies that are providing support;
- the support of as many of the staff as possible;
- awareness among as many of the staff as possible of the benefits the innovation can bring;
- training and support for staff;
- coordination of activities throughout the school and community;
- a health education curriculum of high status.

In addition she adds that alliances and partnerships are a successful means of sustaining action.

### Evaluating the health education component of health promotion for specific topics

Notwithstanding the active developments of health promoting schools it would probably be accurate to conclude that a major proportion of the evaluation of health promotion in schools has, in fact, been of classroom-based health education interventions. In some cases these have been interventions set within multi-component programmes implemented on a community-wide basis but the majority have been confined to schools. Early evaluations tended to focus on knowledge, attitudes and relatively simple behaviours. Comments on effectiveness betrayed some optimism. In 1981 Bartlett concluded that the best developed programmes were successful in developing knowledge, somewhat successful in improving knowledge and infrequently successful in achieving lifestyle change. Four years later Mason and McGinnis (1985), reporting on the SHEE referred to earlier, said:

*The study unequivocally demonstrates that school health education is an effective means of helping children to improve their health knowledge and develop healthy attitudes. It also shows that school health education can decrease the likelihood that children will adopt behaviours that are hazardous to health, such as cigarette smoking.*

In the ensuing period it is not clear that classroom health education activities on their own have become a great deal more effective. In spite of the development of more sophisticated interventions informed by psychological theory there is recognition that effectiveness is increased when such activities are complemented by activities linked to other health promotion components (policy; environmental support, etc.) or where school inputs are a component of the community-wide interventions to be discussed in the final chapter. Given the analyses of the factors influencing health behaviours as discussed earlier in relation to the *Health Action Model* it is common sense to expect that interventions that address more of the influences on behaviours stand a better chance of success. Nonetheless, it is important to have some sense of what school health education interventions taken alone can achieve for specific individual competencies and attributes. In many situations the policy changes and environmental supports for health promotion are not yet in place but schools are keen to make as effective a contribution as possible to preparing children for healthy futures.

It is not possible to review all topic areas of health education but some indications of potential effectiveness can be drawn from illustrative examples. There are a large number and range of individual studies together with reviews of studies within specific health topic areas and the 'review of reviews' to which we have referred (Lister-Sharp *et al.*, 1999). We will draw on the systematic review evidence with due acknowledgment to the limitations in such evidence as discussed earlier, but will draw on further studies in the course of general discussion. Thirty-two pre-existing reviews met the inclusion criteria for the 'review of reviews' and the following topic areas were included:

- substance use (9);
- nutrition and exercise (8);
- sex and family life (4);
- accident prevention (3);
- personal safety (3);
- personal hygiene (2);
- psychological aspects of health (2);
- environment (1).

One hundred and eighty other existing reviews were excluded for the reasons listed in Box 10.

**Box 10** Reasons for Exclusion

| | |
|---|---|
| No systematic search | 133 |
| No study details | 99 |
| No details of intervention's content | 56 |
| No study design assessment | 95 |
| No experimental studies included | 20 |
| No results presented | 42 |

Note: most reviews were excluded for several of the above reasons; no review was excluded solely because of a lack of experimental studies.

Two of the topics in this 'review of reviews' will be discussed to illustrate the nature and extent of achievements. The topics selected are ones which are important for children and young people in all countries and are also important in the context of attention to redressing inequalities in health. They are substance use, with particular reference to the prevention of smoking, and sexual health. The main conclusions for other topics included in Lister-Sharp *et al.*'s (1999) review of earlier reviews will also be noted. The extent to which their conclusions might be challenged were the literature as a whole to be reviewed will be commented on. The section will be concluded with some discussion of particular approaches used in health education interventions drawing on systematic reviews and also on individual studies not included in such reviews.

## Smoking prevention

Prevention of smoking is chosen for a number of reasons: it is a global health issue and was selected as one of two key ones, together with malaria, for special emphasis by the WHO in 1999. Smoking is a behaviour established during school age and has long-term and major implications for health. It is also one where there have been considerable efforts to apply theory to the development of interventions and to identify the most effective combinations of activities and timing of intervention. It is also a topic where there was, in the 1980s, considerable optimism when psychosocial interventions were developed and evaluated in classrooms. A number of reviews of effectiveness have been undertaken, including both systematic and thorough commentary reviews.

In Lister-Sharp *et al.*'s (1999) review smoking and tobacco-related interventions were included within those for substance use as a whole. They identified 82 reviews of substance use and included nine in their 'review of reviews'. These nine were: all types of substance use (2), alcohol alone (3), drugs alone (2), tobacco alone (1) and one of a single drugs programme, DARE. Eighty per cent of the programmes included in the reviews involved classroom teaching alone and the remainder were combinations of school ethos and environment/curriculum or curricu-lum plus family/community The educational components of the studies included in the reviews are of interest:

- 80% had an information component;
- 52% involved the development of resistance skills;
- 34% decision making skills;
- 21% lifeskills development;
- 18% values clarification;
- 15% norm setting;
- 13% stress management and self -esteem development;
- 11% alternatives to tobacco use;
- 10% pledge;
- 7% assistance;
- 6% goal setting.

The most common interventions were two-component programmes combining education and resistance skills. Half the programmes were teacher led, a quarter peer led and a quarter were expert led. We have earlier noted the importance of ensuring that programmes are theory driven and the theory bases be reported. In this area of substance use and misuse there were variations in the extent to which theory was analysed in the individual reviews that were synthesised. That of Foxcroft *et al.* (1995) recorded the theory bases of initiatives and noted that one third of primary studies they included in their review did not mention a theory. A wide variety of theories were used in the remaining studies, mainly derived from social and health psychology.

Four of the nine substance use reviews addressed tobacco-related outcomes (James and Fisher, 1991; Hansen, 1992; Binyet and de Saller 1993; White and Pitts, 1997). Seven of the programmes reported in their reviews where evaluation was by controlled trials using random allocation short-term effects on smoking were reported. All were curriculum-based programmes with an information component, the majority included norm setting and resistance skills and decision making were also frequently included. A further 14 studies which were controlled studies with non-random allocation also reported effectiveness. One programme reported effectiveness with boys but not girls (Armstrong *et al.*, 1990) and that of Clarke *et al.* (1986) reported effectiveness for girls but not boys. Two programmes were deemed to have harmful effects, 13 studies reported no effects and in 12 programmes the results were unclear.

Effects on longer term smoking behaviour was recorded in only three studies. At 6 months Murray *et al.* (1989) reported from a programme which had paper-led, expert-led and media-led versions. This was partially effective at 6 months but not sustained at 6 years. In other studies lifeskills training was effective at one year (Botvin, 1989; Botvin *et al.*, 1989) and the Waterloo smoking prevention programme (Flay *et al.*, 1989) was effective at 2 but not 6 years.

Lister-Sharp *et al.* (1999) also reported on the effectiveness of the 15 programmes which used a peer approach – 13 showed some impact, one had no impact and the last a negative impact. It was concluded that peer-led programmes compared favourably with non-peer-led ones.

A rapid review of evidence on smoking prevention based on existing systematic reviews and update studies using less stringent inclusion criteria than applied in systematic reviews (Tilford *et al.*, 1998) drew six conclusions. Only the first three related to classroom programmes since the purpose of this review was to examine all interventions which might impact on young people's smoking, irrespective of where they were located.

- Multi-component, school-based interventions implemented at the most appropriate age in the smoking career by trained teachers and/or peer leaders incorporating between six and twelve 45 minute lessons with a later booster can reduce smoking prevalence with programme effects lasting up to 5 years.
- While better results can be obtained with smoking-specific than general health education initiatives, such as lifeskills prgrammes, the wider uptake of the latter can create greater impact overall.
- While peer leaders can be as effective as teachers in delivering school-based and community-based

interventions there is insufficient evidence on which to make strong recommendations on prioritising their use in interventions.

- The effectiveness of school-based programmes is enhanced if they form part of a combined intervention with community-based elements and mass media.
- There is evidence of success in reducing illegal sales and criteria for elements of interventions associated with success can be specified.
- Mass media interventions in isolation have an agenda-setting effect and there is evidence of success in securing attitude change. Effects are enhanced in combined interventions.

Finally the most recent systematic review of preventing smoking uptake in young people drew similar conclusions on school-based smoking prevention interventions (NHS Centre for Reviews and Dissemination, 1999).

- The evidence to date for the effectiveness of school-based programmes is limited. However, social reinforcement/social norms type programmes which include curricular components on the short-term health consequences of smoking, combined with information on the social influences that encourage smoking together with training on how to resist the pressures to smoke, seem to be more effective than traditional knowledge-based interventions.
- The training given to teachers that deliver the programmes and how well each component is delivered and implemented are likely to impact on effectiveness.
- The ages of the young people targeted may be an issue. Most programmes were aimed at 11–17 year olds, when attitudes and beliefs about smoking and experimentation may already be established. Programmes before smoking behaviours are formed should be considered.

There is a reasonable measure of consistency in the conclusions that have been reached about the effectiveness of interventions for the prevention of smoking behaviour.

## Sexual health

Sexual health includes the promotion of positive health and the prevention of unwanted teenage pregnancy and sexually transmitted diseases, including HIV/AIDS. As an area of health promotion in schools it presents its own, arguably unique, characteristics. It is an area of the health education curriculum which, traditionally, teachers have been reluctant to undertake and one where requirements set within national curricula have been limited. There have been common tendencies to restrict attention to biological content and to avoid the holistic treatment that is called for in any efforts to achieve positive sexual health. Teachers have not been prepared adequately for their roles in sexual health education. In many societies cultural pressures make the discussion of sexual health matters difficult, although the provision of family life education has been a means by which aspects of this difficult topic have been addressed. There have been gender-related contradictions – expectations that much of the responsibility in sexual relationships lies with girls but, at the same time, girls are subjected to sanctions when they exercise responsibility in sexual encounters. Boys have mostly been provided with less sexual health education.

We are interested in sexual health-related behaviours and while we can assess those such as assertiveness, social interaction, skills in condom use (using models) in the classroom, we do not have access to the real situations where these have to be practised. The social pressures to engage in early sexual activity are not within the immediate control of the school and the economic pressures on young women to engage in early sexual activity in many countries of the world are ones that schools cannot easily change. Unrealistic expectations should not be placed on schools. The more, however, that sexual health education can be provided within an understanding of and commitment to the health promoting setting notion the more likely we may expect to achieve successes. As with the case of smoking prevention we will draw, initially, on the systematic review evidence.

Twenty-five reviews of sex and family life education were identified by Lister-Sharp *et al.* (1999), of which only four met inclusion criteria (Oakley and Fullerton, 1994; Dicenso, 1995; Kirkby, 1995; Peersman *et al.*, 1996). Forty-nine primary studies were included in these four reviews. Thirty-three appeared in one review only, 11 in two reviews and five in three, the differences in part being related to the differing foci of the reviews. Twenty-two were of curriculum-based approaches, 16 combined curriculum with other health promoting schools elements and four were of environmental interventions alone.

The components of the programmes were as follows:

- 30 involved an information component and 10 were information only;
- 17 resistance skills;
- 12 life skills training;
- 10 values clarification;
- 10 decision making;
- 7 self-esteem;
- 4 norm setting;
- 5 other.

Full information about the delivery of programmes was not always reported. Where it was indicated 15 programmes were led by teachers, 14 by outside experts, seven involved group work, three were peer led and three involved the media. The theoretical bases of programmes were rarely reported but when they were programmes were largely based on social psychological theories. Low income and minority groups were well represented in studies and boys and girls were considered separately in one review. The majority of studies were from the USA. Conclusions drawn were:

- the quality of reviews and primary studies was variable;
- a small number of interventions had a positive impact on outcomes predictive of safe sexual behaviour;
- effective interventions frequently included provision of services such as special clinics or were specifically focused on AIDS;
- of the few studies that involved parents or

peers none demonstrated that these approaches increased effectiveness;

- knowledge gains were reported in all studies where assessed and a desirable effect on attitudes in most studies;
- insufficient information was provided on theoretical bases of programmes;
- information on the process of implementation was lacking;
- in this area it may be important to assess how comfortable teachers feel with the material they are required to teach.

In both the areas of smoking prevention and sexual health we can identify some common factors and some differences. In both subject areas interventions with more than one component are provided but there are many which are information only. The theoretical bases of interventions are more clearly reported in substance use interventions than in the sexual health area and peer education has been pursued more frequently in the substance use studies. Clearly there are many studies that have not been included in the reviews because of the methodological criteria which govern inclusion of studies. It is important to be aware of other studies which might point to what may be new and, possibly, effective alternatives to existing approaches or address aspects which have not been fully covered in the systematic reviews. In the area of smoking we would particularly like to be able to identify studies which fully address the gender differences in smoking behaviour and develop effective interventions to address these differences. There are a growing number of studies which have analysed in detail smoking from a gender perspective and this work provides a foundation for developing new types of interventions (Allbut *et al.*, 1995; Michell, 1997). A 1998 review (Tilford *et al.*, 1998) reported that while there were some interesting studies available which increased knowledge about initiation of girls to smoking, the effectiveness literature did not yet provide much evidence from interventions which have carefully and fully addressed gender issues in planning and implementation. This could be the fault of reporting in papers where more

detail is frequently given to the evaluation methodology than to intervention details but we can suggest that this is also evidence of lack of attention to gender issues. Similar comments can be made with reference to ethnicity, although in the USA it appeared that this had been addressed rather more than gender.

In the area of sexual health education a comprehensive review by Grunseit (1993) incorporated a much wider range of studies that in the systematic review of reviews. The review is useful for bringing together those studies which have taken gender into consideration. Their observations about the availability of studies, the methodological limitations of many that were found and the lack of studies from many parts of the world are similar to those made by those completing systematic reviews. Their conclusions about what makes for the more successful classroom programmes did not differ significantly from those of Lister-Sharp *et al.*'s (1999) review. The recommendations to policy makers based on this review are useful to note:

- education on sexual health and/or HIV does not encourage increased sexual activity;
- good quality programmes help delay first intercourse and protect sexually active youth from STD, including HIV, and pregnancy;
- responsible and safe behaviour can be learned;
- sexual health education is best started before the onset of sexual activity;
- education has to be gender sensitive for both boys and girls;
- young people's sexual health is informed by a wide range of sources;
- young people are a developmentally heterogeneous group and not all can be reached by the same techniques.

Conclusions were drawn for the other areas of health education included in the Lister-Sharp *et al.*'s (1999) review of reviews. Key points are provided for three of the topics in order to indicate some of the similarities between the areas and also differences (Box 11).

*Box 11*

---

**Nutrition and Exercise**

- School-based healthy eating programmes which target school lunches can improve their content.
- School-based fitness programmes can increase pupils' levels of fitness.
- Knowledge gains were found in all studies where this variable was reported.
- There is reasonable evidence that it is possible to change dietary intake and improve physiological measures of cardiovascular health.
- Experimental studies have demonstrated impact on the consumption of various nutrients.
- Interventions have used more restricted classroom approaches than substance use/misuse programmes and peer involvement is rare. Parental involvement in addition to classroom programmes and school environment changes was common. Evidence suggested that parental involvement in school healthy eating programmes was important.
- All programmes combining a classroom component with environmental change had positive outcomes.
- Many studies included only short-term follow-up.
- Lack of information on implementation makes it impossible to assess whether this affected effectiveness.

**Accident Prevention**

- High proportion of interventions included changes to school or community environment.
- Interventions involving environmental change were more likely to be effective in changing behaviour.
- Classroom components were unsophisticated when compared with those for substance use and sex education.
- Personal autonomy and self-esteem are relevant to the area and interventions might benefit from including resistance skills or self-efficacy components.
- The majority of road safety interventions were effective or partially effective.
- Reviews provided sufficient information for distinctions to be made about features of effective and ineffective programmes.
- One review reported that when children and young people are actively involved and programmes concentrate on one or two specific messages they are more effective.

**Psychological Aspects of Health**

- Interventions were almost entirely confined to the classroom, led by mental health professionals rather than teachers and none aimed to influence the hidden curriculum or school ethos.
- Interventions were designed to increase knowledge and lifeskills at the individual level and were unlikely to influence the school as a whole as required in the health promoting school ethos.
- About half showed an impact on outcomes related to mental well-being. Gains in knowledge were found when it was a variable of interest and some attitude changes were reported.
- Programmes which included stress management were effective in improving coping skills, anger management, anxiety and self-esteem. Positive programmes were also found for self-concept.
- None of the studies reported on long-term outcomes.

---

The brief summaries from conclusions for other areas reviewed indicate that there is variability across subject areas in the extent to which classroom activities use interventions based on theory. Theory, when reported, is largely derived from social psychology. There is variation in the use of elements additional to classroom ones. There is a general lack of longer term follow-up.

It has to be emphasised again that Lister-Sharp *et al.*'s (1999) synthesis of existing reviews is inevitably not fully current as no updating was applied to each of the review areas. We also have to ask if the constituent reviews, in confining themselves to studies which met methodological criteria – although not, in most cases restricted solely to randomised controlled trials – paint a biased picture of activities taking place in schools and their impacts. The only way to comment robustly on this would be to review all the reviews excluded from the synthesis of reviews and also to review all the studies excluded from each of the specific reviews.

Insights can best be achieved when reviewers have made some attempt to examine systematic review evidence and combine this with evidence from other interventions which do not meet systematic review criteria. A rapid review of smoking interventions (Tilford *et al.*, 1998) attempted to look at the full range of interventions reported in the literature together with those taking place in a health region. There was little evidence in the published literature of interventions offering promising new ways of working in this area. In the detailed mapping of the interventions taking place in the study region there was little evidence of school-based interventions significantly different from those already addressed in the literature, although there were innovations in the community setting. Where innovations were occurring these were not always being evaluated thoroughly or the evaluations reported. Innovations were often low budget ones and the percentage of funds for evaluation would not permit rigorous evaluation.

## Specific health education outcomes and approaches

In 1981 Bartlett, in his assessment of school health education, said that its effects on such pupil outcomes as decision making and social interaction abilities have seldom, if ever, been measured. Since that time such outcomes have been central ones in many health education programmes and have been assessed in the context of a number of preventively oriented programmes and in the context of general lifeskills programmes. Their integral nature to health education was emphasised in a health education initiative which was built entirely around a lifeskills-type programme (Anderson, 1986):

> ...*the need for personal growth and skill enhancement, leading to the development of responsible, autonomous and assertive young people capable of making rational and informed decisions about their health is the foundation of successful health education.*

We will comment on two specific health-related attributes and one type of approach.

### Self-efficacy and self-esteem

These are two core concepts held to be centrally important within the broader concept of empowerment. Independently they are also claimed to be associated with readiness to adopt health behaviours. In the case of the former there is probably little to challenge. In terms of associations of self-esteem with health behaviours the picture is a little more complex, although this is not necessarily reflected in some of the discussions in the literature.

With reference to smoking, studies of the attitudinal factors have included attitudes to self as well as attitudes to smoking as an activity. Low self-esteem has been linked to smoking in young people (Goddard, 1990; Conrad *et al.*, 1992). The strength of this link between smoking and self-esteem has also been challenged. Michell (1997), in an interpretivist study of 11–13 year olds, found that smoking was not particularly related to low self-esteem. Although a few marginalised girls took up smoking in order to gain entry to more popular groups, the largest number of smokers were the 'top' girls recognised as more independent, more mature, more rebellious, more fun and more street-wise than their peers.

Effectiveness in achieving self-esteem changes has been gathered from interventions directed specifically towards psychological health and from studies across a number of other health areas. In pulling evidence together from the various reviews Lister-Sharp *et al.* (1999) reported on self-esteem achievements. The health promoting schools review reported a rise in levels of self-esteem in the *European Network* (Jamison *et al.*, 1998) in most schools during the study, whether intervention or comparison schools – on the evidence of self-reports derived from a longitudinal questionnaire some pilot schools showed a greater rate of improvement than reference schools. This was the only one of the four individual health promoting schools projects reviewed that reported on social and psychological effects, including self-esteem. Within the specific health topic areas in the reviews there were some reports on this variable.

- *Substance use/misuse.* Lifeskills training had positive effects on self-concept but no effect on self-esteem.
- *Healthy eating and exercise.* A *Know Your Body* study found no effects on self-esteem or locus of control. A positive effect on locus of control but not self-efficacy was found in a controlled trial of the same programme. Four other controlled trials assessed self-efficacy with gains reported in one of them.
- *Sexual health.* Self-esteem was reported in one study only but no effect was found. Self-efficacy was addressed in three studies and one evaluated use and refusal self-efficacy separately. This was in the *Youth AIDS Prevention Project* which had positive effects on use self-efficacy but uncertain effects on refusal. Positive effects were also found in a controlled study evaluating *AIDS Prevention for Adolescents in Schools* (Walter *et al.*, 1993). Results in the third study were unclear.
- *Psychological aspects of health.* This review provided the most direct reports on self-esteem. Of the four studies reporting on self-esteem two reported positive effects; one short-term gains which were not sustained while in the second study no statistical data were available to support reported success. This was a programme (*Developing Understanding of Self and Others*) which emphasised learning through active participation by the child, parent and teacher.

From the review of reviews there is not, therefore, a great deal of evidence on the effective development of self-esteem – a curriculum component that was specifically checked for. This does not mean to say that there may not have been mentions in the primary studies included in each of the reviews. The earlier reviewers may not have chosen to report on all indicators included in an evaluation, although they could be expected to have done so. Lister-Sharp *et al.* (1999) commented on the attention to psychological aspects of health:

> *Although programmes could not be relied on to do so, many of those designed to impact on psychological health were successful, at least in the short term. This was true of programmes which focused on psychological health and those whose primary aim was to change health related behaviour but included a psychological component on the grounds that psychological health is necessary to achieve behaviour change. The aspects most amenable to change were self concept and self efficacy.*

As was noted in Box 4, improvements in self-esteem were seen to be rarely or not achievable. It can be suggested that we need further analyses of the concept of self-esteem and more reference in developing interventions to those studies which are examining the construction of self-esteem in young people's social contexts. The study by Michell (1997) is one useful example.

### Peer teaching

There has been enthusiasm for the adoption of peer teaching in programmes with young people in both school and community settings. We will comment on community-based ones in a later chapter. In the systematic reviews evidence we noted the variable use of peer led interventions – most often used in the substance use area and to a somewhat lesser extent in sexual health and relatively little in other subject areas. This is generally in line with subjective impressions of the literature as a whole. Various claims have been made for the use of peer approaches and the rationales have been summarised by Turner and Shepherd (1999). The 10 points they brought together were:

- peer education is more cost effective than other methods;
- peers are a credible source of information;
- peer education is empowering for those involved;
- it utilises an already established means of sharing information and advice;
- peers are more successful than professionals in passing on information because people identify with their peers;
- peer educators act as positive role models;
- peer education is beneficial to those involved in providing it;
- education presented by peers may be acceptable when other education is not;
- peer education can be used to educate those who are hard to reach through conventional methods;
- peers can reinforce learning through ongoing contact.

One of the problems in assessing whether peer-delivered programmes are more effective than those which are teacher led arises from the various ways that peer education is conceptualised and implemented. An early review of school-based peer education (Devin-Sheehan *et al.*, 1976) reported wide variation in participants, aims and methods. In a later review Milburn (1995) suggested that evaluators of peer approaches in general education, prior to the popularity of such methods in health education, limited their claims for success to direct and measurable outcomes resulting from carefully structured and targeted programmes. Peer approaches were initially actively adopted in health education as a component of smoking education programmes and more generally in substance use and were built on social psychological theory. As such they were also used in a structured way. Peer approaches have also been used in the context of *Empowerment Models* using a Freirian dialogue method (Wallerstein and Bernstein, 1988).

When the structured approaches were transferred from the USA to Europe questions were raised about the transferability of the methods to the UK with its differing peer culture. After transfer the interventions tended to be used in less structured ways in the UK, which raised questions about whether effectiveness was, as a result, reduced. Some positive conclusions have been drawn, as noted earlier, about peer methods in the areas of substance use and sex education. Others have been more reluctant to claim any superiority of these methods. For example, West and Michell (cited in Milburn, 1995) concluded that the evidence of effects was fairly limited. Much of the rationale for peer education assumes an uncomplicated influence of peers and West and Michell argue that the case for coercive peer pressure as an influence on adolescent behaviour is more complex than studies indicated and that influence may operate differently with respect to different health behaviours.

Given the diversity of ways that peer education has been conceptualised and used it becomes difficult to draw any conclusions about the method as a whole. The theoretical underpinnings of peer approaches have been varied, although social psychological theories have been drawn on most often. In their review Turner and Shepherd (1999) examined a selection of theories and assessed their value and relevance in relation to the 10 claims for peer education listed above. They concluded that most theories had something to offer towards an explanation of why peer education might be effective but most theories were limited in scope and there was little evidence in practice to support them. While there is little evidence that peer approaches are damaging there is also not a great deal of evidence, to date, to support their wholesale promotion. If young people like learning by the use of these approaches and if they are more or less as effective as teacher-led ones then that is a good case for using them. The costs associated with training for the more structured approaches do, however, have to be taken into consideration.

### Efficiency
It is useful to be able to identify the most efficient way to reach health promotion goals even if such ways are not those of first choice. In school settings in which health education is provided resources may be scarce and competition for them acute. Whatever one's political stance on the deci-

sions taken at the national and international levels which leave schools in such difficult situations it would be naïve to think that educators can avoid the need to be able to justify expenditure on using more expensive strategies.

There is plentiful evidence that the use of multi-component classroom strategies in the field of drug education yields the greatest success but there is the need to understand the relative contributions of the separate components. It may not be important to include all in some complex programmes and attention to efficiency demands the identification of not only what is necessary, but also sufficient. At the same time, it may not be sensible to adopt relatively complex smoking prevention programmes, even though they do have a sound theoretical base, if resources are not available to train teachers to implement them with fidelity or to support the initiatives in other ways required. Teachers, of course, may not wish to implement highly prescriptive programmes with complete fidelity, even if this prejudices overall effectiveness, preferring to introduce modifications in accordance with the local context and young people's needs and interests (Bolam, 1984; Wilcox and Gillies, 1984). In the smoking prevention area the more efficient way would probably be to use simpler and less intensive classroom-based interventions in the context of a school policy on smoking together with a range of community support activities, such as action on illegal sales, advertising, etc.

Some approaches to health education are popular with pupils and while this is clearly one important justification for their use in cost-conscious times it may also be necessary to spell out the superior educational gains from such use. A particularly good example is the use of drama and in particular the use of *Theatre in Education* groups specialising in health-related productions. An evaluation by McEwan *et al.* (1991) examined the costs of using TIE in HIV/AIDS education and concluded that:

*the costs of TIE may be too high where the programme objectives are to impart information, but may be justified in programmes which seek to empower young people or to change their attitudes.*

In all countries of the world the educational process has, at one time or another, been dominated by formal, highly structured and teacher-controlled approaches to learning. In some countries active learning methods are well established but have yet to be adopted in others. We noted earlier the contribution of the *Child to Child* project in introducing active learning methods to schools. The *Geneva Consultation Document* (WHO/UNESCO/UNICEF, 1992) recommended that health education should be based on participatory learning and should engage children in community action projects. It is important to consider how active methods can be effectively and efficiently developed. Promoting the use of activities in schools which are already embedded in the life of specific cultures can be one way to gain acceptance of educational changes that some teachers are reluctant to make. Use of drama, puppets and songs are all examples of ways to introduce more active participation of young people in health education in schools. The use of story telling is a further example which is now quite widely used in health education – not only with children.

The efficiency of those activities known to be effective is reduced if programmes are not tailored to the specific needs of young people, provided at the times in the 'health career' when they are most likely to have impact and carried out by facilitators who have an understanding of the theory and practice of health promotion. The health promoting schools developments are more likely to work well where their complexities are understood and appropriate structures, such as a school-based coordinator, and alliances are in place. As we will discuss in the last chapter, working to develop effective and efficient healthy alliances is a challenge and there are no simple prescriptions for success.

There are many things that can be undertaken which ensure that the resources, often limited, which are available for health promotion are used to best effect. For example, ensuring that all partners have an understanding of the goals of health promoting schools from the outset is generally agreed to be important (Aggleton *et al.*, 2000). Teachers need to be prepared through initial and in-service training for their health promotion roles if they are to be effective and efficient. Such preparation needs to include development of a commitment to evaluate and the skills to do so in ways appropriate to schools. Evidence of the impact of training of teachers on classroom effectiveness is reported by Nyandini *et al.* (1996) in a study of oral health education. Effectiveness of teachers was assessed before and after training. Children taught by teachers in the intervention groups had better knowledge of oral health, reported reduced consumption of sugary snacks, increased toothbrushing frequency and better chewing stick making skills than children taught by teachers in the reference group.

### Addressing inequalities

A purpose of this book is not simply effectiveness but also equity. We have to ask about equity in access to effective health promotion programmes and the achievement of outcomes which are more equitable. In the case of the former we need to consider whether resources for health promotion are, at least, spread evenly but we might also need to ask whether they should be distributed disproportionately to areas of greater need. We noted earlier the *Acheson Report* proposal that health promoting school initiatives should firstly be implemented in disadvantaged areas. It will be interesting to note the extent to which this actually happens. Quite often new initiatives are tried out in less challenging contexts and, to some extent, this can be understood. With new initiatives it is often important to see if success can be achieved in favourable contexts before implementing more widely.

We need to ask whether issues of gender and ethnicity and other areas of inequality have been addressed in developing programmes and in their implementation. We have noted occasional mention of tailoring of programmes to meet girls' and boys' needs but general impressions from the literature are that these issues are insufficiently

addressed. For attention to health inequalities to be appropriately addressed in health promotion in schools there needs to be a general awareness of the social determinants of health. The review of teacher training noted above (Walsh and Tilford, 1998) found that only a minority of courses addressed such issues. The Lister-Sharp *et al.* (1999) review also commented on the lack of studies on the social determinants of health. They noted that they themselves had brought together a large amount of literature and felt confident that the gaps they identified actually were gaps.

One approach to inequities has been the provision of pre-school programmes such as *Head Start*, designed to offer compensatory education in order to enable children to benefit from education in the formal school sector. Positive achievements have been recorded in evaluations from the USA. In the American literature, but to a lesser extent in other countries, there are interventions designed to support and enable children and young people cope with major life events which can contribute to health inequalities, and evidence of successes have been noted (Tilford *et al.*, 1996).

While this chapter has been about schools we need to recall the fact that throughout the world as a whole a very large number of children either have no schooling at all or have to drop out after a few years. Others, because of armed conflict situations, miss out on schooling. Children can also be excluded from schools because of behavioural problems. All these children and young people are particularly vulnerable as far as most aspects of current and future health are concerned. We might expect that fully developed health promoting schools initiatives with strong school–community links might reach out to the young people not in school and it will be interesting to note whether this happens. In the near future it is more likely that community-initiated programmes using community development strategies may address the needs of young people not in schools.

In 1989 Combes criticised the overall approach to health education as highly individualistic in its emphasis on individual responsibilities, attributes and skills necessary for achieving health. In the context of class inequalities (referring to Britain) the individualistic approach was seen to be irrelevant to many children. In the last 10 years the evolution of health promotion from health education has broadened thinking about the nature and purposes of work in schools oriented towards health. It is not yet possible to say that the health promoting schools development or classroom-based health education activities have made a significant impact on inequalities.

## CONCLUSIONS

A major change from health education in schools towards the health promoting school is under way. A health promoting school is one which has an organised set of policies, procedures, activities and structures designed to protect and promote the health and well-being of students, staff and other members of the wider community (Rowling, 1996; WHO, 1998). There is visionary thinking associated with the health promoting school and considerable effort in some countries is being given to progressing this development which, in some cases, is seen to have the potential to enable countries to deal with major social change. Swart and Reddy (1999) have had the following to say about the health promoting school concept in South Africa:

> *South Africa has adopted and commenced with implementing the HPS concept in an attempt to address the historical imbalances and consequences. The challenge is for all these different initiatives to act synergistically so that a strong network of HPSs is developed at local, provisional and national levels. Ultimately the benefits of Health Promoting Schools Networks must be regarded as a worthwhile long term investment in the future of South Africa.*

To be effective the health promoting school needs the ideas which inform it to be understood and accepted. For example, enabling young people to play a fully participatory role is not a change that all in education are necessarily eager to accept. An early evaluation of the *National Healthy School Standard* in England (Aggleton *et al.*, 2000) has said that there is clear evidence that some schemes do not involve young people systematically. Ensuring that the school becomes a health promoting setting also requires inter-sectoral working and the formation of strong alliances. Schools have always had linkages with other sectors, particularly with the health sector, but the nature and strength of these links need to be developed in ways most appropriate to achieving the goals of the health promoting school. In tune with the thinking about evaluation in health promotion the health promoting schools developments are providing an excellent opportunity to develop and refine appropriate models for evaluation. The preferred style may be a mix of quantitative and qualitative methods or a single methodological approach in some instances. The unsuitability of experimental styles for evaluating health promoting schools is widely endorsed. It will be interesting to see whether *Realist Models* of intervention are taken up as they have been in health sector evaluations. Whatever the preferred ways of evaluation they need to be carried out rigorously. However laudable the ideology informing health promoting schools there are ethical challenges to be made if we do not have an accurate and in-depth understanding of the processes and achievements of these developments.

Although it feels as if working towards schools as health promoting settings is the future for developments we have continued to review the effectiveness of classroom-based health education activities. Health education is, of course, one element of the health promoting school but very often still takes place outside the context of health promoting schools developments. There is a large body of literature reporting on these activities. Because of this, in seeking to present a general picture of achievements we have drawn quite heavily on systematic reviews evidence. Given the reservations about such reviews this approach can, of course, be challenged. However, many recent reviewers have been sensitive to the limitations of these reviews and have set their conclusions against a background knowledge of the full breadth of interventions and studies which are taking place and this enhances confidence in the generalisations that are being made.

There are successes in school health promotion and it is important to note these since schools are being expected, in many parts of the world, to make a real contribution to reducing major health problems. There are also shortcomings which have been identified from systematic and commentary reviews. A key one is the lack of attention to theory in planning and/or reporting implementations. There also appears to be a dominance of psychological theory rather than sociological theory but this may partly be because of the criteria which govern selection for many reviews. A development of a framework which combined both psychological and social theory as a framework for sexual health promotion is welcomed and this merits close attention (Wight *et al.*, 1998). While there are many aspects of health promotion in school that require ongoing and comprehensive evaluation it is necessary to ensure that the knowledge that is already available about effective ways to work in health education is disseminated and put into practice. This requires teachers and others involved in school health promotion to be trained and given the appropriate resources to access and apply evidence. We also need to see schools taking a more active role in evaluating their health promotion activities and ensuring that children and young people are given full opportunities to participate in such evaluation.

## References

Acheson, D. (1998) *Independent Inquiry into Inequalities in Health Report*. The Stationery Office, London.

Agerbaek, N., Melsen, B., Lind, O. P. *et al.* (1979) *Effect of regular small group discussion per se on oral health status of Danish school children*. Community Dental and Oral Epidemiology, 7, 17–20.

Aggleton, P., Rivers, K., Mulvihill, C., Chase, E., Downie, A., Sinkler, P., Tyrer, P. and Warwick, I. (2000) *Lessons learned: working towards the National Healthy School Standard*. Health Education, 100 (3), 102–110.

Allensworth, D. D. and Wolford, C. A. (1988) *Schools as agents for achieving the 1990 health objectives for the nation*. Health Education Quarterly, 15, 3–15 and 491–505.

Allott, R., Paxton, R and Leonard, R. (1999) *Drug education: a review of British Government policy and evidence of effectiveness*. Health Education Research, 14 (4), 491–506.

Anderson, J. (1986) *Healthskills: the power to choose*. Health Education Journal, 45 (1), 19–24.

Arbeit, M., Johnson, C., Mot, D. *et al.* (1992 ) *The Heart Smart cardiovascular school health promotion: behaviour correlates of risk factor change*. Preventive Medicine, 21, 18–32.

Armstrong, B. de Klerk, N. Shean, R. *et al* (1990) *Influences of education and advantage on the uptake of smoking by children*. Medical Journal of Australia, 152, 117–124.

Arora, C. M. J. (1994) *Is there any point in trying to reduce bullying in secondary schools. A two year follow up of a whole school anti-bullying policy in one school*. Educational Psychology Practice, 10, 155–162.

Backett-Milburn, K. and McKie, L. (1999) *A critical appraisal of the draw and write technique*. Health Education Research, 14(3), 387–398.

Barnett, E., de Koning, K. and Francis, V. (1995) *Health and HIV/AIDS Education in Primary and Secondary Schools in Africa and Asia*. Overseas Development Administration, London.

Bartlett, E. E. (1981) *The contribution of school health education to community health promotion: what can we reasonably expect? American Journal of Public Health*, 17, 1348–1391.

Binyet, S. and de Saller, R. (1993) *Efficacy of smoking prevention campaigns in adolescents: critical review of the literature*. Sozial- und Praventivmedizin, 38, 366–378.

Bolam, R. (1984) *Recent research on the dissemination and implementation of educational innovations*. In G. Campbell (Ed.) *Health Education and Youth: A Review of Research and Developments*. Falmer Press, London.

Botvin, G. (1989) *School based smoking prevention: the teacher training process*. Preventive Medicine, 18, 280–289.

Botvin, G., Baker, E. and Filazzola, A. *et al.* (1989) *A cognitive behavioural approach to substance abuse prevention: one year follow up*. Addiction Behaviour, 18, 280–289.

Buller, M., Loescher, L. and Buller, D. (1994) *Sunshine and skin health: a curriculum for skin cancer prevention education*. Journal of Cancer Education, 9, 155–162.

Clarke, J., MacPherson, B., Holmes, D. *et al.* (1986)

*Reducing adolescent smoking: a comparison of peer lead, teacher led and expert led interventions. Journal of School Health*, 56, 102–106.

Coates, T., Barofsky, I., Saylor, K. *et al.* (1985) *Modifying the snack consumption patterns of inner city high school students: the Great Sensations study. Preventive Medicine*, 21, 18–32.

Colquhoun, D. (1997) *The health promoting school in Australia: a review. International Journal of Health Education*, 35 (4), 117–125.

Cooke, T. D. and Walberg, H. J. (1985) *Methodological and substantive significance. Journal of School Health*, 55, 301–304.

Combes, G. (1989) *The ideology of health education in schools. British Journal of Sociology of Education*, 10 (1), 67–79.

Conrad, K. M., Flay, B. R. and Hull, D. (1992) *Why children start smoking cigarettes: predicting young adult smoking outcomes from adolescent smoking patterns. British Journal of Addictions*, 87, 1711–1724.

Davis, J. and Cooke, S. (1998) *Parents as partners for educational change. The Ashgrove Healthy School Environment Project.* In B. Atweh, S. Kemmis and P. Weeks (Eds) *Action Research in Practice. Partnerships for Social Justice in Education.* Routledge, London.

Denman, S. (1999) *Health promoting schools in England – a way forward in development. Journal of Public Health Medicine*, 21 (2), 215–220.

Department of Education (1994) *Education Act 1993: Sex Education in Schools*, Circular 5/94. HMSO, London.

Department for Education and Employment (1997) *Building Excellence in Schools Together.* The Stationery Office, London.

Department of Health (1992) *Health of the Nation.* HMSO, London.

Department of Health (1999) *Saving Lives: Our Healthier Nation.* The Stationery Office, London.

Devin-Sheehan, L., Feldman, R. S. and Allen, V. C. (1976) *Research on children tutoring children: a critical review. Review of Educational Research*, 46, 355–385.

DiCenso, A. (1995) *A Systematic Overview of the Prevention and Predictors of Adolescent Pregnancy.* University of Waterloo, Waterloo, Canada.

Dorn, N. and Nortoft, B. (1982) *Health Careers.* Institute for the Study of Drug Dependence, London.

Dushaw, M. L. (1984) *A comparative study of three model comprehensive elementary school health education programmes. Journal of School Health*, 54, 397–400.

Her Majesty's Government (1988) *Education Reform Act.* HMSO, London.

Elliott, J. (1991) *Action Research for Educational Change.* Open University Press, Milton Keynes.

Flay, B., Koepke, D., Thompson, S. *et al.* (1989) *Six year follow up of the first Waterloo school smoking prevention trial. American Journal of Public Health*, 79, 1371–1376.

Foxcroft, D., Lister-Sharp, D. and Lowe, G. (1995) *A Review of Effectiveness of Health Promotion Interventions: Young People and Alcohol Misuse.* University of York, York.

Goddard, E. (1990) *Why Children Start Smoking.* HMSO London.

Grant, J. (1995) *The State of the World's Children.* Oxford University Press, New York.

Greenberg, J. S. (1985) *Comments from the field. Journal of School Health*, 55, 350–352.

Grunseit, A. (1997) *Impact of HIV on Sexual Health Education on the Sexual Health Behaviour of Young People: A Review Update.* Joint United Nations Progamme on HIV/AIDS, Geneva.

Gunn, W. J., Iverson, D. C and Katz, M. (1985) *Design of the School Health Education Evaluation. Journal of School Health*, 55, 301–304.

Hagquist, C. and Starrin, B.(1997) *Health education in school – from information to empowerment models. Health Promotion International*, 12 (3), 225–232.

Hansen, W. (1992) *School-based substance abuse prevention: a review of the state of the art curriculum, 1980–1990. Health Education Research*, 7, 403–439.

Hubley, J. (1998) *School Health Promotion in Developing Countries: A Literature Review.* Leeds Metropolitan University, Leeds.

Hurrelmann, K., Leppin, A. and Nordlohne, E. (1995) *Promoting health in schools: the German example. Health Promotion International*, 10 (2), 121–131.

James, J. and Fisher, J. (1991) *A Review of School Based Drug Education in Australia.* National Centre for Research into the Prevention of Drug Abuse, Curtin University of Technology, Perth.

Jamison, J., Ashby, P., Hamilton, K. *et al.* (1998) *The Health Promoting School. Final Report of the ENHPS Evaluation Project in England.* European Network of Health Promoting Schools/Health Education Authority, London.

Kalnins, I., McQueen, D., Backett, K. S., Curtice, L. and Currie, C. E. (1992) *Children, empowerment and health promotion: some new directions in research and practice. Health Promotion International*, 7, 53–59.

Kirby, D. (1995) *A Review of Educational Programs Designed to Reduce Sexual Risk Taking Behaviour Among School Aged Youths in the United States.* ETR Associates, Santa Cruz, CA.

Koo, H., Dunteman, G., George, C. *et al.* (1994) *Reducing adolescent pregnancy through a school and community based intervention: Denmark, South Carolina revisited. Family Planning Perspectives*, 26, 206–211.

Lister-Sharp, D., Chapman, S., Stewart-Brown, S. and Sowden, A. (1999) *Health Promoting Schools and Health Promotion in Schools: Two Systematic Reviews.* NHS Centre for Reviews and Dissemination, York.

Luepker, R., Perry, C. and McKinlay, S. (1996) *Outcomes of a field trial to improve children's dietary patterns and physical activity: the Child and Adolescent Field Trial for Cardiovascular Health (CATCH). Journal of the American Medical Association*, 275, 768–776.

Lynagh, M., Schofield, M. J. and Sanson-Fisher, R. W. (1997) *School health promotion programs over the past decade: a review of the smoking, alcohol and solar protection literature. Health Promotion International*, 12 (1), 43–61.

Macgregor, S. T., Currie, C. E. and Wetton, N. (1998) *Eliciting the views of children about health in schools through the use of the draw and write technique. Health Promotion International*, 13 (4), 307–318.

Mason, J. O. and McGinnis, J. M. (1985) *The role of school health. Journal of School Health*, 15, 14–18.

McEwan, R. T., Bhopal, R. and Patton, W. (1991) *Drama on HIV and AIDS: an evaluation of a theatre in education programme. Health Education Journal*, 50 (4), 155–160.

McWhirter, J. M., Collins, M., Bryant, I., Wetton, N. M. and Newton Bishop, J. (2000) *Evaluating 'Safe in the Sun' for primary schools. Health Education Research*, 15 (2), 203–217.

Michell, L. (1997) *Loud, sad, or bad: young people's perceptions of peer groups and smoking. Health Education Research*, 21 (1), 1–14.

Milburn, K. (1995) *A critical review of peer education with young people with sepcial reference to sexual*

health. *Health Education Research*, 10, 407–420.

Moon, A. M., Mullee, M. A., Rogers, L., Thompson, R. L., Speller, V. and Roderick, P. (1999) *Helping schools to become health promoting environments – an evaluation of the Wessex Healthy Schools Award. Health Promotion International*, 14 (2), 111–121.

Morrow, V. and Richards, M. (1996) *The ethics of social research with children: an overview. Children and Society*, 10, 90–105.

Murray, D., Pirie, D., Luepker, R. *et al.* (1989) *Five and six year follow up results from four seventh grade smoking prevention strategies. Journal of Behavioural Medicine*, 12, 207–218.

Newman, I. (1985) *Comments from the field. Journal of Schools Health*, 55, 343–345.

NHS Centre for Reviews and Dissemination (1999) *Effective Health Care, Preventing the Uptake of Smoking in Young People*, Vol. 5 (5) The University of York, York.

Nutbeam, N. (1992) *The health promoting school: closing the gap between theory and practice. Health Promotion International*, 7 (3), 151–153.

Nutbeam, D., Clarkson, J., Phillips, K. *et al.* (1987) *The health promoting school: organisation and development in Welsh secondary schools. Health Education Journal*, 46, 109–115.

Nyandini, U., Milen, A., Palin-Palokas, T. and Robinson, V. (1996) *Impact of oral health education on primary school children before and after teachers' training in Tanzania. Health Promotion International*, 11 (3), 193–201.

Newman, I. (1985) *Comments from the field. Journal of School Health*, 55, 343–345.

Oakley, A. and Fullerton, D. (1994) *Risk, Knowledge and Behaviour: HIV/AIDS Education Programmes and Young People.* Institute of Education, University of London, London.

Parsons. C., Stears, D. and Thomas, C. (1996) *The health promoting school in Europe: conceptualising and evaluating the change. Health Education Journal*, 55, 311–321.

Parsons, C., Stears, D., Thomas, C., Thomas, L. and Holland, J. (1997) *The Implementation of the European Network of Health Promoting Schools in Different National Contexts.* Summary Centre for Health Education and Research, Christ Church College, Canterbury.

Peersman, G., Oakley, A. and Oliver, S. (1996) *Review of Effectiveness of Sexual Health Promotion Interventions for Young People.* Epicentre, Institute of Education, London.

Porcellato, L., Dugdill, L., Springett, J. and Sanderson, F. H. (1999) *Primary school childrens' perceptions of smoking: implications for health education. Health Education Research.*, 14 (1), 71–83.

Pridmore, P. and Bendelow, G. (1995) *Images of health: exploring beliefs of children using the 'draw and write' technique. Health Education Journal*, 54, 473–488.

Rowling. L. (1996) *The adaptability of the health promoting schools concept: a case study from Australia. Health Education Research*, 11 (4), 519–526.

Rowling, L. and Jeffreys, V. (2000) *Challenges in the development and monitoring of Health Promoting Schools. Health Education*, 3, 117–123.

Rutter, M., Maughan, B., Mortimore, P. and Ouston, J. (1979) *Fifteen Thousand Hours*. Open Books, London.

Schools Council/HEC (1982) *Health Education*. Forbes Publications, London, pp. 13–18.

Sobczyk, W., Hazel, N., Reed, C. D. *et al.* (1995) *Health Promotion Schools of Excellence: a model programme for Kentucky and the nation. Journal of the Kentucky Medical Association*, 93, 142–147.

Smith, S., Roberts, C., Nutbeam, D. and Macdonald, G. (1992) *The health promoting school: progress and future challenges in Welsh secondary schools. Health Promotion International*, 7, 171–179.

St Leger, L. (1998) *Australian teachers' understandings of the health promoting school concept and the implications for the developments of school health. Health Promotion International*, 13 (3), 223–235.

St Leger, L. H. (1999) *The opportunity and effectiveness of the health promoting primary school in improving child health – a review of the claims and evidence. Health Education Research*, 14 (1), 51–69.

Swart, D. and Reddy, P. (1999) *Establishing networks for health promoting schools in South Africa. Journal of School Health*, 69 (2), 47–49.

The World Bank (2000) *Entering the 21st Century: World Development Report 1999/2000*. Oxford University Press, Washington, DC.

Thomas, M., Benton, D., Keirle, K. and Pearsall, R. (1998) *A review of the health promoting status of secondary schools in Wales and England. Health Promotion International*, 13 (2), 121–129.

Tilford, S., Delaney, F. and Vogels, M. (1996) *Effectiveness of Mental Health Promotion Interventions: A Review*. Health Education Authority, London.

Tilford, S., Godfrey, C., White, M., Nicholson, F. and South, J. (1998) *Evidence Based Health Promotion: Commissioning Interventions for the Prevention of Smoking in Young People*. Centre for Health Promotion Research, Leeds Metropolitan University, Leeds.

Tones, B. K. (1999) *The health promoting school: some reflections on evaluation. Health Education Research*, 11, i–viii.

Turner, G. and Shepherd, J. (1999) *A method in search of a theory: peer education and health promotion. Health Education Research*, 14 (2), 235–247.

Vincent, M., Clearie, A. and Schlucter, M. (1987) *Reducing adolescent pregnancy through school and community-based education. Journal of the American Medical Association*, 257, 3282–3286.

Wallerstein, N. and Bernstein, G. (1988) *Empowerment education: Freire's ideas adapted to health education. Health Education Quarterly*, 15, 379–394.

Walsh, S. and Tilford, S. (1998) *Health education in Initial Teacher Training at the secondary phase in England and Wales: current provision and impact of Government reforms. Health Education Journal*, 57 (4), 1–14.

Walter, H. and Vaughan, R. (1993) *AIDS risk reduction among a multi-ethnic sample of urban high school students. Journal of the American Medical Association*, 270, 725–730.

White, D. and Pitts, M. (1997) *Health Promotion with Young People for the Prevention of Substance Misuse*. Health Education Authority, London.

Wight, D., Abraham, C. and Scott, S. (1998) *Towards a psycho-social theoretical framework for sexual health promotion. Health Education Research*, 13 (3) 217–228.

Wilcox, B. and Gillies, P. (1984) *Some issues concerning the implementation of health education projects in schools*. In G. Campbell (Ed.) *Health Education and Youth: A Review of Research and Developments*. Falmer Press, London.

World Health Organization (1951) *Technical Report Series 30, Expert Committee on School Health Services*. WHO, Geneva.

World Health Organization (1954) *Technical Report Series 89, Expert Committee on Health Education of the Public*. WHO, Geneva.

World Health Organization (1966) *Planning for Health Education in Schools*. WHO, Geneva.

World Health Organization (1977) *The Health Needs*

of Adolescents, Report of a WHO Expert Committee, Technical Report Series 308. WHO, Geneva.

World Health Organization (1978) Primary Health Care: Report of the Conference on Primary Health Care. WHO, Geneva.

World Health Organization (1979) The Child and Adolescent in Society, Report of a WHO Conference. WHO European Regional Office, Copenhagen.

World Health Organization (1983) Expert Committee on New Approaches to Health Education in Primary Health Care. WHO, Geneva.

World Health Organization (1986) Young People's Health: A Challenge for Society, Report of a WHO Study Group and Young People and 'Health For All by the year 2000', Technical Report Series 731. WHO, Geneva.

World Health Organization (1989) The Health of Youth. WHO, Geneva.

World Health Organization (1990) Enabling School Age Children and Adults for Healthy Living, Report Prepared for the World Conference on Education For All, Jontien, Thailand. WHO, Geneva.

World Health Organization (1993a) The European Network of Health Promoting Schools: a joint WHO (Europe) and Commission of the European Communities and Council of Europe Project. Commission of the European Communities and Council of Europe, Brussels.

World Health Organization (1993b) The Health of Young People: A Challenge and a Promise. WHO, Geneva.

World Health Organization (1995) The Overall Progress of the European Network of Health Promoting Schools. WHO European Regional Office, Copenhagen.

World Health Organization (1996) Promoting Health Through Schools: WHO's Global Initiative, WHO/HPR/HEP/96.4. WHO, Geneva,.

World Health Organization (1997) Promoting Health Through Schools. Report of a WHO Expert Committee on Comprehensive School Health Education and Promotion. WHO, Geneva.

World Health Organisation (1998) WHO's Global School Health Initiative: Health Promoting Schools, WHO/HPR/HEP/98.4. WHO, Geneva.

WHO/UNESCO/UNICEF (1992) Comprehensive school health education: suggested guidelines for education. Hygie, XI (3), 40–44.

Young, I. (1993) Healthy eating policies in schools: an evaluation of effects on pupils knowledge, attitudes and behaviour. Health Education Journal, 52, 6–9.

# 6 HEALTH CARE SETTINGS

## INTRODUCTION

In many countries of the world health care institutions are beginning to adopt the settings approach to health education as a more appropriate way to contribute to the promotion of community and individual health. This chapter will examine health promotion in primary care and hospital settings around themes addressed in earlier chapters:

- the conceptions of health promotion held in these contexts and the relationships between health promotion and related activities;
- debates on the philosophical approaches to health promotion in these contexts;
- the organisation and delivery of health promotion;
- issues concerning evaluation and the methodological approaches adopted;
- health promotion achievements.

Primary care describes all those health services provided outside the hospital sector. Globally the term primary health care is associated with the *Alma Ata Declaration* from which originated the goals of *Health For All 2000* (WHO, 1978). In those countries which have long had systems of first line care outside the hospital sector these have traditionally been what is better described as primary medical care.

Traditionally hospitals have been concerned with treatment of ill health and with rehabilitation and have not been particularly concerned with the promotion of positive health in the sense that it is portrayed in the *Ottawa Charter*. As a context for health promotion they present some considerable challenges. There are examples of hospitals playing a somewhat different role in relation to health. For example, in the early stages of implementing primary health care in Tanzania very small district hospitals fulfilled a treatment function but this was carried out by workers who had received a brief training to undertake a limited range of procedures. The more highly trained doctor was expected to prioritise a community-wide preventive function. Johnson (in Poland *et al.*, 2000) has more recently noted developments in countries of the South where hospitals have adopted a community-wide health promotion role. Hospitals came within the health promoting settings development with the publication of a WHO document in 1991 and an international network of health promoting hospitals was subsequently set up. Hospitals have to meet specific criteria to belong to the network but there will be other hospitals influenced by the ideas but which are not part of the network. Whether or not they have a formal link with the health promoting hospitals initiative hospitals have been identified as a key setting for health promotion in national health documents. For example the English *Health of the Nation* (Department of Health, 1992) affirmed that hospitals exist to provide treatment and care but they also offer unique opportunities for more general health promotion of patients, staff and all who come into contact with them. Prior to this focus on general health promotion policy there had been a slow development of specific health promotion policies in the hospital setting – nutrition and smoking being examples in some countries, breast feeding in others (Donovan, 1992). The health promotion developments in hospitals represent a broadening out from the long-term focus on patient education. We will discuss these developments later in the chapter.

## CONCEPTIONS OF HEALTH PROMOTION AND RELATED ACTIVITIES

The diversity of terms and some inconsistencies in their use continue to be characteristic of 'health promotion' in primary care and hospital settings. The term health promotion may be used to describe the totality of health education, health care and policy and environmental actions. Alternatively, and quite frequently, it can be used as an interchangeable term for health education. The terms patient education or alternatives such as patient teaching, patient counselling and client education are also widely used. There will be some who would not wish to consider patient education as part of health promotion since it is not typically undertaken within the broad philosophy described in the *Ottawa Charter*. For the purposes of this chapter we will mainly use health promotion to describe the totality of provision. We will use the terms patient education and health education for work undertaken on an individual basis in health care settings. When, however, studies cited do use the term health promotion to signal what is in effect health education we will retain the writer's term but clarify usage if this appears to be necessary. In the same way that we did in the schools chapter we can distinguish between health promoting settings, in this case hospitals and primary care and health education activities within hospitals, and primary care. The types of activity that fall within health promotion can be seen in Box 1.

The language used in this chapter requires some comment. The term patient is widely used but is also a term with which there is dissatisfaction. As a term it is said to reflect a particular relationship between individuals and health care providers – a passive recipient of services rather than an active partner. The term client is frequently used and can be appropriate where a consumerist relationship is in place. In many countries this term does not reflect the true nature of the relationship that exists and is also not fully consonant with the ideas of health promotion. Service user is used in some countries but is also subject to reservations. There still appears to be an

**Box 1**  Health Promotion in Hospitals and Primary Care

> **Health promotion policy:** general and specific. Policies can be oriented towards the health care sector alone or to sectors in combination, e.g. health care and social care.
>
> **Environment:** actions designed to create health promoting environments in hospitals and primary care and in their communities.
>
> **General health education:** aimed at primary prevention and the promotion of positive health and education to support the achievement of policy development and implementation and healthy environments.
>
> **Patient education:** condition-specific education with patients, their families and other support providers. Frequently focused on tertiary levels of prevention but can also include secondary and primary prevention.

unfulfilled need for a term to replace patient. We share reservations about the language of 'patient' but in this chapter we will incorporate the terms used in the literature which has been drawn on.

### The development and organisation of health promotion in health care settings

#### Primary care

Primary care describes all those services provided outside the hospital sector. Globally the term primary health care is associated with the *Alma Ata Declaration*, from which originated the *Health For All* concept (WHO, 1978). Alma Ata laid down principles for the development of comprehensive primary health care (PHC) as the means by which the goal might be achieved. PHC was to be acceptable and accessible health care for individuals and their families, involving full community participation and at a cost that families, communities and countries could afford. It was intended that PHC should provide preventive, curative and rehabilitative services and include eight essential components, of which health education was to be the central one. The others were to be:

- basic sanitation and an adequate source of safe water;
- healthful nutrition and a secure food supply;
- maternal and child care, including family planning;
- immunisation against the major infectious diseases;
- prevention of endemic diseases;
- appropriate treatment of common ailments;
- a supply of essential medications.

This first level of primary care would depend on the activities of community health workers, nominated by communities and given some basic training to enable them to deal with a limited range of activities and the skills to refer upwards to a next level of care. The community or village health workers would not typically be paid for their services, although support in kind would be provided by their communities and their health work would be undertaken alongside other community responsibilities. There were variations in the way that the PHC programmes were put into effect and differing emphases on the eight essential components. Initially such developments failed to acknowledge and incorporate the contributions that traditional systems of health care did, and could, make to health care services. Later, ways of forming alliances between the systems were developed. What set out as free provision of services in primary health was later modified in many countries in the context of the decline in economic situations from the late 1980s. Payments were imposed for drugs in many countries as part of cost recovery programmes.

The ideas enshrined in Alma Ata were not new and represented, it has been said, *less a birth than an endorsement of an idea, whose time had come* (Mull, 1990). While the slogan of *Health For All* has become a universal one the 'primary health care' ideas from Alma Ata were not seen to be so relevant in those countries with well-established primary care provision for their populations. It can be suggested that because the key elements of primary health care noted above did not appear immediately relevant to countries which had basic infrastructures the underlying principles of Alma Ata were not adequately acknowledged. Green (1987) has argued that the UK, although a signatory to Alma Ata, had failed to provide an adequate framework for a PHC strategy and much remained to be done if the principles of primary health care were to be fully met.

The relations between primary and secondary care vary between countries. In the UK, for example, primary care services deal with nine out of 10 contacts with the health care services and most of these contacts are patient initiated. Except in emergencies hospital care is accessed by referral from primary care. Since space precludes discussion of primary care arrangements in a number of countries we will frequently use the UK or its constituent countries as an illustrative example in this chapter, but some studies will be drawn from elsewhere. For those unfamiliar with the UK, general practitioners (GPs) are private contractors who provide primary health care for patients in exchange for a capitation fee paid by the government. These primary care services include the management of illness and a variety of activities with the well population who are registered with a particular practice. Ninety per cent of GPs work in practices employing some ancillary staff and most practice in groups. The membership of primary care teams varies but it is common to have a number of other professions, including community nurses, practice nurses, midwives and health visitors. As a result of recent changes in health strategy primary care is assuming central stage in health care with the formation of *Primary Care Groups* (PCGs). Over the years health education has been recognised as a key element of primary medical care, although not given the same pivotal role as in PHC. The place that health education and promotion take within primary care will vary from country to country but the development within the UK National Health Service (NHS) will reveal issues around provision and implementation many of which should be relevant elsewhere.

Over the years a series of reports, official documents and organisational arrangements have addressed the provision of health education and health promotion. From the 1980s onwards they were generated by professional bodies and government sources (Department of Health and Social Security (DHSS), 1981, 1986, 1987; Royal College of General Practitioners, 1981a, b). The 1986 consultative document on primary care (DHSS) identified as key objectives the promotion of health and the prevention of illness as key objectives and the subsequent *Promoting Better Health* (DHSS, 1987) stated that the government wished to strengthen the GPs role in health promotion by:

- paying special fees to encourage doctors to provide health checks and necessary follow-ups to patients registering for the first time with a doctor;
- considering incentives to achieve specified levels for vaccination, immunisation and screening, as well as to meet the costs of call and re-call;
- considering amendments to doctors' terms of service to clarify their roles in the provision of health promotion services and the prevention of ill health.

A subsequent government document *Working For Patients* (DHSS, 1989) enabled GP practices to hold their own budgets. A new contract for general practitioners was introduced with the aim of:

> *increasing consumer choice and bringing health promotion and disease prevention within the general medical services.*

The contract included a number of specific measures designed to encourage health promotion, including payments for specified preventive activities, including health promotion clinics. Clinic activities could include well person screening, anti-smoking groups, clinics for the management of stress, diabetes and menopause and self-help groups for weight loss, hypertension and asthma.

The first strategy document for health in Britain, *Health of the Nation* (Department of Health, 1992), placed particular emphasis on disease prevention and on health promotion. This document took up the idea of settings and emphasised the formation of alliances between settings in order to progress prescribed health targets. It

asserted that primary and community health care services would have a major role in achieving successes and that ways would be explored for developing the existing health promotion arrangements in primary care. In 1993 modifications were made to the GP contract to create bandings where the highest priority and highest payments were to be given to activities linked to the achievement of the health goals specified within *Health of the Nation*. Effectively this encouraged activities to be directed largely towards coronary heart disease and stroke prevention. Nationally 90% of practices achieved the highest level of payment. There was dissatisfaction with the bureaucracy involved and the associated workload.

Further changes occurred in 1996, when a new contract for GPs was introduced. From that point individual practices could choose health promotion activities in line with *Health of the Nation* goals, local health priorities and patient needs and submit these to a local *Health Promotion Committee* for approval. Approval was necessary in order for practices to receive payment for health promotion work.

Over this period of 10 years or so there was evidence of a growing recognition of the place of health promotion in primary care but, equally, it was informed by a *Medical Model* and consisted mostly of preventive activities and health education. There were various criticisms of the ways in which this health promotion provision was conceived and the organisational requirements associated with it. The 1993 changes were a response to some of the earlier dissatisfactions but criticism continued. Gillam *et al.* (1995) stated in a *British Medical Journal* editorial:

> *In the absence of either a strategic or an evidence based approach to health promotion in primary care, many important items have been lost while others have been inappropriately retained.*

Their view was that financial incentives for health promotion, if they were to be retained, should be linked to evidence-based interventions with people at higher risk.

A change of government in 1997 introduced significant changes in thinking about determinants of health and the ways that the health services should be organised. As part of modernisation plans in the health services primary care has now become the focus of the NHS, with primary care practices being linked into groups. The major health strategy document, *Saving Lives: Our Healthier Nation* (Department of Health, 1999), has stated that the PCGs are expected to play a leading role, working closely with local communities, in improving health and reducing inequality. In effect they are to take on a wider public health role than hitherto. Primary care is coming closer to the ideas about health promotion which are contained within WHO statements. While expecting the PCGs to continue to offer preventive services, such as screening and smoking cessation advice, they are expected to go beyond this and:

> *over time they will forge powerful local partnerships with local bodies – schools, employers, housing departments – to deliver shared health goals.*

The PCGs and hospitals will be working within an action plan that has health improvement as a key goal for the NHS achieved through working in partnership with other agencies and with communities. *Health Improvement Programmes* will have agreed aims, priorities and targets, evidence-based actions and they will record the involvement of local organisations in the development and implementation of plans. There will be a performance scheme to recognise the achievements of communities that are making progress from a low base of health. The expectations for the new PCGs are ambitious and it is too early to comment on progress towards achieving those specific goals which, to date, have been less central to primary care. The potential for health promotion within this changed structure is considerable. The boards which run the PCGs will be multi-disciplinary but to operate effectively will need, as noted by Lucas and Bickler (2000), to have a common vision of their priorities and functions. Currently little is known about differences between board members

in their views on the relative importance of the three key functions of primary care or how representative these views are of all the members of primary care teams. In order to gain some early insights into these questions Lucas and Bickler undertook a postal survey of GPs and practice nurses and structured telephone interviews with PCG board members in one district in the south of England. The results were interesting, although not surprising.

- There were large differences between GPs and nursing colleagues on the ways that board members should determine priorities.
- There were marked differences in the priorities of board members of PCGs (the majority of whom are GPs) and those GPs who are not board members.
- Two thirds of PCG board members believed that improving health generally and, specifically, a reduction in inequalities were their most important tasks, a view not shared by most GPs in the board localities.
- The suitability of PCGs to achieve the tasks assigned to them was also in doubt and there were differences between respondents. Even a quarter of the board members considered PCGs relatively unsuited to reducing inequalities in health.

This exploratory study also exposed differences between practice nurses and GPs, the former being, in general, more public health and health promotion focused than the GPs, who appeared to be more focused on service development. If GPs who are not members of boards do not attach high importance to health promotion and a reduction in health inequalities this is going to reduce the likelihood of these goals being achieved. In terms of *Communication of Innovations Theory* board member GPs appear to be different from the non-board GPs. This study pointed to the nature of the work that will be needed if the range of PCG functions are to be equally and fully addressed by the non-board members who, as the front line people, are those who have to progress the PCG goals. This study identifies the needs for PCGs to work on ideas about inequalities and their roles in reducing them.

## Hospitals

We noted earlier that hospitals have been identified as a health promoting setting and as a context for health education activity. With reference to the former a network of health promoting hospitals was established in Europe in the late 1980s in affiliation with the *Healthy Cities* network and by 1991 this included 224 hospitals in 12 countries (Ashcroft and Summersgill, 1993). There has also been the related WHO/UNICEF *Baby Friendly Hospitals Initiative* (Donovan, 1992). In 1991 the WHO issued a *Health Promoting Hospitals Declaration*. The constituent elements of a health promoting hospital were:

- creation of a healthy environment for staff and clients;
- integration of health promotion into all the activities of the institutions (prevention, treatment, education, rehabilitation, etc.);
- creation of healthy alliances between the hospital and other institutions resulting in a 'health promoting community' in which all institutions are health promoting. (Spiros and Sol, 1991.)

Five main principles were proposed for use in assessing whether or not a hospital was health promoting (Ashcroft and Summersgill, 1993).

1 Health must appear on the agenda of policy makers in all sectors and at all levels of the hospital.
2 Work carried out in the hospital must be organised so as to create a healthy hospital environment.
3 Hospital personnel and patients must be empowered and enabled so that together they can have control of the elements that influence their health while in the hospital.
4 Personal and life skills of personnel and patients must be developed.
5 The hospital must extend its activities in the health care system beyond merely providing clinical and curative services.

The health promoting hospitals initiative is a major broadening out from what has traditionally taken place in the hospital setting. There has, of course, been a long-standing commitment to patient education in hospitals in a number of countries, the USA being a particular example. In 1974 The President's Committee on Health Education emphasised the importance of reorienting the health care system to the maintenance of good health and prevention rather than primarily to the treatment of illness. At the same time there were demands for health care systems to improve their effectiveness and efficiency and, while assuring quality of health care services, to contain rising health care costs. The cost effectiveness of patient education was noted and this has been a recurring theme in the patient education literature. There was also reference to the idea of the 'active patient' seen in the 1972 American Hospital Association statement:

> *patient education services should enable patients and their families, when appropriate to make informed decisions about their health, to manage their illnesses, and to implement follow up care at home.*

## The nature of health care settings and approaches to health promotion

As in other settings a number of approaches to education exist in health care contexts. As we have noted, until comparatively recently health promotion in hospitals was largely a condition-specific activity focusing on education with patients. This work was strongly influenced by the *Preventive Medical Model* and, to some degree, by the *Educational Model*. Most health education in primary care was also oriented towards achieving lifestyle changes and also dominated by use of the *Preventive Model* or simple *Educational Model*. There have been advocates of both preventive and educational models throughout the history of patient education. Early demands for education of patients fitted neatly within a *Preventive Model* and were in response to the acknowledged lack of compliance with prescribed medical regimens and also to wishes to secure behavioural change in order to prevent infectious and, increasingly, chronic diseases. Education was also seen to be important in preparation of people for hospitalisation and treatment. The frequently used term 'compliance' fitted in with the classic Parsonian model of the patient role – passive, dependent, cooperating with the doctor and an unequal partner in the relationship (Parsons, 1951).

Health services, especially in the USA, were first persuaded of the value of patient education because of its reported successes in improving compliance, increasing patient satisfaction and contributions to reducing costs of care. With the recognition that in many conditions, especially chronic ones, which had emerged as the major threats to health in developed countries, the individual needed to be more fully involved in the working out of lifestyle changes and in planning adherence to complex regiments there was a development from what was termed the guidance/cooperation model towards a mutual participation model (Szasz and Hollender, 1956). This model is couched in rather more patient-centred language but it could be argued that the underlying subtext is one where the patient will agree with professional recommendations.

From the 1960s onwards a number of social movements, particularly the women's, self-care and consumer movements, stimulated challenge to many aspects of formal health care and especially to ideas of passive patients and compliance with professionals.

Although the focus of these movements varied as far as health was concerned they shared a commitment to the ideas of self-determination and active participation in health care activities. Rights to information and to an active role in health decision making were central concerns and the language of compliance was broadly rejected. The strengthening of conceptions of the patient as an active rather than as a passive participant in health care led to activities informed more fully by *Educational* and also *Empowerment Models* alongside continued use of preventive model ideas. Fahrenfort (1987) summarised the situation in patient education as follows:

*In sum the call for patient education or information comes from two different directions –*

*a patient centred one in which autonomy is the key word and a medico-centred one in which compliance still reigns.*

Some would say that not a great deal has changed. The language of compliance and adherence are still well represented in the literature alongside considerations of ways of achieving active participation of patients. The training of some professionals, nurses most particularly, has been extended to incorporate an emphasis on positive health and health promotion. The health promoting hospitals and health promoting primary care settings are informed by holistic ideas of health promotion and the conceptions of individuals as active participants in the process of health care. To the extent that this initiative has been taken up widely ideas about health promotion should have begun to change in health care settings. We will assess the impact of these developments later in the chapter.

An ongoing commitment to ideas associated with the *Preventive Model* is clearly understandable given the raison d'etre, over a long period of time, of most health care arrangements. Changing to include more activity associated with the *Educational Model* as described in Chapter 1 also makes sense for the reasons already noted.

The extent to which there has been, and can be, a wider acceptance and adoption of *Empowerment Models* to guide practice is a key question. This was discussed by Fahrenfort (1987), who identified a gap between the promotion of patient emancipation and self-empowerment in theory and the possibilities of achieving these goals in practice. She found examples of humanistic patient-centredness, more commonly in nurses than in doctors, but saw this as a long way from incorporating what Freire described as dialogue. Dialogue implies not simply two-way communication in which doctors took notice of patients and their needs but required a conviction on the part of doctors that the patient's own knowledge was as relevant in the situation as medical knowledge. In actual practice, Fahrenfort contended, medical knowledge remained the norm in the hospital situation and this was consolidated in two ways: through the assumption that it was medical knowledge that was to be disseminated to patients and through patients' own efforts to gain power in the situation by appropriating medical knowledge. In this process patients became 'lesser' doctors but the real doctors remained the guardians of the knowledge that was imparted in efforts to educate. Considerable practical barriers also existed, she argued, in the establishment of true dialogue. For example, sufficient time can be difficult to secure in the context of competing demands in hospital settings and because of the relatively short periods of time for which many people were admitted. Were success to occur, Fahrenfort suggested, it could not survive sanctions from medical practitioners towards truly autonomous patients. She concluded that patient education was not the royal road to emancipation. Roter (1987), in an examination of models for patient education used a 2 × 2 model (Figure 6.1) which addressed, in particular, decision making and responsibility in client–provider relations. Of the four possible positions she viewed the 'active participation' one as best meeting ethical and philosophical concerns and also meeting the realities of therapeutic encounters.

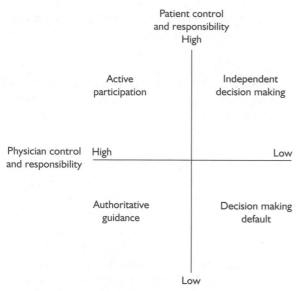

**Figure 6.1**  Decision Making Control and Responsiblity Dimensions of Client–Provider Relations

There is often an assumption that all people do wish to take on an active role. Steele *et al.* (1987) concluded that patients in general wanted to be informed about their illnesses and the treatment options open to them. They argued, however, that while there was evidence that some patients desired an active role in decision making and may benefit from such a role, there was little evidence that this was sought by most patients in most situations.

In a recent paper Gwyn and Elwyn (1999) said:

> *studies which have investigated patient preferences for involvement in decision making have found wide variation between different groups as distinguished by age, educational status, disease type and severity. As a general guide the older the patients and the more severe their illnesses, the less they wanted to be involved in decision making.*

A model for differentiating the forms of decision making between doctors and patients has been developed (Charles *et al.*, 1997, 1999). They have differentiated paternalistic, informed and shared decision models of decision making. The three models are compared with reference to the activities of information exchange, deliberation and decision on treatment (see Box 2).

Charles *et al.* defined shared decision making with reference to treatment decisions as meeting four requirements.

1  At a minimum both the physician and patient are involved in the treatment decision making process.
2  Both the physician and patient share information with each other.
3  Both the physician and patient take steps to participate in the decision making process by expressing treatment preferences.
4  A treatment decision is made and both the physician and patient agree on the treatment to implement.

A number of points about this framework of different ways of decision making in the doctor–patient encounter and its practical applications were made by the researchers.

**Box 2**   Models of Treatment Decision Making

| Analytical stage | Model | | |
| --- | --- | --- | --- |
| | **Paternalistic** | **Informed** | **Shared** |
| Information exchange | | | |
|   flow | Largely one-way | Largely one-way | Two-way |
|   direction | Doctor–patient | Doctor–patient | Doctor–patient |
|   type | Medical | Medical | Medical and personal |
|   amount | Minimum legally required | All relevant for decision making | All relevant for decision making |
| Deliberation | Doctor alone or with other doctors | Patient (plus potential others) | Doctor and patient (plus potential others) |
| Decision on treatment | Doctors | Patient | Doctor and patient |

- It can be used as an educational tool with professionals in practice and in training and as a framework which doctors can use with patients to explain how decision making can be progressed.
- The model makes explicit that the form of decision making model can shift within interactions in the light of what emerges. However, it should also be clear that some forms of switching are easier than others. For example, from paternalistic to shared decision making is easier than the reverse since the nature of information exchange in the former would not have been adequate as a basis for the latter.
- That these are ideal types and are best conceived as points on a continuum.
- There are costs associated with the shared decision making model – time costs in facilitating it or, on the other hand, costs associated with failure to adopt it on repeat visits.
- The framework provides a guide for evaluation.

In addition to asking to what extent patients do want an active role in decision making the realities of pursuing this in differing situations have been raised. Charles *et al.* (1997) identified some questions.

- Whose views of the meaning of shared decision making should count: those of academics and researchers or those of doctors and patients in clinical settings? The two sets of views might be different.

- If a patient and doctor both prefer a paternalistic approach is there anything wrong with adopting this?
- If a doctor prefers the use of an informed model should a patient be 'forced' to comply?
- Given the power, status and informational asymmetry between doctors and patients is it realistic to expect even informed patients to hold their own in negotiations about treatment preferences?
- What is the most effective strategy available to doctors to elicit patient preferences for involvement in treatment decision making?

The actual role in shared decision making, which is a key activity in empowering patients, has been analysed and its realism in differing situations assessed. For example, Gwyn and Elwyn (1999) suggest that a situation of *equipoise*, where options really are options, must exist for a shared decision to be possible. They give the example of demand for antibiotics to treat viral conditions as one where equipose does not exist. Although a shared decision might seem to be reached this would be inaccurate and would best be described as an informed decision engineered in accordance with doctor preference. The difficulties in reaching shared decision making have also been explored with reference to kidney disease treatment. Lelie (2000), on the basis of a qualitative study of 59 interactions between nephrologists and patients where dialysis therapy was discussed, raises the question about what decisions are appropriate for shared decision making and which aspects of treatment should be discussed. In the interactions she studied there were two central decisions – the first about the type of dialysis therapy and the second about the time to start therapy. The first of these was a shared decision, she reported, while the second was not. In the case of the former decision she noted some important omissions in practice. Not all important value assessments were made explicit in the interactions – for example, the value being assigned to life in relation to age. In respect to information about dialysis only certain information was shared – the personal consequences of therapy but not the shortage of organs for transplant. One alternative for dialysis might be presented in more attractive terms which could influence patient choice. The study raised for Lelie the important question of identifying those decisions where shared decision making was relevant. That of sharing the decision about when to start therapy *should* be such a decision. She argues that important non-medical assessments strongly and often influence a medical decision about when to start dialysis and practice should change so that these become shared decisions. At the same time she suggests that doctors cannot and need not discuss all health-related decisions and aspects of decisions with their patients. It is practically impossible, she argues, to discuss all underlying value assessments. She also questions whether to attempt to do so would really satisfy the needs of patients or doctors. She suggests that the usual practice is to explore all health-related values, but not more general values, although this ideal was difficult to fulfil. What should especially be discussed were decisions and aspects that give rise to uncertainty.

A further study by Stevenson *et al.* (2000) used Charles *et al.*'s (1997, 1999) model in examining shared decision making in doctor–patient communication about drugs. They studied 62 interactions between doctors and patients and carried out interviews. They focused on the first two criteria for shared decision making: that both doctor and patient are involved and both parties share information. They found little evidence that doctors and patients both participated in the consultation as defined in the model and, as a

consequence, there was no basis on which to build consensus about treatment preference and to reach agreement. Some GPs did not think people needed information and others did not provide it. Even when information was shared, patients' beliefs were not taken seriously, a finding in line with Tuckett *et al.*'s earlier work (1985). They raised the question of why the doctors in the study (who were self-selected and likely to have had an interest in communication) weren't sharing information and getting patients to share information with them. They suggested that GPs may not agree with sharing information and also do not actually agree with shared decision making. The study results were shared with GPs, who identified barriers to shared decision making and provided some reflections on the researcher's questions. In a first feedback group GPs did not appear to be aware of what the concept of shared decision making entailed. In a second session Charles *et al.*'s framework was used and applied to transcripts of consultations. A number of barriers to shared decision making were identified. Time to address all four characteristics was especially emphasised, although it was suggested that the task could be spread over a number of consultations. Medical training, especially the dominance of hospital-based training, encouraged paternalistic practice rather than shared decision making. In the consultation increased emphasis on opportunistic health screening interrupted the flow of discussion and made shared decision making more difficult. On the other hand, changes towards more team working were felt to increase the opportunities for shared decision making. A number of observations were made about GP roles and patient behaviours which could also reduce the likelihood of shared decision making. These included patient expectations that problems should be solved and the solution involved receiving a prescription, a point supported by other literature (Britten and Okoumunne, 1997; Cockburn and Pitt, 1997). GPs felt they were expected to judge the information patients actually wanted and could cope with and also queried patients' abilities to understand medical language. Interestingly, pressures in their own lives were also reported to influence their ability to participate in shared decision making. Finally, those who attempted shared decision making queried the extent to which this was possible and whether patients really only agree to decisions made by GPs. The participants in the study were interested to examine their consultations in relation to the ideas of shared decision making.

An important study which continues to be of relevance is that of Tuckett *et al.* (1985), who studied 1302 consultations between doctors and patients. Their aim was to explore the extent to which ideas were shared in the medical consultation and they started from the view that the consultation was a meeting between experts; the doctor with scarce specialist knowledge and the patient, by dint of experience, immersion in a culture and past experience, having a set of ideas about the issue of concern. The researchers examined the information that doctors chose to seek from and give to patients and the information that patients sought from or volunteered to doctors.

A main finding of the study was that the consultation was a one-sided affair: doctors and patients did not achieve a full dialogue and did not exchange ideas to any great extent. Doctors spent a fair amount of time sharing what they thought but much less time trying to share what patients thought. Doctors did little to encourage patients to present their views and often actually inhibited them, evaded what they did say and did not tailor information to the known details of patients' lives. The few efforts that were made to establish patients' ideas and explanations were brief to the point of being absent. On the other hand, patients offered little which would have triggered dialogue and, as they neither made clear nor were helped to make clear their ideas, they could not receive explanations in reaction.

The extent to which hospitals, in particular, as they currently operate can move fully towards the ideas incorporated in a health promoting setting has been debated. That so many hospitals have signed up to the health promoting hospitals idea is an indication of an openness to the idea of change, but the barriers may be very considerable to the full achievement of health promotion goals.

Barriers can include the existence of many professional groups each with individual interests. There are also power relationships, particularly the long-standing dominance of the medical profession, which could be threatened by adoption of health promotion ideology. Some of the traditional power of medicine has been reduced with managerial developments in some health care systems but its privileged position is still apparent. Hospitals main function as seen by workers and by communities is to treat ill health. While a fuller attention to health promotion may well be accepted it is not likely that this would be accepted if it threatened traditional functions. The role of the hospital will change as treatments involve less intervention and more is carried out on a day basis and the place of hospitals may eventually be seen fully as secondary to primary care – which will not simply be primary as first call but primary as in 'main' care. The social situation of health care settings as places for health promotion has been discussed fully by Johnson (2000). As a discussant of this contribution Mullen and Bartholomew (2000) argue not against the ideas of health promotion but for the need for hospitals to carry out, in the first instance, their prime function. This would involve meeting treatment goals and providing patient education on the lines of what is known to be effective. While to some degree all these things might happen within a health promoting hospitals initiative there are some possible conflicts. If patient education is to be fully effective it might need to be informed by the ideas associated with the preventive model, which fits uneasily, if at all, with health promotion ideology. We can argue some fit, perhaps, on the grounds that an autonomous patient can agree to hand over autonomy, if only temporarily, in an illness episode.

## Evaluation in health care settings

Of all the settings discussed in this book it is within the health care ones that the application of scientific models of evaluation have been most consistently applied and sustained. There has been widespread use of RCTs to assess the effectiveness of treatments and systematic reviews of evidence have been conducted for many areas and efforts made to implement evidence in practice. There are strong pressures to practise evidence-based health care in many countries While there is a growing acceptance that evidence is an important consideration in planning practice and there is widespread use of standard systematic review evidence, universal acclaim for evaluation confined to scientific approaches does not exist. In the UK health promotion specialist services are typically provided from within the health care system and this group of professionals have expressed considerable reservations about the use of RCTs and positivistic evaluation as we discussed in Chapter 3. With reference to primary care Mathers and Rowland (1997) have this to say about systematic review evidence:

> *... those of us who work in the 'swampy lowlands' of everyday practice rather than the 'sunny uplands' of academia realise that this is fine as far as it goes. However, this is not very far, and such an approach has a very limited application in our day to day work, concerned as it is with managing illness in context. This can create very real difficulties for both doctors and students as they struggle to apply such a model that does not very often or necessarily fit.*

They go on to say that RCTs, while they can be high quality scientific work, can sometimes be used to answer only trivial questions in primary care. And in some cases the questions asked have been severely constrained or even driven by the methodology. Reservations have also been expressed with reference to a specific area of nursing, that of health visiting (Kelsey and Robinson, 1999). They noted that the impact of evidence-based practice had, to date, been greater on medicine than on nursing but that systematic reviews were beginning to be disseminated. For example, systematic reviews of child health surveillance were generating questions about the effectiveness and cost effectiveness of aspects of health visiting to detect developmental or sensory problems. They point out that some components of child health surveillance work have not been addressed

in systematic reviews. While some elements of surveillance might be judged ineffective on the basis of reviews the undertaking of the activity as a whole *does provide an opportunity for the whole child to be seen by a professional worker*. There was a danger of the review evidence being used as a basis for discontinuing what was, in total, a worthwhile activity. Qualitative methods, they claim, applied rigorously, enabled better knowledge claims to be made. Nurses are the health professionals who have taken on major responsibilities for health promotion. There is a history of qualitative research in nursing and it might be expected that nurses would embrace qualitative approaches in evaluating their health promotion activities.

Even where there is commitment to RCT style evaluations some practical and methodological difficulties in implementing such studies in primary care have been raised (Ward *et al.*, 1999). People, for understandable reasons, are not always willing to accept randomisation and a study by Llewellyn Thomas (1991) reported that the people who refuse are those who want more participation in decision making. Patients may also have a preference for one arm within a trial and if not randomly assigned to this may experience negative feelings which influence motivation to comply or, alternatively, lead them to make special efforts – in both cases there are potential impacts on the trial outcomes.

Although qualitative evaluations studies have been less common in health care settings than other kinds these are increasing – in the production of case studies of health promoting hospitals and also in some studies of patient education activities. Action research studies have also often been used in nursing research. The reader will be aware of a contrast between the balance of studies undertaken in health care contexts, methodologically speaking, and those discussed in the later chapter on the community.

Some of the issues in evaluating health promotion in primary care have been examined by researchers with experience of evaluation in this sector (Shiroyama *et al.*, 1995). Some of the points made were:

- undertaking research and evaluation may be new for some or all members of the primary health care team;
- evaluation may be 'bought in' and the need to understand the process fully is not acknowledged;
- if there is collaborative research together with primary health care providers there may be unfamiliarity with some research methods and this can pose threats;
- poor communication or relationships between primary care team members;
- changes in practice organisation and management and external demands on practices can impact on health promotion activities and the evaluations of them; evaluators need to address the economic and political environment in which primary care operates;
- the existence of multiple players and vested interests;
- evaluators can be seen as a threat; there may also be more than one evaluation going on at the same time, creating difficulties;
- the importance of articulating roles and relationships in relation to a project implementation are needed;
- if enthusiasm drops recruitment to studies may drop; forgetfulness and time pressures are also reported as causes of failures to recruit;
- issues of ownership can arise between primary health care team, project implementation teams (where these exist) and evaluation teams;
- aims presented for projects can be vague and the evaluators have a role in making these more specific; differing aims and objectives may also be present in a project and need to be harmonised.

Familiarity with experimental designs and comfort with quantitative data in health care settings will make the introduction of process evaluation and the use of qualitative methods something that has to be addressed carefully where these are important to an evaluation. At the same time we have noted some reservations about experimental design in primary care . There is also a traditional tendency to focus on outcome measures rather than gaining an understanding of the process of an intervention. Many health promotion projects in primary care can be low cost ones and the WHO recommended 10% allocated to evaluation may be too small to undertake any significant evaluation. Selecting certain activities to evaluate thoroughly and teasing out implications for others is one strategy in response to limited resources. There are also difficulties in assessing the cost benefits of health promotion interventions, when this is required, especially with respect to the more diffuse outcomes of health promotion.

An atmosphere needs to be generated which facilitates the discussion and acceptance of project evaluation findings and their wider dissemination when appropriate.

It is with respect to evaluation in health care that some active debates about the use of RCTs have taken place, especially with reference to obtaining informed consent. Such concerns can be seen as a response to the need to practice defensive medicine in some countries, as well as from an active concern for patients. Much of the debate has centred on studies of treatment in health care. RCTs of health education interventions in these settings have also been common and general concerns about experimentation have been expressed about them.

Shiroyama et al. (1995) drew up a number of recommendations for evaluators of health promotion in primary care and these are presented in Box 3.

**Box 3** Recommendations for Evaluators of Health Promotion in the Primary Health Care Setting

At the design stage of an evaluation, evaluators should consider the following:

*The Primary Health Care Setting*
- background, skills and experience of primary health care staff
- coordination and communication within the practice setting
- assessment of the culture and context of the practice

- history of the practice and other relevant organisations
- recent primary health care policy and funding changes

*Roles and Relationships*
- clarification of roles of key parties
- ongoing monitoring of roles and activities undertaken by the project team and evaluator
- the role of the primary health care team in recruitment
- ownership of data and nature of outputs, contractual issues

*Aims and Objectives*
- clarity of aims and objectives
- translation of project statements into tangible evaluation objectives
- value of qualitative as well as quantitative objectives and outcomes

*Research Methods*
- appropriateness of method
- research tools
- potential for replication and/or adaptation

*Ethical Concerns*
- code of conduct
- acceptability of project to patients
- ethical clearance if required

*Costings*
- realistic assessment
- extent to which cost effectiveness and value for money can be determined

*Ongoing Feedback and Dissemination*
- modus operandi between project teams and evaluation team
- feedback and review mechanisms
- nature, frequency and volume of outputs

In hospital settings evaluations of patient education interventions have tended to be localised and many of the above factors may also be relevant. Prioritising the aims of an evaluation over ongoing work can pose problems.

Evaluations of health promoting hospitals can generate a wide range of issues:

- the extent to which there is a shared concept of the health promoting hospital idea and its processes and agreement of the purposes of evaluations;
- differing methodological preferences held by the wide range of stakeholders and the need to establish some consensus around methodology;
- safeguarding adequate resources for evaluation;
- ensuring that there is acceptance of the importance of process as well as outcome evaluation.

The WHO (1991) stated that The Health Promoting Hospital seeks to:

- develop documented and evaluated examples of good practice for the use of other institutions;
- identify areas of common interest in which to develop programmes and evaluation procedures.

Pelikan *et al.* (1998a p17) propose that the *Health Promoting Hospital European Pilot Project* can be judged according to the following criteria:

- Feasibility – has it been possible to carry out the project plan?
- Quality – has it been possible to conduct the project according to pre-defined standards?
- Effectiveness – cost effectiveness and efficiency might be included if a project's aims and design asks for this.
- Sustainability – are the effects proving stable/sustainable?

Case studies of health promoting hospitals are revealing the use of some innovative data collection methods in evaluation. Particularly to be noted is the use of a story dialogue method developed by Labonte and used in evaluating the Pilot Health Promoting Hospital in Preston (Taylor, in Pelikan *et al.*, 1998a). This is a qualitative technique built around the story telling process. The process is structured and the stories are used as triggers to raise probing questions about what had been done in a project, why it was done, what it accomplished and what lessons could be learned.

The practitioner reflects on a process and through structured dialogue with each member having a defined role the story is rigorously analysed. A written record of insights into practice is produced. The process is repeated with other members of a group and themes are drawn out.

## Indicators

A wide range of indicators have been used to evaluate health promotion in health care settings reflecting the diversity of activities and the approaches to health promotion in practice. These are illustrated in Table 6.1. As emphasised in an earlier chapter indicators can be intermediate ones in one approach but outcome ones in others. For example, beliefs and attitudes can be outcomes in an educational approach but in a preventive approach they are intermediate to achieving behavioural outcomes of adherence.

We will now assess the effectiveness of health promotion in health care settings. We will look at some assessments of overall effectiveness of health promotion primary care and hospitals before examining successes of interventions at the individual level in both sectors.

## GENERAL EFFECTIVENESS OF HEALTH PROMOTION IN PRIMARY CARE

We have noted the growing attention in policy documents to health promotion in primary care. We can attempt to assess the extent to which primary care as a whole responds to policy documents and provides health promotion activities. Health education has taken place opportunistically in the contacts between health providers and patients but there are expectations in some countries, as explained for the UK, that there will also be formalised provision.

The views of professionals about health promotion and their professional skills are mediating factors between any policy and actual practice. Where payment is attached to an activity there may a greater likelihood of it occurring than where this is not the case, although this does not necessarily ensure quality of activity unless this is also audited. A number of studies have recorded primary care professionals views of health promotion and give us some indirect evidence of the extent to which health promotion is occurring.

A survey using a postal questionnaire with 1291 GPs (79% response rate) in the Oxford region in England (Coulter and Schofield, 1991) found very positive attitudes towards preventive

*Table 6.1*   Health Promotion Outcomes in Health Care Settings

| Outcomes | Intermediate indicators | Indirect indicators |
|---|---|---|
| Behaviours: adherence to medication; smoking and dietary change, etc. | Beliefs | Patient education libraries |
| | Attitudes | CCTV provision |
| | Decision making skills | Uptake of leaflets |
| Active participation | CCTV use | Shared records |
| Campaigning for services | Self-esteem | Professional collaboration |
| Development and implementation of health promotion policy | Self-efficacy | Health promotion in professional training |
| Cost savings | Knowledge | Planned programmes of patient education |
| Health measures: mortality, morbidity or subjective health | Informed consent | |
| | Behaviours: advocacy skills; | Coordination of patient education |
| Medication use | Patient satisfaction | Patient use satisfaction |
| Self-esteem; locus of control; efficacy | Anxiety | |
| Empowerment | | |
| Primary care–community links | | |

and health promotion roles. When respondents were asked to indicate, using open questions, difficulties they had encountered in the past or expected to encounter in the future in developing these activities 82.5% mentioned at least one. The most common was lack of time (49.8%). Other barriers mentioned were: patient's lack of interest in lifestyle advice (16.2%), lack of interest on the part of the doctor (11.8%), too few practice staff (10.5%), inadequate registers and records (10.1%), inadequate premises (6.4%) and lack of a computer (4.3%).

A forceful critique of health promotion in primary care up to the introduction of new arrangements was provided by Gillam (1996). Following the 1990 contract he records that uptake of clinic payments was initially most extensive in larger, well-organised practices which tended to serve healthier populations. This was, he states, a classic example of the 'inverse care law'. There were lessons to be learned from the 1992 arrangements. The first was the limitations of using financial incentives to stimulate health promotion activity. Doctors were effectively paid, he claims, for collecting information rather than acting on it or auditing the impact of their work. Incentives were insufficiently focused on activities of proven effectiveness. In addition, the contractual changes highlighted the limitations of clinic-based and over-medicalised approaches to health promotion. He stated:

> General practitioners and other members of their primary health care teams need encouragement to think beyond the surgery door, to forge links with those in community seeking the same ends whether in schools, workplaces, pharmacies or other settings.

He looked forward with some reservations to the new arrangements. While the Health Promotion Committees could approve a wider range of activities, including community development, he expected that the composition of committees and efforts to reduce bureaucracy would lead to rubber stamping of existing activities. He concluded by asking about the development of health promotion in general practice:

> Has anyone sought the views of the public on this bizarre episode? Where health promotion is concerned, they are the experts and it is hard to believe that more productive use could not have been made of some half a billion pounds so far spent in this area.

It is interesting to see if the changes introduced in 1996 have been reported on more positively. An interview-based study using a structured and unstructured questionnaire in Nottingham examined the impact of the changes (Coppel and Davis, 1997). Nineteen of the 117 general practices in the city were selected for participation and the study was interview-based using a schedule with structured and unstructured questions. Interviews were undertaken with people most involved in health promotion. Interventions focused on cardiovascular disease continued to predominate in health promotion activity – in line with the earlier banding arrangements. Where broadening out of activities had occurred it was not clear that changes were related to need. There was a marked decrease in health promotion clinic work and greater value placed on health promotion in the consultation. The study also highlighted wide variations in involvement in health promotion activities within and across practices. A number of barriers were reported, lack of resources including computers, staff, money and time being the leading one (eight practices), while five practices gave poor interest from patients and reluctance of patients to help themselves and two practices reported no barriers. The change in arrangements for health promotion had not reduced the barriers. Twelve of the 19 practices had made no attempt to monitor or evaluate their health promotion activities and eight said they would not know how to do so. Six of these wanted assistance. Of the remainder all had some ideas about evaluation but most would only use quantitative methods. Needs were identified for guidance and support in implementing and evaluating health promotion activities. The writers suggested that such support could be crucial to the developments of health promotion in primary care.

A further study in Northern Ireland (Bradley and McKnight, 1997) examined the perceptions of GPs of their roles as health promoters, their educational and training experiences to date and training needs. The study used information from a database on the patterns and uptake of health promotion training, a questionnaire-based survey of 357 doctors (57% response rate) and six focus group discussions. The training sessions offered were categorised as disease management (48%), service management (32%) and health promotion (20%). The mean duration of health promotion attended was 1 day, compared with 1.8 days for service management and 2.8 for disease management. The perceptions of GPs about the extent of health promotion roles were interesting. In ranking their duties curative care was first followed by health promotion, although exactly what was being understood as health promotion is not specified. Approximately two-thirds agreed or strongly agreed with the statement that the GPs role in health promotion should be limited to advice in consultation but one-third agreed that GPs should play the widest possible role in promoting the health of the communities in which they worked. There were negative reactions to the prevailing requirements around recording of health promotion activity (78%). The GPs reported a relative under-provision of educational activity for GPs. However, a recurring comment for the GPs was that they required evidence for the effectiveness of health promotion as a health activity and also for the efficacy of different patient motivational strategies.

It is clear that there have been mechanisms in place for the provision of health promotion in primary care but what is required has been relatively circumscribed. There has been more pressure on recording activity than on demonstrating that programmes have been evidence based and responsive to need. Routine evaluation of health promotion activity is not common, although researcher-initiated activities do take place.

There is generally weak evidence for the effectiveness of health promotion if we take primary care as a whole, although there is evidence of effectiveness for specific interventions, such as smoking advice, as noted in an earlier chapter (Russell *et al.*, 1979, 1988). If health promotion is to be effective across primary care as a whole it needs to be provided routinely by relevant health workers. Activities need to be theory based, take into account needs and priorities of the practice population and those areas where there is evidence of effectiveness and be implemented with attention to quality. There can be tensions between providing health promotion in response to expressed need and incorporating activities where there is evidence of effectiveness. In practice some balance between the two is achievable and expressed needs and proven effectiveness can, on occasion, be fully in tune. For example, there are people who want to give up smoking and there is evidence that smoking cessation can be achieved with support of nicotine replacement therapies.

Although primary care can be effective in health promotion it can only be so if people access the service. Young people, for example, do not readily use primary care in relation to some of the targets that have been set in health strategies. For example, Kari *et al.* (1997), in a school-based questionnaire survey, examined adolescents' attitudes to primary care and to sex and health education. Seventy-four per cent had consulted their GP in the previous 12 months so the potential for reaching this age group is there. Where information was concerned the main sources of information on contraception were books and leaflets (66%) and friends (44%). Only 33% consulted their GP on this subject – 60% knew what was meant by emergency contraception but only 33% knew they were entitled to ask their GP for it. Most of those in the study said they would like a drop-in clinic to discuss personal issues. The writers concluded that adolescents should be provided with more information in a form they can use, a choice of quicker GP appointments when crises occur and a more teenager-friendly health environment. Efforts have been made to respond to teenage concerns in some health authorities. There are also well-documented incidences of low uptake of primary care services by some minority communities (Ahmad, 1993; Benzeval *et al.*, 1995).

Effectiveness of health promotion in primary care will also depend on the motivation of professionals to acquire and put into practice proven strategies. While health promotion is, in many countries, a core component of nurse training it plays a small part in the initial training of doctors. A study of a representative sample of GPs in England (Killoran et al., 1993) recorded that 26% of their sample had received no health promotion training. Of the 72% who had received training only 37% had received it through medical education. At the time practice nurses were undertaking a substantial proportion of health promotion work as they carried out the health promotion clinics. Sixty-two per cent of the practice nurses said that they wanted more training and the following areas were mentioned: personal counselling skills, planning health promotion, knowledge of risk factors and use of computers. This study identified five sets of factors that were seen to be significant in determining the level and quality of health promotion in general practice and which would have to be met if primary care was to contribute effectively to achieving health strategy goals.

1 Training in planning and organising health promotion audits and evaluation and counselling skills. Multidisciplinary training was recommended.
2 Motivation and commitment.
3 Practice capacity for planning and organising health promotion.
4 Audit, evaluation and research.
5 The amount of support from health authorities.

## Hospitals

There are two ways to go about assessing the overall impact of health promotion in hospitals:

• success in achieving health promoting hospital developments at individual hospital level, throughout regional or national health systems;
• assessing the effectiveness of health promotion interventions in the hospitals and the extent to which widespread implementation of effective activities has been achieved.

It is still relatively early to draw firm conclusions on the impact of the health promoting hospitals initiatives as a whole, although there are reported evaluations that can be referred to. We can draw some limited conclusions from recording the growth in the number of hospitals seeking involvement since such hospitals have to meet criteria for involvement: If hospitals want to be accepted into the *Health Promoting Hospitals Network* they have to meet a number of conditions. The hospital management needs:

• to accept the *Ottawa Charter* and the elements of the 1991 *Budapest Declaration* (see Box 4) and staff must support any necessary organisational changes;
• the hospital needs to develop at least five subprojects to run for 5 years which either build on existing work or form new developments;
• there must be a link with an independent institution for research and evaluation purposes;
• the hospital is expected to form alliances with other health care units and with agencies outside the health care system.

**Box 4**  Budapest Declaration: *Criteria for Health Promoting Hospitals*

1 Provide opportunities throughout the hospital to develop health oriented perspectives, objectives and structures.
2 Develop a common corporate identity within the hospital which embraces the aims of the Health Promoting Hospital.
3 Raise awareness of the impact of the environment of the hospital on the health of patients, staff and community. The physical environment of hospital buildings should support, maintain and improve the healing process.
4 Encourage an active and participatory role for patients according to their specific health potentials.
5 Encourage participatory health gain oriented procedures throughout the hospital.
6 Create healthy working conditions for all staff.
7 Strive to make the health promoting

hospital a model for healthy services and workplaces.

8  Maintain and promote collaboration between community based health promotion initiatives and local governments.

9  Improve communication and collaboration with existing health and social services in the community.

10  Improve the range of support given to patients and their relatives by the hospital through community based social and health services and/or volunteer groups and organisations.

11  Identify and acknowledge specific target groups within the hospital and their health needs.

12  Acknowledge differences in value sets, needs and cultural conditions for individuals and different population groups.

13  Create supportive, humane and stimulating living environments within the hospital especially for long term and chronic patients.

14  Improve the health promoting quality and the variety of food services in hospitals for patients and personnel.

15  Enhance the provision and quality of provision, communication and educational programmes and skill training for patients and relatives.

16  Enhance the provision and quality of educational programmes and skills training for staff.

17  Develop in the hospital an epidemiological database specially related to the prevention of illness and communicate this information to public policy makers and to other institutions in the community.

(WHO, 1991)

The comprehensive set of criteria laid out in the *Budapest Declaration* provide a framework around which health promoting hospitals can be evaluated. Plans and the implementation of interventions are to be documented and evaluated according to appropriate locally predefined standards. The hospitals in the pilot phase of the project also agreed to get expert support to safeguard evaluation standards. Of the 149 sub-projects within the pilot hospitals 93 had been evaluated by 1998. In reporting on effectiveness of the sub-projects positive conclusions were drawn about implementation. As to whether they had achieved stated outcomes, Pelikan *et al.* (1998b) report that quantitative answers couldn't be provided at that point in time. On whether the projects had had a positive impact on population health they had the following to say:

> here again we have to draw attention to the fact that this has not been a multi-centre basic science research project with the necessary limitations in the design and sufficient funds to conduct this thorough enquiry. One cannot expect systematic results or answers in this area and in most cases we also would think that they are not necessary.

At the local level most pilot hospitals had attempted to address health promotion in four areas: patients, staff, community and the hospital as an organisation. On the regional/national and international level the project was reported to have been a big success. Cost effectiveness and efficiency had not been part of original agreements and only a few sub-projects had incorporated such measures. A number of factors reported as decisive for the success and also factors that had proved problematical were also reported by Pelikan *et al.* (1998b):

**Success**

a. *Involvement of the WHO as an initiating partner*

- Reputation and credibility of the WHO legitimised the vision of the *Ottawa Charter*;
- provided experiences and support through the *Healthy Cities Project*;
- recruited a coordinating centre for project management.

b. *Combination of an open vision, concrete example and concrete methodology*

- Vision stated in the *Budapest Declaration*;
- the concrete example of the WHO model project hospital in Vienna;
- agreed methodology for standards of local projects.

### Some problem areas

- An open vision creates difficulties in developing evaluation criteria;
- 20 hospitals is a large number to work with in meetings;
- the heterogeneity of projects was an obstacle to work in specific content areas;
- the heterogeneity of hospitals and health care environments restricted possible exchange;
- the project's lack of ability to raise international funds was disappointing;
- there was low political support in some countries;
- support by the WHO and the coordinating centre could have been more extensive.

They concluded that the *Pilot Hospital Project* had proved that it made sense for health promotion to invest in cooperation with the hospital even thought the hospital is a complex and difficult system.

At the *5th Conference of the Health Promoting Hospitals* reports were provided on the general developments in each of the pilot hospitals, the sub-projects and conclusions reached on achievements (Pelikan *et al.*, 1998a, b). The case studies provided illustrate the differing emphases in the projects and the variety of sub-projects. Some hospitals more clearly linked projects to the four areas of development (patients, staff, community and the hospital as an organisation) – in other cases sub-projects could be linked to such areas but the links were not made so explicit. Examples of pilot projects and their evaluation findings are provided in Boxes 5 and 6.

**Box 5** Health Promoting Hospitals Pilot Projects

*Altnagelvin Area Hospital, Londonderry*

**Aims of project**
- To develop the hospital into a healthier organisation by incorporating health promotion criteria into all decision making processes and into the culture of the hospital
- To offer additional health promoting services for patients and adopt the role of model within the community and health care system

**Sub-projects**
1 CPR (cardio-pulmonary resuscitation)
2 Children's education programme
3 Accidents at work
4 Breast feeding promotion
5 Workplace alcohol
6 Smoking and health policy

**Project outcomes after 4 years**
- In 1993 the hospital was a 'smoking hospital' – smoking was no longer the norm
- Alcohol only allowed on premises with special permission
- Healthy eating is encouraged and partnerships with supermarkets have been initiated
- Full-time resuscitation training officer for CPR has been appointed
- Percentage increases in breast feeding each year
- *Accidents at Work Team* formed relationships with all major employers and joint attitude surveys carried out
- Child Education project continues and is popular with schools

**Importance of the project to the hospital**
- Encouraged examination of the hospital from the health promoting point of view and development of relevant policies
- Encouraged exchange of ideas and good practice

- Increased communication between the hospital and the community
- Cemented relationships with other hospitals
- Gave an international focus to the hospital and opened up avenues to diverse cultures

**Box 6**   Pilot Health Promoting Hospitals Project

*The University Hospital, Linkoping, Sweden*

### Objective
- To reorient health services towards health
- Included two overarching projects: the development of decentralised organisation with an outcome orientation towards Health Gain and the introduction of Total Quality Management (TQM)

Ten sub-projects addressed the three broad areas of the health promoting hospitals:

*a. Health Gain for Patients*
- A Swedish Health Care meeting with refugees
- Psychological and social support to patients, relatives and staff suffering from crisis
- Caring for patients with alcohol problems identified in the emrgency ward
- The smoke-free hospital

*b. Health Gain for Personnel*
- Early active rehabilitation for University Hospital personnel

*c. Health Gains for the Society Served*
- Hospital accident analysis and the prevention of accidents
- Shops for a better life
- Osteoporosis prevention project
- Environment protection and pollution control

### Outcomes reported after 5 years
- Orientation towards health gain and TQM had continued despite budget cuts

- Health outcome accounts for three diagnoses per clinic were reported in 1997
- Ongoing projects for health gain measurement and patient-centred outcome measures
- Experiences from the project of early rehabilitation and from the TQM projects were that empowerment of the personnel by deeper participatory involvement in decision making had a strong influence on the well-being of personnel
- Community-oriented projects had strengthened collaboration between local community and regional health authorities
- The hospital was smoke free
- A unit for tobacco use prevention and a health-related information centre had been set up
- The hospital was a member of the Swedish network of health promoting hospitals

### Conclusions
Health gain for patients required adjustment of hospital focus. Regular measuring and reporting of health outcomes were needed in aiming for health gain

Health gains for personnel: making the hospital vision clear, setting goals for activities and making them visible and explicit created confident and assured personnel

Health gains for society: the hospital's knowledge of the state of health in the community together with the expertise and prestige of the hospital made initiation of preventive projects possible

Problems encountered included lack of time and fear of bureaucracy. All ongoing developmental projects needed to be interlinked.

Pelikan *et al.* (1998a) have concluded that the Health Promoting Hospital concept supports hospitals in coping with the challenges they are facing in initiating a developmental process directed at health as a highly valued goal, but open enough to enable necessary local adaptations. This variety is well evidenced in the diversity of sub-projects selected by the various hospitals. It is premature to draw strong conclusions about the long-term effectiveness of these initiatives as there is not as yet sufficient evidence reported.

A caution has been expressed earlier (Tones, 1995) about the main focus of the health promoting hospital developments:

> *it might be wise to beware the inappropriate territorial imperative. There are signs that, in the grip of commendable enthusiasm the hospital might be guilty of goal displacement in venturing too far in the community. ... It is important that the major focus of attention should be the hospital per se. It would be inappropriate at a time of cost cutting, rationing and staff shortages if hospital staff whose credibility rests on degree of contact with the patient were to trespass on the preserves of others such as school teachers and community workers.*

In the hospital setting much health promotion-related activity is undertaken outside formal involvement in health promoting hospitals initiatives. A great deal of this is educational activity with patients. If we are wanting to assess the effectiveness of hospital systems as a whole in providing health promotion a number of factors have a bearing on overall effectiveness. Activities which can be shown to be successful need to be achieved not only within a few selected areas of health or for a restricted range of outcomes but across all aspects of hospital care. For institution-wide successes to be achieved the following are likely to be required:

- policies which specify educational activity as a component of care and specify the mechanisms by which this can be achieved;
- health workers who are appropriately trained to undertake the educational component of care;
- organisational arrangements which maximise the possibility of educational success;
- the wide scale adoption of educational activi-

ties in line with patient and client needs;
- the implementation of interventions known to be effective and efficient;
- full availability of appropriate supporting resources.

We will comment selectively on the extent to which there is evidence of the above being in place.

We commented earlier on a selection of policy documents which have emphasised the importance of health promotion in health care settings. Evidence from various countries on the extent of patient education has been reported from time to time. Bartlett and Jonkers (1990) reported that 37% of hospitals in Canada had health promotion policies but also that 21% of hospitals stated that health promotion was not part of their role. From Australia, Degeling *et al.* (1990) reported that most hospitals surveyed:

> *recognised the importance of patient education but support was based on individual efforts resulting from efforts taken in specialty areas rather than reflecting overall hospital policy.*

With reference to patient education in the USA, Green (1990) reported that budgetary constraints were impacting on the work of patient education coordinators and the capacity to implement the factors known to be effective in programmes. He commented that *hard times have forced a more systematic, coordinated, strategically planned and evaluated patient education program.*

### Organisation of patient education

A first stage in ensuring that health promotion aspects of care are met is to ensure that these are identified and noted in care plans. A second stage is ensuring that needs are met appropriately and activities evaluated. In any period of hospital care people encounter various professionals, ancillary workers, other patients and their families. All can make contributions to health education, formally or informally. In order to achieve coherence between the various contributions some coordination is desirable. At the level of individual patients health education activity can be recorded alongside all other aspects of care. The mean length of hospital stay is declining and it therefore becomes increasingly desirable that there is coordination between hospital and primary care. In addition to coordination of activities for the individual patient, coordination needs also to take place at other levels – the level of specific conditions, for particular client groups such as older people, and as a general hospital-wide activity.

The institution of patient education coordinators first developed in the USA but has spread more widely. An early study (Pack *et al.*, 1983) reported on the effectiveness of programmes in relation to the existence of patient education coordinators. Eighteen criteria for patient education were incorporated into a survey of subject-based programmes in Michigan, USA. Of 281 programmes reported, 219 (78%) had either a full-time or a part-time coordinator. The mean number of criteria met when there was either a full- or part-time coordinator were 13.8 and 12.7, respectively, but only 8.3 where there was no coordinator. There was some variation in the number of criteria met according to the type of coordinator. Where education was considered to be their prime responsibility more criteria were likely to be met than where responsibilities were diverse. Programmes also tended to be more comprehensive where coordinators had received further training.

The development of the patient education coordinator has been reviewed in The Netherlands (Fahrenfort, 1990). By this date 60% of Netherlands hospitals had coordinators. Fahrenfort reported on a five hospital project in which participating hospitals had to meet specified criteria:

- agreement to appoint a patient coordinator for the duration of the project;
- have demonstrated an interest before applying for available grants;
- hospital management had to be supportive to the experiment and agree external monitoring, advice and evaluation.

Monitoring and evaluation were expected to address a number of areas:

- the benefits of coordinator appointment to the development of patient education; qualifications for the coordinator role and the tasks to be performed;
- the changes in the hospital as a result of the coordinator presence;
- organisational barriers and supports to development;
- the long-term necessity of the coordinator function.

At the project outset two views of the coordinator role were in evidence. Hospital administrators tended to stress the public relations aspect of the coordinator while the coordinators themselves were more interested in exploring organisational change. The coordinator posts were not defined in detail and the people in post had to negotiate their roles and this task took up to 2 years. The project reported success in combining aspects of organisational change and education of medical staff about communication with patients.

Fahrenfort noted the development of two trends – the emergence of and belief in patient's rights to autonomy and the development of a greater market orientation to the provision of health care. Patient education was seen to be compatible with both, but she noted:

*the government support for patient emancipation veered towards supporting emancipation as consumerism.*

She made a number of observations on the development of the coordinator role:

- easily visible promotion aspects of the role can take priority over the slower and more difficult but also more important work of organisational development and change;
- organisational change can lead to improved procedures for professional–patient contact, a better understanding of the patient education process and support for professionals in changing aspects of their image, as well as enabling patients to achieve real autonomy;
- the use of patient education counters in a hospital can indicate good intentions towards

patient education without actually changing the way that patients are informed about their health;

- the skills of the coordinator will include those of balancing demands for quick and visible results with the need for longer term organisational change, recognising that the former can trigger support for the latter.

Whether or not hospitals appoint specialist patient education or health promotion coordinators it is important to monitor progress in meeting individual educational needs. The period in hospital is typically only a proportion of a patient career, which begins with consultation in primary care followed by referral to hospital and subsequent admission and followed by further contact with primary care. The educational needs begin from the first point of contact and it makes sense to record activity from this point. This is a key example of the need for 'joint' action. There has also been discussion over the years of the importance of patients holding their own records which could document health promotion activity (Dickey, 1993).

In the next sections we will discuss evaluations of individually focused education with patients in hospitals or in primary care.

## Health education interventions

At the individual level education in health care contexts has addressed a variety of outcomes; knowledge, attitudinal and behavioural outcomes. In some cases information and knowledge have been addressed as outcomes in their own right – at other times with the intention that they will impact on behavioural intentions or specific behaviours. Where behaviours are concerned there has been a long-term emphasis on interventions designed to increase adherence and compliance with treatment regimes. There has also been a range of interventions directed at preventive behaviours and, to a lesser extent, positive health promoting behaviours. We will discuss interventions focusing on information and subsequently those addressing behaviours.

## Knowledge and information

An early case for providing patients with information about treatment that they were to receive was made on the basis that this was related to a number of measurable outcomes: less pain, reduced anxiety, reduced drug need and reductions in hospital stay. Such interventions were theory based and informed by the idea that providing people with anticipatory guidance allowed for rehearsal of feelings and necessary skills, with consequent gains for patients in terms of less pain and reduced length of stay

Ensuring people have information is integral to all models of health promotion. There has for a long time been evidence from across health areas that people want information (Cassileth *et al.*, 1980; Fallowfield *et al.*, 1994). At the same time there has been well-documented evidence of a lack of satisfaction with the nature and amount of information in health care situations. People can have a variety information needs, including:

- information on the existence, causes and prognosis of specific diseases;
- information as anticipatory guidance for hospitalisation;
- information to support rehabilitation;
- information about sources of support.

People also have preferences about sources of information. These are exemplified in a survey of patients in primary care (McGredy, 2000) and a focused study of cancer patients undertaken by James *et al.* (1999). In McGredy's study a large number of patients registered with practices in the North East of England were asked about their information needs:

- the information they did receive;
- the information they would like to receive;
- the people who were seen as sources of health-related information;
- who they would prefer to receive information from;
- the preferred format for receiving information.

There were 4544 respondents in the survey. The top 10 listed areas of health information received together with expressed needs are shown in Box 7.

**Box 7**    Top 10 Areas of Health Information Received and Needed

| Received | | Needed | |
|---|---|---|---|
| Healthy eating | 541 | Stress management | 1404 |
| Family planning | 478 | Relaxation | 1403 |
| Stopping smoking | 434 | Weight management | 1374 |
| Weight management | 434 | Healthy eating | 1258 |
| Breast/testicular awareness | 375 | Becoming more active | 994 |
| Sensible drinking | 360 | Breast/testicular awareness | 979 |
| Becoming more active | 356 | Stopping smoking | 961 |
| Holiday health | 271 | Living on a limited budget | 913 |
| Cancer | 261 | Cancer | 754 |
| Stress management | 261 | Illegal drugs | 660 |

Note: respondents could provide multiple responses to this question.

There are some interesting similarities between the two lists in Box 7. Recorded information need is high compared with the number of people who reported receiving information. Aspects of mental health topped the list of informational needs but were at the bottom of the list on information received. On the other hand, information around healthy eating was high on need and also high on information received. The number of people seeking information on living on a limited budget indicates a need in line with the widened role of primary care in addressing inequalities. In stating who were seen as credible sources of information (where more than one could be given) the top five mentions were as follows: male GP (2883); practice nurse (2645); female GP (2253); pharmacist (1534); health visitor (1238). When patients were asked who they would like to receive information from the same ordering was obtained: male GP (2514); practice nurse (2181); female GP (2090); pharmacist (943); health visitor (640). The preferences for GPs and practice nurses stands out clearly from these results. However, when asked how they would like to receive information a slightly different picture emerged. The GP consultation received the highest number of mentions (2120) but was almost equalled by leaflets (2100) and then followed by practice nurses (1092), clinics (896) and posters (702). The study did not allow conclusions to be drawn on the combination that people preferred, for example, consulta-tion supported by leaflets rather than one or the other in isolation.

The second study was an opportunistic sample survey of patients and their friends and relatives about cancer information support and was carried out in an English hospital (James *et al.*, 1999). All respondents said that they wanted as much information as possible and there were few differences between the three categories of people participating in the study. TV and print media were the most frequently cited sources of general information in all groups (professionals were not listed alternatives). Audiotapes and computers were little mentioned – a situation which would probably have changed in the period since the study was conducted given the rapid adoption of the use of the Internet for health information.

The failure to meet informational needs satisfactorily can happen for many reasons:

- conscious or unconscious omission and oversights;
- disruption from competing activities;
- inappropriate timing of informational inputs;
- inadequate provision of written materials;
- poor professional communication;
- denying informational needs or knowingly withholding information.

We noted earlier in discussing the concept of shared decision making that there were limitations in the sharing of information in the consultation. It is on the basis of detailed studies of inter-actions that interventions leading to more effec-tive communication can be achieved.

As is well documented in the literature, infor-mation alone has a limited impact on variables other than knowledge and beliefs but these are nonetheless important variables to influence and there is, anyway, good evidence, as noted above, that patients do actually want information. In order to be effective a number of criteria need to be met:

- relevant professionals need to acknowledge that informational needs exist and should elicit these using the most appropriate methods with particular clients;
- patients need to recognise and be able to com-municate their information needs;
- attitudes of professionals towards the sharing of information need to be positive and contexts provided which facilitate sharing;
- understanding of the ways that information sharing can be constrained in health care con-texts needs to be enhanced;
- effective and efficient means of sharing infor-mation which are also satisfactory for recipi-ents need to be identified.

Evaluations of success in information exchange have reported on interventions using inter-per-sonal methods alone, various forms of media alone or combinations of the two. For example, an evaluation of a patient education booklet which dealt with 40 common ailments and advice on actions to take was carried out by Milewa *et al.* (2000). Ten thousand copies of the booklet were distributed and the effects on self-referral and self-behaviour were assessed on the basis of self-report. Random sample postal surveys were carried out before the booklet was sent out and 6 months later ($n = 495$) and also in a control area where the booklet was not distributed ($n = 509$). In addition, 85 structured interviews were under-taken in the intervention area. The survey data were analysed according to the availability of information in the households The results sug-gested that acquisition of the booklet exerted a small influence on patient help-seeking behaviour when no comparable publications were possessed. The interviews explored in greater detail some of the reasons for the modest impact. It was con-cluded that understanding the ways that patient education was perceived had to focus on the ways that sub-groups processed and attributed meaning to official and unofficial sources of advice. The education booklets were simply one element in the complexity of factors, individual and social, that impact on individual decisions around help-seeking behaviour.

A situation where written information may provide a useful contribution to achieving uptake in screening is the case of colorectal cancer. This cancer is the second leading cause of malignant disease in Britain. For screening programmes to be effective participation rates need to be increased. The common reasons identified in studies for non-participation have included lack of awareness of the frequency of colorectal can-cer, failure to appreciate the concept of asympto-matic illness, unpleasantness of the screening procedure and fear of further investigations and surgery (Hynam *et al.*, 1995; Hart *et al.*, 1997). Hart *et al.* (1997) assessed the effectiveness of an educational leaflet in increasing the intention to participate in colorectal cancer screening. Their hypothesis was that if the reasons for non-partici-pation were addressed participation overall could be increased. The effectiveness of the leaflet was assessed by its ability to raise awareness of the dis-ease and of asymptomatic illness and screening and increase intentions to take up colorectal screening. The study was based on interviews before and after reading a leaflet with 50 men and 50 women accompanying patients to medical and surgical clinics (other than colorectal cancer investigations) at a large hospital. The leaflet sig-nificantly increased knowledge and understand-ing. It also impacted on people's stated intention to accept screening. Fifty-five per cent of men and 50% of women reversed earlier decisions. The study did not, however, follow up actual behav-iour. Participants actually read the leaflet in the hospital context – not the situation which would prevail if the leaflet had to be picked up in a GP surgery or came through the post. Hart *et al.*

(1997) discussed other studies where there had been mixed results in using leaflets to increase screening. In one study people were sent a letter about colorectal cancer and the purpose of the test 2 weeks before being sent an invitation. Acceptance of screening was raised from 38 to 47%. There were no reports of success by age and sex. Another study had found no differences between people who received educational materials and controls and in a further study compliance fell after receiving educational material. Hart *et al.* concluded that a RCT to quantify the effect of their leaflet was justified. Leaflets are cheap and if distributed widely can have a demonstrable effect on screening even if percentage increases are smaller than in the use of more intensive one-to-one methods.

A systematic review of the literature on written information for a different screening procedure – cervical screening – has been completed and detailed evidence-based criteria developed for each stage of the screening process (Davey *et al.*, 1998). They concluded that information is most effectively communicated verbally by a health professional and supplemented and reinforced by the written information. Improving the quality of written information should, they say, be matched with quality assurance of smear taking and effective comunication skills of the smear taker. This study progressed to the development of three leaflets to be used in the *National Screening Programme*.

Improving the availability of information to ethnic minority groups, especially where there are language barriers, has been identified as a significant issue across all aspects of health and is one where there are a growing number of interventions (Bhopal and Donaldson, 1988; Ahmad, 1993).

## Behaviours

A major part of education in health care settings has addressed behaviours and, as noted earlier, a preoccupation has been to seek to achieve compliance with medical regimens and success has been measured in terms of the percentages of people who have complied. Earlier studies were often about compliance with drug or other aspects of treatment but as the importance of prevention was recognised attention was also directed towards preventive health or lifestyle variables. Preventive health behaviours have been proportionately more important in primary care than in hospital settings but as hospitals take a broader view of health this difference is less clear. Increasingly, evidence of effectiveness for specific educational areas has been brought together in systematic reviews. Examples of these will be discussed.

A number of systematic reviews of patient education have been undertaken (Devine, 1992; Mullen *et al.*, 1992, 1997; Simons-Morton *et al.*, 1992). These have included interventions in both primary and hospital care except where the location to one or other location is specifically stated. All reviews have reported, for a range of acute and chronic conditions, a number of positive outcomes, in knowledge, attitudes, behaviours and clinical outcomes. Two reviews using a different procedure were carried out as part of the *International Union for Health Education and Promotion Project* – one of patient education in hospitals and one outside. They provide detailed analyses of a selected small number of projects applying the detailed review tool mentioned earlier (Chwalow, 1994; van Ballekom, 1994; van Driel and Keijsers, 1997). Two systematic reviews have focused on a range of preventive health behaviours (Simons *et al.*, 1992; Mullen *et al.*, 1997).

### Preventive behaviours

The Simons *et al.* (1992) review focused on patient education interventions for preventive health behaviours delivered in clinical settings from 1971 to 1989. The studies met true or quasi-experimental design criteria and were for seven areas: contraceptive use; breast self-examination; exercise and physical activity; injury prevention; nutrition; smoking; stress management; weight loss and management. Sixty-four of the 121 studies they identified met the inclusion criteria. One-third of the studies were for smoking cessation followed by education on specific nutrients, contraceptive use and weight control. The writers concluded from the review that enough rigorous studies had been reported for us to be able to determine what types of educational approaches were most effective in general and also for certain specific behaviours. They also noted the gaps in the literature, where evidence for some preventive behaviours for effective approaches to education and counseling was sparse.

The more recent review, an extension of the earlier study (Mullen *et al.*, 1997), will be described in more detail. It examined the patient education and counselling literature to estimate the overall magnitude of effectiveness of patient education and counselling and to determine which approaches produced the largest effects. Meta-analysis of findings from primary studies was carried out. This review was directed towards primary prevention. It looked for published and unpublished studies that measured the effect of any education or counselling intervention in apparently healthy individuals seen in clinical settings in a developed country. Settings included those where clinical care was provided in main health care settings or places such as school clinics and workplaces, community health care centres and nursing homes where it was delivered by health care workers. Studies covered the period 1972–1993. The following prevention areas were included:

- contraceptive use;
- breast and testicular self-examination;
- exercise and physical activity;
- injury prevention;
- nutrition;
- stress management;
- substance abuse;
- weight control.

Details of the methodology of the review can be followed up in the paper. Seventy-four studies met the criteria for inclusion. In extracting data from the studies the characteristics of the intervention, the type of behaviour addressed and evaluation study characteristics were recorded. The characteristics of interventions were described as shown in Box 8.

***Box 8*** Characteristics of Interventions

---

*Principles of Education*
- Relevance to patients by tailoring to needs and abilities;
- individualisation of instruction through opportunity for questions or self-pacing;
- feedback about changes in behaviour or health status indicators;
- reinforcement or reward for positive behaviour change;
- facilitation of behaviour change by provision of supplies or materials;
- multiple communication channels.

*Orientation*
This described whether the intervention relied on cognitive or behavioural approaches or both.

*Number of Patient Contacts*
The number of patient contracts were recorded as one or more than one.

*Channel of Communication*
- Use of personal communication or media or both combined;
- profession of communicators.

---

The areas addressed in the studies were combined into three groups: 39 studies on smoking/alcohol, 17 on nutrition/weight control and 18 other studies from a variety of areas. All areas that were sought were represented except testicular self-examination, illicit drug treatment, stress management by coping techniques and certain specified nutritional areas where no studies met the inclusion criteria. A number of problems in undertaking meta-analysis had to be addressed and careful details are provided of techniques used.

The conclusions from the review were that patient education and counselling contributed to behaviour change for disease prevention. They also calculated the percentage improvement for the average member of the experimental group over the average member of a control group. Their estimates were that the average member of the experimental group was 44% better off in the smoking/alcohol studies, 38% for nutrition and 42% for other behaviours. They observed:

> *It is obvious that the answer to population risk cannot be found exclusively in patient education but the evidence suggests that patient education and counseling, along with other individual as well as environmental approaches, is useful. Thus, a reasonable message for physicians and other clinicians, pending further studies, is to provide patient education and counseling for preventive behaviour change. When doing so they should use behavioural techniques, especially self monitoring and should include personal communication and written and other audiovisual materials. These approaches appear to be more important when the recommended behaviour change involves subtracting an existing behaviour.*

There have been calls for education to be a part of every contact between a patient and a health provider and a fully integrated part of health care. If this were to happen, we might not wish to focus, in any detail, on each and every health condition. In general, however, developments have tended to be condition specific rather than general ones with good planning and incorporation of education in some conditions but relative neglect in others.

The relative numbers of studies for selected areas of patient education can be seen in Table 6.2.

There has, however, been a stage of hospital care where general education provision has been well developed – that of preparation for hospitalisation and surgery. It was, as noted earlier, successes in these areas of patient education which were persuasive in campaigns to insititutionalise education as a part of health care. The impacts of education are seen to be both physical and psychological for this stage of care and a range of measures have been used, including: reductions in pain, medications, anxiety, length of stay and satisfaction. Many studies have been carried out under experimental conditions and have tested the relative impact of alternative educational and counselling strategies.

The successes have been associated with the provision of consistent education which meets patients actual needs (Breemhaar and van den Borne, 1991; van den Borne, 1998). Pre-surgical education has consisted broadly of three types of input used singly or in combination: information about procedures to be undergone and sensations to be expected; development of mental strategies to reduce threatening cognitions; coping behaviours – relaxation, breathing, coughing and turning. Theoretical models have been drawn on as bases for structuring educational inputs and for providing explanations. A particular feature of discussions has been the relationship between educational input and the development of control, and Breemhaar and van den Borne (1991) reviewed this link. They concluded that positive effects of pre-surgical education could be explained by increases in perceived control with consequent reductions in stress experiences and the ways it was managed. The positive effects of actions to increase perceived control were related to individual locus of control and the opportunities to exercise control.

Such conclusions serve to remind us that quick fixes of pre-surgical education applied uniformly are unlikely to be uniformly successful. Assessments are required of the need in specific situations for patients to exercise control and of the actual opportunities for doing so. At the same time assessments of patients' wishes to exercise control and their beliefs in their efficacy to do so also need to be carried out. As Breemhaar and van den Borne point out, if a situation does not require control and/or the patient does not wish to exercise it, it is better to leave out the provision of detailed information and behavioural instructions and simply provide assistance in regulating emotions. In those situations where some active contribution is required patients will need to be convinced of the value of the behaviours suggested and of their abilities to carry them out. Recently van den Borne (1998) has reported on the effect sizes obtained in meta analyses of pre-surgical education together with those for other areas of patient education. The areas of patient education where effect sizes over 0.40 were obtained are listed in Table 6.2. An effect size of

0.20 is generally considered small, one of 0.50 as reasonable and one of 0.80 as large.

Lower effect sizes were reported for coping with arthritis pain, depression and handicap and exercise advice for heart disease patients. The average effect size for all studies was 0.49. Table 6.2 illustrates the large number of studies that have been undertaken in the areas of pre-operative education, compliance weight loss and diabetes.

Reviews of this type provide us with a particular kind of evidence derived from particular studies about what can be achieved for interventions informed by preventive and educational models. If such interventions were delivered systematically and implemented fully, significant changes in health behaviours could be achieved. While it is important to seek more efficient ways of achieving desired goals it is equally important to apply existing knowledge promptly.

Health promotion interventions which work within the parameters of the empowerment model have also been assessed although they feature less in systematic reviews of patient education. Steele *et al.* (1987), after reviewing the 'active patient' concept and research, studies drew the following conclusions:

- because the active patient concept has been defined and operationalised in various ways it

is difficult to know if apparent differences in the participation preferences of patients are genuine or reflections of assessment procedures;
- sample sizes in studies have been small, nonrepresentative and cross-sectional. Future research needed to focus on the various determinants of information needs and the preferences for active involvement;
- there was no coherent theory guiding research and an orienting framework was.

So far we have drawn rather heavily on studies informed by a positivist approach for the reason that they are predominant in the health care setting. We will now discuss two studies which have used different study methods and provided evidence on achieving goals associated with empowerment. The first is an interesting study of an action research project working towards empowerment of older people described by McWilliam *et al.* (1997). This was part of a larger project with older people with chronic medical problems and repeated admissions to acute care for conditions which could have been managed at home The overall aim of the project was to enable frail people to manage better at home and decrease need for hospital admissions. A process based on adult education theory described as educative transformation was undertaken. This consisted of a structured process

**Table 6.2** Summary of Meta-analyses in Secondary Prevention and Patient Education, Giving Average Effect Sizes and Number of Studies in Each

| Topic/subject group | Effect size | No. of studies |
|---|---|---|
| Patient education for the chronically ill | 0.52 | 27 |
| Compliance with medical treatment of all types | 0.47 | 58 |
| Patent education, compliance, prevention | 0.74 | 23 |
| Pre-operative information/advice; recovery | 0.46 | 11 |
| Pre-operative information/advice; outcome | 0.44 | 68 |
| Pre-operative information/advice; anxiety | 0.40 | 23 |
| Pre-operative information/advice; pain | 0.38 | 82 |
| Pre-operative information/advice; distress | 0.36 | 80 |
| Patient education for the chronically ill | 0.37 | 55 |
| Pain management for children | 0.52 | 21 |
| Information advice for diabetics; diet | 0.62 | 12 |
| Information/advice for diabetics; self-monitoring | 0.50 | 10 |
| Patient education for diabetics; compliance | 0.43 | 82 |
| Weight loss in cases of obesity | 1.06 | 80 |

of reflective dialogue over 12–16 1 hour home visits. This had the following aims:

- to enable older persons to act as partners in their own care;
- foster a self-help philosophy;
- enhance active decision making;
- improve morale, self-esteem, self-care agency, inter-personal dependency, locus of control and desire for information.

A research nurse and the study participant worked together to assess, plan, enact and evaluate critical reflections on the person's life and health and on the meaning of these reflections. Five health promotion strategies were identified in the intervention.

- *Building trust and meaning:* participants tell their stories and their understanding of the meaning of these is facilitated.
- *Connecting and caring:* participants unload negatives, discover strengths and feel understood and the facilitator role is of one active listening and reflection and providing positive regard.
- *Mutual knowing:* developing conscious awareness of participants, own patterns and strengths.
- *Mutual creating*: rethinking ways of doing things and of seeing one's self such that self-esteem is enhanced and an outcome of empowerment is achieved.

The processes did not occur in a linear fashion but built on each other in a way which enhanced personal health.

McWilliam *et al.* (1997) provide a case study of the process and their conclusion for one person, Mrs X, was:

*over time Mrs X published several columns in the local newspaper. In keeping with the phases of perspective transformation, she had created competence and self confidence in a new role and relationship with the outside world, reintegrating into her life a sense of being a valued and connected part of society. Her frequent visits to emergency and telephone calls to home care services stopped. Continuity of the relationship over time had permitted mutual knowing which evolved the client's knowledge of herself, creating a greater conscious awareness of her own strengths and new images and expectations of life. This self knowledge, promoted and positively reinforced by the nurse, enhanced her self esteem and facilitated mobilisation of personal resources for everyday living even though her physical experience of her chronic illness did not change. Empowerment and ultimately being healthy despite the chronic illness was the outcome.*

Interestingly, this intervention has also been assessed in the context of an RCT (McWilliam *et al.*, 1999). Results for the intervention group compared with a group who received usual home care included:

- significantly greater independence and perceived ability to mange their own health;
- significantly less desire for information immediately post-intervention.

The pattern persisted at one year follow-up but significant differences were limited to independence and desire for information. The researchers concluded that critical reflection had the clinical potential to enhance the health of chronically ill older persons and suggested further work on less frail populations.

The second study is an example of a growing number of studies designed to develop active participation in users of services. These have been particularly common in the area of mental health. Service users have been involved in national policy development and service development at local level. The experiences of user involvement and its impact on services have been examined (Barnes and Wistow, 1994). Barnes and Shardlow (1997) report on a study of three mental health service user groups was undertaken in the context of a wider study of the way user groups seek to influence health and social services within the public sector. The case studies examined groups operating within three different models:

1 working in partnership with officials;
2 acting as pressure groups – including advocacy;

3 entering the market as providers or direct purchasers.

Data collection was through interviews together with some observation in groups and the analysis of documentation. The three groups were:

1 an umbrella group for user groups with an advocacy service and links with the health services and planning and service delivery levels;
2 users and ex-users within MIND, a national mental health voluntary organisation;
3 a drop-in facility for younger people with mental health problems.

A variety of themes were addressed in the qualitative analysis, including aspects of social exclusion and citizenship and what was achieved through participation.

Barnes and Shardlow reported that participation in a group gave people:

> *a voice and as confidence develops they are able to play a role in organising the group, in planning forums involving service purchasers and providers, and in representing the group at conferences and seminars. Acquiring new skills can provide a boost to confidence and self esteem and can be a spring board to opportunities outside the movement.*

None of the groups claimed that involvement had led to shifts in the balance of power in the mental health system but the challenges to the system had led to things being looked at in different ways. In some cases the nature of relationships between providers and users had been changed and this enabled users to play a part in defining and constructing services. In short, it was proposed that groups of people who have used mental health services can be active agents in controlling their own lives but also in providing services to each other and as participants within decision making networks. Finally the groups:

> *have a role to play in revitalising the relationship between users and the service provided within the welfare state in a way which views recipients as partners in the produc-*

> *tion of welfare, rather than as competitive consumers of it.*

## Facilitating the educational process

Educational and counselling needs can, and arguably always should be, defined through dialogue with patients and their families. In arriving at a decision, account has to be taken, in addition to needs, of other characteristics of patients and facilitators and the particular constraints of the context in question. Where education begins in a hospital it is important, as the length of hospital stays is reduced, that this education is part of an ongoing process which continues after discharge. People may frequently not be ready for educational activity in the time they are actually in hospital so a major responsibility rests with primary care to ensure that the educational and counselling process is initiated and sustained. Timing of activities is important. It is a truism to say that education and counselling are most effective if provided as near as possible to the time when need arises. In a study by Wallace (1988) patients expressed a consistent need for preparation (including booklets) prior to hospitalisation rather than after admission. With the use of individualised care plans and the encouragement of active participation of patients in their own care, there are structures and processes for the continued monitoring of educational need and the organisation of appropriate responses.

Earlier meta analyses generated educational principles for use in achieving effectiveness (Mullen *et al.*, 1985; Simons-Morton *et al.*, 1992). These were as follows.

1 Relevance. The relevance of content and educational methods to learner's interest should be ensured.
2 Individualisation. The educational programme should provide opportunities for patients to set the pace of their own learning and to receive answers to personal questions.
3 Facilitation. Behaviour should be facilitated by providing the means for patients and their families to take action or reduce barriers to action.
4 Feedback. The degree to which the patient is achieving progress should be demonstrated.

5 Reinforcement. The patient should be given encouragement for progress towards goals and objectives.

Mullen *et al.* (1985) demonstrated that for adherence to long-term medication, use of these principles was the strongest predictor of outcomes. Clearly these are well-known educational psychological principles but not necessarily always recalled when providing patient education activities. Training health care workers for their educational roles is not routine in professional training in many countries, although it is more common for nurses than for doctors.

## Equity

We have noted varying degrees of success in health promotion activities in the settings discussed. The capacity to translate such findings from what are often small-scale studies to the population as a whole is a challenge. Ensuring that programmes which have been shown to be effective reach all who may benefit is a still greater challenge. The *Acheson Report* (1998) on inequalities in health in England stated:

> communities most at risk of ill health tend to experience the least satisfactory access to the full range of preventive services, the so called 'inverse prevention law'. Prevention services include cancer screening programmes, health promotion and immunisation.

It can be argued that priority should be given to the achievement of equity in the planning, implementation and delivery of health promotion services. The *Acheson Report* noted that ring fenced funding for HIV/AIDS prevention which was allocated on a needs-based formula had achieved some success in allocating resources where they are most needed and that this procedure could be used more extensively. This report also included recommendations with reference to ethnicity and gender which if implemented could reduce health inequalities related to these factors.

We noted earlier that some health topic areas are better provided with patient education than others. An equitable policy for patient education needs to ensure that educational needs are identified for all health topics areas and met appropriately. Responding to needs requires access to interpreting services for some people. If it was accepted that education is a component of every episode of care health areas currently neglected might not be so easily overlooked.

Some health conditions that are chronic can also be associated with social isolation for people. Van den Borne (1998) reported on an ongoing study of interventions designed to reinforce the social network and support for patients with rheumatic disorders. He also indicates the need for support for people living with a stigmatised condition:

> A better understanding of such processes of exclusion, including thorough patient education, can influence the patient's social environment to combat stigmatisation and encourage pro-social behaviour. It may, for example, be important for someone with a certain condition to know who they should tell that they are sick and just what they should actually say.

## CONCLUSION

There is evidence available of effective patient education activities which if implemented fully in hospitals and primary care could make a contribution to promoting health and preventing ill health at the various levels of prevention. Education has been a long-standing component of health care even if not always particularly well done or adequately matched to people's needs. People do want information and counselling and development of new skills as a component of care and it is important that this is available for all health conditions. The growing emphasis on hospitals as health promoting settings is a welcome development and there is interesting work being undertaken in a large number of countries to develop this concept and emerging evidence of successes. In some cases more rigorous evaluation is, perhaps, needed. With reference to patient education the statement made by Bartlett (1985) still holds good:

*The answers to many research questions remain cloudy and other questions remain to be formulated. Yet a considerable body of knowledge now exists on which effective, practical and acceptable patient education programmes can be developed More research now needs to be directed to the question, 'Why aren't we applying the knowledge we already have?'*

Where the new developments of health promoting hospitals are concerned it has been commented earlier (Tones, 1995) that the most significant move towards the health promoting hospital would be to implement what we already know about empowerment through effective communication and education.

# REFERENCES

Acheson, D. (1998) *Independent Inquiry into Inequalities in Health.* The Stationery Office, London.

Ahmad, W. I. U. (Ed.) (1993) *'Race' and Health in Contemporary Britain.* Open University Press, Buckingham.

American Hospitals Association (1972) *A Patients Bill of Rights.* American Hospital Association, Chicago, IL.

Ashcroft, S. and Summersgill, P. (1993) *Perpetual promotion. Health Services Journal,* 103 (5349), 29.

Barnes, M. and Shardlow, P. (1997) *From passive recipient to active citizen: participation in mental health user groups. Journal of Mental Health,* 6 (3), 289–300.

Barnes, M. and Wistow, G. (1994) *Learning to hear voices: listening to users of mental health services. Journal of Mental Health,* 3, 525–540.

Bartlett, E. E. (1985) *Editorial: at last a definition. Patient Education and Counseling,* 7, 323–324.

Bartlett, E. E and Jonkers, R. (1990) *Editorial: Patient education – an international comparison. Patient Education and Counseling,* 15, 99–100.

Benzeval, M., Judge, K. and Whitehead, M. (1995) *Tackling Inequalities in Health: an Agenda for Action.* Kings Fund, London.

Bhopal, R. S. and Donaldson, L. J. (1988) *Health education for ethnic minorities, current provision and future directions. Health Education Journal,* 47 (4), 137–140.

Breemhaar, B. and van den Borne, H. W. (1991) *Effects of education and support for surgical patients: the role of perceived control. Patient Education and Counseling,* 18, 199–210.

Bradley, T. and McKnight, A. (1997) *The educational needs of GPs for health promotion in primary care. International Journal of Health Education,* 35 (4), 126–128.

Breemhaar, B. and van den Borne, H. W. (1991) *Effects on education and support for surgical patients: the role of perceived control. Patient Education and Counseling,* 18, 199–210.

Britten, N. and Okuoumunne, O. (1997) *The influence of patients' hope of a receiving a prescription on doctors' perceptions and the decision to prescribe: a questionnaire survey. British Medical Journal,* 315, 1506–1510.

Cassileth, B. R., Zupka, R. V., Sutton-Smith, K. and March, V. (1980) *Information and participation preferences among cancer patients. Annals of Internal Medicine,* 92, 832–836.

Chwalow, J. (1994) *Patient Education Outside Hospitals. A Review of the Effectiveness of Health Education and Health Promotion.* Dutch Centre for Health Education and Health Promotion and UHPE/EURO, Utrecht.

Charles, C., Gafni, A. and Whelan, T. (1997) *Shared decision making in the medical encounter: what does it mean? (or it takes at least two to tango). Social Science and Medicine,* 44, 681–692.

Charles, C., Gafni, A. and Whelan, T. (1999) *Decision making in the physician-patient encounter: revisiting the shared treatment decision making model. Social Science and Medicine,* 49, 651–661.

Cockburn, J. and Pitt, S. (1997) *Prescribing behaviour in clinical practice: patients' expectations and doctors' perceptions of patient expectations: a questionnaire study. British Medical Journal,* 315, 520–523.

Coppel, D. H. and Davis, P. (1997) *Health promotion in general practice: has the 1996 GP contract inspired or hindered effective health promotion by GPs in Nottingham? Health Education Journal,* 56, 128–139.

Coulter, A. and Schofield, T. (1991) *Prevention in general practice: the view of doctors in the Oxford region. British Journal of General Practice,* 41 (345), 140–143.

Davey, C., Austoker, J. and Jansen, C. (1998) *Improving written information for women about* cervical screening: evidence based criteria for the content of letters and leaflets. *Health Education Journal*, 57, 263–281.

Degeling, D., Salkeld, G., Dowsett, J. and Fahey, P. (1990) *Patient education and practice in Australian hospitals. Patient Education and Counseling*, 15, 127–138.

Department of Health (1992) *The Health of the Nation: a Strategy for Health in England.* HMSO, London.

Department of Health (1999) *Saving Lives: Our Healthier Nation.* The Stationery Office, London.

Department of Health and Social Security (1981) *Care in Action: A Handbook of Policies and Priorities for the Health and Personal Social Services in England.* HMSO, London.

Department of Health and Social Security (1986) *Primary Health Care: An Agenda for Discussion.* HMSO, London.

Department of Health and Social Security (1987) *Promoting Better Health: Government Programme for Improving Primary Health Care.* HMSO, London.

Department of Health and Social Security (1989) *Working for Patients.* HMSO, London.

Devine, E. C. (1992) *Effects of psychoeducational care for adult surgical patients: a meta analysis of 191 studies. Patient Education and Counseling*, 20, 37–47.

Dickey, L. L. (1993) *Promoting preventive care with patient held mini-records: a meta analysis of patient held mini-records: a review. Patient Education and Counseling*, 20, 37–47.

Donovan, P. (1992) *Leading the way to a baby friendly world. Hygie*, XI (2), 8–10.

Fahrenfort, M. (1987) *Patient emancipation by health education: an impossible goal. Patient Education and Counseling*, 10, 26–37.

Fahrenfort, M. (1990) *Patient education in Dutch hospitals: the fruits of a decade of endeavour. Patient Education and Counseling*, 15, 139–150.

Fallowfield, K., Ford, S. and Lewis, S. (1994) *Information preferences of patients with cancer. The Lancet*, 344, 1576.

Gillam, S. J. (1992) *Provision of health promotion clinics in relation to population need: another example of the inverse care law? British Journal of General Practice*, 42, 54–56.

Gillam, S. (1996) *Health promotion in general practice – financial follies, new opportunities. Guest Editorial. Journal of Institute of Health Education*, 34 (4), 103.

Gillam, S., McCartney, P. and Thorogood, M. (1995) *Health promotion in primary care – even less coherent than before. British Medical Journal*, 312, 324–325.

Green, A. (1987) *Is there primary health care in the UK? Health Policy and Planning*, 2 (2), 129–137.

Green, L.W (1990) *Hospitals and health care providers as agents of patient education. Patient Education and Counseling*, 15, 169–170.

Gwyn, R. and Elwyn, G. (1999) *When is a shared decision not (quite) a shared decision? Negotiating preferences in a general practice encounter. Social Science and Medicine*, 49, 437–447.

Hart, A. R., Barone, T. L. and Mayberry, J. F. (1997) *Increasing compliance with colorectal cancer screening: the development of effective health education. Health Education Research*, 12 (2), 171–180.

Hynam, K. A., Hart, A. R., Gay, S. P., Inglis, A., Wicks, A. C. B. and Mayberry, J. F. (1995) *Screening for colorectal screening: reasons for refusal of faecal occult blood testing in a general practice in England. Journal of Epidemiology and Community Health*, 49, 81–86.

James, C., James, N., Davies, D., Harvey, P. and Tweddle, S. (1999) *Preferences for different sources of information about cancer. Patient Education and Counseling*, 37, 271–282.

Johnson, J. L. (2000) The health care institution as a setting for health promotion. *British Journal of General Practice*, 47, 109–110.

Kari, J., Donovan, C., Li, J. and Taylor, B. (1997) *Adolescents attitudes to general practice in North London. British Journal of General Practice*, 47 (415), 109.

Kelsey, A. and Robinson, M. (1999) *Editorial: 'But they don't see the whole child. British Journal of General Practice*, 49(438), 4–5.

Killoran, A., Calnan, M., Cant, S. and Williams, S. (1993) *Pacemaker. Health Services Journal*, 103 (5340), 26–27.

Lelie, A. (2000) *Decision making in nephrology: shared decision making? Patient Education and Counseling*, 39, 81–89.

Llewellyn-Thomas, H. A., McGreal, M. J., Thiel, E. C. et al. (1999) *Patients willingness to enter clinical trials: measuring the association with perceived benefits and preference for decision participation. Social science and Medicine*, 32, 35–42.

Lucas, K. and Bickler, G. (2000) *Altogether now? Professional differences in the priorities of primary care groups. Journal of Public Health Medicine*, 22 (2), 211–215.

Mathers, N. and Rowland, S. (1997) *General practice – a post modern specialty. British Journal of General Practice*, 47, 177–179.

McGredy, K. (2000) *Finding common ground between normative and expressed health promotion needs across 24 Tees side GP surgeries*, M.Sc. dissertation, Leeds Metropolitan University, Leeds.

McWilliam, C. L., Stewart, M., Brown, J. B., McNair, S., Desai, K., Patterson, M. L., Del Maestro, N. and Pittman, B. J. (1997) *Creating empowering meaning: an interactive process of promoting health with chronically ill older Canadians. Health Promotion International*, 12 (2), 111–123.

McWilliam, C. L., Stewart, M., Bell Brown, J., McNair, S., Donner, A., Desai, K., Coderre, P. and Galadja, J. (1999) *Home based health promotion for chronically ill older persons: results of a randomised controlled trial of a critical reflection approach. Health Promotion International*, 14 (1), 27–41.

Milewa, T., Calnan, M., Almond, S. and Huner, A. (2000) *Patient education literature and help seeking behaviour: perspectives from an evaluation in the United Kingdom. Social Science and Medicine*, 51, 463–475.

Mull, J. D. (1990) *The primary care dialectic: history, rhetoric and reality*. In J. Coreil and J. D. Mull (Eds) *Anthropology and Primary Care*. Westview Press, Oxford.

Mullen, P. D., Green, L. W. and Persmyer, M. S. (1985) *Clinical trials of patient education for chronic conditions: a comparative analysis of intervention types. Preventive Medicine*, 14, 753–781.

Mullen, P. D. and Bartholemew, K. (2000) *Commentary*. In B. D. Poland, L. W. Green and I. Rootman (Eds) *Settings for Health Promotion. Linking Theory and Practice*. Sage, London.

Mullen, P. D., Mains, D. A. and Velez, R. (1992) *A meta-analysis of controlled trails of cardiac patient education. Patient Education and Counseling*, 19, 143–162.

Mullen, P. D., Simons-Morton, D., Ramirez, G., Frankowski, Green, L. M. and Mains, D. A. (1997) *A meta-analysis of trials evaluating patient educaiton and counseling for three groups of preventive health behaviours. Patient Education and Counseling*, 32, 157–173.

Nichols, S., Koch, E., Lalemand, R. C., Heald, R. J., Izzard, L., Machin, D. and Lmillee, M. A. (1986) *Randomised trial of compliance with screening for colorectal cancer. British Medical Journal*, 293, 107–110.

Pack, B. E., Hendrick, R. M., Murdock, R. B. and Palma, L. M. (1983) *Factors affecting criteria met by hospital based patient education programe. Patient Education and Counseling*, 5, 76–84.

Parsons, T. (1951) *The Social System*. Free Press, New York, NY.

Pelikan, J. M., Krajic, K. and Lobnig, H. (1998a) *Feasibility, Effectiveness, Quality and Sustainability of Health Promoting Hospital Projects*. Ludwig Bolzmann-Insitute for the Sociology of Health and Medicine, Vienna.

Pelikan, J. M., Garcia-Barbero, M., Lobnig, H. and Krajic, K. (1998b) *Pathways to a Health Promoting Hospital. Experiences from the European Pilot Project 1993–97*. Ludwig-Boltzmann-Institute for the Sociology of Health and Medicine, Vienna.

Poland, B. D., Green, L. W. and Rootman, I. (2000) *Settings for Health Promotion Linking Theory and Practice*. Sage, London.

Pye, G., Christie, M., Chamberlain, J. O., Moss, S. M. and Hardcastle, J. D. (1988) *A comparison of methods for increasing compliance within a general practitioners based screening project for colorectal cancer and the effect on practitioner workload. Journal of Epidemiology and Community Health*, 44, 66–71.

President's Committee on Health Education (1974) *Report of the President's Committee on Health Education*. Department of Health Education and Welfare, New York, NY.

Roter, D. (1987) *An exploration of health education's responsibility for a partnership model of client provider relations. Patient Education and Counseling*, 9, 25–31.

Royal College of General Practitioners (1981a) *Health and Prevention in Primary Care: Reports from General Practice*. RCGP, London.

Royal College of General Practitioners (1981b) *Prevention of Psychiatric Disorders in General Practice*. RCGP, London.

Russell, M. A. H., Wilson, C., Taylor, C. and Baker, C. D. (1979) *Effects of general practitioners advice against smoking. British Medical Journal*, 2, 231–235.

Russell, M. A. H., Stapleton, J. A., Hajek, P. *et al.* (1988) *District programmes to reduce smoking: can sustained interventions by general practitioners affect prevalence? Journal of Epidemiology and Community Health*, 42, 111–115.

Shiroyama, C., McKee, L. and McKie, L. (1995) *Evaluating health promotion projects in primary care: recent experiences in Scotland. Health Education Journal*, 54, 226–240.

Simons-Morton, D. G. Mullen, P. D., Mains, D. A., Tabak, E. R. and Green, L. W. (1992) *Characteristics of controlled studies of patient education and counselling for preventive health behaviours. Patient Education and Counseling*, 19, 173–204.

Speros, C. I. and Sol, N. (1991) *Health Promotion in Hospitals*, WHO Regional Publications, European Series 37, pp. 267–281. WHO, Geneva.

Steele, D. J., Blackwell, B., Guttman, M. C. and Jackson, J. C. (1987) *Beyond advocacy: a review of the active patient concept. Patient Education and Counseling*, 10, 3–23.

Stevenson, F. A., Barry, C. A., Britten, N., Barber, N. and Bradley, C. P. (2000) *Doctor–patient communication about drugs: the evidence for shared decision making. Social Science and Medicine*, 50, 829–840.

Szasz, T. S. and Hollender, M. H. (1956) *The basic models of the doctor patient relationship. Archives of Internal Medicine*, 97, 587–592.

Tones, B. K. (1995) *Editorial: the health promoting hospital. Health Education Research*, 10 (2), i–v.

Tuckett, D., Boulton, N., Olson, C. and Williams, A. (1985) *Meetings Between Experts*. Tavistock, London.

Van Ballekom, K. P. and van de Ven (1994) *Patient Education in Hospitals. A Review of the Effectiveness of Health Education and Health Promotion*. Dutch Centre for Health Promotion and Health Education and IUHPE/EURO, Utrecht.

van den Borne, H. W. (1998) *The patient from receiver of information to informed decision maker. Patient Education and Counseling*, 34, 89–102.

van Driel, W. G. and Keisjers, J. F. E. M. (1997) *An instrument for reviewing the effectiveness of health education and health promotion. Patient Education and Counseling*, 30, 7–17.

Wallace, L. M. (1988) *Psychological studies of the development and evaluation of preparatory procedures for women undergoing minor gynaecological surgery*, Ph.D. thesis, University of Birmingham, Birmingham.

Ward, E., King, M., Lloyd, M., Bower, P. and Friedli, K. (1999) *Conducting randomised trials in general practice: methodological and practical issues. British Journal of General Practice*, 49, 919–922.

World Health Organization (1978) *Primary Health Care: Report of the Conference in Primary Health Care*. WHO, Geneva.

World Health Organization (1991) *The Budapest Declaration on Health Promoting Hospitals*. WHO, European Regional Office, Copenhagen.

# 7 HEALTH PROMOTION IN THE WORKPLACE

## THE WORKPLACE, HEALTH PROMOTION AND A SETTINGS APPROACH

> *Love labor: for if thou dost not want it for food, thou mayest for physic. It is wholesome for thy body and good for thy mind.*
>
> (William Penn, 1693)

The workplace provides an interesting challenge to health educators – a challenge which has been accepted rather more readily in North America than in Europe. Knobel (1983) has estimated that it is possible to reach 85% of the US population via the worksite and, for this reason alone, delivering health education to the workforce is of great strategic importance within the grand overall design of health promotion. Apart from this intrinsic merit, workplace health promotion has been included in the book because it exemplifies rather well two main propositions. First it illustrates conflicting philosophies rooted in the often different needs of key participants – workers and bosses. For management success will normally be judged by hard economic indicators while for many radical health promoters well-being may actually be incompatible with the profit motive! The workers' perceived needs are likely to be located somewhere between these two extremes.

Second, the workplace offers a tangible example of the ways in which success, however defined, is dependent on the synergy of individual behaviour and structural/organisational factors. For instance, smoking cessation programmes will be facilitated by a comprehensive workplace smoking policy. Similarly, the teaching of stress management skills without prior examination of the inherent stress-generating nature of work itself is neither efficient nor ethical.

At one level, the definition of workplace health promotion is simple enough. Davis *et al.* (1984) pro-

vided an operational definition as a guide for determining whether or not a given firm had a health promotion programme. They argued that *A company was considered to have a HPDP (health promotion and disease prevention) programme if it provided health screenings, classes or preventive health services on an ongoing basis.* On the other hand, Parkinson *et al.* (1982), foreshadowed the 'settings approach' when they refer to a ... *combination of educational, organisational and environmental activities designed to support behaviour conducive to the health or employees and their families.*

We have already discussed the 'settings approach' and referred to WHO's role in popularising a strategy that adopts an ecological approach to health promotion – an approach that takes account of the whole environment and ethos of a given setting rather than merely considering a setting as a convenient location in which to deliver health education. Eakin (2000) provides an illuminating definition (Box 1).

**Box 1**

> *The setting of health promotion is critical to the form, content, and outcome of practice. Perhaps in no field of health promotion is this more true than in the workplace. The setting refers to the immediate physical and built environment (e.g., the building, the work process) and the psychosocial environment (e.g., the organizational, economic, legal, and political environments...). Importantly, the setting also includes the ideological context of work and industrial organization, the assumptions and beliefs embodied in laws and social practices, such as the employment relationship, the rights of private enterprise, and labor–management customs. The notion of setting thus includes both material and sociopolitical context.*
>
> (p171)

Eakin's reference to the ideological context of work is timely. We mentioned above the possibility of conflicting philosophies; we will elaborate on and illustrate this observation throughout the rest of this present chapter. We will also seek to address the following questions: why deliver health education in the workplace? It is clearly assumed to be worthwhile (at least in North America!) but who are the real beneficiaries? What can we expect from work-based health promotion? How successful is it? What is its potential for enhancing well-being and preventing disease? What are its limitations? What should be its main focus and how does this focus relate to such issues as achieving equity?

## WORK AND HEALTH

The relationship between work and health is paradoxical. It stimulates vigorous debate and strikes a sensitive political nerve. On the one hand, those of a Marxist persuasion may view work as a capitalist device to exploit the proletariat. At the risk of cheapening this point of view we might pose an oft-quoted rhetorical question: if work is so good, why don't the very wealthy do more of it? Bosquet (1977) has expressed the point with some force:

> So deep is the frustration engendered by work that the incidence of heart attacks among manual workers is higher than that in any other stratum of society. People 'die from work' not because it is noxious or dangerous ... but because it is intrinsically 'killing'.

**Box 2**

> To crush, to annihilate a man utterly, to inflict on him the most terrible of punishments so that the most ferocious murderer would shudder at it and dread it beforehand, one need only give him work of an absolutely, completely useless and irrational character.
>
> (Dostoevsky, The House of the Dead, 1862)

Reference was made in Chapter 1 to the work of Marmot (see for example Marmot, 1994) in identifying work as a risk factor for diseases such as CHD, and the ideological and practical importance of addressing 'new' workplace 'pathogens' will be further discussed later in this chapter.

A more common (and better documented) standpoint is that unemployment rather than work is health damaging. Indeed, the evidence has been so extensively and comprehensively assembled and presented that the relationship between unemployment and mental, physical and social disease will be taken as axiomatic for present purposes. However, in terms of the models of health education outlined earlier, both the above perspectives would favour a radical approach which sought to raise consciousness and stimulate social and political change in order to remedy what are viewed as serious social problems. Measures of success would therefore relate to the extent to which such social and political change actually occurs.

Less common but no less radical in its way is a third approach to the issue of health and work. It is concerned with the nature of work in a 'post-industrial society' (Hopson and Scally, 1981) which is characterised by chronic unemployment, reduction of the working week, job sharing, early retirement, part-time employment and an increase in discretionary time and leisure. Preparation for a post-industrial society requires the same skills and competencies needed to handle 'Future Shock' (Toffler, 1970). In other words, the task of health and social education is not merely to provide an extensive preparation for greater leisure but will also involve fundamental questioning of the work ethic and the new, or rather rediscovered, enterprise culture. Since the futurologists' predictions of the nature of work will require a variety of social and personal skills associated with flexibility, resilience and proactivity, the appropriate health education model is that which develops self-empowered decision making.

Ironically, though, the problem is not necessarily one of coping with the demands of unanticipated leisure but rather with an increasing workload that has deleterious effects on family life and health. As Platt *et al.* (2000) note, in a review of changing labour market conditions and health,

> *In general, working hours have been reduced (in Europe), mainly as a result of the shift in employment from agriculture and manufacturing to services and the growth of female employment. The exceptions to this trend are Ireland and the UK; the latter holds the record for the highest average weekly hours worked by employees in the 12 country European Union (43.7 hours in the early 1990s).*

Polanyi *et al.* (2000) comment on a similar situation in Canada, noting that many workers are unhappy with the situation.

**Box 3**

> *Although one third of Canadians feel they are "constantly under stress" and one in four consider themselves "workaholics", more than 25% of Canadians want to work less with less income.*
>
> (Swift, 1995)

In the context of the hard and pragmatic concerns which are typically associated with workplace health promotion an approach which centres on personal and social development and seeks to facilitate empowered decision making might seem somewhat fanciful. However, the importance of considering fundamental questions of this kind was acknowledged by a conference on *Health Promotion in the Working World* organized by WHO (1987). This postulated several futuristic scenarios.

- *Business as usual.* Assumes full employment will once again be achieved and this will be the predominant form of work with the associated consumption of goods and services and the centrality of paid work to individual self-esteem.
- *Hyperexpansionist.* Postulates chronic unemployment as described earlier. Society will consist

of two groups – employed and unemployed. The former will consist of a cadre of elite professionals using capital-intensive technology.

- *Sane, humane, ecological.* Again, assumes chronic unemployment but posits a radical change in values which allows other useful activities to receive appropriate recognition and payment in addition to traditional paid work. Paid and unpaid work will be equally divided between men and women. Households and neighbourhoods will be the workplaces and production centres in society.
- Variations on some of these themes were also proposed including '*Eco-Utopia*' (small decentralised, self-sufficient eco settlements) and '*Findhorn*' (characterised by spirituality and inner growth). In contrast '*Chinatown*' postulated a population explosion with multimillion metropolises; alternatively the '*Dallas*' scenario predicted a western-dominated competitive Darwinistic imperialism in which, presumably, the North American rationale for worksite health promotion would be even more popular!

Returning to the present, the more conventional analysis of work and health sees the workplace as a source of pathogens of one kind or another ranging from general work-produced stress to specific industrial hazards such as accidents, cancers and the like. Stress is of particular interest because it illustrates so well the conflicting perspectives of more radical health educators and the employers whom they accuse of 'victim blaming'. The number of identified work stressors is legion. The WHO (1987) lists poor physical working conditions, shift work, job overload and job underload, role conflict, role insecurity, promotion blockage, two-career families, lack of opportunity for participation in decision making, etc.

A study by Braun and Hollander (1987) examined job stress among employees in the Federal Republic of Germany. They showed that high job demands and low job decision latitude were related to stress. The study implications could be either to teach stress management skills or to alter the structure of the work situation. Although not in principle incompatible, the choice of one or other of these alternatives is, as we shall see, likely to reveal ideological differences in approach to workplace health promotion. A successful 'victim blaming' strategy would be revealed by the acquisition of, say, relaxation skills or a reduced level of stress on an appropriate scale; the success of a more radical approach would be measured by actual environmental changes or intermediate indicators of progress towards such change.

## DIFFERENT PERSPECTIVES ON SUCCESS

As will have been apparent from the discussion of health and work, successful worksite health promotion will be interpreted differently by the various actors: academics, futurologists, community physicians, public health workers and social scientists will have different value systems from employers and workers, although doubtless common ground exists. The health promoter's perspective may well be dominated by the prospect of gaining access to a substantial proportion of the adult population. The choice of strategies will in part be dictated by the two principles of access and availability of skilled and credible health educators. Access to a generally hard-to-reach population is an outstanding feature of the workplace. It has been estimated that in the USA some 85% of the population may be contacted in this way, a proportion which compares very favourably with the 75% contact which the practice population has with a general practitioner every 3 years and the 15,000 hours spent by students in school. The question of credibility and competence is, however, a different matter. Logically we would look to the occupational health service to deliver health education but this, of course, depends on the existence of such a service! McEwen (1987) noted that in 1977 about ... *85% of all firms (in the UK), employing about 34% of the workforce, had no occupational health service other than first-aiders employed less than ten hours a week ... .*

Buck (1982), after a small scale survey of firms in a district health authority in northern England, was more optimistic. Occupational health staff reported that their two most frequent types of health work were, first, treatment and, second, environmental visiting. Fifty-five of the 59 respondents recognized the existence of opportunities for health education in the treatment situation and 29 commented that opportunities arose 'often' or 'sometimes' in their visits to the working environment. Clearly recognition of opportunity did not mean that they actually took advantage of the situation to provide health education. Moreover, since the response rate was only 47%, it would not be unreasonable to expect a distinct lack of commitment in the non-respondents!

A national survey in the USA by Vojtecky *et al.* (1985) provides a useful indication of the involvement of occupational health services in health promotion. A sample of 1953 was drawn from a sampling frame of 11,000 occupational health professionals. Again there was a low response rate of 34%, so observations should be treated with caution. Five categories of health professional were identified: industrial hygienists, doctors, nurses, health educators and others. The proportion of total work time which the groups claimed to spend on health education was, respectively, 33, 22, 38, 89 and 23%. Major programme categories were health promotion, accident prevention and hazard protection. The proportion of each professional group having involvement with broader health promotion work ranged from 31 (industrial hygienists) to 98% (nurses). A wide range of teaching methods was used, with the health educators using the broadest spectrum (50% using 10 of 13 listed methods). Interestingly, when the groups were asked to say whether their objectives were primarily changes in knowledge, attitude or practice, it was the health educator group which seemed more determined to change behaviours (80%) whereas 50% of nurses were concerned only to provide knowledge. Whether this indicates a difference in philosophy or whether nurses tended to assume that knowledge would automatically lead to behaviour change is not clear. Notwithstanding the relatively small response rate, the situation appears distinctly more healthy than in Europe, although the researchers lament the fact that only 62% of the occupational health professionals delivering health education had had any specific training in doing so.

## THE MANAGEMENT PERSPECTIVE

It is worth reiterating the point that the USA has led the way in workplace health promotion. Programmes operate in some 80% of US workplaces (Biener *et al.*, 1994) – a situation that is, in part, explained by the peculiar health care system in that country. In general, though, it would not be unfair to summarise the motivation of workplace managers and employers in two words: economic self-interest.

This viewpoint is sharply illustrated by a comment attributed to Xerox top management that the loss of one executive from preventable illness would cost the organization $600,000 (Cooper, 1985). It should be noted that the received wisdom that health promotion in the worksite will in fact save money has not gone unchallenged. Walsh (1988) cites three sceptics (Russell, 1986; Schelling, 1986; Warner, 1987) in her own critique of work place programmes. Nonetheless, the general feeling appears to be that appropriate educational and promotion programmes will result in increased productivity and sales and generate a reduction in costs. The rationale for these programmes in terms of productivity and cost reduction is summarized in Table 7.1.

Clearly some of these arguments are peculiar to the US health care delivery system, with its emphasis on private health insurance. It is, however, worth noting that according to Conrad (1988a, b) costs had been rising by up to 20–30% a year in the USA. Polanyi *et al.* (2000) consider that costs of health benefits amount to 9% of corporation payrolls – a rise from 3% in the 1980s (Northwestern National Life Insurance, 1994).

We are reminded of the significance of these costs by Alexander (1988):

> *During the past decade, large corporations have become increasingly concerned that providing health care benefits no longer con-* *stitutes an incidental cost of doing business. In 1961, such benefits were 25.5% of payroll. By 1981, they were 41.2%. Between 1987 and 1980 corporate health insurance premiums escalated markedly from $43 billion to $63 billion. The most notable impact on the manufacturing sector was documented for General Motors, which in 1977 was believed to have added $176 to the cost of every car and truck to offset the $825 million it spent during the same year for employee benefits. A recent survey of a sample of Fortune 500 companies and the largest 250 industrials suggested that health insurance costs will equal profits after taxes in about 8 years.*

The attractiveness of an effective health promotion service and the victim blaming nature of the programmes become understandable in the light of these statistics. The economic motivation of managers is thus hardly surprising and is supported by Davis *et al.*'s (1984) investigation of worksite health promotion in Colorado. Companies surveyed which had established programmes were asked to provide reasons for having started health promotion activities; companies interested in starting were also asked to indicated their motivation for so doing. Survey results are shown in Table 7.2. The economic motivation underlying decisions is self-evident, particularly for those companies contemplating adoption.

## THE WORKER PERSPECTIVE

The worker perspective has probably received less consideration than that of management, presumably because of an assumption that workers might welcome interventions designed to enhance their well-being whereas managers would have to be subjected to a 'sales pitch'. It is doubtless true that trade unions will welcome moves which can be shown to be for their members' benefit and workers will respond to the same initiatives, particularly if these happen in 'management time'!

However, Polanyi *et al.* (2000) strike a cautionary note about union involvement in Canada

**Table 7.1** A summary of the main benefits of worksite health promotion programmes in North America in relation to productivity and cost reduction

Increased productivity
1. Reduction in sickness absence
2. Reduced absenteeism
3. Increase in worker morale
4. Presentation of a good corporate image*
5. Attracting competent staff in a competitive market situation

Reduction in costs
1. Decrease in accidents and associated compensation claims
2. Decline in health insurance costs as a result of lower demand for in-patient care, reduced treatment costs and fewer disability and death benefits
3. Decline in staff replacement and training costs as a result of lower staff turnover

*According to Conrad (1988a) this desirable image is acquired by **capitalizing on cultural wellness!**

**Table 7.2** Reasons given by companies for starting health promotion and disease prevention programmes (from Davis et al., 1984)

| Reason | Companies with existing programmes (%) | Companies interested in starting programmes (%) |
|---|---|---|
| To improve health and reduce health problems | 82 | 68 |
| To improve employee morale | 59 | 52 |
| To reduce health care costs | 57 | 67 |
| To reduce turnover and absenteeism | 51 | 57 |
| To improve productivity | 50 | 64 |
| Response to employee demand or interest | 33 | 20 |
| To be part of innovative trend | 32 | 11 |
| To improve public image | 20 | 18 |

– and one that applies equally to Britain. They point out that health activists seeking to improve health conditions for the work force

> ... *have been set back by the conservative political climate of the 1980s (Sass, 1989) and the steady decline in unionization levels in the United States (to 15% of the work-force; Walker, 1993). Unions have had to be concerned with opposing layoffs and increases in the pace of work, leaving little time to address broader psychosocial issues related to work organization.*

Several studies in North America have sought to ascertain the reasons for worker participation.

For example, Conrad (1988a, b) identified a major concern with fitness and weight control. Spilman (1988) noted gender differences in motivation which were consistent with generally recognised views about women's health; for instance, a general high participation rate, concern with weight loss for cosmetic reasons and concern with their nurturant roles as unpaid family health care workers. Kotarba and Bentley (1988) described motivation to participate in a workplace wellness programme in terms of either a ... *commitment to wellness, or as a vehicle for experimenting with or establishing a new style of self, the identity of a "well person" so highly valued in contemporary western culture.* This latter observation will serve as a further cautionary note: worker motivation is clearly culture bound and will reflect general health norms. There can be no guarantee that the UK workforce will identify with the North American 'healthist' pursuit of 'high level wellness'! Indeed, suspicion about management motives might well predominate. Moreover, in the context of our earlier discussion of health and work the workforce in Britain is more likely to be concerned about unemployment than even exposure to hazardous substances, let alone participation in the pursuit of fitness in order to reduce management overheads!

## WORKPLACE HEALTH PROMOTION: BLAMING THE VICTIMS?

Polanyi *et al.* (2000) provide a revealing discussion of the victim blaming tendency in workplace health promotion that is highly relevant to one of the major themes in this book. The author comments that notwithstanding the rhetoric for addressing organisational determinants of health and illness, radical approaches in both small workplaces (Eakin and Weir, 1995) and large (Hollander and Lengermann, 1988) are noticeable by their absence. *Workplaces remain primarily focused on changing individual worker lifestyles with little consideration of the conditions that shape such behaviors.* As Syme (1994) remarks, individually targeted interventions are ineffective because they ... *do nothing about those forces in society that cause our problems in the first place, and that will continue to provide a fresh supply of at-risk people, forever.*

Alexander (1988), in an article on the 'ideological construction of risk', points out this philosophical underpinning. Not only is health promotion predicated on a need by ... *the American state and almost all sectors of capital to curtail their share of the social wage* ... but ... *corporate managers choose selectively from a body of theoretical knowledge regarding illness and disease etiology in a way that restores sanctity to the individual, eschews history and social complexity and legitimates existing social relations.* No apology is made for making a further reference to the inherent tendency for workplace

health promotion to focus on the individual at the expense of general social structures and particular organisational influences on health and illness. McEwen (1987) is also concerned to make this point and cites Navarro (1976), who not only asserted the economic and political aetiology of alienation of the individual in society, occupational diseases generally and cancer in particular, but also pointed out how the power balance in western industrialised society inevitably favours the individualistic approach of traditional health education (Box 4).

**Box 4**

> ... *one of today's most active state policies at the central government level in most western capitalist countries is to encourage and stimulate these health programs, such as health education, that are aimed at bringing about changes in the individual but not in the economic or political environment.*
>
> *It is interesting to note that while much of the disease affecting the working class in Engels' time was supposedly due to the poor moral fibre of the workmen and their families, today the poor health conditions of that class and the majority of the population are assumed to be due to the lack of concern for their own health and their poor health education. In both cases, the solution to our public lack of health is individual prevention and individual therapy.*

Walsh (1988) notes the 'healthist' aspect of the American fitness programmes. *Could it be*, she asks, *that health promotion is a lifestyle enclave in the worksite and if so is it deflecting energy from collective efforts to improve the quality of worklife for all?*

Gordon (1987) also notes the victim blaming tendency but in addition comments on the possibility of ethical difficulties relating to confidentiality and trust in work-based medical practitioners and, more importantly for our purpose here, the intrinsic tendency to exert explicit or implicit pressure on workers to participate in health promotion programmes. Such coercion, however benevolent, together with an associated 'top-down' approach, is not only inconsistent with WHO's principles of health promotion but militates against the spirit of the *British Health and Safety at Work Act* (Howells and Barrett, 1975), which emphasizes responsibility, self-regulation and participation, all of which processes are consistent with WHO's view of health promotion.

Polanyi *et al.* (2000) cite as evidence of US concern with lifestyle factors Tully's (1995) comment that ... *the programs winning the 1995 Everett Koop health promotion awards in the United States still focus on urging individuals to renounce their high-risk behaviors.* With reference to the workplace, Tully identifies a number of verbs characterising the award winning companies' programmes as follows: 'systematically pursue; prod; advise; motivate'...'stubborn; secretive; crotchety' workers to change their habits!

**Box 5**  The Lifestyle Focus of the Everett Koop Awards

*To the extent we encourage people of all ages to adopt healthier habits, we address health care and the attendant costs at their roots ... (people) are being invited to check their own health risk levels under health risk assessment programs. The point is that awareness of the consequences of high risk health behavior ... smoking, substance abuse, cholesterol ... are the road signs pointing to their solution.*

(Health Project, 1994, pp1 and 5–6)

We will now turn to a brief consideration of different approaches to or categories of workplace health promotion. This classification includes occupational health *per se* together with the sub-category of '*Employee Assistance Programmes*' (EAPs); we will then compare and contrast the lifestyle focus of traditional workplace health education and health promotion with radical and empowering alternatives. Polanyi *et al.*

(2000) provide a useful basis for this discussion with a three category system of programme definition. This is summarised in Table 7.3.

Table 7.3 needs little explanation. Clearly, the authors contrast traditional workplace health promotion with strategies that address the fundamental determinants of health in the workplace, i.e. to use the model advocated in this book, a radical empowering approach. Such an approach would, of course, not merely be offered as a more effective – and equitable – alternative to what is described in Table 7.4 as 'traditional workplace health promotion' but would apply equally to 'traditional occupational health and safety'. We will note later that a radical approach to occupational health and safety will involve inter alia redefining contemporary workplace 'pathogens'.

## Occupational health services: new threats to health

Traditional health and safety education is concerned to identify and educate those at high risk – either for personal health problems such as CHD or in the context of a specific occupation.

More recently, broader based health promotion programmes have focused on general health and fitness. All three approaches are consistent with agreed goals of an occupational health service as McEwen (1987) points out in these terms:

- protecting the workers against any health hazard which may arise out of their work or the conditions in which it is carried on;
- contributing towards the workers' physical and mental adjustment, in particular by the adaptation of the work to the workers and their assignment of job for which they are suited;
- contributing to the establishment and maintenance of the highest possible degree of physical and mental well-being of the workers.

Examples of such programmes are readily available. For instance Ippolito-Shepherd *et al.* (1987) describe an agricultural occupational health education programme in Latin America; Schenk *et al.* (1987) present results of research

**Table 7.3**   Strategies to improve workplace health

| Strategy | Stimulus | Goals | Examples |
|---|---|---|---|
| Traditional occupational health and safety | Physical hazards of heavy industrial labour | Reduce toxicity of environment<br>Reduce physical demands of work | Industrial hygiene<br>Modification of equipment and practices<br>Protection |
| Traditional workplace health promotion | High absenteeism and benefits costs | Reduce individual risk of illness through education, skills development and support programmes | Fitness programmes<br>Smoking cessation courses<br>Counselling<br>Weight reduction programmes |
| Promoting workplace determinants | Recognition of relationship between 'job strain' and ill health | Reduce workplace psychosocial demands<br>Increase social support<br>Increase worker participation in decision making | Flexible hours and holidays<br>Job redesign<br>Job rotation<br>Worker decision making<br>Supervisor training |

From Polanyi et al. (2000, p. 141).

into rubber industry workers' beliefs and attitudes about safety which might be used to devise risk reduction health education interventions.

There are still numerous examples of traditionally hazardous work conditions contributing to accidents and 'old type' chronic diseases. For instance, Platt *et al.* (2000), in their review of changing labour market conditions and health in Europe, cite a study by Paoli (1992) that demonstrates that some 30% of respondents to a EU survey in 1991–1992 considered their health and safety at risk while at work. This perception was substantially associated with exposure to noise, air pollution, handling dangerous substances and working in painful positions.

On the other hand, it will be increasingly necessary for health promotion in the 21st century – at least in the Western World – to address a number of new conditions or new perspectives on old health problems. Polanyi *et al.* (2000) provide a catalogue of the pathological features of the contemporary workplace in the USA and these are listed below.

- The drive for competitiveness undermines worker rights and creates worsening work conditions.

- In the interests of cost reduction and flexibility, firms cut wages and lay off full-time staff (especially those belonging to unions and having better pay and benefit conditions) and contract out work.

- Increasing government debts have resulted in cuts to income support and social programmes.

**Box 6**   Inequity and the Dual Economy

*Technological and economic change do seem to be encouraging the development of a "dual economy", with a small stratum of well-paid professionals and a large group of unskilled workers with little job security. In the 1980s, the top 5% of U.S. wage earners saw their salary increase by 23% … while the bottom 20% experienced a slight decline.*

(Rifkin, 1995, cited in Polanyi *et al.*, 2000 p151)

From a European perspective, Platt et al. (2000, op.cit.), characterised the current situation as follows:

- participation rates (total labour force as a percentage of the working population) have tended to increase – as a whole;
- participation rates among the under 25 year old group have declined (reflecting the growth of tertiary education and training);
- participation rates among older workers, especially males, have fallen;
- participation rates among women have increased;
- working hours have been reduced (with exceptions – as noted earlier);
- there has been a move from the agricultural and industrial sectors into service industries;
- there has been a demand for flexibility (i.e. the ability to adapt rapidly to changes in conditions and technology with a consequent increase in 'precarious' employment and a decline in 'standard' full-time permanent employment.

The authors categorise the major sources of the health challenges of changing occupational circumstances thus:

- *workplace reorganisation*: downsizing, reorganisation and job insecurity;
- *moving into and out of the new labour market*: redundancy, early retirement and re-employment;
- *new technology*: especially video display terminals (VDTs);
- *features of the work environment*: job satisfaction, involvement and demand-control.

An extended discussion of these circumstances is not possible here but Platt *et al.*'s conclusions, from four review papers and 18 empirical papers, about the impact on health of VDTs are worth summarising (Box 7).

**Box 7**   The Impact of VDT Use on Health

- *Lower paid, less skilled computer users are more psychologically distressed than higher paid, more skilled computer users.*
- *The stress associated with the move to new technology is greater among lower paid, less skilled and older employees than*

*among higher paid, more skilled and younger employees.*
- *Seven job factors tend to produce high stress [across a range of job categories (Smith, 1997)]: high job demands; lack of control over the work process and/or inability to participate in decisions; high level of task difficulty coupled with inadequate skills; monotony, lack of variety or lack of task content; poor supervisory relations or lack of supervisory support; technology problems, e.g. computer breakdown; a fear of job security.*

(Platt *et al.*, 2000 para. 8.5)

The health promotion implications of the phenomena described in Box 7 doubtless need little explication – for instance, in respect of inequity the need for careful targeting of population groups and tentative intervention strategies.

Again, because of our discussion in Chapter 1 about the need to broaden analysis of risk factors for chronic diseases such as CHD and because of implications for empowerment, some further discussion of Platt *et al.*'s fourth category above is appropriate. Two features of the work environment are of particular interest: job satisfaction and what has been called the '*Job Demand-Control Model*' (Karasek and Theorell, 1990). Six studies revealed job satisfaction to be positively associated with various health conditions – including sick building syndrome and neck and shoulder symptoms, various health perceptions, satisfaction with co-workers and, to a lesser extent, with autonomy, pay and the work itself.

The essence of the *Job Demand-Control Model* is the assertion that a combination of heavy demands and limited decision latitude to moderate these demands results in job strain. Job strain leads to various negative health consequences (of which the most dramatic – identified in Japan – is *Karoshi*, 'death from overwork' or 'stress death').

For example, after a review of 36 studies of the relationship between 'job strain' and cardiovascular disease, Schnall *et al.* (1994) argued that a sufficient body of literature had accumulated to accept a robust causal relationship had been established.

Platt *et al.*'s conclusions from their review was that evidence supported the model – but only among those *...who experienced high self efficacy in their work. Among people with low(er) self-efficacy, increasing control may exacerbate the stress of demanding jobs.* Yet again, the need for subtle and sophisticated analysis of psychosocial determinants – followed by equally subtle and sophisticated interventions – is demonstrated by these observations.

## Traditional workplace health promotion

The traditional – and not infrequently – victim blaming approach to health promotion in the workplace requires little further comment here. The selective review that follows later in this chapter is comprised largely of such studies. We will, however, comment on one particular variety of programme which is both popular (at least in terms of prevalence) and problematical. It is usually described as an EAP.

## Employee assistance programmes

Although there is considerable overlap between the two, health promotion programmes may be distinguished from one well-recognised category of worksite intervention, particularly in North America. This category is usually referred to as an EAP. Roman and Blum (1988) provide a useful comparison between EAPs and *Health Promotion Programmes* (HPPs). They offer two definitions of EAPs:

> *... mechanisms to increase the chances for continued employment of individuals whose job performance and personal functioning are adversely impacted by problems of substance abuse, psychiatric illness, family difficulties or other personal problems.*
>
> (Roman and Blum, 1987)

> *... job-based programs operating within a work organization for purposes of identifying 'troubled employees', motivating them to*

> *resolve their troubles, and providing access to counselling or treatment for those employees who need these services.*
>
> (Sonnenstuhl and Trice, 1986)

It is immediately clear from these definitions that EAPs are concerned with secondary prevention whereas other health promotion programmes would tend to focus on primary prevention. Roman and Blum also observe that whereas trade unions (in the USA) are probably suspicious of HPPs, they almost unanimously support EAPs. They additionally note that both HPPs and EAPs are 'mission driven' (*The zealotry that accompanies many HPPs is often matched by the zeal with which EAP practitioners view the urgency of recovery from alcoholism ...*)! A key difference between both types of programme centres on the potential stigma associated with EAPs compared with HPPs. Clearly EAPs require confidentiality and a conviction by workforce and unions that admitting to problems will not lead to job loss. This latter point is of especial importance for the implementation of alcohol policies in the workplace. Indeed the development of worksite policies may be considered a separate category of health promotion exercise, at least in the UK.

## Radical health promotion: the empowerment imperative

The critique of the workplace concentration on individualistic, 'victim blaming' health promotion has been examined above – and, extensively, in Chapter 1. Apart from ethical and equity concerns, it is a general rule that the lifestyle focus of individualistic programmes will frequently be ineffective – due, of course, to their failure to tackle underlying problems and causes.

Polanyi *et al.* (2000) identified a number of such failures:

> *Behavioural changes tend to be short-term in nature without concurrent changes to the social and cultural context that shapes individual behavior ... and some 90% of smokers who quit resume smoking within a year (Benowitz and Henningfield, 1994) ... only 10% of people continue to use stress man-*

*agement skills over the long term (Aaron, 1995); and weight loss and fat reduction success rates are low. (Syme, 1988)... .*

The authors also comment on the failure of the MRFIT in the USA to achieve improvements in cardiovascular outcomes, ... *despite highly motivated participants, a well-designed behavioral intervention plan, very generous resources, and excellent staffing* (MRFIT Research Group, 1982).

***Box 8*** Limits to Lifestyle Change

> *One's capacity to modify potentially pathogenic behaviors and to "stick with it" is directly related to one's wealth, power and education – in short the degree of control one has over one's future ... one's "will to change" is largely predetermined by one's social environment.*
>
> (Renaud, 1994 p321, cited in Polanyi *et al.*, 2000)

Not all individually focused programmes can be classed as fundamentally victim blaming. For instance, in the UK a general health and fitness programme originally developed by the Health Education Council for adult learners has been translated into the workplace. This '*Look After Yourself*' (LAY) programme involved teaching about exercise, relaxation, healthy eating and other lifestyle health factors (Dames *et al.*, 1986). It was made available to the workplace on request; its goal was to train tutors within the work situation so that the programme becomes routinised. The programme in question operated largely as an adult education initiative which just happened to be located in the workplace. However, although it examined a wide range of health issues and topics, the emphasis was still on individual behaviour change. More importantly, it did nothing to address the fundamental question of the damaging effect of the workplace and certain aspects of work in general.

Following our arguments in earlier chapters about the centrality of empowerment and taking account of the nature of the workplace health haz-

ards identified above the most effective and ethical workplace health promotion should ideally be concerned with critical consciousness raising. Freudenberg (1981) described three consciousness-raising initiatives involving community mobilisation; one of these was located in the workplace. The focus was occupational safety and health and involved formation of the Carolina Brown Lung Association. The programme set out to explain safety procedures to workers and taught them how to monitor dust levels in the workplace. They were also trained in ways of taking action when legal standards were violated.

Further details of the programme will be discussed in our selective review below.

## Health impact assessment

A major part of the radical health promotion agenda – in addition to and associated with the consciousness-raising function – is the strategy of *Health Impact Assessment*. The principle is clear even though the practice might be difficult to implement. In short, as WHO has observed (WHO, 1992), the development of any national or local policy – no matter what the subject – should routinely involve a process of assessing the likely impact of that policy on health – and, hopefully, take steps to minimise any deleterious effects. Regrettably, of course, the pursuit of wealth may frequently not be reconcilable with the pursuit of health – witness the mendacious manoeuvrings of the tobacco industry over decades (Pollock, 1999). Accordingly, any serious move towards health impact assessment (let alone acting on the results of that assessment) will, in accordance with the *Empowerment Model* outlined in Chapter 1, depend on mobilising the full and combined forces of advocacy, critical consciousness raising and public pressure.

## An empowerment perspective

We have mentioned Freudenberg's (1981) sterling efforts to generate a radical approach to workplace health promotion but must acknowledge that in the context of capitalist economies such ventures must be rare indeed – and unlikely to gain the willing cooperation of management!

311

Radical challenge must come at a more macro level and from outside the workplace. On the other hand, an empowering strategy is generally consistent with a radical approach and stands a much greater chance of gaining acceptability from all key stakeholders. Following our earlier assertion that empowerment in general is conducive to the achievement of preventive goals, we might add here that an empowerment approach to workplace health promotion might well be consistent with the profit motive! However, education designed to empower the workforce is relatively rare, for obvious reasons! It is, therefore, worth reporting on a Canadian mental health initiative (Novick, 1987). The *Mental Health and Workplace Project* is unusual in that it acknowledges the importance of environmental variables both within and without the workplace. The programme philosophy is fundamentally concerned with self-empowerment. Novick, chairperson of the project, describes a 'New Work Agenda into the Nineties' based on the following assumptions:

- employment is a form of work which is done for remuneration as well as for psychological and social benefits;
- persistently high levels of unemployment are detrimental to the health and well-being of Canadian citizens and an unacceptable waste of human resources;
- a lack of more secure, stable, quality employment opportunities is increasing the stress and anxiety of working Canadians.

It acknowledges the 'future shock scenario', noting that groups ... *previously excluded or only marginally employed (e.g. women, youth, disabled people) are making their claim for fair access to the workplace.* Wide income disparities between high paid and low paid workers and the polarisation between a low skilled underclass and a high skilled elite must be taken into account by a programme concerned to educate about work. The importance of balancing employment with family life, life in the community and personal development must be recognised.

Six propositions are finally made by Novick:

- employment should be structured and organised in ways that are compatible with and reinforcing to the quality of Canadian family life;
- working life should include opportunities for continuing learning for job advancement, work skill development, retirement and general personal betterment;
- there should be recognition of the importance of alternative forms of work, such as household, voluntarism, recreational and cultural activities as well as paid forms of work;
- all Canadians should have access to a fair share of meaningful and dignifying employment during their adult lives;
- people should have more worklife choices in terms of how they arrange their employment time weekly, monthly and yearly in order to complement other pursuits and interests which they have;
- real worklife choices must entail provisions for both income security and employment stability within a framework for economic renewal.

The approach of 'Worklife Education' is perhaps summarised in the view that *The workplace is a community*. All of its members should be empowered to care better for themselves and for each other. This self-empowerment approach is substantially different in emphasis from mainstream workplace programmes in which disease prevention and health protection provide the main justification for intervention (with or without the cost–benefit implications) – even though it might lack the radical muscle of Freudenberg's more fundamental challenges.

## PLANNING THE PROGRAMME

Whatever the ideology, it is quite apparent that workplace programmes must be properly designed and planned if Type 3 errors are to be avoided. In this respect health promotion in the workplace is no different to health promotion in any other context or setting. Therefore, at the very least, if the programme is to be health promotion rather than health education the inclusion of supportive policy is a *sine qua non*. As a matter of fact, the development and implementation of health policies has for many years been a feature of health promotion in the workplace – especially with respect to safety policy and, more recently, policies on smoking. Indeed, on occasions it has appeared that policy has been implemented without the benefits of supportive *education*!

Typically policy development has centred on alcohol, smoking, fitness and nutrition (often in the context of preventing CHD) and, less often, stress reduction. The elements of a workplace smoking policy will be briefly adumbrated below prior to considering implications for indicators of effectiveness (for further details see Jenkins and McEwen, 1987).

First, a smoking policy would have the following environmental goals; a ban on smoking in areas where special safety or health hazards exist; at least 50% of cafeteria areas would be designated non-smoking provided that smoke did not affect the non-smoking zone; all common areas would be non-smoking; smoking areas would be provided for smokers; smoking cessation facilities would also be made available. Appropriate signs would be displayed; information would be disseminated to the management and workforce; the policy would apply to all members of staff; there would be no discrimination against anyone exercising their rights under the policy.

Second, generally agreed steps are involved in implementing policy as follows:

- establishment of a working party;
- definition of objectives;
- survey of employee attitudes and request for suggestions for policy implementation;
- construction of draft policy;
- consultation exercise;
- adoption of agreed policy by senior management;
- implementation;
- creation of non-smoking environments;
- provision of help for smokers;
- institution of measures for policing and maintaining policy provisions.

With reference to systematic programme planning in general, Sorenson *et al.* (1990) argue for treating each workplace as a separate community having its own corporate culture but identify six essential steps for effective programme implementation, as listed below.

- *Build community support.*
- *Assess community norms, culture, and activities.*
- *Establish community advisory board.*
- *Assess work-site culture and social norms.*
- *Capitalize on opportunities to facilitate the program.*
- *Identify and modify existing barriers.*
- *Solicit top management and union support.*
- *Use employee input in planning.*
- *Conduct employee surveys.*
- *Appoint employee steering committee.*
- *Appoint work-site liaison.*
- *Provide ongoing programming with environmental and social supports.*
- *Conduct periodic programme evaluation.*

(Sorensen *et al.*, 1990 p160)

The planning model is characteristic of the US approach to community organisation – central to which is an emphasis on inter-sectoral working, i.e. via 'community coalitions'.

An integral part of the approach is to establish a 'community board' involving management, unions and labour leaders and health promotion workers. A task force might well be created having a number of special functions:

- a catalyst *for the support and involvement of local business and labor leaders;*
- a source *of information on ways to tailor programs to community needs;*
- a liaison *between employers and community service providers (e.g. American Heart Association, and the American Cancer Society; the YMCA and other nonprofit organizations) and service vendors (e.g. hospitals, employee assistance programs, health clubs);*
- a clearinghouse of information *for employers on health information, community resources, and effective implementation models of health promotion;*

- a *coordinator* in sponsoring community wide health promotion activites and
- a *support* for ongoing program implementation.

(Sorensen *et al.*, 1990 p161)

Perhaps the most comprehensive and systematic planning model of all, Green's *Precede–Proceed Model*, has been applied to the workplace setting (Green and Kreuter, 1999 Ch. 9). Its major advantage, apart from its thoroughness, is its ecological orientation. Bertera (2000) describes four studies based on *Precede–Proceed* in the DuPont Company. Reference is made to the results in the selective review section below.

This planning approach described by Sorensen has yielded successful outcomes in various settings and contexts. We should, however, note that the strategy involves *community organisation* rather than *community development*. Accordingly, the focus of those employing such a model will be with traditional behaviour change.

## EFFECTIVENESS OF HEALTH PROMOTION IN THE WORKPLACE

We will complete this chapter with some discussion on general aspects of evaluating workplace health promotion initiatives and present a selective review of studies. First, it is worth reiterating some observations about indicators.

### Devising indicators of success

Before offering a selective review of examples of apparently successful interventions in the workplace it may be useful to reiterate earlier observations about effectiveness and efficiency and the kinds of indicator used to assess these.

First of all, interpretation of success will depend on the philosophical and ideological underpinning of the project. A major contention of this chapter thus far has derived from observations about the importance of addressing the fundamental workplace-related determinants of health. In short, the vast majority of interventions have been focused on individual behaviour change – typically because this is thought to result in the achievement of such goals as increased pro-

ductivity, reduction in absenteeism and avoidance of litigation (an important reason for banning workplace smoking!). Again, although an altruistic motive may be detected in terms of a concern for the workers' health, the focus is still normally individualistic. The cynic, of course, may well argue that the apparent concern for individual and family well-being is, at the very least, likely to enhance the 'brand image' of the particular firm or organisation and may result in retaining skilled workers. Outcome indicators of success, therefore, might include incidence of disease (an inappropriate indicator – see comments in Chapter 2) or (more appropriately) the adoption of behaviours believed to reduce risk and disease incidence.

As discussed in Chapter 2, a number of intermediate indicators may be used when behavioural outcome measures are difficult to secure. It would also be appropriate to devise indirect indicators, e.g. of training courses for occupational health staff. With reference to the achievement of policy goals, the use of indirect, intermediate and outcome indicators of behaviour change would be paralleled by measures of the successful development and implementation of policy initiatives together with indicators that provide evidence of the effect of implementation on behavioural outcomes, e.g. the effect of implementing a smoking policy on (1) adherence to the policy and (2) general cessation or reduction in individual smoking outside the workplace. The seven steps involved in implementing policy (see above) would, of course, be indirect indicators of ultimate success but could be regarded as 'milestone' process indicators by simply asking whether the steps have actually been achieved. And, of course, if the 'milestones' have been attained, process evaluation should also be used to illuminate and assess the efficiency and quality of the activities involved, e.g. the efficiency of the communication with the workforce, the extent to which key criteria for effective inter-sectoral working have been met.

As for a radical approach to workplace health promotion, the ultimate measures of success would be couched in terms of national legislation about harmful practices and/or changes within the workplace, e.g. rather than providing (effective) counselling and stress management training, successful health promotion would be judged by the extent to which the organisation itself has been changed structurally to reduce the causes of stress. As with the assessment of initiatives concerned with producing individual behaviour change, indirect, intermediate and outcome measures of success can be identified together with measures of process used as 'milestones' or, formatively, to influence and enhance the quality of the health promotion input.

A variety of such indicators will be observed in the selective review which follows our discussion of 'effectiveness reviews' below.

## EFFECTIVENESS REVIEWS OF WORKPLACE HEALTH PROMOTION

In recent times we have witnessed a veritable explosion of effectiveness reviews – doubtless following the economic imperative that clinical and health services be firmly rooted in evidence that they will actually achieve a health gain (an issue discussed earlier in Chapter 3). The normal procedure involves a systematic trawl through published sources of data based on a clearly defined set of criteria about what kinds of data are 'good enough' to be included. 'Good enough' typically centres on a determination to avoid Type 1 error wherever possible and, therefore, frequently involves reference to the 'gold standard' of the RCT.

Reference will be made below to three reviews with the aim of extracting a number of issues and principles rather than merely listing specific cases.

### Changing labour market conditions and health

We have already referred to Platt *et al.*'s (2000) systematic literature review of the relationship of changing labour market conditions and health – especially in the context of making observations on the determinants of health and illness. One particular section of this review is concerned with 'Workplace health promotion interventions'.

Three sub-sections are identified: stress reduction, absenteeism and health behaviours.

### Stress reduction

Two literature reviews were appraised (Burke, 1993; Murphy, 1996), together with three empirical studies on the effects of workplace interventions on stress (Arnetz, 1996, 1997; Barrios-Choplin *et al.*, 1997; Reynolds, 1997). Platt *et al.* (2000) interpret the evidence from these various studies as follows:

> ... the findings from these studies, taken together with the conclusions of the two field reviews, suggest that stress management interventions targeted at individuals can be effective in reducing physical and psychological symptoms.

More importantly, though, in the light of our discussion of radical health promotion, the authors conclude that *Organisational outcomes, however, require to be tackled using interventions which address the sources of stressing the total work setting* (Section. 5.2).

### Absenteeism

Five studies were reviewed (Jeffery *et al.*, 1993; Kerr and Vos, 1993; Schi, 1993a, b; Michie, 1996; Lechner *et al.*, 1997). Platt *et al.*'s interpretation was as follows: ... *all the findings point to a major impact of workplace health promotion activity on absenteeism* (Section 5.4).

### Health behaviours

Two reviews of the effects of workplace health promotion in respect of topics such as nutrition, weight control and exercise were analysed by the authors (Griffiths, 1996; Wilson *et al.*, 1996) together with eight specific studies on cardiovascular risk factors, smoking and alcohol misuse (Broder *et al.*, 1993; Glasgow *et al.*, 1993; Brenner and Fleischle, 1994, 1997; Jeffery *et al.*, 1994; Murza *et al.*, 1994; Conrad *et al.*, 1996; Cook *et al.* 1996).

Platt *et al.* draw the following pessimistic conclusion:

*The only conclusion that can be stated with any confidence is that the regulation of smoking in the workplace appears to modify the amount of smoking among smokers but to have little effect on the overall prevalence of smoking.*

What is, arguably, the most important conclusion has to do with methodological weakness (probably of the original intervention design, the research articles and, perhaps, the effectiveness review process itself). In short, Platt *et al.* refer regularly to *methodological weaknesses*, the difficulty of *drawing definitive conclusions ... in view of the methodological limitations of many of the empirical studies* and the fact that *The empirical studies ... varied considerably in terms of the soundness of the adopted research design ...* and *... given the lack of uniformity among the interventions on offer, there must be some question about which particular elements within an overall intervention actually produce the* (reported) *effect.*

The general conclusions of Platt *et al.*'s review are worthy of note (see Box 9).

**Box 9**  Changing Labour Market Conditions and Health

*Despite concerns about the methodological quality of the studies included in this review, we conclude that there is substantial evidence of significant health impacts associated with current labour market conditions. Our findings suggest that workplace reorganisation, redundancy, new technology and features of the modern work environment are likely to be associated with deficits in physical and/or psychological health among a wide range of employees. This suggests that European governments should subject their labour market policies to routine health impact assessment, both prospectively and retrospectively, and consider how negative consequences of current labour market change can be reduced or offset through countervailing mechanisms. Employers (of companies of all sizes) should*

*be encouraged or required to pay more attention to the health and human resources aspects of their business decisions, even in times of economic and financial instability. The health sector should be challenged to ensure that in all aspects of its work (promotion and prevention as well as treatment) close attention is paid to the link between employment, unemployment, health and well-being. Health promotion will need to consider how best it can fulfil its mission in the workplace setting, in particular addressing the question of the appropriate level (individual or organisational) at which interventions can most profitably be implemented.*

(Platt *et al.*, 2000 Section 8.7)

## Effectiveness review of health promotion interventions in the workplace (HEA)

The English Health Education Authority commissioned a review of workplace interventions (Peersman *et al.*, 1998). Its main findings are summarised below.

First, it is interesting to note that the inclusion criteria for the review explicitly searched for studies based on participatory methods and studies that included not only outcome but process measures. Of 139 studies, 50 matched the inclusion criteria and of these 15 were considered to be methodologically sound (i.e. employed control or comparison groups). Two broad generalisations were made: first, an attempt was made to identify those programme characteristics that were related to effective outcomes and, second, a number of recommendations were made about evaluation research. As for the first of these, a number of general principles underpinning effective health promotions '*to effect individual behaviour change*' (our emphasis) were identified. Not surprisingly, many of these would apply to interventions in any setting. These features of effective programmes are listed in Box 10.

**Box 10**   Characteristics of Effective Workplace Programmes

- Visible and enthusiastic support for, and involvement in, the intervention from top management;
- involvement by employees at all organisational levels in the planning, implementation and activities of the intervention;
- a focus on definable and modifiable risk factors which are a priority for the specific worker group to make an intervention more acceptable and increase participation;
- interventions should be tailor made to the characteristics and needs of the recipients;
- optimal use of local resources should be made in organising and implementing the intervention;
- evaluation should be included as an integral part of any new intervention programme and include a range of outcome and process measures.

Yet again, a cautionary note is struck about generalising from effectiveness reviews due to the methodological weaknesses of most published studies. On the basis of their review the authors summarise their views about the effectiveness of the programmes they assessed. These are listed below.

- Comprehensive programmes combining screening and risk assessment with a choice of education programmes and/or environmental changes have been effective; however, with few sound studies to draw on, replicating these interventions cannot guarantee success.
- Least effective were weight control programmes combining education and financial incentives; sustained weight loss appears particularly difficult.
- There is no conclusive evidence for the effectiveness of social support provided by peers or group leaders as part of broad educational interventions.

- The effect of interventions incorporating a skill development component is inconclusive with equal numbers of effective and ineffective interventions; however, combining skills training with social support in interventions targeting a specific risk behaviour is more likely to be effective than skills training as part of broad, complex interventions.
- Healthier eating has been encouraged by targeted provision of information such as point-of-purchase labelling of healthy food choices in workplace cafeterias and computer-generated personalised nutrition advice.
- Two complex interventions addressing healthy eating were considered ineffective: one operated at the level of individuals, organisations and communities; the other involved presentations, computerised data analysis, supermarket tours, take-home activities and group walks.
- Individualised delivery of information appeared effective in a range of interventions. This finding was also supported by a process evaluation of a complex intervention suggesting that engaging the 'eager' employees into wellness programmes was easy if programmes were provided on site. Engaging the 'reluctant' employees requires one-to-one approaches.
- The importance of healthy alliances was supported by a number of studies showing success in controlling blood pressure, smoking and alcohol consumption, as well as improving knowledge and changing behaviour related to cancer prevention, however, other studies involving healthy alliances had disappointing results.

It should by now be apparent that the difficulties involved in drawing conclusions about designing effective programmes are legion – and substantially due to limited and/or inappropriate research design. The implications for the efficient design of evaluation research drawn by Peersman *et al.* are eminently sensible – although perhaps occasionally liable to challenge. In their view, evaluation research should seek to incorporate the principles below.

- Interventions with multiple components should be clearly described in terms of what these components are, how they are implemented and by whom.

- Workplace health promotion interventions should have fully integrated evaluation components initially focusing on the delivery and acceptability of the intervention and ultimately addressing its effectiveness.
- Appropriate quantitative and qualitative procedures, as well as statistical techniques for analysing effectiveness, should be used.
- Whenever possible studies of effectiveness should employ the design of a randomised controlled trial, although quasi-experimental approaches with adequate control or comparison groups should also be considered.
- Evaluation of workplace health promotion interventions should include systematic information on cost effectiveness where possible.
- The need for methodological rigour must be recognised among evaluators of health promotion activities and among peer reviewers and editors of journals to raise publication standards, including the importance of publishing studies reporting 'negative' results.
- The widespread lack of methodological rigour requires commissioners and providers to inform their planning of services from systematic review or from critically appraised primary studies.
- There is a need to develop research methods appropriate for evaluating the role of healthy alliances and other complex interventions with the aim to assess their effectiveness and to identify their active components.

## The IUHPE review series

In 1994 the European Regional Office of the International Union for Health Promotion and Health Education (IUHPE) initiated a project designed to contribute to improving the effectiveness of health promotion. Systematic reviews of 16 subject areas in health promotion were published. They included topics (such as sexual behaviour and nutrition), target/at-risk groups (such as elderly and socially deprived groups) and settings (such as patient education in hospitals and school health). Reference will be made below to one of these settings-based effectiveness reviews: *Promoting Health at Work* (Veen and Vereijken, 1994). One of the strengths of the whole venture was the emphasis it placed on trying to provide not just a brief label of effective/ineffective, with a note about statistical significance, but rather to offer systematic insight into the nature and quality of the interventions.

The general strategy and inclusion criteria that were applied to the series can be consulted in Appendix 7.1.

After trawling five databases and consultation with experts the review of workplace interventions finally identified 21 studies deemed to be of reasonably sound methodology and generally fitting the selection criteria detailed in Appendix 7.1. Six of these were from Europe. The topic areas reviewed were quite representative of 'typical' workplace interventions – as seen in our selective review below and preceding discussions in this chapter. The topic areas are listed below and in some instances refer to more than one topic or outcome. They are:

- smoking prevention;
- reducing risk factors for cardiovascular disease;
- stress management;
- managing lower back pain/preventing musculoskeletal disorders;
- cancers;
- substance abuse;
- noise and hearing loss;
- dental health;
- integrated approaches to several types of health problem.

In addition to a general description of the interventions, the instrument used for analysis provided information on the following:

- target group;
- place and mode of contacting target group and sampling;
- nature of objectives;
- theoretical underpinning;
- intervention content, strategies and methods;
- duration of intervention and intensity of contact;
- evaluation design: summative or formative;

- nature of measuring instruments used;
- outcomes, including details of attrition rates and general assessment of effectiveness.

In the context of our earlier observations about the importance of theory it is interesting to note that five publications referred explicitly to their theoretical base; a further six publications could be adjudged to have some implicit theoretical dimension, e.g. use of 'positive reinforcement' might be mentioned. Most of the studies selected employed a quasi-experimental design; six studies utilised random allocation. Formative evaluation figured to some extent in six studies but these tended to be informal or incidental – rather than being prominent features as would be essential for illumination and generalisation.

A general indication of overall effectiveness was provided for each of the studies appraised. Bearing in mind the selection criteria for this review, it is revealing to note that the reviewers were prepared to rate only four studies as *'effective'*. Two were judged to have been *'ineffective'*; the remainder were considered to have been *'partially effective'*. Further reference to those rated as 'effective' will be made in the selective review below.

## HEALTH PROMOTION IN THE WORKPLACE: A SELECTIVE REVIEW

In 1970 in the USA an *Occupational Safety and Health Act* was enacted *... to assure so far as possible every working man and woman in the nation safe and healthful working conditions and to preserve our human resources ... .* The achievement of this goal was to be ensured by *inter alia ... education and training programs in the recognition, avoidance, and prevention of unsafe or unhealthful working conditions ...* (Vojtecky *et al.*, 1985). In Britain similar legislation in the form of the *Health and Safety at Work Act* was introduced in 1974. Symington (1987), in a conference on *Health Promotion in the Workplace*, commented on this Act and the *Employment Protection Act* which followed it in 1975 and argued that while they were primarily concerned with health and safety issues, *... this new awareness ... provides a climate and a platform from which health promotion activities of a general nature can thrive.* He went on to point out that while not required by the Acts, screening programmes together with alcohol and smoking policies emerged as a useful by-product. While this is undoubtedly true, the fact is that developments in Britain have not kept pace with those in North America. Indeed, it is interesting to note an assertion by Webb at the same conference that after 20 years of decline in work related diseases and injuries *... figures for recent years show an alarming rise from 70.4 per 100 000 employees in 1981 to 87.0 per 100 000 in 1984.* He goes on to speculate that *... some workers are paying in health terms for the economic changes of recent years.*

At the time of writing no comprehensive survey of UK workplace health promotion activities is available. However, examples of good practice in Scotland were presented in the conference report referred to above: these included programmes operated by seven commercial organisations, various district councils on alcoholism, trade unions, health education departments, the employment medical advisory service and local health boards. Topic areas discussed were safety, alcohol, exercise, nutrition, smoking, mental health, women's health and heart disease.

It will by now be clear that the situation in North America is very different. Fuchs *et al.* (1985) commented on the escalation of interest between 1975 and 1985. They provided a selective review of 11 key textbooks, referred to 30 journal articles on general health promotion at work and listed 101 topic-specific articles together with 25 exemplars of more popular magazine pieces. The distribution of topics by popularity is as listed in Table 7.4. If these figures are representative it is clear that the impact of safety legislation has been less than the more general health promotion movement – with, of course, its implications for cost containment!

Davis *et al.* (1984) recorded an even greater range of topics in their survey of Californian workplaces. Between 16 and 72% of companies provided a wide range of screening services.

**Table 7.4**  The most popular worksite health promotion programmes (after Fuchs et al., 1985)

| Rank order | Topic | No. of references |
|---|---|---|
| 1 | Exercise programmes | 33 |
| 2 | Hypertension and coronary heart disease | 19 |
| 3 | Drugs and alcohol | 17 |
| 4 | Stress management | 12 |
| 5 | Smoking | 8 |
| 6 | Weight reduction | 5 |
| 7 | Safety | 4 |
| 8 | Cancer screening | 3 |

These were, in ascending order of popularity: cervical cancer; colon/rectal cancer; diabetes; pulmonary function; annual medical examination; work-related problems; height and weight; general risk appraisal; high blood pressure; pre-employment medical examination.

Between 30 and 78% offered a wide range of information programmes. Again in ascending order of popularity, these were: seat belt use; cervical cancer; breast self-examination; cancer prevention; work-related injury; low back pain; high blood pressure; alcohol and drug abuse; nutrition; smoking; stress; exercise.

Various services (e.g. group instruction, individual counselling and referral to community resources) were on offer with provision ranging from 28 to 80% of firms. Services provided were: industrial alcoholism programmes; employee assistance; self-defence for women; low back pain; smoking cessation; weight management; stress management; exercise.

Hollander and Lengermann (1988) carried out a systematic survey of Fortune 500 companies (i.e. the 500 largest US firms) to determine the nature and extent of health promotion provision (in 1984). The response rate was approximately 50%. Of these, two thirds had a worksite programme and two thirds reported plans to expand these. One third of those not having programmes planned to initiate health promotion activities. In general, the larger firms were more likely to have programmes which also tended to be more extensive. The number of health promotion activities reported ranged from 5.7 to 8.9.

Walsh (1988) cited an unpublished manuscript of the Office of Disease Prevention and Health Promotion which reported a 1985 national survey of private sector employers having 50 or more personnel. This recorded at least one health promotion activity at nearly 66% of establishments; larger establishments tended to have many more programmes.

It would seem unlikely from the survey data presented above that health and safety legislation alone would be responsible for the accelerating provision of health promotion programmes in the USA. A more realistic estimate would be based on the general cultural pressure towards fitness and wellness along with the belief in the cost effectiveness of interventions. Doubtless further impetus has been provided by the particular reference to worksite health promotion in the Surgeon General's report *Healthy People* (US Department of Health, Education and Welfare, 1979), which comments on the worksite as a locus for health education and health promotion.

**Box 11**

> *When work is a pleasure, life is a joy. When work is a duty, life is slavery.*
> (Maxim Gorky, *The Lower Depths*, 1903)

The worksite may provide an appropriate setting for health promotion as well as health protection activities. A number of companies have already shown leadership in providing employee fitness programs and encouraging worker participation, but more can be done.

The report also urged advertisers to be aware of their key role in influencing consumer behaviour and noted that advertising, ... *particularly for food products, over-the-counter drugs, tobacco, and alcohol – has generally not been supportive of health promotion objectives.*

The report was published in 1979 and aspects of worksite health promotion were subsequently incorporated into the influential *Objectives for the Nation* (US Department of Health and Human Services, 1980) in 1980. Since then the appropriateness of the setting has indeed been increasingly recognised. But what of success? To what extent has the faith of employers been justified?

First, there is little doubt that if appropriate educational techniques are used the impact of particular interventions can be positive, even in behavioural terms. For instance, Street (1987) describes two safety education interventions (Foster, 1983; Denyer, 1986). The first revealed a pre-post programme difference in knowledge, beliefs and attitudes towards wearing hearing protection. Moreover, after the intervention fewer people stated that they 'never used hearing protection'. However, the familiar gap between attitude and practice was noticeable in the reported results: Whereas some 80% of the group agreed that it was important to protect their hearing, only 65% stated that they actually wore protectors most of the time.

The second programme was concerned with eye protection. It employed relevant precursor 'educational diagnosis' of the target group and added a 'policy element' to the education in the form of threatened disciplinary action for non-compliance. Actual injuries fell over an 8 week period from 72 to six.

However, rather more substantial and extensive justification for large-scale investments of money and effort in workplace programmes would be expected if programmes were to continue. Davis et al.'s (1984) study indicates that those employers operating health promotion programmes think that they work.

Further to the data provided in Tables 7.1 and 7.2, additional details of employers' perceptions of benefits are provided in Table 7.5. Of course employer perceptions may well have been biased by wishful thinking! However, their views on reduced absenteeism may well be justified if Blair et al.'s (1986a) study is generally applicable. After an intensive 10 week programme of fitness teaching there were not only significant differences in physiological and clinical characteristics in the 3846 participants receiving the instruction but there were also, on average, 1.25 days less absenteeism in the group. The researchers calculate that the programme had therefore resulted in savings of $149,578!

Many other reviews have reported similar kinds of success. Knobel (1983) reported a reduction in disability costs for each $1000 of total wage payments from $13.28 in 1976 to $9.43 in 1978 at Southern Bell. This cost saving was ascribed to a coordinated prevention and promotion programme.

Knobel also commented on the Campbell Soup Co. programme which resulted in the removal of approximately 20 polyps each year at a cost of $6500 with estimated annual reductions of $100,000 in direct insurance payments.

The company detected and treated between 60 and 90% of hypertensives, thus avoiding over a 10 year period an estimated $130,000 in hospitalization, rehabilitation and disability costs.

Northern Natural Gas reported a reduction in absenteeism of approximately 5 working days a year after a fitness programme. School administrators and teachers, according to Knobel, had 17% reduced absenteeism after a programme of exercise, stress management and nutrition teaching. A nine component health promotion programme, which cost New York Telephone approximately $2,800,000 in 1980, generated savings of $5,500,000 from reduced absenteeism and treatment costs.

Blair et al. (1986b) described the programme at Johnson and Johnson whose 'Live for Life' scheme includes health risk appraisal, fitness, diet and nutrition, smoking cessation, hypertension control, stress management, weight control

**Table 7.5** Employer's perceptions of the benefits of worksite health promotion programmes (after Davis et al., 1984)

| Category | Perceived as benefit by (%) |
| --- | --- |
| Improved morale | 81 |
| Improved health | 52 |
| Improved productivity | 46 |
| Reduced illness and injury | 46 |
| Reduced staff turnover and absenteeism | 40 |
| Reduced medical care utilisation | 30 |
| Reduced health care costs | 23 |
| Attracted better calibre applicants | 17 |

and general health education. Over a 2 year period 20% of women and 30% of men had adopted vigorous exercise compared with 7 and 19% of a control group of company employees. Overall fitness and sense of well-being had also apparently improved. And again, the 'bottom line' calculation: there were fewer hospital admissions and in-patient days for Johnson and Johnson employees and an estimated annual in-patient cost increase of $43 compared with $76 for non-programme employees (Bly *et al.*, 1986).

The Canada Life Assurance Company's *'Fitness and Lifestyle Project'* (Shephard *et al.*, 1982) provided similar evidence of success. A saving of more than 0.5 hospital days per employee was claimed which was associated with a financial saving of $84.5 per employee year.

Sloan (1987), in reviewing several of the projects mentioned above, presents a critique of the prevailing paradigm in North America. He reminds us again that ... ***some obvious alternative and complementary approaches are overlooked***. In particular, he mentions the psychological and organisational climate of work. It should, perhaps, also be noted that there are instances where the worksite does not appear to generate successful results! For instance, smoking cessation programmes may well achieve worse results than alternative modes of delivery and Klesges *et al.* (1987) reported only 17% mean success rate at six months. Jason *et al.* (1987) reported that work-based support groups increased the effectiveness of a smoking cessation programme using television and self-help manuals but reported only 7% continuous abstinence at 12 months, admittedly utilising stringent criteria.

It is worth reiterating at this point the general assertion that any given programme will be more effective when it is part of a general integrated programme of education and policy and when it is supported by a consistent and integrated approach within the wider community – witness for example the *'Pawtucket Heart Health Program'*.

**Box 12**   Weight Loss in the Pawtucket Program

---

*As part of the Pawtucket Heart Health Program, worksite volunteers implemented a weight control campaign with 512 employees from 22 companies. At the end of the program, a total of 1818 pounds had been lost at an average of 3.55 pounds per person and a cost of $0.81 per pound lost.*

(Nelson *et al.*, 1987).

---

Bertera (2000) describes the DuPont company's *'Integrated Health Service Scheme'* and cites four studies that were considered to have been successful. As noted earlier, Green's planning model was used as a basis for programme design. The studies briefly described below addressed absenteeism, lifestyle risks and illness costs.

- Two pilot programmes demonstrated a decline in absenteeism that averaged 6.8% per year over a four year period in one work site and 7.9% per year over a six year period in another site. The reduction recorded in a control site averaged only 2.1% (Bertera, 1990a).

- A second investigation into programme effectiveness in reducing absenteeism had as its population 29,315 employees at 41 different intervention sites. There was a 14% decline over a 2 year period compared with a 5.8% decline in control sites (*n* = 14,573 employees). The initiative was deemed to yield a more than satisfactory cost–benefit result: the net difference between intervention and control sites of 11,726 fewer disability days provided a return of $2.05 for every dollar invested by the end of the second year (Bertera, 1990b).

- An investigation of the impact of behavioural risk factors on absenteeism and estimated health care costs revealed that employees with any of six risks had levels of absenteeism between 10 and 32% higher than those without such risk levels (Bertera, 1991). The calculations are intrinsically interesting but serve to illustrate the particular attractions of effective workplace health promotion for US industry. Clearly, the same level of motivation does not exist in other countries – though the excess costs are of course of great concern to the national health services (Box 13).

**Box 13** Excess Illness Costs Per Person/Year – the DuPont Program

| | |
|---|---|
| Smoking | $960 |
| Overweight | $401 |
| Excess alcohol | $389 |
| Raised cholesterol | $370 |
| High blood pressure | $343 |
| Low seat belt use | $272 |
| Lack of exercise | $130 |

The total cost to the company was estimated at some $ 70.8 million annually.

Given the cost calculations mentioned above, a third intervention (Bertera, 1993) that assessed the impact of a programme designed to modify individual unhealthy behaviours was of especial interest. The programme's impact on 7178 participants over a 2 year period was as follows: the number of employees with three or more behavioural risks declined by 14%; there was also a 12% decrease in the mean number of (self-reported) days of absence. The changes in the various targeted behaviours ranged from seat belt wearing (78.9% increase in utilisation) to overweight (0% change).

This latter study by Bertera was one of the interventions deemed effective by Veen and Vereijken (1994). They did, however, strike a cautionary note. Because the DuPont company was committed to running the programme at successive worksites as soon as it was ready, there were no baseline measures for the comparison group – which limits generalisability. This observation is, of course, quite legitimate, but it underlines observations we have made earlier about the importance of not relying on traditional research designs for making decisions about effectiveness. Fortunately, in this particular case the reviewers

had sufficient information about the programme itself to reach a conclusion that the programme had indeed been effective. For instance, the variety of methods employed in the workplace had been fully specified:

- self-instruction/self-help kits;
- workshops/role play/games;
- lifeskills training;
- smoking policy implementation;
- cafeteria offering health food;
- blood pressure machine availability.

In such a situation the construction of appropriate intermediate indicators together with other kinds of triangulated evidence (including process data) would, following the 'judicial principle', have led to a firm conclusion of effectiveness without feelings of anxiety about a lack of controlled trial.

A *'Worksite Wellness'* programme described by Erfurt *et al.* (1991) also merits attention. It was judged 'effective' in the IUHPE review (Veen and Verrijken, 1994). It was designated a *'Worksite Wellness Program'* and was actually concerned with addressing unhealthy lifestyle dimensions. In the case of the programme under discussion these were hypertension, obesity and cigarette smoking. The effectiveness review was able to provide quite thorough details of the intervention, which used a community organisation approach that included a task force ('wellness committee') having client representation and participation. Mass media support (in the form of exhibitions, educational broadcasts, written materials) was developed for inter-personal counselling and education. The specific methods included:

- self-instruction/self-help kits;
- one-to-one counselling;
- group discussions;
- workshops/role play and games;
- lifeskills training;
- health communication networks;
- peer support groups;
- plant-wide health promotion activities

(together with various 'learning resources' such as records of screening).

The intervention lasted 3 years and a number of

'health educators' and 'wellness counsellors' were involved, together with external providers of health promotion. The evaluation involved three study groups of 500 people and one of 400 people. Each group had increasingly intensive interventions starting with screening only together with referral for those at risk. The maximum intervention group had in addition health education/information and classes, routine follow-up counselling and 'social organisation' within the plant.

Major improvements in risk-related behaviours were found: more hypertensives were treated and showed greater reductions in blood pressure; participation in weight loss and smoking cessation programmes increased. Success was greatest with maximum health promotion input together with lowest relapse.

Limitations described by the reviewers included: difficulties in assessing the contribution of a major public anti-smoking programme that happened during the period the programme was operating; difficulty of separately assessing the effect of multiple educational inputs in the highest impact group from the level of on-site staffing (out-reach element); the self-report nature of measuring smoking prevalence.

Again, these limitations re-assert the importance of including in the evaluation appropriate intermediate and process indicators to increase confidence in the relative effectiveness of particular programme components.

Another programme judged 'effective' by Veen and Vereijken (1994) centred on promoting 'wellness' in respect of major lifestyle-related health problems. Indicators of success were defined by the following changes:

- knowledge/beliefs/awareness;
- attitude;
- trial adoption of behaviors;
- biomedical risk;
- availability of services, facilities or preventive infrastructures;
- legislation/regulation;
- incidence or prevalence of illness.

The following methods were used in the intervention:

- group lifeskills training (menu of nine);
- feedback of biometric results;
- written materials and 'incentives' such as T-shirts, mugs, gym bags;
- environmental facilities were made available: choice of healthy food; fitness room with showers and lockers; space and computer facilities for providing the educational interventions.

A steering group, with administrative support, organised the programme and activities were provided by a doctor, a nurse, a psychologist with student involvement and 'sex consultants'(!). The programme was designed to operate for several years.

No comparison group was involved in the evaluation which assessed changes in the characteristics listed in the 'indicators' above. Some 1500 workers were randomly selected and invited to join the programme. Significant changes were shown by all indicators. Important process measures showed support for the programme by 40% of upper management; adequate funding and support were provided; relevant staff training was introduced; a doctor worked with the programme for 16 hours a week (Harris and Ewing, 1989).

The limitations identified by the reviewers centred on the evaluation's failure to provide enough detail about the exact content of the courses, a lack of process evaluation for illumination and formative development, aa lack of detail about the reliability and validity of measurement instruments and, of course, the lack of a comparison or control group.

It is not clear whether the final study described as 'effective' by the IUHPE study (Veen and Vereijken, 1994) should be regarded as dealing with an occupational hazard! However, its concern was with the promotion of dental health in a Danish chocolate factory (Peterson, 1989). The programme lasted 2 years and the intervention consisted of 3–4 consultations a year lasting approximately 70 minutes in the first year and an additional 40 minutes in the second. The methods employed were:

- self-instruction/self-help kits;
- one-to-one counselling;

- group skills training;
- offer of clinical preventive care and prophylaxis (service provision);
- continuing presence of a dental hygienist in the factory.

Indicators were:

- clinical: visible plaque index; gingival bleeding; calculus index;
- educational/learning: dental knowledge, attitudes and dental health behaviour;
- social network activities (resulting in worker discussion about programme).

Despite the lack of a control group, the intervention was considered to have been successful in effecting changes in all relevant measures – as well as worker and management satisfaction. The reviewers' observations about limitations were that the study should be regarded as a demonstration project to be followed by a replication using comparison groups in order to refute the possibility of a rival hypotheses for explaining the changes in health status and related measures.

As we noted earlier in relation to Platt *et al.*'s (2000) review, a majority of workplace evaluations can be criticised for inadequate designs and lack of detail on which to judge the inner workings of projects. Several reviewers, such as Chen (1984), have rightly concluded that proper experimental or quasi-experimental research design were relatively rare, although we have questioned the appropriateness of actually using such designs in the first place. All in all though, on the evidence of the studies cited above, it would be reasonable to conclude that many programmes actually had an impact. Indeed, the general view in North America appears to be that worksite health promotion is actually successful. Impact evaluation of the kinds described above is virtually non-existent in Britain. However, where a company has initiated a comprehensive programme there seems to be a view that it was worth the effort. For instance, the personnel manager of Polaroid UK argued that for an outlay of £16,000 there had been a significant effect on people's lifestyles (Fuchs *et al.*, 1985) in relation to diet and exercise

and a claimed reduction in absenteeism from 6.3 to 3.7% over a 4 year period.

One of the more thorough and comprehensive workplace endeavours in the UK was the 'Look After Yourself' (LAY) programme developed by the Health Education Council. An evaluation of a pilot programme revealed evidence of effectiveness. First, in relation to indirect indicators, 73% of the 60 initial recruits attended all eight sessions. Additionally, various intermediate measures gave evidence of heightened awareness of stress together with a positive attitude towards and competence in controlling it. Outcome measures of changes in eating, exercise, alcohol consumption and smoking demonstrated lifestyle changes: between 26 and 89% of 85 participants recorded a change in one or more of these behaviours. Changes were also observed in various physiological indicators, namely aerobic capacity, body fat, blood pressure and lung efficiency. Programme participants also expressed satisfaction with and interest in the programme as a whole (Denyer, 1986).

The research designs of these programmes would doubtless not impress those favouring 'proper' experimental techniques which might allow us, in Chen's (1984) words, to ... *be better able to prove that health education indeed is worthwhile*. However, it is worth reiterating the contention made above that although rigorous research design is often eminently desirable in order to generate internal validity, in general such designs are not essential. Indeed in the interests of external validity, illuminative evaluation will often be more useful provided that it is based on sound theory and utilizes relevant intermediate and indirect indicators.

Cost–benefit analysis, although doubtless attractive to many decision makers in the UK, is clearly of much greater relevance to North America and its peculiar system of health care delivery and payment. Nonetheless, the behaviour changes which generate cost savings and increased productivity are in most cases the same changes which will enhance well-being and can thus justify both the inclusion of health promotion in British workplaces and the use of less rigorous measures of programme effectiveness in evaluation.

**Box 14**

> *One of the saddest things is that the only thing a man can do for eight hours a day, day after day, is work. You can't eat eight hours a day nor drink for eight hours a day, nor make love for eight hours.*
>
> (William Faulkner, 1958)

## Some recent developments

A number of significant recent initiatives have occurred in developing workplace health promotion (see for instance Chu *et al.*, 2000). In 1996 a *'European Union Network for Workplace Health Promotion'* was formed (Federal Institute for Occupational Safety and Health, 1996) and WHO has launched its *'Global Health Work Approach'* (WHO, 1997). The European Network listed five key priorities for action in the Luxembourg Declaration on 28th November 1997. They are:

- an increase in awareness of workplace health promotion and promote responsibility for health with regard to all stakeholders;
- identification and dissemination of models of good practice;
- development of guidelines for effective workplace health promotion;
- to ensure commitment of the member states to incorporate principles of workplace health promotion in respective policies;
- to address the specific challenges of working effectively with small and medium enterprises.

(after Chu *et al.*, 2000)

Amongst other things, the Project aims to identify examples of good practice – such as Volkswagen (see Box 15).

**Box 15** Volkswagen – a Model of Good Practice

- Innovative working time models (working time accounts);
- introduction of new forms of work organisation;

- corporate regulations to prevent sexual discrimination and mobbing;
- ergonomic job design which involves the employees and health specialists with investment decision procedures including the planning of new equipment.

Strategies used to achieve the above goals:

- health circles (problem solving groups with the task of identifying health-related problems and possible measures for improvement);
- extended job inspection routines involving employees;
- regular employee surveys on health matters;
- special training modules for health and safety education.

(after Chu *et al.*, 2000)

Chu *et al.* (2000) also describe the emergence of networks in the Western Pacific Regional Network of WHO (WHO, 1997) and the development of guidelines (WHO–Western Pacific Regional Office, 1998). They also cite Queensland's Steering Committee on Workplace Health Promotion (Allen and Dwyer, 1994). The following 'principles and guidelines' reflect many of the key features of effective programme design together with ideological commitments consistent with the *Ottawa Charter*. The following should, therefore, be the basis for collaboration between employers, workforce and health professionals. They are, in order of priority:

- cost effectiveness;
- support for workplace health and safety;
- managed by the workplace (rather than central intervention);
- proper needs assessment;
- voluntary participation;
- training in health promotion principles and practice;
- sustainable;
- based on principles of social justice;
- includes evaluation;

- uses mixed strategies;
- should, where appropriate, involve family members;
- considers structures, cultures, laws and policies of the workplace.

(after Queensland Health, 1996)

The Municipal Health Bureau, the Chinese Government and WHO collaborated to develop a pilot workplace health promotion project involving 21,613 workers in four workplaces. This has been considered to offer a model of good practice and the evaluation of this 'Shanghai Project' is worth noting (see Box 16).

**Box 16** Evaluation of the Shanghai Project (1995)

- Reduced incidence of work-related injuries by 10–20%;
- reduced diseases and related health care costs (e.g. pharyngitis from 16 to 10%);
- improved health and safety knowledge and practices (use of safety devices or protective equipment increased from 20–30 to 70–90%);
- reduced risk behaviour (reduction of salt consumption, cigarette smoking);
- reduced levels of sick leave by 50%.

(after Chu et al., 2000)

Before leaving this brief discussion of developments in the Western Pacific it may be helpful to note the framework for workplace health assessment developed by Griffith University (Chu et al., 1997). It derives from an approach that, following Hawe et al. (1990), emphasises process, impact and outcomes (as we noted in an earlier chapter, 'impact' refers to the immediate effects of an intervention and is typically assessed by what we have called 'intermediate indicators'). An abbreviated version is given in Table 7.6.

## Workplace health promotion: the radical dimension

The discussion of behaviour change and economic indicators of success has, in this chapter, perhaps appeared almost obsessive! This is due to the excess of data of an economic kind and the dearth of evidence of effectiveness in other domains of a more radical nature. It is perhaps naïve to expect truly radical initiatives in the workplace and the kinds of participation to which reference was made above in the context of the Volkswagen model scheme may be the best we can expect. However, in accordance with the principle of equity espoused in this book, we will conclude this chapter by reporting Freudenberg's (1981) account of successful examples of consciousness raising and community action. He reminds us of the 'traditional' hazards facing workers (Box 17).

**Box 17** Traditional Hazards Facing Workers

*Work-related diseases afflict at least 4 million people a year; as many as 400 000 Americans die annually from these diseases. ... In addition, 9 million workers are injured on the job each year and 13 000 people die from these injuries. ... 20% of all cancers are related to work place exposure to carcinogens.*

(Freudenberg, 1981)

He cites examples of consciousness-raising health education designed to provide a radical response to the situation described above. The case of the *Carolina Brown Lung Association* was mentioned earlier. This radical health promotion programme provided workers with understanding and skills to monitor health hazards and take action in the case of violations. It also incorporated the broader health promotion tactics of lobbying and advocacy – for instance in order to achieve fair compensation and ensure the availability of proper health care for the victims of industrial disease.

The *New York Committee on Occupational Safety and Health* is also cited as an exemplar of radical health promotion. This group has sponsored educational forums on health hazards and has lobbied vigorously in order to achieve 'Right-to-Know' legislation. It also provides technical assistance and advice for trade unions and spon-

**Table 7.6** An integrated framework for workplace health assessment (Griffiths University)

| Category | Indicators |
| --- | --- |
| Organisational features | Workplace culture, management style, division of labour, work group cohesion, worker autonomy, shift work, award structure, defined career paths, workload, worker involvement in decision making, communication channels, power/control versus responsibility, job satisfaction and morale, equity issues, relationship with outside communities |
| Physical environment | Hygiene and environmental conditions, exposure to hazards (noise, dust, heat, chemical, etc.), built environment (lighting, aesthetics, space, etc.) |
| Health and safety data (industry and workplace specific) | Absenteeism, worker compensation, sick leave, injuries and disability, lost time frequency rate, specific OH risk factors, OHS mortality and morbidity, health services utilization |
| Nature of work | Work tasks, routinised activities, manual handling, design or work setting, ergonomic measures, repetitive motions |
| Demographic, lifestyle data and worker–client base | Number of workers, income, education, ethnicity, socio-economic status, gender, age distribution, tobacco/alcohol use, nature of client base |

*After Chu et al. (1997).*

sors lectures at union meetings in addition to producing educational materials.

Criteria for success are readily defined: outcome indicators might include the achievement of legislation which will improve safety standards. Intermediate indicators could document the increasing level of awareness in a community and different degrees of social action. In a later article Freudenberg (1985) provides further instances of radical health promotion. Indicators of success have been extracted from these and are categorised in Table 7.7.

These last examples of workplace health promotion are very different from many earlier examples: not only do they adopt a radical approach which is philosophically and ideologically distinct from the narrower individually focused and frequently 'healthist' programmes, but they also have moved us outside the bounds of the worksite and into the community. The final strategic approach which will be discussed in this book also focuses on the community. At one level

of analysis it will examine the notion of community-wide approaches and consider integrated programmes which would incorporate worksite health promotion as one element in a broader but, hopefully, coherent strategy. At another level it will concern itself with a much narrower and geographically more limited approach having a very particular philosophy. This strategy is termed community development: its rationale and ideology and the methods it employs to achieve its goals have much in common with the radical formula for workplace health promotion delineated by Freudenberg.

**Box 18**

> *Work spares us from three great evils: boredom, vice, and need.*
>
> (Voltaire, *Candide*, 1759)

**Table 7.7**  Indicators of 'radical' health education

| Inhibitors of success | Examples of process involved |
| --- | --- |
| *Outcome* | |
| January 1981, Philadelphia enacted the nation's first municipal Right-to-Know law | Results from several years of community and workplace education by Delaware Valley Toxics Coalition |
| *Intermediate* | |
| United Automobile Workers produce a handbook *A manual for Cancer Detectives on the Job* which ... **teaches members across the country how to conduct an investigation, file an OSHA complaint and bargain for health and safety.** | Stimulus from an organised coalition of tenants' associations, environmental groups and Vietnam veterans |
| Tenants' associations develop a flair for creative use of media (skills acquisition) | Learning how to produce reports, hold demonstrations, organise public meetings |
| A mortality study is produced by workers which identifies potential carcinogens. Improvements are made to ventilation | Workers approach National Union for help |

# REFERENCES

Aaron, T. (1995) *Stress Management Approaches for Small Business: A Comprehensive Review from a Health Promotion Perspective*. University of Toronto, Toronto.

Alexander, J. (1988) *The ideological construction of risk: an analysis of corporate health promotion programs in the 1980s. Social Science and Medicine*, 26, 559–567.

Allen, J. and Dwyer, S. (1994) *The workplace project – organisational change in Queensland workplaces*. In C. Chu and R. Simpson (Eds) *Ecological Public Health: From Vision to Practice*. Centre for Health Promotion, University of Toronto, Toronto and Institute of Applied Environmental Research, Griffith University, Brisbane.

Arnetz, B. B. (1996) *Techno stress – a prospective psychophysiological study of the impact of a controlled stress reduction program in advanced telecommunication systems-design work. Journal of Occupational and Environmental Medicine*, 38 (1), 53–65.

Arnetz, B.B. (1997) *Technological stress: psychophyiolgocial aspects of working with modern information technology. Scandinavian Journal of Work Environment and Health*, 23 (suppl. 3), 97–103.

Barrios-Choplin, B., McCraty, R. and Cryer, B. (1997) *An inner quality approach to reducing stress and improving physical and emotional well-being at work. Stress Medicine*, 13 (3), 193–201.

Benowitz, N. L. and Henningfield, J. E. (1994) *Establishing a nicotine threshold for addiction: the implications for tobacco regulation. New England Journal of Medicine*, 331, 123–125.

Bertera, R. L. (1990a) *Planning and implementing health promotion in the workplace: a case study of the DuPont Company experience. Health Education Quarterly*, 17 (3), 307–327.

Bertera, R. L. (1990b) *The effects of workplace health promotion on absenteeism and employment costs in a large, industrial population. American Journal of Public Health*, 80, 1101–1105.

Bertera, R. L. (1991) *The effects of behavioral risks on absenteeism and health care costs in the workplace. Journal of Occupational Medicine*, 33 (11), 1119–1124.

Bertera, R. L. (1993) *Behavioral risk factor and illness day changes with workplace health promotion: two-year results. American Journal of Health Promotion*, 7 (5), 36–73.

Bertera, R. L. (2000) *Commentary on Polanyi* et al. *(op.cit.).* In B. D. Poland, L. W., Green and I. Rootman (Eds) *Settings for Health Promotion: Linking theory and Practice*. Sage, Thousand Oaks, CA.

Biener, L., DePue, J. D., Emmons, K. M., Linnan, L. and Abrams, D. B. (1994) *Recruitment of worksites to a health promotion research trial: implications for generalizability. Journal of Occupational Medicine*, 36, 631–636.

Blair, S. N., Piserchia, P. V., Wilbur, C. S. and Crowder, J. H. (1986a) *Health promotion for* educators: impact on absenteeism. *Preventive Medicine*, 15, 166–175.

Blair, S. N., Piserchia, P. V., Wilbur, C. S. and Crowder, J. H. (1986b) *A public health intervention model for work-site health promotion. Journal of the American Medical Association*, 255, 921–926.

Bly, J. L., Jones, R. C. and Richardson, J. E. (1986) *Impact of worksite health promotion on health care costs and utilization. Journal of the American Medical Association*, 256, 3235–3240.

Bosquet, M. (1977) *Capitalism in Crisis and Everyday Life* (trans. J. Howe). Harvester Press, Hassocks.

Braun, S. and Hollander, R. (1987) *A study of job stress among women and men in the Federal Republic of Germany. Health Education Research*, 2, 45–51.

Brenner, H. and Fleischle, B. (1994) *Smoking regulations at the workplace and smoking behavior: a study from southern Germany. Preventive Medicine*, 23 (2), 230–234.

Brenner, H., Born, J., Novak, P. and Wanek, V. (1997) *Smoking behavior and attitude toward smoking regulations and passive smoking in the workplace. A study among 974 employees in the German metal industry. Preventive Medicine*, 23 (2), 138–143.

Broder, I., Pilger, C. and Corey, P. (1993) *Environment and well-being before and following smoking ban in office buildings. Canadian Journal of Public Health*, 84 (4), 254–258.

Buck, A. (1982) *Promoting Health and Safety at Work*. University of Nottingham/Nottingham Health Education Unit, Nottingham.

Burke, R. J. (1993) *Organizational level interventions to reduce occupational stressors. Work and Stress*, 7 (1), 77–87.

Chen, M. S. (1984) *Proving the effects of health promotion in industry: an academician's perspective. Health Education Quarterly*, 10, 235–245.

Chu, C., Driscoll, T. and Dwyer, S. (1997) *The health promoting workplace: an integrative perspective. Australia and New Zealand Journal of Public Health*, 21, 377–385.

Chu, C., Breucker, G., Harris, N., Stitzel, A., Gan, X., Xueqi, G. and Dwyer, S. (2000) *Health-promoting workplaces – international settings development. Health Promotion International*, 15 (2), 155–167.

Conrad, K. M., Campbell, R. T., Edington, D. S., Faust, H. S. and Vilnius, D. (1996) *The worksite environment as a cue to smoking reduction. Research in Nursing and Health*, 19 (1), 21–31.

Conrad, P. (1988a) *Worksite health promotion: the social context. Social Science and Medicine*, 26, 485–489.

Conrad, P. (1988b) *Health and fitness at work: a participant's perspective. Social Science and Medicine*, 26, 545–550.

Cook, R. F., Back, A. S. and Trudeau, J. (1996) *Preventing alcohol use problems among blue-collar workers: a field test of the Working People program. Substance Use Misuse*, 31 (3), 255–275.

Cooper, C. L. (1985) *The road to health in American firms. New Society*, 73, 335–336.

Daines, J., Gralian, B., Brown,. G., Edmondson, R. E. and Atkins, M. (1986) *'Look After Yourself' 1978–86: Innovation and Outcomes*. Department of Adult Education for Health Education Council, Nottingham.

Davis, M. F., Rosenberg, K., Iverson, D. C., Vernon, T. M. and Bauer, J. (1984) *Worksite health promotion in Colorado*, Public Health Reports 99, pp. 538–543.

Denyer, B. (1986) *Reducing the incidence of eye injuries. Occupational Health*, 38, 112–114.

Eakin, J. M. (2000) *Commentary on Promoting the determinants of good health in the workplace*. In B. D. Poland, L. W. Green and I. Rootman (Eds) *Settings for Health Promotion: Linking Theory and Practice*. Sage, Thousand Oaks, CA.

Eakin, J. M. and Weir, N. (1995) *Canadian approaches to the promotion of health in small workplaces. Canadian Journal of Public Health*, 86, 109–113.

Erfurt, J. C., Foote, A. and Heirich, N. A. (1991) *Worksite wellness programs: incremental comparison of screening and referral alone, health education, follow-up counselling, and plant organization. American Journal of Health Promotion*, 5 (6), 438–448.

Federal Institute for Occupational Safety and Health (1996) *European Network Workplace Health Promotion, 1st Meeting of the Member States, Reports of the Workshop on 21 June, 1995 in Dortmund*, Conference Report Tb72. Wirtschaftsverlag NW, Bremerhaven.

Foster, A. (1983) *Hearing protection and the role of health education. Occupational Health*, 35, 155–158.

Freudenberg, N. (1981) *Health education for social change: a strategy for public health in the US.*

*International Journal of Health Education*, XXIV, 1–8.

Freudenberg, N. (1985) *Training health educators for social change. International Quarterly of Community Health Education*, 5, 37–52.

Fuchs, J. A., Price, J. E. and Marcotte, B. (1985) *Worksetting health promotion – a comprehensive bibliography. Health Education*, 16, 29.

Glasgow, R. E., Hollis, J. H., Ary, D. V. and Boles, S. M. (1993) *Results of a year-long incentives-based worksite smoking-cessation program. Addictive Behaviors*, 18 (4), 455–464.

Gordon, J. (1987) *Workplace health promotion: the right idea in the wrong place. Health Education Research*, 2, 69–71.

Green, L. W. and Kreuter, M. W. (1999) *Health Promotion Planning: An Educational and Ecological Approach*, 2nd edn. Mayfield, Mountain View, CA.

Griffiths, A. (1996) *The benefits of employee exercise programmes. Work and Stress*, 10 (1), 5–23.

Harris, S. L. and Ewing, J. W. (1989) *The total life concept transplanted from AT&T to Sandia National Laboratories. American Journal of Health Promotion*, 4 (2), 118–127.

Hawe, P., Degeling, D. and Hall, J. (1990) *Evaluating Health Promotion: A Health Worker's Guide.* Maclennan and Petty, Australia.

Health Project (1994) *1994 Everett Koop Awards Programs Highlight the Rising Tide of Demand Reduction to Cut Health Costs*, press release, October 17.

Hollander, R. B. and Lengermann, J. J. (1988) *Corporate characteristics and worksite health promotion programs: survey findings from Fortune 500 companies. Social Science and Medicine*, 26, 491–501.

Howells, R. and Barrett, B. (1975) *The Health and Safety at Work Act. A Guide for Managers.* Institute of Personnel Management, London.

Hopson, B. and Scally, M. (1981) *Lifeskills Teaching.* McGraw-Hill, London.

Ippolito-Shepherd, J. I., Feldman, R., Acha, P. N. *et al.* (1987) *Agricultural occupational health and health education in Latin America and the Carribbean. Health Education Research*, 2, 53–59.

Jason, L. A., Gruder, L., Buckenberger, L. *et al.* (1987) *A 12 month follow-up of a worksite smoking cessation intervention. Health Education Research*, 2, 185–194.

Jeffery, R. W., Forster, J. L., Dunn, B. V., French, S. A.,

McGovern, P. G. and Lando, H. A. (1993) *Effects of work-site health promotion on illness-related absenteeism. Journal of Occupational Medicine*, 35 (11), 1142–1146.

Jeffery, R. W., Kelder, S. H., Forster, J. L. and French, S. A. (1994) *Restrictive smoking policies in the workplace: effects on smoking prevalence and cigarette consumption. Preventive Medicine*, 23 (1), 78–82.

Jenkins, M. and McEwen, J. (1987) *Smoking Policies At Work.* Health Education Authority, London.

Karasek, R. A. and Theorell, T. (1990) *Healthy Work: Stress, Productivity, and the Reconstruction of Working Life.* Basic Books, New York, NY.

Kerr, J. H. and Vos, M. C. H. (1993) *Employee fitness programs, absenteeism and general well-being. Work and Stress*, 7 (2), 179–190.

Klesges, R. C., Glasgow, R. E., Klesges, L. M. Merray, K. and Quale, R. (1987) *Competition and relapse prevention training in worksite smoking modification. Health Education Research*, 2, 5–14.

Knobel, R. J. (1983) *Health promotion and disease prevention: improving health while conserving resources. Family and Community Health*, 1, 16–27.

Kotarba, J. A. and Bentley, P. (1988) *Workplace wellness participation and the becoming of self. Social Science and Medicine*, 26, 551–558.

Lechner, L., de Vries, H., Adriaansen, S. and Drabbels, L. (1997) *Effects of an employee fitness program on reduced absenteeism. Journal of Occupational and Environmental Medicine*, 39 (9), 827–831.

Marmot, M. (1994) *Work and other factors influencing coronary health and sickness absence. Work and Stress*, 8 (2), 191–201.

McEwen, J. (1987) *Health and work.* In I. Sutherland (Ed.) *Health Education: Perspectives and Choices*, 2nd edn. National Extension College, Cambridge.

Michie, S. (1996) *Reducing absenteeism by stress management: valuation of a stress counselling service. Work and Stress*, 10 (4), 367–372.

MRFIT Research Group (1982) *Multiple risk factor intervention trial: risk facto changes and mortality results. Journal of the American Medical Association*, 248 (12), 1465–1477.

Murphy, L. R. (1996) *Stress management in work settings: a critical review of the health effects. American Journal of Health Promotion*, 11 (2), 112–135.

Murza, G., Annuss, R. and Dickersbach, M. (1994) *'Hab ein Herz fur Dein Herz' (Have a Heart for*

*Your Heart) – a worksite health promotion programme on cardiovascular risk factors. Irish Journal of Psychology*, 15 (1), 191–202.

Navarro, V. (1976) *Medicine Under Capitalism.* Croom Helm, London.

Nelson, D. J., Sennett, L., Lefebvre, R. C. *et al.* (1987) *A campaign strategy for weight loss at worksites. Health Education Research*, 2, 27–31.

Northwestern National Life Insurance Company (1994) *Back to Work: Managing Disability, Recovery and Re-employment.* Employee Benefits Division, Minneapolis, MN.

Novick, M. (1987) *The new work agenda into the nineties. Work and Well-Being Quarterly*, Fall, 26–30.

Paoli, P. (1992) *First European Survey on the Work Environment 1991–1992.* European Foundation for the Improvement of Working and Living Conditions, Dublin.

Parkinson, R. S., Beck, R. N. and Collings, G. H. (Eds) (1982) *Managing Health Promotion in the Workplace.* Mayfield, Palo Alto, CA.

Peersman, G., Harden, A. and Oliver, S. (1998) *Effectiveness of Health Promotion Interventions in the Workplace.* Health Education Authority, London. (See also Summary of Main Findings at http://www.hea.org.uk/research/download/review13.htm.)

Peterson, P. E. (1989) *Evaluation of a dental preventive program for Danish chocolate workers. Community Dental Epidemiology*, 17, 53–59.

Platt, S., Pavis, S. and Akram, G. (2000) *Changing Labour Market Conditions and Health: A Systematic Literature Review (1993–1998).* European Foundation for the Improvement of Living and Working Conditions, Dublin. (See also http://www.EuroFound.ie/files/html/EF9915EN_8.shtml.)

Polanyi, M. F. D., Frank, J. W., Shannon, H. S., Sullivan, T. J. and Lavis, J. N. (2000) *Promoting the determinants of good health in the workplace.* In B. D. Poland, L. W. Green and I. Rootman (Eds) *Settings for Health Promotion: Linking Theory and Practice.* Sage, Thousand Oaks, CA.

Pollock, D. (1999) *Denial and Delay: The Political History of Smoking and Health, 1951–1964.* Action on Smoking and Health, London.

Queensland Health (1996) *Better Health for Working People: Guiding Principles.* Queensland Health, Brisbane.

Renaud, M. (1994) *The future: Hygeia versus Panakeil?* In R. G. Evans, M. L. Barer and T. R. Marmor (Eds) *Why are Some People Healthy and Others Not? The Determinants of Health of Populations.* Putnam, New York, NY.

Reynolds, S. (1997) *Psychological well-being at work: is prevention better than cure? Journal of Psychosomatic Research*, 43 (1), 93–102.

Rifkin, J. (1995) *The End of Work: the Decline of the Global Labor Force and the Dawn of the Post-market Era.* Putnam, New York, NY.

Roman, P. M. and Blum, T. C. (1987) *The relation of employee assistance programs to corporate social responsibility attitudes: an empirical study.* In L. E. Preston (Ed.) *Research in Corporate Social Performance and Policy.* JAI Press, Greenwich, CT, pp. 213–235.

Roman, P. M. and Blum, T. C. (1988) *Formal intervention in employee health: comparisons of the nature and structure of employee assistance programs and health promotion programs. Social Science and Medicine*, 26, 503–514.

Russell, L. (1986) *Is Prevention Better than Cure?* Brookings Institute, Washington, DC.

Sass, R. (1989) *The implications of work organization for occupational health policy: the case of Canada. International Journal of Health Services*, 19 (1), 157–173.

Schelling, T. (1986) *Economics and cigarettes. Preventive Medicine*, 15, 549–560.

Schenck, A. P., Thomas, R. P., Hochbaum, G. M. and Beliczty, L. S. (1987) *A labor and industry focus on education: using baseline survey data in program design. Health Education Research*, 2, 33–44.

Schnall, P. L., Landsbergis, P. A. and Baker, D. (1994) *Job sharing and cardiovascular disease. Annual Review of Public Health*, 15, 381–411.

Shephard, R. J., Porey, P. and Cox, M. H. (1982) *The influence of an employee fitness and lifestyle modification program upon medical care costs. Canadian Journal of Public Health*, 73, 259–263.

Shi, L. (1993a) *Worksite health promotion and changes in medical care use and sick days. Health Values: Journal of Health Behavior, Education and Promotion*, 17 (5), 9–17.

Shi, L. (1993b) *Health promotion, medical care use, and costs in a sample of worksite employees. Evaluation Review*, 17 (5), 475–487.

Sloan, R. P. (1987) *Workplace health promotion: the North American experience.* In H. Matheson (Ed.) *Health Promotion in the Workplace.* Scottish Health Education Group, Edinburgh.

Smith, M. J. (1997) *Psychosocial aspects of working with video display terminals (VDTs) and employee physical and mental health. Ergonomics*, 40 (10), 1002–1015.

Sonnenstuhl, W. and Trice, H. (1986) *Strategies for Employee Assistance Programs: The Crucial Balance*. IRL Press, Ithaca, NY.

Sorensen, G., Glasgow, R. E. and Corbett, K. (1900) *Involving work sites and other organizations*. In N. Bracht (Ed.) *Health Promotion at the Community Level*. Sage, Newbury Park, CA.

Spilman, M. A. (1988) *Gender difference in work-site health promotion activities. Social Science and Medicine*, 26, 525–535.

Street, C. G. (1987) Unpublished MSc dissertation, Department of Community Medicine, University of Manchester.

Swift, J. (1995) *Time and work. Canadian Forum*, 74 (841), 9–12.

Syme, S. L. (1988) *Social epidemiology and the work environment. International Journal of Health Services*, 18 (4), 635–645.

Syme, S. L. (1994) *The social environment and health*. In *Proceedings of the 11th Annual Honda Foundation Discoveries Symposium*. Canadian Institute for Advanced Research, Toronto, pp. 59–64.

Symington, I. (1987) *Health promotion in the workplace: legislative aspects*. In H. Matheson (Ed.) *Health Promotion in the Workplace*. Scottish Health Education Group, Edinburgh.

Toffler, A. (1970) *Future Shock*. Bodley Head, London.

Tully, S. (1995) *Fortune: America's healthiest companies. Fortune Magazine*, 98–100.

US Department of Health and Human Services (1980) *Promoting Health/Preventing Disease: Objectives for the Nation*. US Department of Health and Human Services, Washington, DC.

US Department of Health, Education and Welfare (1979) *Healthy People: The Surgeon General's Report on Health Promotion and Disease Prevention*. US Department of Health, Education and Welfare, Washington, DC.

Veen, C. and Vereijken, I. (1994) *Promoting Health at Work: A Review of the Effectiveness of Health Education and Health Promotion*. IUHPE/NIGZ, Woerden.

Vojtecky, M. A., Kar, S. B. and Cox, S. G. (1985) *Workplace health education: results from a national survey. International Quarterly of Community Health Education*, 5, 171–185.

Walker, C. (1993) *Workplace Stress*. Canadian Autoworkers Union, Willowdale, Ontario.

Walsh, D. C. (1988) *Toward a sociology of worksite health promotion: a few reactions and reflections. Social Science and Medicine*, 26, 569–575.

Warner, K. E. (1987) *Selling health promotion to corporate America. Health Education Quarterly*, 14, 39–55.

Wilson, M. G., Holman, P. B. and Hammock, A. (1996) *A comprehensive review of the effects of worksite health promotion on health related outcomes. American Journal of Health Promotion*, 10 (6), 429–435.

World Health Organization (1987) *Health Promotion in the Working World*. WHO European Regional Office, Copenhagen.

World Health Organization (1992) *Health Dimensions of Economic Reform*. WHO, Geneva.

World Health Organization (1997) *WHO's Global Healthy Work Approach*. Education and Communication and Office of Occupational Health, WHO, Geneva.

World Health Organization–Western Pacific Regional Office (1998) *Regional Guidelines for the Development of Healthy Workplaces*. WPRO, Manila.

# 8 THE MASS MEDIA AND HEALTH PROMOTION

*Advertising has always been wreathed in metaphysical mists. From the time of the first medicine-man selling snake oil from the back of the stagecoach, to the self-induced hypnosis created by so-called 'subliminal' advertising, to the about-to-be wonders of global commercials via satellite, there has always been a need on the part of some people, at least, to believe in the talismanic properties of advertising and its supposed power to 'manipulate' its audience.*

Torin Douglas (1984)

In this chapter the mass media are viewed in the same strategic way as, for instance, community development, patient education or schools. Just as schools have particular characteristics and may thus make a qualitatively different impact from, say, informal education in the community, mass media have their peculiar strengths and weaknesses. Ideally they would be used as part of a comprehensive programme which employs the range of strategies and agencies described earlier in this book. All too frequently they have been used in far from splendid isolation – either because the prospect of a fully coordinated programme has been too daunting or, more likely, because they have been assumed to possess a power akin to that of a kind of educational 'magic bullet'. The view expressed below is not unique to Dr Goebbels!

**Box I**   The Power of Propaganda

*Nothing is easier than leading the people on a leash. I just hold up a dazzling campaign poster and they jump through it.*

(Joseph Goebbels, cited in Rhodes, 1976)

It should by now be clear that to ask whether health promotion works is to ask a meaningless question. This tenet certainly applies to the analysis of mass communication campaigns which, over the years, have been the cause of much heated debate about effectiveness and efficiency. Rather than asking whether mass media work, we should be asking what kind of effect we might expect from different kinds of media used in different situations and contexts to present different sorts of message about different subjects to different target groups. We must also ask questions about both the intended and unintended or incidental effects of mass media and examine the extent to which such effects should be taken into consideration or even deliberately manoeuvred as a tool of health promotion.

We are faced with a complex picture and yet it is possible to provide valid generalisations both at the level of communication theory and at the more pragmatic level of guidance for users. This chapter will, then, seek to illuminate certain key issues in the use of mass media. It will examine the peculiar features of the media and their different forms; it will consider the incidental and unplanned effects of media; it will discuss the essential elements of different theories and models of mass communication and their pragmatic application in social marketing; it will ask what lessons might be learned about marketing health and will place particular emphasis on pre-testing. Given our interest in equity, we will also note how mass media can be guilty of victim blaming in a brief review of the contribution they might make to remedying inequalities in health. We will subsequently emphasise the importance of mass media's political role in promoting healthy public policy by means of the techniques of agenda setting and media advocacy. The chapter will conclude with a sampler of health education programmes having a major mass media component, reinforcing

the general – and perhaps stunningly obvious –
point that a successful community programme
incorporates mass media as a subsidiary but important element within the programme as a whole.

## THE MEANING OF MASS MEDIA

As the words suggest, the two key features of mass
media are their mass audience and the fact that
there is no inter-personal communication
between the originator of the message and the
mass audience: the message is mediated. It is the
mass audience which is so enticing to the communicator since it offers the seductive but illusory
prospect of instant influence.

**Box 2**  Potential Benefits of Mass Communication

> *... nothing but a newspaper can drop the same
> thought into a thousand minds at the same
> moment.*
>
> (de Tocqueville, cited in Paisley, 1981)

Goebbels experienced a similar but more ambitious optimism for his propaganda ministry! With
the advent of radio and television the possibility of
wholesale change at national or even international
level created joy in the minds of those seeking to
manipulate population behaviours and alarm in the
minds of those who wished to preserve the integrity
of individual freedom to think and decide. However, although it is certainly possible to contact a
mass audience, the second major characteristic of
mass media makes it extremely unlikely that the
population might be manipulated at the whim of the
propagandist. In other words, the fact that the message is mediated makes it impossible to gain immediate feedback of the results of the communication
and thus provide a tailor-made communication
which is responsive to the needs, personality and
moods of the audience.

## Mass media: limits to communication

As has so often been noted, the blunderbuss
attributes of mass media are inconsistent with
offering the 'different strokes for different folks'

which are a component of an efficient influence
process. Figure 8.1 makes this important point
about feedback and reminds us of the difference
between communication and education.

In inter-personal communication the communicator effectively codes a message for transmission to an audience (typically one person or a
small group of people). The format of the message
will most often be symbolic (e.g. written or spo-
ken speech) but may be iconic, in which case pictures may be used to clarify the message.
Alternatively, because it is considered likely to
produce certain learned outcomes, an enactive
format could be employed. This would require
some form of audience participation to communicate the message and achieve the communicator's
purpose. For example, role play might be used to
increase awareness of a social issue or to change
audience attitudes. Non-verbal communication is
an important component of the whole communication package.

It is of course apparent that mass media may
simulate some of the features of this communication process – the presenter of a television programme may be specially chosen to be credible to
the audience and may seek to ensure that his or
her non-verbal communication is consonant with
the programme goals. Again, a variety of iconic
messages may be used on television or other visual
media. Some attempt may be made to achieve
audience participation. However, there is no way
of knowing whether or not the audience has participated, has responded to the pictures or the
charm of the presenter or whether, indeed, the
audience has even understood the various messages let alone acted upon them. Although feedback may be provided for media producers – in
the form of audience research, return of newspaper coupons, measures of population behaviour
before and after programmes – there is no instant
and observable response from the individuals
comprising the audience. Audience phone-ins
during radio programmes probably provide the
closest approximation, but the encounter is typically very short and excludes the majority of the
listeners. Delayed feedback is no substitute for
immediate feedback if anything other than the

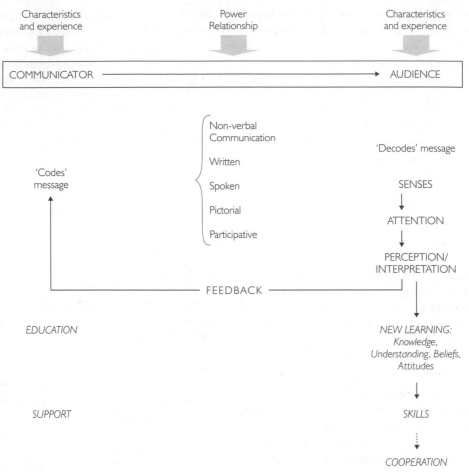

**Figure 8.1** The Communication Process

communication of relatively simple messages is to be achieved comprehensively and efficiently. Moreover, immediate feedback not only allows the communicator to repeat, clarify and vary the message, it enables him or her to look for unwanted side-effects such as the arousal of excessive anxiety, a point of some ethical importance.

Clearly with the prospects of dramatic developments in interactive electronic communication via the Internet, the lack of immediate media feedback may be rectified. However, it is more likely that Internet programmes will have more in common with programmed learning (see below) than with mass media *per se*.

Most communication attempts are concerned to do more than ensure that the message has been correctly interpreted and understood. In reality their purpose is to generate some learned outcome: the acquisition of new information or understanding; a change in belief and attitude; the learning of a new skill and even the adoption of a new practice or change in lifestyle. As noted in Chapter 2, it is usually acknowledged by media workers that there is a 'hierarchy of effects': it is relatively easy to 'agenda set' and communicate simple information; it is increasingly difficult to change attitudes, teach complex skills and persuade people to adopt new behaviours, especially where these involve exertion, discomfort or the abandoning of pleasure! The various intermediate indicators of programme success which were described in Chapter 2 and the model underlying these relate to this communication dilemma for the mass media. In order to achieve the more difficult and often long-term outcomes, the requirements of immediate feedback and the personalising of approaches make it difficult for mass media to compete with interpersonal education.

Before proceeding to clarify further the capabilities of different forms of media, we should note the distinction between mass media and the various media devices used as adjuncts to inter-personal communication and education.

***Box 3*** Mass Media and Learning Resources

> The strengths and weaknesses of mass media are inherent in the words themselves.
>
> *Mass* implies potential access to very large numbers of people in one instant in time.
>
> *Media* implies that the message is mediated and, consequently, there is a lack of immediate feedback potential in the message transmitted.
>
> There is a fundamental difference between mass media and superficially similar devices used as audio-visual aids to inter-personal education.

The film used as an audio-visual aid to a lecture or as a trigger for group discussion may appear superficially similar to a mass media television programme. In effect the film is a learning resource which is part of the iconic and enactive format of the communication; it is directly controlled by the communicator without loss of the important feedback principle. A good example of such use is provided by the work of Evans and McAlister based on McGuire's *Inoculation Theory* (McGuire, 1973; Evans *et al.*, 1978; McAlister and Hughes, 1979). These studies utilised film or video as part of a programme designed to inoculate young people against social pressures to smoke. By and large, film was effective in producing behavioural outcomes only when accompanied by other techniques such as peer-led teaching and structured role play. McAlis-

ter *et al.* (1980) were able to claim that students receiving this media-aided inter-personal teaching were recruited to smoking at less than half the rate of controls not receiving the programme. Similar results using lifeskills training in the field of substance misuse provide evidence of the importance of inter-personal education in the problematical arena of persuading the young ... *to eschew deeply satisfying activities which are validated by peer and other social pressures*. The effectiveness of mass media-based smoking programmes should be judged against this alternative – or rather complementary – approach (Botvin *et al.*, 1980).

Given a recent interest in 'tailoring' media or computer programmes to individual needs, it is important to note that tailoring can merely involve the design of, say, videos incorporating precise specification of target group characteristics. Insofar as such videos are used to enhance the effectiveness of professional education and counselling, they should be considered as an efficient learning resource (see for instance Eakin *et al.*, 1998). If they are to be provided to clients or patients without inter-personal education and support they should be considered as mass media – albeit media that has benefited from proper pre-testing (see later observations about the importance of pre-testing programmes).

It is interesting in this general context to consider the special case of programmed learning (or in the more up-to-date version, CAL – computer assisted learning). At first glance a programmed text or programme designed for use in audio-visual form would appear to have characteristics of a resource to be used as part of inter-personal education and at the same time share some of the features of mass media. A programme could, for instance, be used totally outside the inter-personal encounter, either on a self-access, student-centred basis or through mass distribution as a book. Since properly validated programmes are highly efficient teaching devices, this would appear to give the lie to earlier assertions about the limitations of mass media. The fact is, of course, that a programmed text or related device has (i) been designed for a specific audience (cf. the notion of audience segmentation below) and (ii) through the proper process of validation and standardisation, incorporates the principle of immediate feedback in its construction (providing the student with 'IKR' – immediate knowledge of results). The dissemination of such programmes with their intrinsic capacity to interact with the audience might well combine the advantages of inter-personal education with the attractions of reaching a mass audience. The implications for open learning and distance learning are self-evident, although a discussion of these is beyond the scope of this book. Reference to this tactic does, however, remind us of the heterogeneous nature of mass media, a fact we must consider before seeking to make generalisations.

## Media varieties

It is apparent that mass media vary considerably in their potential and capabilities, despite the common characteristics discussed above. They differ in form and format: leaflets and posters are substantially different from the electronic media of television and radio. They differ in their potential for reaching audiences and in the nature of the audience they reach: local radio listeners have different characteristics from readers of quality national press; in the UK, Open University and Channel Four documentaries will appeal to viewers who may not be addicted to soap opera. They differ in their credibility and trustworthiness.

Fuglesang (1981) offered a salutary reminder that modern media technology is relevant only to about 20% of the world population who can read and write and have access to electronic media. Folk media using, for example, puppets and the oral tradition of proverb and storytelling replace the technology and mass audience of western society. However, the focus of this book is primarily on developed countries and three examples will illustrate the different potential of various forms of media.

The first example illustrates the superiority of cinema advertising compared with what many would regard as the most powerful medium – television. Douglas (1984), in a guide to advertising, reminds us that cinema not only offers higher quality sound and image definition than television but also differs in audience composition and involvement (in addition to the fact that it is possible to advertise 'illicit' products in the cinema which it is not possible to present on television, at least in many countries). Douglas cites Marplan research which compared recall of a hitherto unknown product after exposure to cinema and television advertising. Young women who had seen the commercials were interviewed on the following day. Recall of the main point of the commercial by the cinema audience was 26%, compared with 9% by the television audience. In the context of discussion about what we might expect from media exposure, it is interesting to note that spontaneous recall was only 2% for the television audience (but 8% for the cinema audience). Recall after prompting went up a further 36% for television audiences compared with 56% for cinema audiences. Douglas ascribes this superiority to the greater impact produced by screen size, better sound and image quality and absence of distractions.

The second example offers evidence of the kind of result which might be expected from one of the trusty stock-in-trade media devices of the

**Box 4**   Media: 57 Varieties!

| Television | Radio | Postage stamps | Posters |
|---|---|---|---|
| Leaflets | Documentaries | Carrier bags | Film |
| Books | Newspapers | Sky writing | T-posters (buses) |
| Puppets | Song | Records and tapes | Fragrances and smells |
| Video (mass distribution) | Key rings | Displays and exhibitions | Etc. |

health promoter – the exhibition. Research carried out by the Transport and Road Research Laboratory (TRRL) in 1970 recorded numbers of people attending road safety exhibitions, audience characteristics and their source of information about the exhibition, their progress round the exhibition and the time spent at each exhibit or display. The TRRL adduced a number of important generalisations.

**Box 5**   Generalisations about Exhibitions

> - Attendance at even the best road safety exhibitions is unlikely to exceed 1000 per day. It is often much less than this. The prospects of getting at … (major target group) … are therefore extremely poor.
> - Local press publicity can increase the attendance by at least 50%.
> - The audience at exhibitions appears to be a broad cross-section of the population … it has not been possible to find whether they … are in most need of propaganda.
> - When going round exhibitions visitors tend to spend very short times at exhibits. The average time spent at many exhibits is less than one minute. None of the visitors see all the exhibits, many see less than half. Animated exhibits attract a lot of attention, but often distract visitors from the static displays.

The third example concerns credibility. It is an axiom of *Attitude Theory* that beliefs and attitudes are unlikely to change if the source of the communication is perceived to be untrustworthy, lack expertise or other forms of authority. A similar point is made in *Communication of Innovations Theory* by the principle of homophily. It is therefore interesting to ask whether different forms of mass media are more acceptable than others and whether these are more or less credible than alternative forms of inter-personal communication. Budd and McCron (1979) interviewed 692 adults from Central England and, among other things, invited them to indicate

how far they would trust information about changing one's life for the sake of one's health derived from each of 12 sources. These sources included medical personnel, lay people and media. The family doctor received the highest rating (an average score of 3.51 on a four point scale). The four lowest ratings (1.8, 1.72, 1.69 and 1.68, respectively) were accorded to a magazine articles, television adverts, newspaper articles and, last of all, a friend or neighbour. Radio and television documentaries scored at an intermediate level (2.43 and 2.39) but were boosted by having doctor involvement! Even the humble poster was rated third most credible when displayed in a GP's surgery or waiting room.

A more recent study (Kerr and Charles, 1983) makes a related point. However, while television advertising – especially about health – was treated with scepticism and mistrust, women's magazines and certain television personalities were often considered more credible than some health professionals, at any rate on the subject of feeding a family.

Table 8.1 lists characteristics of the most frequently used media channels.

## Incidental and unplanned effects of mass media

Before considering what the generalisations from *Mass Communication Theory* have to offer for health promotion practice we must note a further dimension to the classification of mass media effects. Whereas the main concern of health education is the development of programmes deliberately designed to influence audience characteristics, it is important to recognise that mass media may well have incidental and often unpredicted effects. Rather like the hidden curriculum in the school setting, these incidental effects may have to be taken into account as possibly unhealthy pressures or canalised in the interests of health promotion.

The fact that mass media can have a dramatic and unforeseen impact has been fully recognised since Cantril (1958) documented the sizeable panic produced among the citizenry by Orson Welles' production of H. G. Wells' *War of the Worlds* in the 1930s.

339

***Table 8.1***     Characteristics of mass media channels

*Television*
- Potentially largest range of audiences, but not always at times when public service announcements (PSAs) are most likely to be broadcast.
- Deregulation ended government (US) oversight of station broadcasting of PSAs and public affairs programming
- Opportunity to include health messages via news broadcasts, public affairs/interview shows and dramatic programming
- Visual as well as audio make emotional appeals possible; easier to demonstrate a behaviour
- Can reach low income and other audiences not as likely to turn to health sources for help
- Passive consumption by viewer; viewers must be present when message is aired; less than full attention likely; message may be obscured by commercial 'clutter'
- PSAs can be expensive to produce and distribute; feature placement requires contacts and may be time consuming

*Radio*
- Various formats, offering potential for more audience targeting than TV (e.g. teenagers via rock stations); may reach fewer people than TV
- Deregulation ended government oversight of station broadcasting of PSAs and public affairs programming
- Opportunity for direct audience involvement via call-in shows
- Audio alone may make messages less intrusive
- Can reach audiences who do not use the health care system
- Generally passive consumption; exchange with audience possible, but target audience must be there when aired
- Live copy is flexible and inexpensive; PSAs must fit station format
- Feature placement requires contacts and may be time consuming.

*Magazines*
- Can more specifically target segments of the public (e.g. young women, people with an interest in health)
- No requirement for PSA use; PSAs more difficult to place
- Can explain more complex health issues and behaviours
- Print may lend itself to more factual, detailed, rational message delivery
- Audience has chance to clip, re-read and contemplate material
- Permits active consultation; may be passed on; can be read at reader's convenience.
- PSAs are inexpensive to produce; ad or article placement may be time consuming

*Newspapers*
- Can reach broad audiences rapidly
- PSAs virtually non-existent
- Can convey health news and breakthroughs more thoroughly than TV or radio and more quickly than magazines; feature placement possible
- Easy audience access to in-depth issue coverage is possible
- Short life of newspaper limits re-reading and sharing with others
- Small papers may take public service ads; coverage demands a newsworthy item

*Adapted from Making Health Communication Programs Work: A Planner's Guide (Information Projects Branch Office of Cancer Communications, National Cancer Institute, Bethesda, MD; http://rex.nci.nih.gov/nci_pub_interface/hcpw/home.htm).*

**Box 6**  The Invasion from Mars

> *... long before the broadcast had ended people all over the United States were praying, crying, fleeing frantically to escape death from the Martians. Some ran to their loved ones, others telephoned farewells or warnings, hurried to inform neighbours, sought information from newspapers or radio stations, summoned ambulances and police cars.*
>
> *At least six million people heard the broadcast. At least a million of them were frightened or disturbed.*
>
> (Hadley Cantril, 1958)

Less dramatic but more insidious is the way in which press and television report health issues. Even the recording of a cancer cure is likely to be couched in terms which reinforce the general alarm and pessimism conjured up by the very term. Wellings (1986) makes a similar point about the public's processing of media reporting of the 1983 'pill scare'. Draper and colleagues made related points about the ways in which the very grammar of television reporting tends to introduce bias which, for example, favours the supremacy of high technology medicine at the expense of the less glamorous but potentially more beneficial preventive and health promotion measures (Best *et al.*, 1977) – a point that will be reiterated in a later discussion of media advocacy.

Again the incidental presentation of health issues in entertainment programmes and soap opera may foster misleading images and attitudes. Characterisation may serve to validate images of unhealthy lifestyles as part of a norm-sending process. The portrayal of alcohol on television conveys a norm of heavy drinking and associates consumption of alcohol with benefits rather than costs (Institute for Alcohol Studies, 1985; Hansen, 1986).

The impact of advertising unhealthy products is a highly contentious political issue. Advocates of advertising, not unsurprisingly, stress its social benefits and minimise the negative effect on recruitment (Henry and Waterson, 1981). The effect of cigarette promotion on children has been the subject of research (Chapman and Fitzgerald, 1982; Charlton, 1986; Piepe *et al.*, 1986; Aitken *et al.*, 1987). Although it is not yet possible to demonstrate unequivocally that there is a causal relationship between advertising, sponsorship and smoking recruitment, it seems likely that children who smoke are generally more aware of cigarette advertising and sponsorship than non-smokers and more favourably disposed to the brands. What is clear is that such advertising and sponsorship establishes a hidden curriculum which legitimises smoking and denotes its continuing acceptability.

We will now, however, turn to the deliberate use of mass media to produce desired learning outcomes, focusing particularly on their potential for producing behaviour change and the adoption of approved practices.

## MASS MEDIA THEORY

Throughout this book we have emphasised the importance of theory in making sound decisions about how best to evaluate health promotion programmes: how to be sure about the ideological basis of action; how to select appropriate indicators of success; how to interpret results. Theoretical understanding is especially important in the field of mass media interventions – given their susceptibility to politically inspired wishful thinking. For the reasons mentioned above – the potential of mass communication for providing a quick fix in ensuring rapid adoption of desirable behaviours by whole population groups – mass media are frequently treated as panaceas. The fact that action is frequently undertaken in apparent ignorance of existing, well-established theory merely reiterates the value of making clear just what theoretical alternatives are available. Accordingly, a number of key theoretical perspectives will be explored below.

**Box 7**  Models of Mass Media Effect

- Hypodermics and aerosols.
- Social context and Marxist explanations.
- Uses and gratifications.

## Hypodermics and aerosols

An analysis of research and theory into the effects of mass media suggests a shift in opinion over the years from an apparently magical belief in their omnipotence (fostered perhaps by a mixture of Dr Goebbels and Vance Packard) to an almost totally opposite assertion that mass media will not produce any significant changes in actual behaviour, especially in the difficult domain of health. As McQuail (1994) observes in his classic text,

*... the entire study of mass communication is based on the premise that the media have significant effects, yet there is little agreement on the nature and extent of these assumed effects.*

(p327)

Day, in a foreword to Douglas (1984), describes colourfully the emotion generated by the debate about the effectiveness of media advertising – as may be seen from the quotation at the head of this chapter! He observed,

*I have yet to see the evidence that advertising unsupported by product performance has ever had more than a temporary effect in persuading anyone to do anything against their own best interests.*

This view is consistent with the orthodoxy which came to replace the early '*direct effects*' or '*hypodermic*' models of media influence. According to the latter the community presented itself as a compliant patient for its injection. If the injection did not work either a different medicine was called for or a larger dose! The influence of Katz and Lazarsfeld (1955) and Lazarsfeld and Merton (1975) led to a kind of '*null effects*' model in which mass media were considered to have a minimal impact.

Katz and Lazarsfeld had questioned the power of mass media in their development of a two-step hypothesis of influence according to which the adoption of behaviours by a social group or community resulted from inter-personal interaction with opinion leaders who were (i) more receptive of media information than the mass of people and (ii) were sought out for advice by the community

and were thus relatively influential. Klapper's influential (1960) review consolidated this general view of media limitations. Reinforcement rather than conversion was the prime role of the media:

*Within a given audience exposed to particular communications, reinforcement, or at least constancy of opinion, is typically found to be the dominant effect (of mass media), minor change as in intensity of opinion is found to be the next most common; and conversion is typically found to be the most rare.*

(cited in Wallach, 1980 p15)

Mendelsohn (1968) also challenged a 'direct effects' model of mass media influence. In his somewhat poetic conceptualisation the image of the hypodermic is replaced by that of an aerosol:

*Rather than being a hypodermic needle, we now begin to look at mass communication as a sort of aerosol spray. As you spray it on the surface, some of it hits the target: most of it drifts away, and very little of it penetrates.*

It is worth noting in passing that Mendelsohn does acknowledge the possibility that at least some of the message hits the target even though presumably very little actually results in desired behaviour change.

It is apparent that the media influence process is a complex one. It should by now be clear that it is not enough to say that mass media can or cannot readily influence audience behaviour. One simple fact can, however, be stated: in normal circumstances mass media will not easily change people's behaviour unless individual motivation and normative influences are favourable. McKinlay's lament (1979) on the failure of mass media to promote health is eminently explicable when this simple fact is taken into account.

*How embarrassingly ineffective are our mass media efforts in the health field (e.g. alcoholism, obesity, drug abuse, safe driving, pollution, etc.) when compared with many of the tax-exempt promotional efforts on behalf of the illness generating activities of large-*

*scale corporations. It is a fact that we are demonstrably more effective in persuading people to purchase items they never dreamed they would need, or to pursue at risk courses of action, than we are in preventing or halting such behaviour.*

## The social context and Marxist explanations

A more cautiously optimistic view, based on a more thoughtful consideration of the wide range of mass media and their different usages, is currently prevalent. Indeed, as long ago as 1966 Klapper argued for a less 'black or white' approach to the discussion of whether mass media could in fact provide a new magic bullet (Klapper, 1997). He argues that:

*The old quest of specific effects stemming from the communication has given way to the observation of existing conditions or changes, followed by an inquiry into the factors, including mass communication, which produced those conditions and changes. … In short, attempts to assess a stimulus which was presumed to work alone have given way to an assessment of the role of that stimulus in a totally observed phenomenon.*

Again, Lazarsfeld and Merton (1975) had previously provided a simple explanation of those circumstances in which mass media might be expected to have an effect. One or more conditions must be met: '*monopolization*', i.e. where there are no contrary influences and messages; '*canalization*', i.e. where a particular message or recommendation for action plugs into existing motivations and preferences; '*supplementation*', i.e. where inter-personal efforts supplement media-based messages.

***Box 8*** Three Conditions for Mass Media Effectiveness

*Monopolization*
*Canalization*
*Supplementation*
(Lazarsfeld and Merton, 1975)

Budd and McCron (1979) emphasise that mass media influences cannot and should not be isolated from their social context. These influences:

*… interact and sometimes compete with, other sources of information and influences in complex ways, and that the individual selects, and compares from these diverse sources to construe a meaningful explanation for himself about particular issues which may, or may not, be in line with the intention behind any or all sources of information available to him.*

The social context can also be interpreted in terms of what Dorn and South (1983) refer to as a 'consensual paradigm', i.e. media collude with and encapsulate, in cliché and stereotype, social norms, exemplified by reference to the norm-sending role of soap operas and news reporting. Dorn (1981) further draws our attention to his preferred class cultural model which urges health educators to take account of the sub-cultural constructions of meaning of, for example, different social classes and ethnic groups. Ball-Rokeach and de Fleur (1976) propose a dependency model involving a tripartite relationship between media, audience and society. An interesting implication of the theory is that:

*… when people's social realities are entirely adequate … media messages may have little or no alteration effects. … In contrast, when people do not have social realities that provide adequate frameworks for understanding, acting and escaping, and when audiences are dependent in these ways on media information received, such messages may have a number of alteration effects.*

One particular view of the ways in which social context mediates mass communication messages is grounded in Marxist philosophy. Indeed, it epitomises the Marxist use of the term ideology (*… meaning in the service of power*; Fairclough, 1995). According to this view mass media are one of the means whereby a ruling class controls the masses. McQuail (1994) summarises this view succinctly as follows:

- mass media are owned by the bourgeois class;
- mass media operate in their class interest;
- mass media promote working class false consciousness;
- media access is denied to political opposition.

The validity of at least some of these points may be tested within the context of our later discussion of the barriers to media advocacy.

Berger (1991) also provides a more detailed Marxist analysis. He comments on the essence of this analysis as follows:

> *Marxist thought is one of the most powerful and suggestive ways available to the media analysis for analyzing society and its institutions.* (Chapter 2 of his book) ... *deals with such fundamental principles of Marxist analysis as alienation, materialism, false consciousness, class conflict, and hegemony – concepts that can be applied to media and that help us understand the ways media function.* (Of particular importance is) ... *the role of advertising in creating consumer lust ...* .
>
> (p32)

The various models discussed above tend to present an image of the mass media audience as a relatively passive entity which is more or less difficult to influence – depending on whether it is the hypodermic or the aerosol which is wielded. It is, however, misleading to consider the recipients of the message as either undifferentiated or passive. As was noted in an earlier chapter, *Communication of Innovations Theory* classifies the community into categories in accordance with their relative openness to change. This analysis is useful in that it not only views the audience as a heterogeneous group but also relates readiness to adopt innovations to the perceived characteristics of the new idea or practice and the likely costs or benefits which might result from adoption. In other words, the recipients of mass media messages neither passively accept nor reject the influence but rather analyse and interpret it in an active fashion, typically in the context of inter-personal interactions with family or friends. Clearly, the Marxist perspective would suggest that the analysis and interpretation may well be governed by false consciousness rather than on the basis of rational decision making or pure self interest.

Mendelsohn (1980) makes a distinction between '*Homo mechanicus*' and '*Homo volens*', the latter being an

> ... *active organism who often seeks out usable information – the dynamic individual who uses only that information he or she needs from the media while disregarding the useless stuff.*

This latter approach has elsewhere been referred to as a uses and gratifications model, suggesting as it does that the active recipient of media messages selects from those messages what (s)he needs to gratify current motivation.

As Dorn and South (1983) have pointed out, this interpretation is very acceptable to the promoters of unhealthy products since it denies accusations of manipulation of a naïve and gullible public! They also note how this conflicts with both right and left wing theories of media manipulating the populace. Right wing mass manipulative models view people as being often naïve and feckless and therefore corruptible by unhealthy media influences. Left wing theories view the mass of people as being subjected to control by a capitalist elite which uses its ownership of media to exploit its audience.

A full review of the *Uses* and *Gratifications* provided by mass media is not possible here (for a more complete view see Katz *et al.*, 1974; Rubin, 1983, 1994). To some extent the uses and gratifications approach is an extension of individual psychology in that it notes that human behaviour is goal directed and behaviours are adopted that result in gratifications of one sort or another (see our comments on the *Law of Effect* in Chapter 2). Again, consistent with the principles of selective attention, selective perception and defensive avoidance, media messages are filtered, assessed and selectively used for gratification. McQuail's (1994) revised view of the theory can be summarised in six principles:

*(1) Personal social circumstances and psychological dispositions together influence both, (2) general habits of media use and also, (3) beliefs and expectations about the benefits offered by media, which, in turn, shape, (4) specific acts of media choice and consumption, followed by, (5) assessments of the value of the experience (with consequences for further media use) and, possibly, (6) applications of benefits acquired in other areas of experience and social activity.*

(p319)

Apart from its implications for determining the likely success of media-based programmes with particular audiences, the *Uses and Gratifications Theory* provides an important challenge to those who bewail the corrupting effects of mass media on population values and morality. For instance, the death of one of the most popular and influential British 'agony aunts' – Marjorie Proops – was followed by suggestions (albeit from a minority) that her frank, open (and sensible) advice on sexual matters had contributed to an alleged moral decline in society. This assertion was vigorously challenged by another journalist (see Box 9).

**Box 9**   Dear Marje!

*People knew Miss Proops' views, as surely as they know the views of all journalists who write on a regular basis. ... When they wrote to her, they knew in advance what she would say. ... An estimated three per cent of the population did write to her, comfortable in the certainty that she thought what they thought. Not that she could form their thoughts for them. ... And as one reader said 'You put that so well; it's just what I have been thinking for ages'.*

(Carol Sarler, *Independent*, 15th November 1996)

Berger (1991) provides a comprehensive list of suggested gratifications offered by the media.

- To be amused.
- To see authority figures exalted or deflated.
- To experience the beautiful.
- To have shared experiences with others (community).
- To satisfy curiosity and be informed.
- To identify with the deity and the divine plan.
- To find distraction and diversion.
- To experience empathy.
- To experience, in a guilt-free and controlled situation, extreme emotions, such as love and hate, the horrible and the terrible, and similar phenomena.
- To find models to imitate.
- To gain an identity.
- To gain information about the world.
- To reinforce our belief in justice.
- To believe in romantic love.
- To believe in magic, the marvellous, and the miraculous.
- To see others make mistakes.
- To see order imposed on the world.
- To participate in history (vicariously).
- To be purged of unpleasant emotions.
- To obtain outlets for our sexual drives in a guilt-free context.
- To explore taboo subjects with impunity.
- To experience the ugly.
- To affirm moral, spiritual, and cultural values.
- To see villains in action.

Although a discussion of the above attractions is beyond the scope of this book, their relevance to health promotion – either substantively or as a marketing device – is doubtless obvious.

## On myth and the social construction of health messages

Reference has been made by Tones (1996) to the importance of one of the most useful perspectives on the ways in which mass media can provide gratification for an audience, namely 'discourse analysis' in general and the concept of myth in particular. Chapman and Egger (1983) have provided an especially perceptive review of the way in which cigarette advertising frequently validates prevailing dominant myths. In so doing it often manages to bypass the health implications of the product by emphasising the gains – but not just in terms of 'real' needs such as reducing withdrawal symptoms of tobacco dependency. According to the authors, myth is

*... any real or fictional story, recurring theme or character type that appeals to the consciousness of a group by embodying its cultural ideals or by giving expression to deep, commonly felt emotions.*

(p167)

Smokers, for instance, are *gratified* by advertisements that objectify real or sought after self-identity, attitudes and fantasies.

A glimpse of the mechanics of responding to myth is provided in the following brief summary of the authors' close scrutiny of the appeal of a number of Winfield cigarette advertisements that used the popular comedian and actor Paul Hogan as presenter.

In short, Hogan's real life identity as a social survivor who moved from relatively impoverished circumstances to fame (i.e. the 'rags to riches' myth) embodied an Australian ideal – someone who had not lost his working class roots but successfully negotiated all levels of society with panache and self-confidence. Hogan's 'source credibility' was cleverly supplemented by the message he delivered.

The message incorporated in the 'copy' and dramatisation was economically encapsulated in the linguistic meaning for Australians of the word '*anyhow*', which signifies a fatalistic and almost stoical shrug in the face of adversity. The advertising acknowledges the health problem as a kind of concealed sub-text and responds to the problem by its appeal to myth. As Chapman and Egger put it:

*Frightened of lung cancer? Well, never mind, it won't happen to you* (note the 'personal fable' mentioned in Chapter 2 in connection with faulty risk perception). *Still a little worried – well forget it. We've all gotta die ... . ANYHOW. Have a Winfield!*

(p175)

In contrast, the 'mythical' appeal of 'Marlborough Man' and the cigarettes he endorses is to people who feel *rushed, ordered, powerless, insignificant, lost for words and trapped in urban artifice.* The brand image offers freedom, power and signals one's own inner strength to others.

Interestingly, Chapman and Egger attempted to generate their own health promotion myth in the form of a 30 second TV spot which was based on the common denominator: smoker = loser; non-smoker = winner. It is, however, notoriously difficult to create myths about activities associated with NOT doing something! The problem of marketing healthy activities is, of course, one faced consistently by health promoters and health educators; we will give some detailed consideration to this below in the context of discussing *Social Marketing*.

## MAJOR MASS MEDIA STRATEGIES IN HEALTH PROMOTION

Hopefully, it will be clear that an understanding of the theories of mass media use outlined above should increase the likelihood of the judicious use of mass communication in the promotion of health. We will now consider a number of important mass media strategies that might be used by health promoters. We will start with a critical assessment of *Social Marketing* and subsequently consider the ways in which health promotion needs to address certain actual or potential negative influences of mass media on health by means of '*collaborative consultation*'. We will then argue the importance of *Media Advocacy* – the radical use of mass media to influence healthy public policy.

### Social marketing

The comparison that McKinlay (above) made between commercial advertising and health marketing is particularly apposite at a time when health promoters are urged to learn from the alleged superior expertise of commerce and adopt a marketing approach to influencing health- and illness-related behaviours. The relevance of *Social Marketing* will therefore now be considered. In particular it should be possible to see how recommended approaches articulate with *Communica-*

*tion Theory* as discussed above. Moreover, if we are to make sound judgements about the evaluation of mass media in health promotion, we should understand the kinds of expectations of success inherent in *Social Marketing* as well as noting the rules pertaining to efficient management of educational interventions using media. We must also note its limitations and ways in which the marketing of health differs fundamentally from marketing commercial products (Tones, 1994).

Marsden and Peterfreund (1984) argued that adoption of marketing principles would provide public health departments with a guide and incentive to help them

> *... shed a bureaucratic tradition and a lack-lustre image which compromises their ability to provide services and to function as authoritative sources of health information.*

Others, who have perhaps interpreted health promotion rather narrowly as a profile raising excursion into energetic media-backed publicity, look to commerce for tips on how to sell health (see for instance Docherty, 1981; Player, 1986). However, Bonaguro and Miaoulis (1983) outlined a marketing approach to Green's well-known *Precede Model* (Green and Kreuter, 1991) asserting that the goals of marketing and health promotion are similar. Since one of the major aims of this chapter is to examine what kinds of success we might realistically expect from mass media-based health education, it is clearly important to look critically at these claims for the *Social Marketing* approach. Do we have a new panacea or, more modestly, what insights can we gain from the best commercial practice for the marketing of health?

First of all, we should note that the notion of health marketing is not that recent a discovery. Lovelock (1977) commented on the value of marketing concepts and strategies for health marketers. He also referred the reader to earlier work by Kotler (1975) and Zaltman *et al.* (1972). More recently, Solomon (1989) identified 10 key marketing concepts having relevance for health promotion through public communication campaigns (Box 10).

**Box 10**   Ten Key Marketing Concepts

> - *The marketing philosophy;*
> - *The 'four Ps' of marketing;*
> - *Hierarchies of communication effects;*
> - *Audience segmentation;*
> - *Understanding all the relevant markets;*
> - *Information and rapid feedback systems;*
> - *Interpersonal and mass communication interactions;*
> - *Utilization of commercial resources;*
> - *Understanding the competition;*
> - *Expectations of success.*
>
> (Solomon, 1989)

These 10 concepts will serve as a basis for discussing what we might learn from commercial approaches to marketing but in order to assess their relevance we should be in no doubt about the fundamental differences between the selling of commercial products and the selling of health.

Two outstanding points emerge: (1) in general, people do not actually want to be healthy – or at any rate they prefer to avoid what is involved in getting healthy!; (2) unlike commercial campaigns which, after trying new brand images, abandon an unpopular product and produce something different that people do want, health promotion must continue to pursue its ethical and professional goals.

**Box 11**   Selling Health Like Soap

> *Marketing communications in nonbusiness situations or why it's so hard to sell brotherhood like soap.*
>
> (Rothschild, 1979)

As McCron and Budd (1987) have pointed out, the question of advertising effectiveness is shrouded in myth yet the popular view is not only that advertising is powerful but it must work because businesses spend so much money on it. It is, in fact, salutary to note the difference in expectations of success between businesses and those who look for quick results from health education! This is, however, only one of the distinctions between the commercial and public domains. These differences are summarised below.

- There is clearly a considerable difference in the size of budgets typically available to commercial and public domain communicators.
- Commercial advertisers would normally set much lower standards for success than commissioning health education programmes (see comments made in Chapter 2 about the hierarchy of communication effects and setting realistic standards). Whereas the latter would expect evidence of behaviour change – preferably dramatic – the former would have much lower ambitions and, for example, might not expect any change in sales at all. During the late 1970s a well-known chain of bakers spent some £300,000 on 10 television commercials. These were thought to have been a great triumph even though there had been no increase in volume sales. The firm was content to maintain their market share in the context of a general rise in bread consumption! (Reported in *Daily Mail*, 13 February 1980.)
- A more important distinction between the marketing of health and commercial products is the fundamental difference in the nature of the products on offer. The commercial product offers the customer gratification of some existing need; if the customer does not like the product, the manufacturer will produce something he or she does like or will change its image. The highly successful campaign to sell the chocolate bar *Yorkie* was in the last analysis based on people's liking for chocolate. The campaign's success lay in appropriate manipulation of brand image to appeal to psychological needs other than taste gratification. In contrast, health education frequently seeks to sell a product which commercial advertisers would consider no one in their right mind would buy! Potential customers are not uncommonly urged to stop doing something they find enjoyable and start doing something unpleasant or difficult. Playing with brand

imagery is of course possible (as we note later in our discussion of pre-testing), but this involves the adding of '*psychographic*' icing to an often rather unpalatable cake.

- What is more, the product which is being promoted by health education is frequently intangible and offers gratification at some indeterminate time in the (often distant) future. This almost exactly reverses the pattern of commercial sales techniques which promise immediate gratification, often on credit.
- A further important distinction concerns ethical considerations. While commercial advertising is now constrained to avoid blatant lying, it is by its very nature economical with the truth. Education, by definition, should be concerned with helping people make informed decisions (although there are proponents of a persuasive prevention model who are eager to use advertising techniques to manipulate and coerce). Again, health education should be concerned with avoiding unwanted side-effects such as anxiety or unresolved dissonance. Commercial advertising is also concerned to avoid negative images and connotations which are likely to have an immediate impact on sales figures. However, it is much easier to do this since the basic message is invariably positive: our product will meet your needs and make you feel good. Again, health education cannot, ethically, make a decision to ignore or abandon the equivalent of an unprofitable market. Indeed, disadvantaged groups and other 'resistants' to the sales talk often form the main market.
- Finally, because commercial advertising can rely on the pre-existence of audience motivation, the change in the audience which it seeks to produce is often limited to brand awareness and the creation of a positive attitude to the particular product. The behavioural response is relatively simple – the purchase of a product which in all probability differs from previously purchased products only in its physical or psychological packaging. Health education seeks to change deeply seated attitudes and even values and sometimes to produce the adoption of often complex behaviours.

- The very real differences between the marketing of health and commercial products should, however, not blind us to the lessons to be learned from good commercial marketing practice. Indeed, perhaps the most important lesson is that the products on sale are very different! We will use Solomon's 10 point analysis as a basis for the discussion.

## Market philosophy

The first point worthy of note has to do with the concept of 'market philosophy', which is based on the idea of 'exchange'', i.e. that there should be equity between marketer and consumer: the prime goal is to meet consumer needs (real or imagined); the customer is always right! As Marsden and Peterfreund (1984) reminded us, the cavalier presentation of health services would make the commercial marketer blush. Apart from the obvious need (in the words of the Ottawa Conference) to re-orient health services, the way in which some health educators patronise their clients can be counter-productive. Mendelsohn (1980) makes the point very forcibly (Box 12).

**Box 12**   What We Don't Need!

> Among the 'needs' we all have is not to be bombarded with information we already have or do not have any use for (e.g. information asserting that excessive drinking may be bad for us); not to be commanded to do something that is vague and unachievable without explicit simple instructions regarding its achievement (e.g. 'drive carefully'); not to be unreasonably frightened (e.g. any drinking during pregnancy, no matter how moderate, will surely result in the birth of a monster); and not to be insulted by the health communicator who implies that everyone the communicator is trying to address is (1) ignorant … (2) … sinfully 'irresponsible' in that they don't give a damn about their own lives/or the lives of others; and (3) they are slothfully 'apathetic' in not immediately doing without question what the communicator commands them to do.

An important question concerns the definition of consumer 'needs'. As we will see, community development urges us to base our programmes on 'felt needs'; frequently these needs do not match the epidemiological reality and require a complex negotiation with the client group which is beyond the scope of mass media.

## The four 'Ps': product, price, place, promotion

Solomon's second point was concerned with the four Ps, namely product, price, place and promotion – what others have called the *marketing mix*. There are clear messages for the health educator: the (health) product should be tangible, attractive and accessible. While some health promotions meet all three of these criteria, many others are unnecessarily vague. For example, the sale of condoms or wholemeal bread involves tangible products which are relatively accessible and which may be attractively packaged, but general messages to 'take more exercise' or 'look after yourself' are less tangible and, for a majority of people, inaccessible and downright unattractive. The relative lack of attractiveness of the product has already been noted but the notion of accessibility is of interest. While there may be an element of physical accessibility in health promotions (e.g. access to clinic or availability of healthy food) the question of psychological accessibility may be overlooked. It is clear that many people wish to adopt a healthier lifestyle but lack skills and support to do so. The lack of these facilities effectively renders the desired change inaccessible (see earlier references to the *Health Action Model*).

The matter of price is self-evident. In health promotion the cost is more likely to be psychosocial than financial. It is only necessary to remind the reader of the central part which the notion of costs and barriers plays in the *Health Belief Model* (discussed in Chapter 2).

Place and promotion may be considered together. Place emphasises the importance of distribution of the goods and retail outlets. Promotion reminds us that advertising is only one element of the marketing mix. The relevance of both of these will be taken up later when we consider the seventh of the 10 points.

## Hierarchy of communication effects

The third concept refers to the 'hierarchy of communication effects'. This relates to what we have elsewhere described as a proximal–distal chain between input and output. Commercial marketing acknowledges that success becomes increasingly difficult to achieve as we move from measures of simple market penetration to behaviour change. McGuire (1981) comments on this *'distal measure fallacy'* and illustrates nicely the different criteria of success used by the public and commercial sectors (Box 13).

**Box 13**   The Distal Measure Fallacy

> *All too often the communicator evaluates the campaign or its component parts in terms of a response step early in the chain, quite distant from the later step (no. 10) that actually constitutes the criterion of success. The public communication campaigner should look with horror upon the practice in the commercial advertising industry of buying 50 billion dollars' worth of time and space each year solely on the Step 1 (exposure) criterion of Neilsen ratings or circulation figures as if all that counts is reaching the public.*

Despite McGuire's objection and for reasons stated earlier, because of pre-existing motivations of the public, market penetration may be all that is necessary to sell products.

## Audience segmentation

The fourth concept is that of audience segmentation. The term is peculiar to marketing but is fundamentally similar to the well-recognised concern of health promotion with 'needs assessment' (one of the major research elements in systematic programme planning – as described in Chapter 2). Segmentation is concerned with the idea of market 'aggregation' and argues that media campaigns will be more effective insofar as they can

move towards 'disaggregation'. In other words, if messages and channels can be devised which appeal to different homogeneous subsets of the population, more effective and efficient results will be achieved. It is worth observing in passing that inter-personal communication is based on what would be called total market disaggregation, i.e. the condition achieved by inter-personal approaches which supply *'different strokes for different folks'*.

The criteria for segmentation range from the cruder geographic and demographic variables, e.g. targeting lower social class groups via the popular press, to more sophisticated measures of personality (sometimes referred to in advertising parlance as 'psychographics'). Stein (1986) ascribed part of the success of a cancer information service to its targeting of four groups: smokers who want to quit, persons over 50, cancer patients and their families and blacks. Mendelsohn (1986) described an effective crime prevention campaign which found it impossible to refine its message delivery to reach specific groups. Nonetheless, the blunderbuss approach adopted appeared to work but produced different effects in different segments of the audience. For instance, in relation to demographic variables affluent people (at proportionately lower risk) made greater gains in intention to engage in neighbourhood crime prevention activity than did the higher risk less affluent groups. On the other hand, lower income groups showed a greater readiness to report suspicious looking people to the police. In respect of psychographic criteria the campaign appeared to have resulted in greater overall levels of preventive competence among those who initially believed themselves to be relatively less able to safeguard themselves and their property. The attitudes of those perceiving themselves initially to be less at risk of crime were more likely to have been influenced by the campaign than those perceiving themselves to be more vulnerable. The latter group, however, were more likely to act and follow the specific crime reduction recommendations made by the programme. The distinction made between the reactions of different social groups to media messages – and the implications for developing messages specifically related to lower social groups – will receive further discussion below in the context of mass media and the pursuit of equity.

Lavigne *et al.* (1986) viewed market segmentation as a central feature of their APPLAUSE project (Appropriate Public Presentations for Learning about Alcohol and other drugs Using Segmentation Effects). This illustrates particularly well how pre-testing of population groups and individuals forms an integral part of programme planning. Lavigne *et al.* subdivided their market segment of parents into two further high and low risk groups and listed demographic and psychographic characteristics. For instance, the high risk group were more likely to be blue collar and male, having negative attitudes to legal and social controls over alcohol use and being less likely to believe that parents influence their children's behaviour. They were also more likely to engage in risky drinking behaviours and to have experienced health and social consequences of drinking. This segmentation allowed the project team to develop strategies designed to take account of these inter-group differences.

Apart from the self-evident value of identifying and pretesting key market segments, perhaps the main principle to be extracted from the points made above is the difficulty faced by mass media in achieving precisely tailored programmes; such fine tuning must be left to inter-personal interactions.

We will give further consideration to pre-testing below. At this juncture, though, it is important to comment that there are two kinds of pre-testing: pre-testing people, i.e. identifying their peculiar needs and characteristics in order to develop relevant programmes, and pre-testing mass media messages and programme designs. It is this latter variety that we will discuss below.

## Market understanding

The fifth of Solomon's recommendations is to understand the market. In effect this is an injunction to recognise the existence of secondary markets which might facilitate or inhibit access to and the success of programmes in influencing the primary target groups. On a simple level we might invite media workers to 'look for the gatekeeper'. If a programme depends on the display of posters in clinics and the nurse or doctor in charge is upset by the poster presentation no amount of pre-testing on the target group will prevent disappointment. The poster will not be displayed!

## Feedback

Solomon's sixth recommendation concerns the evaluation process. In short he urges that each programme, in addition to summative, should incorporate formative/process evaluation to allow the programme to be modified through the provision of rapid feedback of results.

## Interaction between inter-personal and mass communication

The seventh criterion for marketing success centres on the interaction of inter-personal and mass communication. It is virtually axiomatic that mass communication may be enhanced by inter-personal education. Commercial practice has recognised this guiding principle in its firm separation of advertising from the broader promotion/marketing function and, more specifically, in its recognition of the importance of the retail outlet in influencing customer purchasing patterns.

## Commercial resources

Here Solomon makes the point that those marketing health should utilise commercial resources where possible. There is readily available commercial expertise (e.g. market research firms) which may have greater expertise than, say, a small health education department. The firm (suggests Solomon) may even provide their services at discount rate or even for nothing – in order to improve their own brand image!

## Competition

When marketing health it is essential to understand the competition and produce a better product! The competition for health education consists primarily of the anti-health lobby and its political supporters. One of the most interesting recent attempts to learn from this maxim is described by Chesterfield-Evans and O'Connor (1986), who reported on the Australian BUGAUP campaign (Billboard Utilizing Graffitists Against Unhealthy Promotions). Chapman's (1986) *Lung Goodbye* offers the would-be subversive a handy set of tactics to combat the powerful Goliath of the tobacco industry – a point that will be further developed in our later observations on *Media Advocacy*.

## Expectations

As we emphasised in discussing the importance of objective setting in Chapter 2, it is necessary to formulate realistic targets, in planning a campaign, and not be cajoled into colluding with unrealistic expectations of success.

## THE SYNERGY OF INTER-PERSONAL AND MASS COMMUNICATION STRATEGIES

One of the most important principles raised by Solomon is the well-established fact that mass media are more effective to the extent that they are supported by *inter-personal* action. Indeed, both practitioners and theoreticians are at some pains to point out that marketing is more than advertising and relies heavily on inter-personal contacts.

Chaffee (1981), in an interesting analysis of political campaigns, makes a similar point about the importance of inter-personal support. He argues that about one-fifth of a community pay little attention to politics; one-third are politically active communicators but about half of the total population follow politics in a relatively passive fashion via the media and ... *are moved to inter-personal discussion only on the occasion of a highly salient, unanticipated or ambiguous political event*. It is the inter-personal discussion which influences political attitudes. Chaffee supports this view with the observation that watching the Watergate hearings on television was less important than discussing them in accounting for any changes in political attitude. He goes on to make a further significant observation: unsupported media are most likely to be effective when:

- there is low audience involvement in the matter under discussion;

- there is little difference in available choices;
- the message is unopposed.

Liu (1981) provides an intriguing examination of mass campaigns in communist China and reminds us that the Chinese have always stressed the importance of training activists to support their mass media campaigns.

We should also note the reciprocal situation: community-wide programmes will be more successful when they have media support. For example, Flay *et al.* (1986, 1987) discuss the synergy of media and inter-personal education from the opposite perspective and show how media in the form of television programmes can boost the effect of school-based education and trigger further inter-personal influence in the form of parental involvement.

Following assertions made in earlier chapters, the achievement of both inter-personal education and mass communication goals may never occur unless appropriate, supportive policy measures are in place!

## THE PRIMACY OF PRE-TESTING

### Assessing audience characteristics

Pretesting must form part of any well-designed health education programme. It is also an integral part of the process of evaluation. As mentioned above, two main pre-testing goals may be distinguished – assessing relevant characteristics of the target population and pre-testing the programme itself and its component parts. The assessment of audience characteristics also serves to provide a baseline or yardstick against which the programme's success may be judged through the application of post-tests as part of the normal function of summative evaluation (as described in Chapter 2). Lefebvre *et al.* (1995) illustrate the first of these two pretesting tasks in their insistence that the target group for health promotion programmes should be 'vivid and personalised'. They argue that good assessment of client characteristics effectively conveys an important message to the target group in question (Box 14).

**Box 14**  An Unspoken Message to the Client Group

> *I know a lot about you; I understand you, your problems, aspirations and needs. I want to tell you something that I believe in, am enthusiastic about and believe that you will be enthusiastic about too – as soon as I give you the facts and let you make up your own mind.*
>
> (Whit Hobbs, quoted in Wells, 1989 pp6–7).

## Steps in developing communication materials: developing and testing materials

The National Cancer Institute in Bethesda, Maryland, USA provides a succinct list of key issues to do with the development of mass communication materials and their pretesting (Box 15). These issues comprise the second stage of a six stage planning process (Figure 8.2).

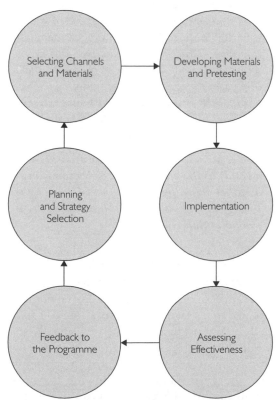

**Figure 8.2**  Pre-testing as Part of Systematic Programme Design

These 'Steps in Health Communication' demonstrate graphically the importance of pre-testing in the development of mass media programmes: 'Developing Materials and Pre-testing' occupies one-sixth of the total programme planning procedure.

**Box 15**  Stage 3 Developing Materials and Pretesting

*Key Issues*
- What are the different ways that the message can be presented?
- How does the target audience react to the message concept(s)?
- Does the audience:
  - ➢ understand the message?
  - ➢ recall it?
  - ➢ accept its importance?
  - ➢ Agree with the value of the solution?
- How does the audience respond to the message format?
- Based on responses from the target audience, do changes need to be made in the message or its format?
- How could the message be promoted, the materials distributed, and progress tracked?

(National Cancer Institute, 1998)

Palmer (1981) provides a useful example of audience pre-testing in formative research in his description of the development of the *Children's Television Workshop Health Minutes* programme – a series of minute long presentations on health topics. Pre-testing focused on 10 measures:

- individual needs and values (to which programmes could appeal as part of the 'canalisation' process);
- barriers to health behaviours;
- family members' involvement in health decisions;
- prior improvements in lifestyle (seeking to associate new health behaviours with prior health promoting decisions);
- subject matter explorations (previous relevant knowledge or ignorance);

- knowledge of symptoms;
- health lexicon (in order to devise an appropriate vocabulary for Hispanic speakers);
- prior influence of television and radio (impact of earlier programmes on health behaviours);
- parents' perceptions of themselves as child trainers.

Clearly the measures of individual characteristics and their immediate socio-environmental situations will depend on programme purposes and may be defined in various ways, technical or non-technical. Romano (1985) describes research into smoker characteristics using focus group interviews which resulted in the development of four psychographic profiles. These were the 'Fatalists', the 'Diligent', the 'Avoiders' and the 'Oblivious'! Subsequently programme materials were developed to take account of these different personality types.

Turning now to the pre-testing of programmes rather than potential audiences, Romano (1984a), in one of the most useful guides available on the subject, identified two major stages: concept development and message execution. The first of these is concerned with the evolution of potential messages and associated rough artwork – often in the form of animatics. These are devised initially as a result of *a priori* decisions about their likelihood of achieving programme goals. The tentative messages are then pre-tested on a representative sample of the target group (Romano, 1984b).

Leathar (1980) provides a classic example of the way in which a message had to be modified in response to evidence of misperception after pre-testing. He describes the reactions to an anti-smoking poster developed to remind people of the link between smoking and ill health. The setting was a graveyard; the cigarette was represented symbolically as a tombstone. A line of copy at the bottom of the picture asked the rhetorical question *Why do you think every packet carries a government health warning?* Although the original version received several awards from professional advertisers, it was misperceived by the primary target group, smokers. This example of selective perception and defensive avoidance is described by Leathar as follows:

> *Smokers, on the other hand, saw things somewhat differently. In general, they showed a high level of psychological defensiveness towards the entire advert. Initially, they claimed to see the cigarette as a variety of unrelated objects: a stick of rock, lipstick, even a telegraph pole. Furthermore, they superficially assumed the bottom line simply to be the conventional government health warning itself, thus failing to see it as a statement relating the visual material to the warning. They thus not only misperceived the symbolic visual presentation of the cigarette tombstone, but saw little, if any, relationship between this and the factual copy line which was intended to be the main theme of the advertisement. This confusion was further compounded by the image presented. Like non-smokers, smokers attributed a certain 'lightness' to the impression created, but this was attractive and pleasant and in no way symbolic of ill health. It reminded them of pleasant and rather idyllic country scenes, of bluebells and daffodils and pretty girls; of sunshine and ploughmen's lunches in 'nice' country pubs.*

> *The scene was subsequently restructured as a result of the pretesting in order to provide a rather more funereal impression and the line 'Ashes to ashes' was introduced as a symbolic link.*

One of pre-testing's major functions is to develop messages and programmes tailored to a given market segment. In commenting on the irrelevance of many messages for lower social class groups, Player and Leathar (1981) underlined the importance of providing socially sensitive advertising. They challenged the advice given to those requiring support in coping with the withdrawal symptoms following attempts to give up smoking – advice such as 'suck a clove', 'doodle with a paper clip' or 'start a new social activity'! In order to avoid such middle class bias at the concept development stage, Leathar (1980) used a projective technique to determine target group reactions to the packaging of two alternative forms of booklet offering advice on how to stop smoking. Working class respondents showed a clear preference for one of the two covers when asked to describe the 'personality' which each of the covers conveyed to them. The preferred cover was associated with a person who drank in typical pubs, was open and friendly and could be relied upon to lend money and help you out. In the words of *Communication of Innovations Theory*, the most attractive cover was more '*homophilous*'!

## Pre-testing methods

The techniques and instruments used in pre-testing are, of course, not fundamentally different from those used in evaluating health promotion programmes generally. The various indicators of success listed and discussed in Chapter 2 could equally be applied to many aspects of pre-testing and it is not difficult, for instance, to relate these to the standard pre-testing questions developed by the US Office of Cancer Communications Health Message Testing Service (Romano,

1984b). Table 8.2 is particularly interesting because it not only provides a pragmatic list of measures related to the pretesting of television public service advertisements (PSAs) but also provides guidelines for interpreting the results.

It will be recalled that establishing meaningful and realistic standards of success is a fundamentally important task for health promotion programming.

Table 8.3 (National Cancer Institute, 1998) also offers a useful list of 'Tips for Developing PSAs' which have been based on research and may thus serve as what were described as 'indirect indicators' of performance in Chapter 2. Indeed, we pointed out in Chapter 2 that the indicators used as benchmarks of pre-test performance would routinely operate as indirect indicators within an overall health promotion programme.

Standard pre-testing techniques comprise: individual in-depth interviews, central location intercept interviews, self-administered questionnaires, focus group interviews, gatekeeper review and readability testing. As may be imagined, these are based on standard quantitative and qualitative research approaches as discussed in earlier chapters.

*Table 8.2*    Guidelines for interpreting responses to standard pretesting questions

|  | High score range (%) | Average score range (%) | Low score range (%) |
|---|---|---|---|
| Attention/recall (per cent remembering seeing message after one exposure) | ≥ 41 | 30–40 | ≤ 29 |
| Main idea (per cent remembering main idea of message after one exposure) | ≥ 36 | 25–35 | ≤ 24 |
| Worth remembering (per cent indicating yes) | ≥ 76 | 60–75 | ≤ 59 |
| Personally relevant (pert cent indicating message is talking to someone like themselves | ≥ 66 | 50–65 | ≤ 49 |
| Anything confusing (per cent indicating yes) | ≤ 9 | 10–20 | ≥ 21 |
| Believable | ≥ 91 | 75–90 | ≤ 74 |
| Well done | ≥ 66 | 50–65 | ≤ 49 |
| Convincing | ≥ 71 | 55–70 | ≤ 54 |
| Informative | ≥ 76 | 60–75 | ≤ 59 |
| Made its point | ≥ 91 | 75–90 | ≤ 74 |
| Interesting | ≥ 66 | 50–65 | ≤ 49 |
| Pleasant | ≥ 66 | 50–65 | ≤ 49 |

***Table 8.3***    Tips for developing TV PSAs

- Keep messages short and simple; just one or two key points
- Be sure every word works
- Repeat the main message as many times as possible
- Identify the main issue in the first 10 seconds in an attention getting way
- Summarise or repeat the main message at the close
- Superimpose the main point on the screen to reinforce the oral message
- Recommend a specific action
- Demonstrate the health problem, behaviour or skill (if relevant)
- Provide new, accurate, straightforward information
- Present the facts in a straightforward manner
- Use a memorable slogan, then music or sound effects to aid recall
- Be sure that the message presenter is seen as a credible source of information, whether an authority, celebrity or target audience representative
- Use only a few characters
- Select an appropriate approach (e.g. testimonial, demonstration or slice-of-life format)
- Make the message understandable from the visual portrayal alone
- Use positive rather than negative appeals
- Emphasise the solution as well as the problem
- Use a light, humorous approach, if appropriate, but pre-test to be sure it works and doesn't offend the audience
- Avoid arousing fear, unless the fear is easily resolved and the message carefully tested
- Be sure the message, language and style are considered relevant by the intended audience
- Use 30 or 60 second spots to present and repeat complete message: use 10 second spots only for reminders
- If the action is to call or write, show the phone number or address on the screen for a least 5 seconds and reinforce orally (phone calls require less effort than writing for most people)
- Check consistency with campaign messages in other media formats
- Use language and style appropriate for the target audience

**Pre-test before final production**

*.... and remember, the most careful message planning won't replace the need for creativity!*

*Adapted from Making Health Communication Programs Work: A Planner's Guide (Information Projects Branch Office of Cancer Communications, National Cancer Institute, Bethesda, MD; http://rex.nci.nih.gov/nci_pub_interface/hcpw/home.htm).*

***Box 16***    Pre-testing Methods

> - Self-administered questionnaires;
> - central location intercept interviews;
> - theatre (or hall) testing;
> - focus group interviews;
> - readability testing;
> - gatekeeper review.

One or two further comments will serve to illustrate the particular flavour of pre-testing approaches.

- *Focus group interview or panel testing.* This seeks to gain insight into the characteristics of given communications and programmes by recording the discussion of a panel consisting of representatives of the target group and noting their reactions to the pilot materials. Conversation, questioning or more specialised tactics – such as the projective technique mentioned above – may be used in this context.
- *The central location intercept interview.* This may also be called a 'hall test' since interviewees, typically identified by quota sampling, will be invited to a hall or other convenient central location for panel testing or indeed any other kind of research into audience reactions. Romano (1984a) also describes a more expensive version of the hall test – 'theatre testing' – which allows larger numbers to respond to visual and electronic communications.
- *Gatekeeper review.* This acknowledges the importance of researching the reaction of key

individuals who will control the target audience's access to given health education programmes.

## Pre-testing written materials

One of the more important and specialist applications of pre-testing involves the analysis of written materials. A detailed discussion of this area is beyond the scope of this chapter but requires some brief review. Since the majority of communication and learning materials in health education are in written form it is clearly important that the target group responses are properly tested. It is of course possible to use any of the techniques discussed above to judge the suitability of written materials. For instance, a 'copy editing' technique could be used in conjunction with individual or group interviews. This involves the respondents actually writing on, say, a pamphlet or leaflet and scoring out offensive items, underlining confusing phrases and writing in alterations or additions. However, the testing of written materials normally comprises three broad approaches: content analysis, typographical analysis and measuring readability. Content analysis has its own technology but in its simpler form consists of systematically sampling written passages or books and categorising content in whatever way is most likely to illuminate the particular research and its goals. For instance, Davison (1983) analysed the questions asked at a series of public cancer education sessions and examined their implications for the content of cancer education. The study of mass media programming by Best *et al.* (1977) was based on a content analysis of news reporting, just as Hansen's (1986) observations on the incidental portrayal of alcohol in the mass media documented references to and depiction of alcohol in advertising, documentaries and entertainment programmes such as soap operas. Redman (1984), in a useful chapter on printed and non-print materials in patient education, reports a content analysis of 27 mental health pamphlets which demonstrated that:

> ... *approximately 60% of the content was in the middle-class cultural mould and that*

> *another 30% consisted of ambiguous platitudes. ... The conclusion of this analysis was that the mental health movement was unwittingly propagating a middle-class ethic under the guise of science.*

Research into the design of print has received rather less attention in health education and tends to focus on the relative legibility of different typefaces, use of upper case compared with lower case letters and the general aesthetic presentation (see for instance Hartley, 1980). On the other hand, the assessment of readability is or should be part of the routine process of developing written communications.

Three main strategies tend to be used in measuring reading ease. The first of these uses a frequency count principle arguing that people will be more likely to comprehend commonly used words. And so vocabulary is checked to see if it forms part of an agreed core of basic, i.e. frequently used, language. Perhaps the best known of these approaches is the Dale–Chall list, which includes the 3000 most commonly occurring words in the American language (Dale and Chall, 1948). A second procedure is based on calculations of the redundancy inherent in particular written passages, i.e. the amount of repetition, overt or covert. The Cloze procedure (Holcomb and Ellis, 1978) removes every fifth word from a passage and invites respondents to estimate the meaning of the missing word. The higher the success rate, the greater the comprehensibility of the passage.

However, the most commonly used approach to assessing readability is based on the empirical finding that the comprehensibility of written material is correlated with sentence length and number of polysyllabic words within the sentence. Short sentences containing words having few syllables tend to be easier to read than long sentences containing a high proportion of long words. Although the most popular of these various formulae internationally is undoubtedly the Flesch formula (Flesch, 1948), a simpler version is the FOG (Frequency of Gobbledegook) formula (Harrison, 1980). The Office of Cancer Communications, on the other hand, uses the SMOG (Subjective Measures of Gobbledegook) formula (McLaughlin, 1969).

It is important to be aware that all of the reading ease measures referred to above do not pre-test a representative sample of the actual target group and are thus not as reliable nor as valid as genuine pre-testing. For instance, the popular Dale–Chall, Flesch, FOG and SMOG formulae were all indirectly derived from results of the McCall–Crabbs Standard Test Lessons in Reading and thus relate to average developmental stages of reading competence in American children. As Pichert and Elam (1985) point out, *Readability formulas may mislead you!* Nonetheless, there are real correlations between these formulae and the intelligibility of written data and they provide valuable pre-testing tools when used with caution. In any case, once we move beyond the realm of checking comprehension and recall into the realm of attitudes and intentions we would be advised to take the results of all pre-testing with the proverbial pinch of salt. Attempts to discover how people will actually react to communications and programmes on the basis of their comments about acceptability, interest, personal preference or stated intention should always be guided by a degree of scepticism. This of course applies even more so when observations are made about other people's likely responses!

Although it is desirable to routinely check the intelligibility of written materials as part of the pre-testing procedure, the results of research and practice make it possible to provide generally applicable advice for promoting reading ease. The check list in Table 8.4 is from the National Cancer Institute (1998).

## COOPERATIVE CONSULTATION

We have been at some pains in the book so far to reiterate the importance of empowerment as both an ideological perspective in its own right and as a strategy designed to achieve any health promotion goal by strengthening individual and community characteristics and capabilities and by removing social, economic and other environ-

mental barriers. We have also argued that programmes which fail to take account of such barriers – and/or are otherwise inadequate – result in Type 3 error.

In the present chapter we have discussed *Social Marketing Theory* as a basis for achieving public health goals. On the one hand, we have made it clear that any mass communication programme should incorporate the acknowledged principles for effective working – for instance by using the checklist for enhancing readability and, in general, taking account of Solomon's key principles – listed above. We might go further and argue that failure to carry out proper pre-testing procedures is not only inefficient but unethical. Indeed, the very characteristics of mass media preclude the possibility of assessing the effect of messages on individuals and this might result in a worst case scenario in which a health education programme had failed to achieve its behaviour change goals (because it was either inadequately designed or an inappropriate strategy for achieving those goals – or both!) but actually produced unwanted side-effects such as guilt or anxiety which could not be reduced by adopting the recommended preventive behaviours. The precept 'at least do no harm' comes to mind!

We have also indicated that, despite the adoption of the techniques of social marketing, there is a basic difference between marketing commercial products that meet customers' felt needs and marketing health outcomes that might not meet clients' perceived needs – or, if they do meet those needs, clients are prevented from accessing them due to their lack of genuine availability, for psychological or social reasons.

Accordingly, in order to meet health promotion's requirement that the healthy choice should be the easy choice, we must consider alternative mass media strategies that might reduce the barriers to choice. The first such strategy has been termed 'cooperative consultation': this involves health promoters working with media organisations in such a way that they are persuaded to change the nature and/or ways in which mass media programmes are delivered. In other words, it is a device to create healthy public policy.

**Table 8.4** Making print materials easier to read

*Text should be:*
- introduced, stating the purpose to orient the reader
- summarised at the end to review major points
- presented in short sentences within short paragraphs
- 'broken up' with visuals placed to emphasise key points and text
- 'bullets' and titles or subtitles to reinforce important points
- written in the active, not passive, voice
- underlined, in bold or 'boxed' for reinforcement
- clarified with the use of examples
- tested for readability
- tested with audience
- explained, if necessary, in a glossary (with key words defined within the sentence)

*Try to avoid:*
- jargon and technical terms or phrases
- abbreviations and acronyms

Just as necessary as clear writing is text that is easy to read and graphics that help the reader understand and remember the text.

*Graphics should be:*
- immediately identifiable
- relevant to the subject matter and reader
- simple, uncluttered
- used to reinforce, not compete with the text

*Try to avoid:*
- small type (less than 10 point)
- lines of type that are too long or too short
- large blocks of print
- 'justified' right margins
- photographs that won't reproduce well
- less than professional quality drawings (they may make your text appear less credible)

*Adapted from Making Health Communication Programs Work: A Planner's Guide (Information Projects Branch Office of Cancer Communications, National Cancer Institute, Bethesda, MD; http://rex.nci.nih.gov/nci_pub_interface/hcpw/home.htm).*

Cooperative consultation is based on three assumptions:

- there is something about particular or general mass media productions that is health compromising;
- it is not politically feasible to legislate for changes to those productions;
- it is possible to achieve a compromise that is satisfactory to both health workers and media professionals and their backers.

For instance, it has recently become evident that although direct advertising of cigarettes on television and certain other media has been banned in many countries, cigarette smoking figures with increasing prominence in an incidental way during programmes. This might, for instance, be in the form of *'product placement'* (e.g. particular brands of cigarettes featured as 'props' in plays) or where cigarettes figure as 'fashion accessories' for models (whose use of smoking in everyday life as a slimming aid may already be very well-known through other media sources). By way of further illustration, Amos *et al.* (1998) not only described this phenomenon but also provided convincing evidence that electronically 'air brushing' cigarettes into photographs resulted in markedly different perceptions of the images.

*Box 17*  Young People's Perceptions of Smoking Images from Youth and Style Magazines

*(The research) ... reports the findings of the first study which has investigated young people's perceptions of non-advertising smoking images in youth magazines. A self completion questionnaire was administered to a total of 987 people from three age groups (12–13, 15–16, 18–19 years). Respondents rated perfectly matched (other than the presence/absence of a cigarette) smoking and non-smoking pictures taken from youth and style magazines on a range of attributes. They also rated their self, ideal and socially desirable images on the same attributes. It was found that the presence of a cigarette affected how the pictures were rated and that the nature of this effect differed between pictures. In general, smoking images were rated as being more druggy, wild and depressed. In contrast the matched non-smoking images were rated as being more healthy, rich, nice, fashionable, slim and attractive. Smokers and non-smokers differentially rated themselves in the same way that they differentiated between smokers and non-smokers in the photographs. It is argued that these magazine images of smoking may be acting to reinforce smoking among young people.*

(Amos *et al.*, 1998 p491)

At the time of writing there is no legislation that will ban 'advertising' of this kind and although in Europe legislation might ultimately be introduced, persuading magazine editors and owners to change their policy offers the only hope of reducing the effects of 'unhealthy' media presentations. The prospects of collaboration, needless to say, are not very hopeful given the variety of political and economic barriers that would have to be overcome. It is for this reason that a more radical approach may be necessary – an approach we will discuss later in the context of reviewing the potential of *Media Advocacy*.

One of the most complete discussions of cooperative consultation is due to Breed and Defoe (1982) and Defoe and Breed (1989). The authors provide two case studies of ways in which pressure from health promoters resulted in policy changes in both television and newspaper representations of alcohol. A four stage process is described:

- research into media content;
- provision of concise materials about alcohol are distributed to relevant media staff;
- 'specific education' is provided face-to-face at production meetings and other similar situations;
- a 'feedback' stage where media personnel discuss the results of modifications to policy with health education 'consultants'.

According to Defoe and Breed the operation was successful and resulted in negotiating a seven point charter in relation to alcohol portrayal in the media (Box 18).

*Box 18*  A Charter for Alcohol Portrayal on Media

- *Try not to glamorize the drinking or serving of alcohol as a sophisticated or an adult pursuit.*
- *Avoid showing the use of alcohol gratuitously in those cases when another beverage might be easily and fittingly substituted.*
- *Try not to show drinking alcohol as an activity which is so 'normal' that everyone must indulge. Allow characters a chance to refuse an alcoholic drink by including non-alcohol alternatives.*
- *Try not to show excessive drinking without consequences, or with only pleasant consequences.*
- *Demonstrate that there are no miraculous recoveries from alcoholism; normally, it's a most difficult task.*
- *Don't associate drinking alcohol with macho pursuits in such a way that heavy drinking is a requirement for proving oneself as a man.*
- *Portray the reaction of others to heavy alcohol drinking, especially when it may be a criticism.*

(Defoe and Breed, 1989)

Given the widespread use of alcohol and the generally recognised problems of changing both policy and behaviour regarding alcohol use, Defoe and Breed's policy development should be regarded as something of a triumph! There are, however, other cases of effective collaboration – including an example of collaboration from the UK in which a positive and major drugs focus was successfully introduced into a popular young person's programme which describes the life and times of a secondary school, *Grange Hill* (Shaw, 1986). When one of the school children became involved with drugs it created widespread interest and, subsequently, the series editors worked with a young people's news programme (*Newsround*) to produce a *Drugwatch Special*. An additional spin-off was the production of a different kind of media – an anti-drug song entitled *Just Say No*. Although, there was no evidence of behaviour change (an entirely unrealistic goal), the whole media event was considered successful – as judged by incoming telephone calls, letters from parents and young people and requests for information.

It is doubtless salutary to observe that enthusiasm for trying to produce dramatic changes in entertainment programmes should be tempered by a recognition that the main, indeed from the producer's perspective the sole, purpose of the programme is entertainment!

Nonetheless, the soap opera has been seen as a prime target for interference by health promoters – and in some instances seems to have been greeted with success. It therefore merits a little further discussion here.

## The soap opera and health promotion

The use of soap opera for educational purposes is one of a number of media tactics based on entertainment appeal (so-called entertainment–education or '*edutainment*').

Soap operas offer an illustration par excellence of *Uses and Gratifications Theory* in action. They are based in reality but do not portray it accurately (for instance the level of alcohol consumption, number of deaths, marital breakdowns and other harrowing events are grossly exaggerated when compared with their objectively defined prevalence in 'real life') in

other words, they trade in myth. Nonetheless, the interest they arouse and level of awareness they create in the viewing public (and even the non-viewing public) can be phenomenal. They provide not only a topic of conversation but produce spin-off stories in magazines and articles in which the characters appear to take on a life of their own. Moreover, they can achieve (typically unplanned) behaviour change. For instance, when a character in the UK television soap *Brookside* was imprisoned for murdering her abusing husband (having buried him under the patio) women's charities apparently received numerous phone calls from angry and despondent women. As a newspaper report put it, *'The word inundated isn't even strong enough to described the number of calls we had last night'* said *Sandra Horley, director of the battered wives' charity Refuge.*

**Box 19**

> BROOKSIDE DEATH VERDICT
> TRIGGERS RUSH FOR REFUGES!

According to Rogers and Singhal (1990) the concept of entertainment and education via soap operas originated in 1974 on a Mexican commercial television network. However, at the risk of lapsing into jingoism, it has been argued that the first ever soap that had a deliberate intention to educate and improve practice was the long-running radio programme *The Archers* (... *an everyday story of country folk*). This programme is currently still running but at its inception shortly after the end of the World War II it was quite unashamedly viewed as a propaganda programme designed to raise the quality of British agriculture. It was – allegedly – successful!

Rogers and Singhal comment that the Mexican soap (*Acompaname*), which promoted family planning, achieved high ratings and ... *convinced half a million Mexicans to visit government family-planning health clinics*. They also report that the success of the Mexican experience inspired India to broadcast *Hum Log*, a series having more ambitious goals, including addressing gender inequality, health generally, alcoholism and family planning (Singhal and Rogers, 1989). This, in turn, apparently persuaded Kenya to move into the edutainment field. The authors describe other programmes in Mexico (Singhal, 1990), Nigeria, (Winnard *et al*, 1987), Egypt and Turkey. On the basis of a range of different indicators these interventions were considered to have been effective.

It seems clear that the incorporation of 'health propaganda' in entertainment programmes must be handled with great care. On the basis of reported failure of programmes that centre on the health issue rather than the entertainment it would be assumed that messages must be subtly nested within the storyline and be consistent with the characters created. In other words, the use of soap opera will involve quite delicate negotiation – and consultative collaboration – if all parties are to be satisfied (Robbins, 2000). However, hospital drama would seem to offer an opportunity to address preventive medicine issues without militating against the main entertainment purpose of the production. Indeed, studies in The Netherlands have demonstrated the kinds of success that can be achieved – in this case *Medisch Centrum West*, a hospital drama that incorporated cardiovascular health messages from The Netherlands Heart Foundation into several episodes (Bouman *et al.*, 1998; Bouman, 1999). As Bouman *et al.* observed,

> *Medisch Centrum West was both entertaining and informative at the same time, although viewers were well aware that the programme included a health message, they did not find it intrusive to their enjoyment of the storyline. It was interesting to learn that fans were more tolerant and positive towards the E & E (entertainment and education) strategy than non fans. Age, sex and education level explained only 5% of the variance.*

(p503)

## CRITICAL CONSCIOUSNESS RAISING, MEDIA ADVOCACY AND CREATIVE EPIDEMIOLOGY

Although edutainment strategies – with or without collaborative cooperation – can achieve suc-

cess, it is hard to envisage how such strategies can seriously address the major health issues discussed in Chapter 1 in such a way that genuinely empowering policies might be implemented. Mass media, however, can make a substantial contribution to such goals *in principle*; in practice, however, their use can be problematical due to often major political barriers.

Reference to the *Empowerment Model* presented in Chapter 1 illustrates the ways in which individual and community empowerment might be addressed – and the potential role of mass media in this enterprise. It may be recalled that central to the task of mobilising radical community support is the strategy associated with Paolo Freire – *critical consciousness raising* (CCR). In our discussion in Chapter 2 of the ways in which empowerment can be translated into practice we offered a variation on the classic Freirean community development technique by, for instance, emphasising the importance of having recourse to 'community coalitions' in order to help redress the power balance between the disempowered and the powerful. We also noted in Chapter 1 two varieties of initiative associated with CCR. These were CCR 'proper' and '*agenda setting*'. Agenda setting referred to an educational process that raised important issues for public consideration – prior to possible policy change. Not infrequently, governments and others holding power will be prepared to implement policy change provided that they believe they can do so without antagonising the public in general and their supporters in particular – and, of course, without risking electoral defeat. Indeed, government might be ideologically committed to certain policies but fear electoral unpopularity by implementing those policies. Accordingly, agenda setting through mass media might sufficiently 'soften up' the public to the point where government comes to believe (after judicious consultation with focus groups!) that people are prepared to have restrictions imposed on their liberty and/or tolerate increased taxation. The situation currently facing the UK government in respect of its plans to achieve full monetary union with the European Community springs to mind in this connection!

As noted elsewhere, the use of mass media to influence the adoption of seat belts achieved only moderate results. However, it is likely that the continuing publicity raised sufficient awareness in the public about the costs of accidents and the benefits of seat belts that the government were able to legislate for their use in the reasonably safe knowledge that the measure would be acceptable.

It is clear that agenda setting is a function that is ideally suited to mass media. During World War II the distinguished journalist Ed Murrow, discussing the influence of radio and newspapers, rightly observed that mass media might not be at all effective at telling people what to think but were stunningly successful in telling them what to think about.

McCombs and Shaw (1972), in an oft quoted article, describe the agenda setting function of mass media as follows:

> ... *in choosing and displaying news, editors, newsroom staff and broadcasters play an important part in shaping political reality. Readers learn not only about a given issue, but also how much importance to attach to that issue from the amount of information in a news story and its position ... the mass media may well determine the important issues – that is, the media may set the 'agenda' ... .*

However, in the context of conviction politics and the harsh reality of *realpolitik* agenda setting may be too innocuous to achieve change. It may prove impossible to gain access to mass media to raise certain issues in order to mobilise community action. A more vigorous approach – which transcends the use of media – will be necessary. This approach is best described in terms of *advocacy*. Advocacy has traditionally been used to refer to the action of those in society who have a relatively high degree of expertise and power on behalf of those who are disadvantaged in some way and are relatively powerless. For instance, patient advocates acted on behalf of patients who lacked the expertise and confidence to challenge the power of the medical system. As Chapman (1994) points out, the meaning of advocacy has

been broadened and extended to include more substantial efforts to challenge social circumstances. As noted in Chapter 1, the *Ottawa Charter* principles emphasised that the achievement of equity was paramount in achieving *Health for All*. Inter-sectoral working and active community participation were seen as goals in their own right but also as instrumental functions that might lead to the ultimate goals of equity and health for all. Advocacy was also seen as a means to achieving the same ends (and, incidentally, apparently contrasted with health education as a relatively ineffectual activity). Our own formulation here is that a particular form of radical health education is an essential component in health promotion; in the present discussion it is an integral part of critical consciousness raising and the general advocacy function.

Wallack *et al.* (1993) refer to *Media Advocacy* as follows:

> *The mass media constitute an important part of the environment in which the selection, presentation, definition, and discussion of public issues occur. Media advocacy seeks to influence the selection of topics by the mass media and shape the debate about these topics. Media advocacy's purpose is to contribute to the development and implementation of social and policy initiatives that promote health and well-being and are based on principles of social justice.*

They also add a caveat:

> *The success of media advocacy, however, may depend on how well the advocacy is rooted in the community.*

(pp73–74)

## The need for *Media Advocacy*: the nature of news

Lupton (1994), in her analysis of news coverage of health issues, provides further support for the *Uses and Gratification Theory*, together with telling arguments why *Media Advocacy* is needed to provide a different social construction on events. Irrespective of any conspiracy theory, the very conventions of news reporting ensure that public health issues are under-reported at the expense of dramatic high technology medical triumphs or associated disasters. Table 8.5 summarises the typical features of news coverage of health and medical matters.

## A matter of framing

Wallack *et al.* (1993) describe framing as ... *the process by which someone packages a group of facts to create a story*. They cite Nelkin's (1987) view that ... *the framing of a story helps to create the basis by which public policy decisions are made*. Wallack *et al.* proceed to make an important point (which is relevant not only to America but applies to capitalist society in general). They comment:

> *Framing social and health problems in the mass media occurs in a predictable way, based in American individualism. As a result, the audience sees problems as individual in nature and disassociated from broader social and political factors.*

These observations about the role of mass media are, of course, entirely congruent with our discussions of 'victim blaming' in Chapter 1 and the importance of political empowerment approaches to health promotion discussed in Chapter 2.

**Box 20**  Alternative Political Frames for Charitable Action!

> *Archbishop Helder Camara of Brazil said, 'When I feed the hungry, they call me a saint. When I ask why they have no food, they call me a Communist'.*
>
> (Quinn, 1991, cited in Wallack *et al.*, 1993)

It is quite apparent, therefore, that the barriers facing those who seek to raise critical consciousness about health issues and the socio-structural causes of illness are not merely restricted to the nature of news reporting. Again, it is not merely the opposition of powerful lobbies such as the tobacco industry – together with the collusion of governments – which have been dramatically exposed in recent years, which militate against the creation of healthy public policy. Rather it is the ways in which the prejudices, aspirations and fears of the ordinary public which have been expertly manipulated by the propagandists employed by those powerful lobbies. For these reasons, dra-

**Table 8.5**  Common characteristics of news coverage of health and medical issues

- Regardless of degree of severity or prevalence, some health issues receive more media attention than others.
- The news media tend to distort information, favouring extreme views over more moderate, considered views.
- Therefore, health risks are often not placed in perspective against other risks to life.
- Media coverage of health risks and treatments is often contradictory and confusing for the audience, e.g. immunisation might be reported in highly positive terms one week, then with suspicion the next.
- Coverage of risks gives a broad view, but often does not report on the reliability of the information used, give background information or give more detailed information about the extent to which health risks might affect the audience.
- As a consequence, coverage of health risks tends to invite panic, but does not provide enough details to enable people to assess their own risk.
- Coverage often focuses on the dramatic nature of biomedical treatment rather than ways of preventing illness.
- The news media have the power to function as a lobby by setting public and political agendas on what is important and worthy of action.
- Commercial advertisers may influence the content of news stories about health risks.
- The source of the news story is important in determining the way in which the story is framed, e.g. medical journal articles will tend to attract more legitimacy than the media releases of a consumer/activist group.
- Greater attention is given to health risks that are relatively serious and rare (e.g. Legionnaires' disease and toxic shock syndrome) than to common, chronic health issues such as diabetes.

*Adapted from Chapman and Lupton (1994, p. 37).*

matic – even daring – measures have had to be used to counter opposition. These measures have inevitably involved the '*re-framing*' of public perceptions. As Wallack (1990) notes:

> *Media advocacy promotes a range of strategies to stimulate broad-based media coverage in order to reframe public debate to public health problems. It does not attempt to change individual risk behaviour directly but focuses attention on changing the way in which the problem is understood as a public health issue. For example, a media advocacy approach might develop a strategy to stimulate media coverage regarding the ethical and legal culpability of alcohol companies that promote deadly products to teenagers. The purpose is to shift attention from defining alcohol problems as solely the property of individuals and highlight the role of those who shape the environment in which individual decision about health related behaviour are made.*
>
> (p376)

Chapman (1994) provides a very detailed analysis of what is involved in the process of 're-framing' in a case study entitled '*garden aesthetics versus children's lives; media advocacy for the prevention of childhood drowning*'. In this he describes the arguments or 'frames' used by those who objected to proposed public health legislation obliging swimming pool owners to put safety fences around their pools and contrasts these with the 'frames' used by the advocates of safety fencing. Some of these are presented in Box 21.

## Creative epidemiology

Creative epidemiology involves the presentation of valid data and statistics but portrayed in an especially dramatic way. Wallack (1990), for example, described a demonstration sponsored by the US National Cancer Institute (the Utica Alvin Ailey Protest). It set out to challenge Philip Morris' strategy of 'buying legitimacy' by sponsoring local dance. A striking message was designed that stated

> *Philip Morris brings you more than art ... it also brings you cancer, heart disease, emphysema, stroke, bronchitis, 135,729 deaths every year.*

Raw *et al.* (1990) also describe a number of similar activities and Chapman and Lupton (1994) provide a detailed '*A–Z of Public Health Advocacy*' that includes some 89 strategies and tactics in a comprehensive armamentarium of advocacy weapons! These include *Creative Epidemiology*. One particular case study is especially impressive in that it was apparently pivotal in gaining the Australian Federal Government's support for a legislative ban on tobacco sponsorship (Box 22).

***Box 21*** Arguments of Pool Fencing Advocates and Opponents

| Pro | Con |
| --- | --- |
| Children are naturally inquisitive, exploratory. It is human for parents to be fallible. Some drownings occur with unsighted 'trespassing' children. | Drownings due to parental negligence. Trespassers should be given little sympathy (blame the victim). |
| There are already many costly safety precedents. | Our homes are our castles; down with Big Brother government and the nanny state. |
| A child's life is priceless. Protecting citizens is an important role for the state. | Fencing will disadvantage those with no children – especially pensioners. What about other waterways? |

(After Chapman, 1994)

**Box 22** A Case Study in Creative Epidemiology

Data were assembled on the cigarette prefer-ences of Australian children smokers in four different states. Their preferences happened to correspond perfectly (and dramatically) with brands of cigarette that sponsored the major football leagues in each of the four states. The data were compiled into a simple graph representing the prevalence of smok-ing with histogram columns consisting of cig-arettes of different length set against a background of cigarette packets representing the different brands advertised in the state. This clearly presented and disturbing evi-dence was distributed to all politicians and the media.

The graph was reproduced on the front page of Sydney's leading newspaper. The Minister for Sport said that the graph was what had influenced her.

(After Chapman, 1994 p162)

## Using mass media to tackle the health divide

In 1998 an Expert Group on Mass Media was estab-lished by the English Health Education Authority (Hastings *et al.*, 1998). Its task was to examine the potential of the mass media for addressing the prob-lem of the 'Health Divide' – a 're-discovered' prob-lem and a matter in which the recently elected Labour Government had declared a serious interest. It is interesting to note the two different and oppos-ing ways in which the problem was 'framed'. First it was agreed that the well-recognised strategies and techniques involved in designing mass communica-tion should routinely be used to address this partic-ular issue – as with any other client group. On the other hand, it was acknowledged that since the more advantaged members of society were more responsive to mass media information than disad-vantaged groups, the result of superior communica-tion strategies would be to actually accentuate the gap between rich and poor.

Accordingly, the importance of audience segmen-tation was reiterated together with the need to pre-cisely target different sectors of society. In other words, specific mass media strokes should be devel-oped for different (disadvantaged) folks. Following best media practice this might best be achieved by:

- Data base and relationship marketing: i.e. utilis-ing a detailed data base which would allow mes-sages to be sent (e.g. by direct mail) ... *that exactly match the needs of the target, cus-tomised for example, to those living in deprived communities in general, or one particular com-munity or even part of that community*. Follow-ing the dictates of relationship marketing, it would also be desirable to ... *build relationships with their customers: to maintain their atten-tion, good will and loyalty*.

- Emotional messages and branding: i.e. devel-oping particular brand images for the health promotion products and utilising appropriate emotional appeals. Apparently, ... *brands are extremely important in consumer marketing because they provide a robust vehicle for satis-fying people's emotional and practical con-sumption needs*.

- More importantly perhaps, *Research into how working class populations use cultural symbols in advertising found that these groups are often poorly informed about the objective merits of different products and therefore tend to rely more heavily than other groups on 'implicit meanings' – context, price, image – to judge products* (Durgee, 1989). Furthermore, ... *peo-ple in deprived communities are less likely to evaluate products on a rational, objective basis, but look for clues as to the product's value in terms of its price or its image. .... the symbolic appeal of brands is particularly effective in tar-geting those individuals who do not have the time, skills or motivation to evaluate the objec-tive attributes and benefits of a particular cam-paign* (de Chernatony, 1993).

It would, of course, be entirely reasonable to view the solutions proposed above for 'getting through to' disadvantaged groups as a quite blatant form of victim blaming! And we did note in Chap-ter 2 how ideology was reflected in both strategy and methods involved in planning health promotion programmes. Apart from the ideological dimension, it seems highly doubtful whether the health promotion 'product' could be effectively marketed in this way – especially bearing in mind earlier observations about the limitations of social marketing. The alternative approaches centre on using mass media to directly address the actually causes of deprivation – namely the social, economic and general material circumstances of disadvantaged groups. And Hastings *et al.* (1998) do indeed offer this approach as an alternative. There are two main variants – and these, again illustrate ideological dimensions discussed in Chapter 1 together with certain strategies discussed above.

They are:

- Tackle directly the anti-health lobbies – and, since the prevalence of smoking is especially high in disadvantaged groups of all kinds, tobacco receives particular attention. The raft of measures undertaken by the UK government in the context of the report *Smoking Kills* (Department of Health, 1999) is clearly relevant to this strategy.
- Use a *Media Advocacy* approach. Interestingly, this approach does not receive the detailed technical analysis devoted to the question of audience segmentation and database marketing. However, sufficient detail about the philosophy and practice of this strategy has been provided above. In the view of the authors of this present book the *Media Advocacy* approach embodies the most appropriate ideology for equity – and the most efficient strategy for change.

**Box 23**  Two Approaches to Using the Media to Combat Inequalities: Victim Blaming or Radical Advocacy?

- Use database and relationship marketing together with emotional appeals to directly persuade disadvantaged groups to adopt healthier practices.
- Use *Media Advocacy* – with optional civil disobedience (see BUGA UP and Chapman's A–Z of advocacy techniques) – to tackle the root causes of deprivation and alienation.

## LESSONS FROM *MASS COMMUNICATION THEORY*

We have in this chapter so far reviewed models and theories of mass media. It is clear that mass media cannot be used as a panacea for achieving planned social change – of any kind. It is equally clear that a substantial body of expertise exists about what mass media can and cannot be expected to achieve. We also have a good understanding of ways in which mass media should be employed to achieve the most effective outcomes. The over-riding lesson is that the best results will be attained when mass media are used to support a wide range of integrated activities, including inter-personal education together with the development and implementation of supportive policy. We have not only reviewed different theoretical explanations of how mass media operate and discussed these in the context of strategies for action, we have also drawn attention to the ideological dimensions. Accordingly, while we have pointed out the fundamental difference (both technical and ideological) between marketing commercial products and 'selling health', we have urged those using mass media for health promotion to make proper use of the particular techniques specified by this approach. On the other hand, we have endorsed the use of *Media Advocacy* in order to address the socio-economic and other environmental barriers to healthy choices and build healthy public policy and the pursuit of equity.

## A SELECTIVE REVIEW OF MEDIA STUDIES: GENERAL OBSERVATIONS

The mass media strategy is, in one important respect, different from the remaining 'delivery strategies' discussed in this book. Although each of these has its own idiosyncracies and flavour, mass media differ fundamentally in the lack of personal contact between educator and audience. The media strategy is therefore of particular interest, especially since it promises so much but, in many people's view, delivers relatively little. This latter part of the chapter will therefore present evidence which should help us decide what we might realistically expect from mass media. In judging this evidence we must, of course, bear in mind the general principles, stated in the first part of the book, that the quality of evidence will depend on (i) the definition of success employed therein, (ii) the extent to which appropriate research designs have been used and (iii) the choice of particular methods based on intelligent use of learning and communication theory. The latter point will not, of course, apply to the mass media strategy except insofar as media are used to represent particular tactics such as face-to-face interaction (e.g. a video of a counselling session) or group work (e.g. a film of a smoking cessation clinic). In such instances learning tactics are being employed at second hand. The only other situation where choice of appropriate teaching methods is important in the context of mass media use is when the latter are supplemented by auxiliary inter-personal methods.

Particular varieties of media do of course have different capabilities and characteristics, as we have seen above, and the review which follows will provide separate evidence of the potential of some of these for achieving different kinds of outcome. More particularly, we will consider the use of posters and leaflets and compare these, implicitly or explicitly, with the arguably more powerful electronic media – radio and television. In addition, we will examine the capabilities of mass media for dealing with some specific health problems, including a particularly problematical issue, that of substance misuse.

What then might we say about mass media efficiency? Can we generalise or must we again say it depends on the type of media, subject matter and target group? As indicated in the Introduction to the 2nd Edition of this book, Gatherer *et al.* (1979) provided one of the first attempts to provide a comprehensive answer to the question 'is health education effective?'

As a result of analysing 49 evaluations of mass media programmes they concluded that mass media were in fact inferior to individual instruction and groups. Seven out of 11 of their cases demonstrated some changes in knowledge (of the order of 6% and typically short lasting); two out

of two studies demonstrated some attitude shift (of between 3 and 6% – though four studies recorded an attitude change in the wrong direction); 20 out of 30 studies showed some behaviour change. As regards this latter category, Gatherer *et al.* note that behaviour change is most likely where a single action is required (e.g. clinic attendance or use of a phone-in service); it tends to be relatively short lived and change is less likely to occur when general changes in behaviour pattern are required.

**Box 24**  An Early Review

| 49 evaluations of mass media programmes were reviewed: | |
|---|---|
| 7 out of 11 | demonstrated some change in knowledge; |
| 2 out of 2 | demonstrated some attitude change; |
| 20 out of 30 | demonstrated some behaviour change. |

Atkin (1981) also offers a review of campaign effectiveness; his analysis was not intended to be the kind of comprehensive catalogue which Gatherer *et al.* compiled but provides a rather more thorough and sophisticated analysis of the reasons why certain campaigns were or were not effective. He commented, for instance, on the failure of a campaign to teach Cincinnati residents about the United Nations. Neither knowledge gain nor effective change resulted from a ... *heavy flow of multi-media messages*. According to Atkin lack of success was due to an excessive quantity of information at the expense of quality. He ascribed other failures to: the use of unpopular media channels and lack of audience penetration; use of vague messages rather than making specific recommendations; poor audience segmentation; generating audience reaction through hard sell techniques; a failure to take account of the audience's latitude of acceptance.

On the other hand, when learning theory and the principles of effective media communication were taken into account, programmes have been demonstrably successful. Atkin cites a programme on sexually transmitted diseases called 'VD Blues' (Greenberg and Gantz, 1976) which attracted a wide audience, increased their perception of the seriousness of the problem, enhanced knowledge levels – especially about mode of transmission and cure – and apparently resulted in thousands of people visiting VD clinics after the programme. He also referred to a successful programme described by Mendelsohn (1973) which utilised a quiz format to communicate information about a *National Driver Test Program*. This had an estimated audience of 30 million viewers, generated over a million letters and ... *stimulated thousands to enrol in driver improvement courses*.

There are other well-documented examples of successful media programmes which should satisfy critics. For instance, Farquhar-Pilgrim and Shoemaker (1981) described a series of campaigns designed to influence Americans' extravagant use of energy. Applying *Communication of Inovations Theory*, they concluded that proper design which took account of audience motivation could produce very acceptable results. They demonstrated, for example, a good level of penetration – their messages reached 83% of city adults an average of 14 times. The target group seemed to be more willing to pay for energy saving devices (the percentage varied between 5 and 17%). Moreover, an increase in sales of such devices was recorded and a higher proportion of the target group undertook various energy saving practices such as installing shower flow control devices than a comparison group: the adoption rate was between 16 and 27% higher than the comparison, depending on the device in question. While this example might not appear to be directly relevant to health education practice, it does illustrate that campaigns which ask people to take action for the collective good can be effective, provided that appropriate appeals are made to self-interest (in this case financial gain).

Bell *et al.* (1985), in their review of research in health education (1948–1983), also report examples of effectiveness. For instance, an assessment of the Glasgow rickets campaign claimed an eight-fold increase in demand for vitamin D supple-ments for older Asian children together with a 33% increase in requests for paediatric drops (Dunnigan *et al.*, 1981). The review also included England and Oxley's (1980) study which reported a halving of the rate of head infestation among a population of 147,385 children after a regional campaign. Again, Bell *et al.* record the success of a programme in increasing the level of rubella vaccination which involved general practitioner support of a national publicity campaign directed at women in the practice population. Within the study population 1187 women responded to a request to attend for screening and 106 of the 133 who were eligible for immunisation accepted this (Hutchinson and Thompson, 1982).

Turning now to the use of educational broadcasting, it is clear that properly constructed programmes can have a wide range of desirable effects. Rogers (1973) showed how the BBC *Merry-Go-Round* sex education programme (when used in the context of classroom teaching – and thus a learning resource rather than media proper) could change beliefs and attitudes. Children who experienced the programmes not only increased their knowledge of sexual vocabulary but also developed different attitudes to nudity, reproduction and toilet habits: in other words, they acquired a greater and more healthy openness in relation to sexuality.

Again, McCron and Dean's (1983) thorough evaluation of a series of programmes produced by Channel 4 Television on health matters (*Well Being*) revealed a wide range of beneficial outcomes. They summarised some of these effective outcomes as follows:

> ... *in television terms, a relatively successful programme attracting a considerable audience, which showed a relatively high appreciation of the programmes ... follow-up activities ... were useful in ... promoting a degree of audience feedback and participation ... programmes promoted thinking and encouraged the development of new understandings.*

A review by Gordon (1967) of a traditional mass media-centred campaign also reveals how a mix of radio, TV, posters and pamphlets can have a behavioural outcome. A mix of 800 posters, 50,000 leaflets, mass mailing of letters to groups and clubs, press releases, press advertising, 11 radio spots and the involvement of three TV stations generated attendance at a Baltimore diabetes clinic on the following 3 days of the following numbers: day one, 512; day two, 790; day three, 1350. Interviews with those attending the clinic seemed to confirm that attendance had been primarily due to media information (64% press; 14% radio; 8% TV; remainder inter-personal contact). As the author notes, ... *large groups of individuals stand ready to take action on any given issue and merely lack the information or cue to make the action possible*.

**Box 25**

> ... *large groups of individuals stand ready to take action on any given issue and merely lack the information or cue to make the action possible.*

Certainly, in the above-mentioned case media triggered action. It would, however, be patently wrong to say that this would happen for any given issue. Indeed, analysis of the examples of the media programmes above will in all cases indicate the presence of key conditions: pre-existing audience motivation; time and professional presentation necessary for communication of complex information; the adjunct of inter-personal pressure; etc. However, it is rather difficult to find an easy explanation of the apparent success of a media-based intervention by the Indian Cancer Society which claimed to have doubled attendances at its six Bombay clinics specialising in the early detection of cancers. This would have been expected *a priori* to have been a difficult task. The journal article provides insufficient detail from which to determine which important preconditions seem responsible for overcoming the important affective barriers which often militate against successful cancer education (Ajit, 1982). Following the 10 points of social marketing, the charita-

ble involvement of an advertising agency might indeed, as claimed, have provided the skills and expertise necessary for a sensitive campaign! On the other hand, it may be the case that developing countries are more susceptible generally to mass media interventions and/or that it is easier to utilise community networks to enhance the impact of mass media. Alternatively, it may be that in Western, urbanised society health education is more concerned with requiring the abandoning of pleasures and addictions associated with affluence whereas the major barriers in developing countries have to do with cultural misconceptions and associated issues. Whatever the reason, there seems to be consistent evidence of successful media interventions in these countries. For instance, Jenkins (1983) reviewed 17 projects: most revealed some significant changes and many of these were behavioural. These included a 3% decline in population growth rate (Costa Rica); an improvement in breast feeding from 25 to over 50% (Yap Islands, Micronesia); 75% of all under fives vaccinated in one day (Nicaragua); an increase from 0 to 24% adding oil to meals to enhance the energy content after a radio campaign (Philippines); an increase from 20 to 59% having latrines (Tanzania).

Evidence of the effectiveness of family planning campaigns has normally come from developing countries. Taplin (1981) reported that six projects improved contraceptive availability, increased sales of products, spread knowledge and stimulated wider use of methods promoted. For instance, *A campaign in Esfahan increased pill accepters by 54% and total contraceptive use by 64% over a six-month period*. Again, the impact of China's family planning programme is legendary and, as Liu (1981) indicated, this combined a blend of media and inter-personal persuasion. By 1972 79% of China's population was using contraception; the rate of population increase was reduced from 23 per 1000 in 1963 to 4.7 per 1000 in 1974.

*The International Quarterly of Community Health Education* (1985, Vol. 5, pp149–166) included a study by Cernada and Lu (1982) in a list of articles, selected by health educators, of the most worthwhile publications of the 1970s. This described a mass media demonstration project which provided evidence of successful penetration, knowledge and attitude change and an increase in low cost contraceptive practice. It could, of course, be argued that it is relatively easy to sell at least some varieties of family planning practice: health educators are offering a tangible product together with real benefits in terms of a reduction in anxiety and economic pressures while minimising loss of gratification. Relatively few thoroughly evaluated studies of family planning education are available for Western countries, possibly because the service does not really need promoting! Those that are available seem to indicate reasonable levels of success. For instance, a study of a press/poster/leaflet campaign in Lambeth in 1972–1973 increased numbers of new patients at clinics by 68%, total attendances by 26% and clinic sessions by 46%. A similar programme in Holland aimed at young people under the age of 18 succeeded in trebling numbers of clinic visitors at a time of year when attendance figures normally dropped. Both studies are reported by Smith (1978).

One final point will be made about the use of mass media in developing countries. It will be recalled that the major single benefit – perhaps the sole benefit – of mass media is their capacity to reach a mass audience and to do so relatively cheaply. Leslie (1981) provides evidence of the effectiveness of mass media and nutrition education (Box 26).

**Box 26** Mass Media Can Be Effective in Promoting Good Nutrition

> *... the most firm conclusion suggested by the evaluations is that mass media health and nutrition education projects can reach large numbers of people (up to several million) in a relatively short period of time. The evaluations also indicate that, although there is a considerable range in costs among projects it is possible to achieve this outreach at a cost as low as $0.01 per person.*

Between 10 and 50% of the audience remember the main nutrition message. When a specific nutrition message has been designed, there is:

> *... a reasonable expectation that the target audience could modify their behaviour accordingly and ... a reasonable expectation that this modified behaviour could bring about an improvement in health or nutrition status ... .*

This chapter will be concluded by considering three situations where particular aspects of mass media or the kind of message they convey will determine the likelihood of success. In this way a major theme of this book will be reiterated: it is of relatively little value making generalisations about effectiveness without a careful analysis of goals, strategies and methodology. First, we will consider the influence of media characteristics by considering and comparing the use of leaflets and posters. Secondly, we will look at a functionally different kind of health education problem – persuading individuals to use seat belts. Thirdly, we will consider goals and content by reviewing particularly problematical issues for health education – the misuse of substances. This will include comments about drugs generally and alcohol and smoking in particular.

## POSTERS AND LEAFLETS

Before considering the potential of these two popular devices we should reiterate the distinction made earlier between the use of media as mass media and the use of media as audio-visual aids or learning resources. It is almost a truism to say that the appropriate use of an audio-visual aid will enhance any given teaching method. For instance, Burt *et al.* (1974) described a successful piece of patient education in which inter-personal education by medical and nursing staff delivered to survivors of acute myocardial infarction was supplemented by written advice and pamphlets. Sixty-two per cent of the smokers in the experimental group had remained non-smokers for between one and three years compared with 27.5% in a control group. This study did not separately quantify the relative contribution of the written materials. However, Russell *et al.* (1979) were able to show that leaflets added a couple of percentage points to the effectiveness of the verbal advice provided by a doctor.

The use of leaflets as mass media – i.e. without inter-personal support – is more problematical. Tapper-Jones and Davis (1985) documented a detailed and comprehensive survey of a sample of Welsh GPs use of leaflets. The study demonstrated clearly that leaflet use was widespread in primary medical care: the vast majority of doctors used leaflets and/or other teaching aids. Of the sample of 176 GPs 91% used diet sheets, 85.5% a variety of hand drawn diagrams, 58.5% various leaflets, 39% preprinted diagrams, 26% plastic models, 19% a patient counselling compendium, 15.5% *'Family Doctor'* booklets and 3.5% *'some other aid'*. The major suppliers of the leaflets were, first of all, various pharmaceutical companies and, second, the Health Education Council. Interestingly, GPs rated television as the most effective means of communication, followed by 'personal advice from doctors' – the reverse of Budd and McCron's (1979) observation of patients' ratings of credibility!

The study by Russell *et al.* cited above led to the development of a specially tailored booklet containing advice on giving up smoking. This was dispatched to all GPs in England and Wales. Its fate serves to illustrate some of the limitations of the leaflet and will now be considered in the context of social marketing's notion of a 'hierarchy of effects'. We should first note that a leaflet must often be delivered to a 'gatekeeper' who will make it available to the prime user. The leaflet must be acceptable to the prime user and its message must then impinge on the consciousness of the target population: people must pick up the leaflets, read them, pay attention to the messages contained therein and, if they have been properly pre-tested, they should understand their content. Following our earlier mention of the *Hierarchy of Communications Effect*, hopefully, they may also believe the message and this belief may in turn contribute towards the development of a favourable attitude to a healthy outcome which

may then predispose the learner to adopt some behaviour or, possibly, to change some unhealthy practice, assuming, of course, that the social and physical environment will support and not inhibit such a course of action!

Spencer (1984) attempted to track the GUS (*Give Up Smoking*) leaflets mentioned above. His survey revealed that 57% of the sample did not remember having received the booklets. Of those who did recall having received them, 72% found them acceptable and 39% had used them. However, only one in three of this user group appeared to have used the booklets in the prescribed fashion, i.e. as a consultation aid requiring the GP to provide a personalised message for the patient in the context of inter-personal advice and exhortation about stopping smoking. Posters accompanied the booklets and 69% of the 43% of doctors who had any recollection of receiving the kit claimed to have displayed the poster in the practice premises.

The ubiquitous and frequently maligned poster has been subjected to many appraisals, most of which demonstrate very low effectiveness when used without inter-personal support. Posters are, almost by definition, designed to convey persuasive messages without such adjuvant support (in contrast to a chart which is meant to be used as a teaching aid). Grant (1972) studied the impact of two differently styled posters urging women to have a cervical smear. These were prominently displayed in a number of clinics and women were interviewed in order to determine what they recalled of the posters. Relatively few could recall the posters (although one designed in a question-and-answer format was superior to the other). Significantly, the women who were most aware of the posters had already had a smear test; their recall doubtless reflected self-congratulatory selective attention! A similar study by Cole and Holland (1980) reported that only 16 out of 198 women could remember accurately two posters displayed in a health centre waiting room. Over 90% did not read available leaflets or take one home.

A particularly optimistic attempt to use posters was described by Auger *et al.* (1972). Both posters and mobiles were used in a hospital setting to influence smoking behaviour. While the researchers did not imagine that a poster could influence smoking habit, they thought that smokers in canteen areas might be persuaded not to smoke in that given situation or perhaps to extinguish their cigarettes. An ingenious form of indicator of success was employed: baseline '*debris indices*' were developed by counting and measuring cigarette butts before and after the poster/mobile display. The result? No change! It should be noted, in passing, that this study pre-dates the substantial normative shift away from smoking and the prevalence of non-smoking policies in hospitals, restaurants and the like. It might well be the case that posters would have some trigger effect if used today in a similar context.

The Transport and Road Research Laboratory has carried out several experimental studies of media impact. One study demonstrated that by taking learning theory into account and sequencing the information presented in a poster, a significant improvement in correct interpretations of safe road crossing practices could be produced in children of various ages. While 36% of all children aged five to seven misinterpreted all messages on a draft poster, only 9% got the messages wrong on the revised 'sequenced' poster. Clearly, as the designers noted, understanding is only weakly related to road crossing behaviour; nonetheless, the same organisation demonstrated that posters used by the roadside could actually influence driving practices. After displaying double crown size posters for a week in six sites the number of overtaking actions fell from 1866 to 1355 and the proportion of risky overtaking declined from 9 to 4.5%. However, posters used in a similar way had no effect on more complex driving behaviours, such as keeping an adequate distance between cars on the M4 at Slough! (Transport and Road Research Laboratory, 1967, 1972).

The final example to be discussed in this section on posters and leaflets is a well-designed and extensively monitored campaign to prevent children's accidents. It is particularly interesting in that: (i) it used booklets in conjunction with a series of television programmes; (ii) its measure of effectiveness encompassed most of the kinds of indicator examined in Chapter 3; (iii) because it appealed to carers of young children, motivation to take action must have been relatively high, certainly by comparison with programmes which required the audience to undertake uncomfortable activities or forgo gratification. The campaign consisted of three components: a 10 programme television series lasting 10 minutes per programme and employing a popular television personality as presenter; a 36 page booklet; a community initiative which sought to establish local *Play It Safe* groups consisting of a variety of lay and professional people concerned with safety. The impact of the programme has been thoroughly documented (BBC, 1982; Jackson, 1983). The effectiveness of the TV programme will be summarised before analysing the separate effect of the booklets. Results will be described in accordance with the 'chain of indicators', ranging from awareness through to behaviour change.

First, audience penetration was good. Some 8,000,000 people on average watched each programme (15.5% of the viewing population over the age of four). By the end of the series 59% of adults and 40% of children had seen at least one programme. The viewing figures indicated a representative social class distribution; as it was hoped to reach lower socio-economic groups, audience segmentation was thus satisfactory.

Second, viewers had a positive attitude to the programmes: 96% of viewers found them interesting, 47% found them '*very helpful*' and a further 37% considered them '*quite helpful*'. More important, however, for the achievement of campaign goals is the audience attitude to the preventive measures which the programmes attempted to promote. In seeking to gain insight into these outcome measures and the intermediate variables which influenced them some 2000 people were interviewed before and after the campaign. A sample of viewers was also compared with a matched group of non-viewers and their beliefs, attitudes and reported changes in practice were compared. The results can be summarised as follows.

- Viewers tended to have more favourable reactions on four measures of six general attitudes to child safety.
- Viewers were more likely than non-viewers to accept the probability of specific accidents occurring in eight out of 11 test situations.
- Viewers were also more likely than non-viewers to believe that parents could do something to prevent the 11 accident situations described in the booklets. Whereas neither of the differences mentioned in the two paragraphs above were statistically significant, two of these efficacy beliefs did meet the criterion of statistical success.

Third, in respect of actions taken, viewers were on average more likely to have translated positive attitude into practice. Of a possible list of 15 specific safety actions viewers took 5.97 actions compared with non-viewers 5.44. Again, this difference was not significant statistically. However, when a separate analysis of viewers who were 'responsible for children every day' was carried out, the differences in this category and in the categories listed above did reach a level of significance. In other words, the section of the target group which perceived the direct relevance of the recommendations was influenced significantly to a greater or lesser extent. Whether a difference of 0.9 safety actions taken is considered a success clearly depends on expectations of a mass media campaign!

Turning next to the contribution of the booklet, the following information was provided by the BBC's research department. Between December 1981 and the end of March 1982 a total of 1,500,000 copies had been distributed, a figure which included 45,000 individual requests. Research into the population reached by the booklet indicated that some 11% of a total of 1926 adults interviewed had seen the publication and 4% claimed to have read it. In comparison, 15% of a sample of 1080 programme viewers had seen the booklet and 6% claimed to have read it. Predictably, the proportion of lower socio-economic groups having written for the booklet, seen it or read it was smaller than middle class groups. Some 75% of the 1080 viewers claimed to have read all of the booklet and 71% of these claimed to have read it thoroughly. Ninety-seven per cent were pleased with the publication and found it useful. Fifty-nine per cent considered it taught them 'a lot of things I didn't know' but 76% believed that 'sensible parents would already follow most of the advice in the booklet'. What of actions taken? Although there may well be overclaiming, it does seem to be the case that the booklet had prompted actions among at least some readers. For example, 16% of booklet readers (which, remember, is 16% of the 4% of the population who claimed to have read it) stated that they now took more precautions in the kitchen; 15% were more careful with medicines and dangerous liquids; 10% took safety action concerning glass; 6% took more fire precautions and checked electrical safety; 4% secured windows, made stairs safer and secured cupboards.

A further interesting observation may be made about the impact of the total campaign. Some 15 local groups had been formed before the TV series was actually shown as a result of advance publicity and liaison work. This additional source of interpersonal support might be expected to maximise the impact of the campaign proper. In fact, a study in an inner city area by Colver *et al.* (1982) showed that 55% of the working class families interviewed did not watch any of the TV programmes and only 9% of a group specially encouraged to watch the series took any of the 15 safety actions. However, when a comparable group received a home visit and were given specific advice some 60% actually took some kind of action.

**Box 27** Adopting Safety Behaviours: Effect of Interpersonal Support

- Nine per cent of a working class group of parents or guardians of young children who watched a number of TV programmes adopted any of 15 possible safety actions.
- In comparison, 60% of a similar group that received a home visit from a health visitor did take some action.

The evaluations of posters and leaflets discussed above clearly make the point that the peculiar features of given media will influence the likelihood of a successful outcome. However, these intrinsic factors will compete with other components of the whole influence process, making prediction difficult if not impossible: for instance the success of the *Play It Safe* booklets was affected by the context of the TV programmes, by the audience's beliefs about children's vulnerability to accident and, above all, by the addition of inter-personal education in Colver's study. Sometimes the anticipated benefits of given media may not materialise. For example, Harris (1983) reported on the failure of a local radio-based campaign to persuade the community to take on responsibility for preventing hypothermia in elderly relatives and neighbours. One of the key indicators – whether or not elderly people living alone had been visited in the previous 7 days – seemed to show that there had been a 9% decline in visits after the programmes! At first glance the 'folksy' nature and community orientation of local radio might have made it particularly suitable for this kind of campaign. Although hypothermia might not seem to be a particularly problematical health topic – most people would not be expected to be hostile to helping old people – the subject matter of many programmes offers an almost desperate challenge to the ingenuity of those seeking to produce change through mass media.

In the next section of this chapter the results of a particularly rigorous study will be presented which seem to the author to indicate just what unsupported mass media can achieve under difficult but not impossible circumstances – promoting the wearing of seat belts. The concluding section of this chapter will review an acknowledged problem area, that of substance abuse in general. It will comment on drug education, identifying the prevention of alcohol misuse as especially difficult compared with tobacco smoking.

## A CASE STUDY OF SEAT BELT USE

In 1973 Levens and Rodnight assembled evidence of the effectiveness of a series of controlled area experiments in the use of mass media to promote seat belt wearing in Britain. The value of the study rests on the following facts:

- evidence of important driver/front seat passenger characteristics is presented;
- precise details of media input and their cost are provided;
- objective evidence of specific behaviours is described;
- we can be as confident as anyone can that the results of media programmes can be ascribed to the input rather than other 'contaminating' events.

First, the pre-testing of driver characteristics revealed the following useful data: drivers already appeared to be motivated to wear seat belts. Some 85% of those interviewed claimed to have a positive attitude to seat belt wearing, believing that this would cut down injuries. It seemed that despite this attitude many drivers did not 'belt up' and it was not possible to rely on reported use of belts since drivers consistently overestimated it. The number claiming to wear seat belts more than half the time was 57% but observed levels of wearing were only 17%. Any measure of programme effectiveness must therefore try to use observation rather than self-report.

Further research into the failure of drivers to use seat belts, despite their generally favourable attitude, suggested that this might be due to beliefs that although belts would reduce accidents, drivers were not susceptible to such accidents in a variety of situations (despite objective evidence to the contrary). In *Health Belief Model* (HBM) terms the target group clearly believed in the effectiveness of seat belts but were ambivalent about susceptibility and seriousness. At all events, a programme was devised which used three appeals: 'appeal to the head', 'appeal to the heart' and 'appeal to the nervous system'. In other words a logical/factual approach compared with an emotional approach and an approach which tried to instil a habit so that seat belt wearing became routinised. Qualitative research indicated that this latter was probably the most effective and the slogan '*Klunk, Klick! Every Trip*', presented by someone having high source credibility, was considered to have provided a mnemonic. The implication of this being that in HBM terms the main perceived cost was merely the effort involved in establishing a routine (apart, of course, from the 15% who were implacably opposed on ideological grounds!).

The programmes were then launched in different regions in Britain utilising different levels of expenditure, mostly on TV advertising but supported by poster displays. The results were carefully monitored by observing levels of seat belt wearing at a variety of sampling points. The rate of wearing increased in each of the regions sampled and to some extent reflected the level of media expenditure. There did seem, however, to be a decay effect with the exception of the final area where the trend seemed to be upward, perhaps indicating the start of a normative shift. The extent of the effect is summarised by Levens and Rodnight as follows (Box 28).

**Box 28** Promoting Seat Belt Use: Expected Success

> *It is possible, within a media expenditure range, corresponding to a national equivalent of from £235,000 to £720,000 (1972 prices) to raise the level of seat belt wearing by a percentage ranging from 3% to 16% (from a basic 14%–15% start point) and to do so within a period of three weeks. The probable cost of bridging the gap between 32% and 75% wearing by persuasive advertising alone … could never be justified in benefit terms.*

The authors concluded that a burst of advertising over 3 weeks followed by supportive posters for a further 3 weeks would be the most cost effective way of proceeding. If we return to our earlier comment about the expectations of commercial advertisers, the changes produced would represent a very high level of success. However, the researchers did observe that having reached such a level any further effects could not be achieved by more mass media work. Using the level of seat belt wearing prevalent in Australian states – where, at the time, legislation had been introduced – as a yardstick (i.e. 75% wearing), they concluded that it would not be cost effective to bridge the gap between 32 and 75% using mass media alone. In Britain the need for such media-based health education disappeared with the advent of legal compulsion. It is, incidentally, worth offering a reminder at this juncture that although education failed to increase the level of wearing much above 30%, its agenda-setting function facilitated the enactment of health policy as described earlier. In other parts of the world health education is still needed to protect vehicle occupants. In this context it is interesting to note how a broad-based media plus community programme in North Carolina followed good commercial practice and offered various incentives to drivers wearing seat belts (in the form of prizes and the opportunity to draw a winning lottery ticket). The programme was successful in raising the level of wearing from 24 to 41% in 6 months and sustaining it at 36% after a further 6 months (Gemming *et al*, 1984). Let us compare this level of success with programmes which seek to modify substance abuse and influence levels of drug and alcohol use and smoking.

## SUBSTANCE ABUSE

In comparison with safety education, family planning and many of the other topics receiving consideration above, attempts to deal with the problems of substance abuse seem to be doomed to failure, especially if the sole mode of attack is mass media campaigns. In short, the task would seem to involve persuading individuals to forsake habits which give them pleasure and to which they may be addicted – in one sense or another – or which meet some important psychological or social need. Moreover, drug education currently operates in a social context in which a substantial majority of people use drugs of one kind or another – in other words, drug use is an established norm. The significance of these motivational barriers will be apparent when we consider examples of campaigns designed to promote smoking cessation and foster sensible drinking.

First, however, we will consider a recent attempt to use mass media to influence illegal drug use.

Despite expert opinion and Home Office policy, the UK government made a decision to launch a mass media campaign costing some £2,000,000 directed at heroin misuse. The amount of money involved may be put into some kind of perspective by noting that the major national health education agency's total budget at the time amounted to some £10,000,000. It is highly probable that the hidden goals of the campaign were to be seen to be doing something to deal with a problem of doubtful magnitude but which created a good deal of moral outrage and indignation. At any rate, an evaluation was commissioned by government. In assessing the results of this evaluation, four questions have to be asked.

- Should £2,000,000 have been spent on the programme?
- Were any real changes detectable in the target audience at the end of the campaign?
- If there were any such changes, could they reasonably be attributed to the campaign?
- In the event of real changes being observed, were these really significant rather than merely statistically significant, i.e. might they make any contribution to the reduction of drug misuse?

Of course, *a priori* the money should not have been spent in that way. First, epidemiologically, the problem of heroin use did not justify such an expenditure. Second, the accepted wisdom of drug education asserted that programmes should not use unsupported mass media nor should they focus on one specific drug. However, to many people's surprise, the evaluation appeared to indicate that, against all the odds, there was a significant and relevant change in beliefs and attitudes (since heroin use was so unusual there was no possibility of measuring any actual behaviour change). It is not possible here to provide a detailed and critical analysis of the research (for fuller discussion see Tones, 1986) but several valuable conclusions for media use generally may be drawn. First, it was apparent that the campaign had been very successful in penetrating the market

(which comprised young people aged 13–20) and in achieving levels of awareness which ranged from 80 to 98%, depending on the assessment criteria used. It thus supported the general axiom that properly constructed programmes can indeed successfully raise awareness. The second point which can be made is that it is increasingly difficult to find adequate control groups for national media programmes and therefore any observed results cannot be unequivocally ascribed to the programme itself. This was unfortunate since there did appear to be statistically significant changes in a series of measures of belief, attitude and intention which appeared to indicate a general hardening of attitude towards heroin use. However, because a control group was lacking and because the perfectly acceptable practice of using randomly selected but separate population sub-samples to measure attitudes, etc. before and after the campaign had been used, it was possible to argue that the observed changes might have been due to pre-existing differences in the samples, even though these should have been removed by the process of random selection. Such an argument would have looked suspiciously like rationalisation on the part of opponents of mass media drug education had it not been for several anomalies in the results. For instance, there seemed to be a tendency for the pre-campaign sample to have a generally less cautious approach to life than the post-campaign samples: the pre-campaign group appeared more likely to argue with parents and a higher proportion claimed that they would 'stand by their friends whatever they did'. These general attitudes could hardly have been influenced by a campaign dealing with a specific drug and the apparent hardening of attitudes could be ascribed to the fact that the post-campaign samples were generally more cautious, god-fearing and already opposed to hard drugs!

However, a much more important point can be made about the heroin campaign. Let us assume that the claimed shift in attitudes and beliefs was genuine. What impact could this be expected to have on the likelihood of a group of young people resisting the offer of hard drugs? Apart from the fact that beliefs about the effect of heroin on the body would probably be challenged when the young people in question actually engaged with a heroin using subculture, such beliefs and associated attitudes would be insignificant in real terms in the context of the various other alleged influences on drug misuse, such as unemployment, social deprivation, home background and socialisation, personality factors, self-esteem, machismo, rebelliousness, curiosity, social interaction skills, peer pressure, cultural norms, availability of drugs and beliefs about the gratifications provided. In the face of these factors the potential of mass media for influencing drug-related behaviour must be small. An alternative government strategy which allocated a similar amount of money to provide for about 100 drug coordinators for education authorities for a year would appear to be much more cost effective, even if it did not cater for the sense of moral outrage of the populace! However, let us move on to consider our most popular drug – alcohol.

## Alcohol

At first blush – and under the influence of a stereotyped view of desperate junkies unable to 'kick their habit' – we might expect alcohol education to offer greater opportunities for effective intervention than the heroin campaign discussed above. In fact, one of the biggest challenges to health promotion is posed by alcohol. The reasons are perhaps self-evident: unlike smoking, the health education message is relatively complex. It seeks to promote '*moderate*' or '*sensible*' drinking and requires the individual to calculate relative strengths of different liquor; it requires judgement and decision making. Moreover, the use of alcohol is strongly supported by social norms while smoking is becoming an increasingly deviant behaviour. The vast majority of smokers acknowledge the negative aspects of their habit and claim that they would like to give up, seeking only a magic formula and appropriate support to help them do so. The tobacco manufacturers are under constant attack while the brewing industry has a much more positive image. On the other hand, like smoking, alcohol consumption provides considerable gratification, both physical and

social. It is thus hardly surprising that examples of effective alcohol education are almost non-existent, particularly in the context of media campaigns and community-wide programmes.

The effectiveness and efficiency of alcohol education programmes have been comprehensively reviewed. In addition to the general reviews of Gatherer *et al.* (1979) and Bell *et al.* (1985), Kinder (1975) analysed some 66 studies on drug and alcohol education published between 1963 and 1973. Blane and Hewitt (1977, 1980) also produced state-of-the-art reviews of mass media. More recently Dorn and South (1983) provided a critical appraisal of 404 publications. The conclusions to be derived from all of these reviews are summarised in Box 29.

***Box 29***  A Resumé of Studies of the Effectiveness of Alcohol Education

- There have been relatively few methodologically sound evaluations (perhaps with the exception of a few studies of drink-driving).
- Expenditure on health education has been completely insignificant compared with the promotion of alcohol. Such campaigns as there have been have tended to be of limited geographical coverage and to have been broadcast at inappropriate times. As Dorn and South observe,

  *For every £1000 which is paid in liquor duty and tax in the UK, 43 pence is spent on education about alcohol and its effects. In 1980 over £76 million was spent on drink advertising.*

- The pro-alcohol messages conveyed directly and indirectly by media indicate both its social acceptability and its high prevalence.
- A social marketing approach incorporating thorough pre-testing should be used by health educators.
- There is a need for locally oriented community programmes having a strong inter-personal education component.

- Alcohol education programmes frequently produce a change in knowledge and occasionally attitude but rarely influence drinking behaviour.

To some extent the above observations about the effectiveness of health promotion in promoting appropriate use of alcohol might be made about most health education issues; it just happens that influencing alcohol consumption is especially difficult. We will now illustrate the points above and other mass media issues discussed earlier by selectively reviewing a few of the plethora of studies in this area. The first of these are concerned with the incidental effects of mass media.

The incidental, 'norm-sending' aspects of mass media were mentioned earlier in this chapter and reference was made to Hansen's (1986) work on media images of alcohol. Several published studies underline the importance of this norm-sending role of the media in relation to alcohol. The following are cited by Dorn and South (1983). Block (1965) described the ways in which press reporting stereotyped and stigmatised the alcoholic. A series of investigations by Breed and Defoe (1978, 1979a, b, 1980a, b, 1981) examined not only the portrayal of alcohol in magazine advertising but also in press reports, prime time TV sitcoms, comic books and campus magazines. Gerbner et al. (1981) pointed out the higher prevalence of alcohol images in top-rated programmes. King (1979) predated Hansen's observations by demonstrating similar types of presentation in British 'soaps'. Finn (1980) reminded us of the wide variety of mass media by reporting a content analysis of greeting cards which again perpetuated the negative stereotyped images of the alcohol abuser.

One of the possible mechanisms whereby these incidental effects may be produced is that of modelling. Both Caudill and Marlatt (1975) and Garlington and Dericco (1979) have argued that media models may influence the drinking rates of male students.

As we noted in our earlier discussion in this chapter about consultative collaboration, the norms conveyed through media presentations are essentially unrealistic. These mythical messages are listed below.

- Everyone drinks heavily (i.e. at a rate per unit time far in excess of real life drinking).
- Drinking is associated with sexual prowess, romance, enjoyable social occasions, power and commercial success and generally occurs in up-market situations.
- Few negative consequences are shown. Drinkers remain clear headed, do not have accidents, stay slim and healthy or, alternatively, may be seen as antiheroes. These latter provide a celebration of cosy self-gratification and folksy moderation in the face of attempts by fanatical zealots who try to impose unattainable ideals of health and fitness on the populace at large.
- 'Problem drinkers' are presented only in the caricatured form of skid row down-and-outs.

Following the theoretical discussion at the start of this chapter, it is not, of course, intended to suggest that this background of 'normative noise' will necessarily have any direct effect on people's drinking. It does, however, following the principles of 'uses and gratifications', provide people with the 'evidence' to justify their current practices and resist the pressures of health education. In the face of this background 'noise' conveying the normality and desirability of heavy alcohol consumption, it is perhaps some consolation that media credibility is relatively low (at any rate when it can be seen to attempt to influence). As indicated earlier, Budd and McCron (1979) demonstrated a low level of trust in health messages generally when delivered by mass media. This situation, not surprisingly, appears to apply to drugs and alcohol also. For instance Dembo et al. (1977) reported that high school students perceived TV and radio as having low credibility compared with other media and with inter-personal sources of information. It is not, however, clear whether the incidental presentation of health-related information is subject to the same degree of sceptical appraisal. It is probably wise to assume that it is not.

The implications of the work described above for health promotion are clear but not necessarily easy to achieve. At the level of policy the controllers of broadcast media must be prevailed upon to ensure that the consequences of alcohol consumption are more realistically portrayed. At the level of individual health education the natural scepticism of the viewing public must be nurtured by increasing awareness of media conventions and developing critical appraisal skills. Given the relative ineffectiveness of mass media in fostering 'sensible drinking' this aspect of health promotion merits increasing emphasis.

Turning now to these more deliberate attempts to influence people's knowledge, attitudes and practices with regard to alcohol, we might first ask about the trade's success in persuading individuals to start drinking and increase their level of consumption. As indicated earlier (Henry and Waterson, 1981), the advertisers of alcohol modestly deny having any effects on recruitment, asserting that they offer a public service by allowing the existing drinker to select from available beverages, i.e. the goal is brand switching. Several attempts have been made to give the lie to this assertion and demonstrate that advertising does have an effect on consumption. While it does seem likely that preferences for different kinds of alcohol (e.g. beer versus spirits) may be influenced (Brown, 1978), it is difficult to find sound evidence that restrictions on advertising will reduce consumption (Ogbourne and Smart, 1980) or show anything other than weak econometric associations. In the absence of such evidence it becomes more difficult to urge governmental action. If there is an effect, it is clearly of a much lower order than the impact of such structural factors as fiscal, economic and legislative measures (Bourgeois and Barnes, 1979). However, even if advertising does not in fact increase total consumption, the norm-sending function should be sufficient to justify pressure for controls.

Again, if it is indeed true that advertisers with their vast advertising budget really cannot influence consumption, the chances for health educa-

tion reducing total consumption would *a priori* appear to be slight. Published research supports this view but also demonstrates the anticipated '*Hierarchy of Communication Effects*' that were discussed earlier (namely that it is relatively easy to create awareness but increasingly difficult to influence recall, attitudes and behaviour). Some indication of this is provided by Maloney and Hersey's (1984) detailed account of an intensive marketing strategy to transmit alcohol public service advertisements (PSAs) nationwide (in the USA). Messages were aimed principally at women and youth. Assessment of the campaign reach (penetration) as measured by the proportion of the target audience likely to be watching TV at a given time of day multiplied by the market share of a particular TV station indicated that the PSAs reached on average 31.8% of all adults, 22% of the female target group and 19% of young people. However, according to the authors, commercial practice suggests that product purchase requires at least three exposures to an advertisement, which in turn means a level of campaign reach of 42% of an audience. Although the average penetration was 22%, there were in fact 13 markets where more than 42% of the primary targets were exposed to the PSAs and three where the exposure was 60% or more.

And so, given a sufficient level of media expenditure, the first goal of awareness can clearly be attained. Two case studies will now be considered in order to illustrate what might be expected from media campaigns which try to surpass this relatively limited goal. The first was launched in the north east of England and the second in California.

The *Tyne-Tees Alcohol Campaign* was piloted in 1974 (Health Education Council, 1983) and, in the view of many people, had unrealistic objectives of producing changes in consumption in a region noted for its heavy drinking. After a series of changes and developments the campaigns continued into the 1980s. At a meeting to assess its effects (Health Education Council, 1982) eight key findings were listed. These illustrate what might realistically be expected from such a campaign (Box 30).

**Box 30** Effects of an Alcohol Campaign: North East England

- People (in North East England) were aware of their regional attitudes to alcohol being 'different'.
- People in the North East were more inclined to believe alcohol was a problem, though they were inclined to think of it as caused by other problems.
- People in the North East were more aware of sources of help.
- More than 70% recalled the campaign and there were significant levels of recall of specific messages.
- One in eight people claimed that it had some influence on their thinking about alcohol.
- Safe drinking levels were believed to be lower in the north east than in Leicester (a comparison region).
- There was more awareness of 'equivalents' (i.e. relative alcoholic strength of different drinks) in the North East than in Leicester.
- There might be some antagonism building up towards health education messages.

The programme in California, which we will now consider, is of special interest because it was designed particularly to take account of known limitations of mass media. It was called the 'Winners' programme (indicating its attempt to promote a positive image) and is described by Wallack and Barrows (1983). It ran for 3 years at a total cost of some $2,500,000. It was located in three sites: one acted as a control, one received a media-only programme and the third received media plus an additional community-based effort (thus seeking to emulate the Stanford Heart Disease Prevention Programme). Programme goals were as follows: awareness raising and provision of information; attitude change and subsequently changes in actual drinking behaviours; medical indicators, namely cirrhosis rates (after an appropriate time lapse); social indicators in the form of drunk driving rates, arrests for disorderly conduct, etc. It was considered that success would

lead to cost benefits and an overall reduction in per capita consumption.

The target was adults aged 18–35 and after the first year it was hoped that other groups might be influenced.

The media programme included: three 30 second TV commercials, three 60 second radio slots; press advertisements; 110 billboard displays. The media mix was calculated to reach 90% of the target group on an average of 35 occasions. The message content emphasised positive advantages of lower consumption, presenting images of the moderate drinker as happy, in control, sociable and macho. Women were depicted as self-assured and in control.

It is interesting to note how political factors almost immediately affected the programme planning. The Wine Institute exerted pressure which delayed the programme to the extent that there was a 40% lower exposure than had been originally planned.

The community programme was designed to incorporate an inter-personal element. Some 14,453 people attended meetings; 67,000 pieces of programme material (balloons, badges, etc.) were distributed; various publicity events were arranged; teacher training programmes were developed. According to the authors, however, the community programme did not meet expectations in that there was little integration with media inputs and a planned recruitment of volunteers who might hold home meetings did not materialise.

The results follow the now expected pattern: good levels of awareness, some attitude change and no behaviour change. For detailed results readers are referred to the original article. However, the following will serve to indicate the nature and scale of the changes achieved (Box 31).

**Box 31** Effects of an Alcohol Campaign: California

- There was a high level of slogan recognition (79% in the adult group, 86% in the youth group). As with many other results these tended to be more pronounced in the media plus community area and greater than in the control community.

- There was a generally high level of correct interpretation of the messages (e.g. 70% adult, 84% youth) and 20% of adults and 30% of youth scored at least eight out of 12 on a scale of overall comprehension. The problem of lack of feedback potential of media was, however, to be observed in that some 25% believed that one of the PSAs was promoting alcohol – even after pre-testing!

- Recall was generally good (50% adults, 72% youth).

- In general there was a disappointing level of change in the *affective* area. For example, awareness of alcohol problems and concern about these problems showed relatively slight increases, as did concern about own level of drinking (e.g. 8% adults, 2% youth). On an attitude scale containing 13 statements relating to advertising of alcohol, drunkenness, etc. there was only one significant change (and that was in the adult group).

- As for behavioural outcomes, 15% of those who recognised the '*Winners*' slogans reported a reduction in drinking or claimed that they intended to do so, but there was no supporting evidence of this. There was no change in other items which attempted to measure quantity and frequency of drinking nor was there any change in a seven category drinking problem scale.

In short, it is clear that even in a very well-constructed and evaluated programme which takes account of the dictates of social marketing there is no evidence of behaviour change. It could, of course, happen that the campaign's impact on knowledge and awareness might, in the context of future developments, make the success of such hypothetical developments more likely. Wallack and Barrows (1983) described the situation thus:

*The California Prevention Demonstration was unique in many ways, but in terms of the types of outcomes that were produced it was quite typical. The major evaluation findings of increased awareness, some gain in knowledge and no attitude or behaviour change is consistent with a myriad of other mass media programs and prevention efforts in general.*

The authors argued that Lazarsfeld and Merton's views (1975) were even more applicable to the current scenario than they were 40 years previously. They strongly assert the points made in Chapter 1 of this book that mass media programmes in difficult areas like alcohol use will only be effective when complemented by significant public policy measures. As it is:

*Mass media campaigns and other kinds of individual-oriented interventions are safe because they virtually never challenge any powerful vested interests. Such interventions implicitly state that the problem is in the person and not in the system. Yet as we have suggested above, the person and the system are inseparable; you cannot address one without also addressing the other.*

The results of workplace interventions, discussed in an earlier chapter, would bear out these views. However, research on mass media work on smoking yields much more impressive results, particularly when combined with inter-personal efforts and based on sound learning theory. The reasons for any such success compared with alcohol interventions were suggested earlier. For the moment we will briefly consider some of the results of evaluations of programmes designed to foster smoking cessation.

## Smoking

Before commenting on the effectiveness of mass media in combating smoking we must note that just as alcohol use and misuse has its own peculiarities as a public health problem, the special characteristics of smoking must be taken into account before judgements are made. First of all, there are two qualitatively different smoking prevention tasks:

the prevention of recruitment differs from the promotion of smoking cessation. The motives which underlie young people's adoption of the habit are not at all similar to the motivation which may prevent adult (or even young people) quitting. For young people tobacco and its pharmacology are largely irrelevant; smoking serves a symbolic purpose and meets instrumental needs, gratifying the values associated with machismo, toughness, precocity and the like. It also provides a valuable adjunct to self-presentation and social interaction. While some of these aspects may also be important to the adult smoker, the cigarette's role in affect control becomes much more prominent.

The educational tasks demanded by these two different prevention goals are thus distinct. In simple terms, the aims of preventing the onset of smoking involve the creation of a negative attitude to the habit and, more importantly, providing substitute gratification in the form of lifeskills, etc. On the other hand, since the majority of smokers already appear to have a negative attitude to their habit, the major preventive goal is to provide a trigger to cessation followed by support to minimise the chance of relapse. The very nature of these different educational objectives means that the mass media have been seen as more appropriate to the smoking cessation exercise rather than to preventing recruitment (although, as we have seen, TV may be a useful supplement to school-based programmes which seek to prevent recruitment to smoking). As we will see, the effectiveness of mass media in stimulating cessation (the only justifiable goal) has depended on the extent to which support can be provided or mobilised and this in turn has meant borrowing inter-personal techniques.

Three kinds of intervention will be described below. The first of these involves mere consciousness raising about the importance of stopping smoking, with or without the provision of more detailed information and mailed supporting literature. The second involves a more thorough TV presentation incorporating several sessions and based on social learning theory. Typical of the former situation is the UK National No Smoking Day.

Reid (1985) describes the relative effectiveness of two successive no smoking days in 1984 and 1985. Apart from providing results which reveal the anti-smoking potential of this sort of publicity tactic, the hierarchy of effects is nicely illustrated. For instance, after pre-publicity designed to coordinate national health education efforts on the day itself some 716 press reports were recorded, together with 424 mentions on TV or radio. Over a 14 day period there were 13 national radio or TV slots and an estimated 134 hours of broadcasting (including in 1985 mentions on the popular 'soaps' *Brookside* and *Coronation Street*).

Public awareness was high and amounted to some 79% of the population. There was local support from over 100 health education units as well as other organisations such as schools, hospitals, etc. In terms of acceptability, 70% of an interview sample agreed that the day was a good idea and only 7% were firmly opposed.

In order to determine the impact on smoking, a survey of 2000 adults was carried out in 130 sampling points throughout the country. The results were as follows: of 2000 adults, 735 were smokers; 95 (13%) reported trying to give up and five succeeded in giving up for the day. A further study of 4000 adults 3 months later provided corroboration of the first survey. Eleven per cent reported they had tried to give up smoking on National No Smoking Day; 9% claimed to have been successful for 2 months before relapsing. However, only three out of the 4000 were still non-smokers after 3 months (and only one of these claimed that this was due to the day itself!).

Was this a success or a failure? The cost incurred was £50,000 and included expenditure on 250,000 posters and 300,000 smokers' contracts. At any rate, it was decided to repeat the day in 1985 with an increased budget (£100,000). Although no information was presented on cessation rates, it was clear that awareness was again high: some 76% had heard of the programme on TV and 6.5% of smokers claimed to have given up for the day. An interesting indicator is provided of the booster effect of local involvement: some 22,000 people used a telephone to '*Dial a Tip*' but 14,000 of these were from Plymouth where two local TV personalities committed themselves to stop smoking during the week.

It is clearly unwise to set unrealistic behavioural standards for a publicity venture such as National No Smoking Day. Rather, it should be viewed as an agenda-setting exercise which might to some degree counteract the norm-sending messages transmitted by the tobacco advertisers and may even act as an ultimate trigger to a small number of individuals who have been screwing up their courage to abandon their habit!

A more extensive but to some extent more abortive media venture was reported by Raw and de Plight (1981). A 15 minute programme was presented at prime time in a regular documentary slot. It had a 'hard-hitting evangelical style' (*... we want to make a frontal attack on smoking ... we're going to send you every known device to make you give it up and stop killing yourself*). That section of the public who were already motivated to quit and were waiting for the 'magic bullet' responded eagerly. Four thousand calls were received in 30 minutes and eventually some 600,000 people wrote in for the kit which was to help them stop smoking. Unfortunately only 20,000 kits were available. The public was not impressed!

Eventually a more limited kit was sent out to a sample of 20,000 applicants together with a questionnaire. The response rate was 12%. Of the 1752 who returned usable questionnaires 1602 said they intended to stop smoking, 747 tried to stop, 57 succeeded for between 2 and 3 months;, 41 were still not smoking after 6 months and 14 were abstinent at 1 year. The success rate among those who returned the questionnaires was thus 0.79%. It should, however, be noted that 46% had found the kit unhelpful.

Other studies of similar ventures have met with greater success: for instance, Cuckle and Vunakis (1984) studied a random sample of 4492 subjects out of 500,000 who requested a postal smoking cessation kit after a TV programme on the hazards of smoking. Compared with a control group, cessation after 1 year was superior in the experimental group (11 versus 16%). Interestingly, but not surprisingly, validation via salivary cotinine measurement revealed lower results but there was still a statistically significant difference (7 versus 9%). These results are not dissimilar to those found by O'Byrne

and Crawley (1981) after an Irish programme. Some 5% of kit recipients claimed to have stopped smoking between 3 and 5 months after the campaign. The superiority of the American figures presumably reflects the greater normative 'push' to non-smoking in the USA compared with Eire. Normative factors would also have to be considered in the comprehensive and well-documented study by Puska *et al.* (1979) in Finland.

In the general context of the *North Karelian Heart Disease Prevention Project* a smoking cessation course was presented on TV in 1978. It was launched at a national press conference and was supported by extensive press reporting. The major voluntary organisations also informed their members about the programme and a serious attempt was made to encourage smokers to follow the programme in organised groups. Lay leaders of these groups were provided with support materials. The programme lasted 4 weeks; there were seven sessions broadcast during the evening and lasting 45 minutes each. The programmes were designed to incorporate inter-personal methods in that a group of 10 smokers were featured in the studio and sessions were led by two experts. The techniques used by smoking cessation clinics were employed. In other words, the mass media strategy was about as thorough as it could be: there was intensive and comprehensive coverage on the one available TV channel; it was supported by additional publicity in the context of a regional programme which had raised awareness of the national heart disease problem; it employed inter-personal methods on screen and encouraged group support in local neighbourhoods. How well did it do? The results showed that 39.5% of men saw between one and three of the broadcast sessions (the figure for women was 38.7%); 4.2% of men and 7.3% of women saw all seven. As for the impact on smoking, a survey carried out 1 year after the final programme revealed that 17% of smokers followed the programme but did not try to stop and 1.4% stopped smoking but started again. Only 0.8% of those who were smoking at the start of the series were non-smokers after 1 year. Analysis of those who followed the programmes in a support group yielded the following results. In North Karelia 404 people were in these organised groups; 320 completed the course. Of those who completed the course, 21% succeeded in stopping smoking for a period of at least 6 months.

One of the most thorough and effective programmes employing mass media to promote smoking cessation is described by Best (1980). This used not only mass media but employed the principles of behaviour modification in the form of 'self-management' components previously used in face-to-face clinics. Six programmes were broadcast on consecutive weeks between 7.00 and 7.30 p.m. The potential audience was some 20,000 adults (in Washington, DC). Viewers were invited to write in for the self-help guide mentioned above and each TV programme was linked to a chapter in the booklet. Those who applied for the booklet served as the subjects of the evaluation.

At the end of the series 86.5% of the survey group returned a completed questionnaire, 64.2% returned a second questionnaire at 3 months and 71.4% returned a questionnaire at 6 months. Cessation rates at these times were 11.5, 14.7 and 17.6%, respectively.

How should we assess the results of both the Finnish exercise and the intervention described by Best? Puska *et al.* made the observation that although the programme achieved a rate of success which was small percentage wise, some 10,000 smokers country-wide might have stopped smoking with the aid of the programme and that is a lot of smokers in absolute terms. Best commented that the spontaneous quit rate (in the USA) was probably 5%; long-term success rates for smoking cessation clinics are of the order of 15–20% (perhaps higher if supplemented by prescription of nicotine chewing gum); face-to-face behaviour modification methods utilised by Best achieved 50% at 6 months. By these criteria the 17.6% achieved by his TV programmes is good. In terms of cost effectiveness he calculated that the face-to-face method cost $200 per success, smoking clinics cost $250 or more while, because of the large audience reached by media, the TV series cost some $48 per documented abstinence (at 6 months).

One final point will be made about the use of mass media and smoking prevention. While it is clear that education about smoking generally and education delivered by mass media in particular are undoubtedly more effective than alcohol education, we should bear in mind Wallack's observations about the importance of structural social change in supporting education. Engleman (1983) describes this synergism between publicity, education and legal/fiscal measures in influencing smoking rates. He argues that not only has education itself had an impact on smoking, but it has also been responsible for such increases in taxation on cigarettes as have been imposed in recent years. He refers to the USA and argues that had it not been for the first *Surgeon General's Report* in 1964 and the subsequent education and publicity, smoking would have been 22% greater than it was in 1975. Since that time the reductions have continued, although it seems likely that as we move into the asymptote further progress will be increasingly difficult and mass media will have an increasing role to play in stimulating policy change rather than persuading individuals to quit. At the same time the main thrust of smoking education must be targeted on young people, mainly in the schools and utilising appropriate inter-personal educational strategies.

More importantly, in the light of our discussion of the centrality of *Media Advocacy* in health promotion, we should remind ourselves of a strategy that scored a major success. The strategy was BUGA UP, an acronym for *Billboard Utilising Graffitists Against Unhealthy Promotions*. The use of acronyms incidentally figures at an early stage in Chapman's 'A–Z' weaponry of advocacy methods (alphabetically speaking). BUGA UP might be described as the militant wing of MOP UP (*Movement Opposed to the Promotion of Unhealthy Products*). Their major activity involved the illegal 're-facing' of outdoor billboards and interrupting media promotions by the tobacco companies (C for civil disobedience). Amongst other things they entered a competition held by Philip Morris (in Australia in 1981) which sought an Australian 'Marlborough Man'. BUGA UP's preferred candidate was Frank, ... *a man confined to a wheelchair who smoked through his tracheotomy air hole.* They also produced a portrait of Frank as a poster for placement on Sydney billboards. This,

385

predictably, attracted a good deal of media attention (and was later used on the cover of the *Medical Journal of Australia*). A similar poster, incidentally, was produced by AGHAST in 1984 in London – ostensibly for inclusion in an exhibition sponsored by John Player Special cigarettes at the National Portrait Gallery. This was entitled *The early death of Jack Filbert*. Not surprisingly, it was considered unsuitable so AGHAST (a Bristol-based activist group) held an alternative exhibition entitled the *Lung Slayer Portrait Award* (D for demonstrations in Chapman's 'A–Z').

BUGA UP also gatecrashed an international conference of advertising agencies at the Sydney Opera House in 1986 (G for gatecrash in the lexicon). They set up a mock '*confessional booth*' and invited advertisers who worked on tobacco accounts to confess their sins! The gatecrashing exercise split Sydney media's coverage of the conference!

BUGA UP provides a clear illustration of the wide variety of tactics and techniques used in *Media Advocacy* – in addition to providing its own radical media displays on 'borrowed' tobacco industry posters. It therefore again demonstrates the fact that mass media interventions, conservative or radical, are enhanced by other face-to-face action. Was BUGA UP successful? Some years ago one of the authors asked a key protagonist what BUGA UP was doing at that time. The response was that it no longer existed – it had won! Clearly it is not possible to provide traditional evidence of success based on such research designs as the RCT. It is, however, possible to provide extensive evidence based on indirect and intermediate indicators of successful processes and changes in individual characteristics. Bearing in mind the comment from the minister of sport mentioned earlier in this chapter, there seems to have been changes in outcome (e.g. the voting patterns of politicians). The fact that Australia subsequently took an international lead in banning all forms of tobacco advertising provides evidence that demonstrates, beyond reasonable doubt, that *Media Advocacy* had, on this occasion, made the major contribution to a healthy outcome!

Because of the controversial nature of mass media this chapter has looked in some depth at the issues involved and the requirements of effective media work. The conclusion to be drawn is that mass media can serve a very useful purpose in health education when properly designed and when their inherent limitations are recognised.

In earlier chapters we emphasised the importance of avoiding Type 3 error, i.e. making inappropriate judgements about the failure of health promotion interventions when those interventions were doomed to fail because of inadequate design and planning. There are, of course, a variety of books on the use of mass media in health promotion and many of these provide both generalisations and recommendations for designing mass media interventions (e.g. Backer *et al.*, 1992). Nonetheless, we feel it is useful to complete this chapter with some relatively succinct generalisations and recommendations about the appropriate design of masse media programmes. Accordingly, Table 8.6 provides a final summary of key principles governing media usage.

**Table 8.6**  Using mass media: some key principles and generalisations

1. Mass media should not be used on their own; they *should* be used to support programmes that centre on interpersonal interactions, e.g. in schools, workplaces and other settings. They should be considered as an integral part of community-wide programmes together with supportive policy measures.

2. The potentially most effective use of mass media is in the form of media advocacy, i.e. creating public awareness of issues. The following variants are in ascending order of potential effectiveness, and radicalism:

   • gaining unpaid advertising opportunities by providing newsworthy information;
   • 'agenda setting' about health issues as a precursor to later action;
   • consciousness raising using 'creative epidemiology' to stimulate actions having a focus on disease and inequalities in health;
   • 'critical consciousness raising' about social, economic and environmental issues in the pursuit of equity, supported by various additional advocacy strategies, such as demonstrations and civil disobedience.

3. Politically speaking, 'consultative cooperation' with media funders and producers may be the only strategy possible for health promotion. It involves use of well-recognised principles of achieving 'inter-sectoral collaboration', such as negotiation and 'reticulist' skills.

4. The use of 'soap opera' and other entertainment programmes have a number of particular advantages. They should be used where possible, provided that it is remembered that their main purpose is to entertain! 'Edutainment' programmes may be more amenable to promoting health messages as part of their function is, by definition, education. Again, expertise in collaborative working is an essential prerequisite for success.

5. Bearing in mind the fundamental difference between marketing commercial products and health products, all mass media work should follow tried and tested marketing principles, in particular the following.

- Audience segmentation, which should be considered as an essential element in the process of identifying target groups and needs assessment: the following are particularly important:
  - use of database marketing, which offers increasing scope for moving beyond the description of general demographic description and identifying 'psychographic' characteristics, i.e. beliefs, values, attitudes and other individual attributes;
  - recognise that it may be necessary to identify another target group of 'gate-keepers' before the primary target group can be reached;
- It is essential to assess the socio-economic and other structural aspects of the target groups that may act as barriers to their responding to the media messages.
- Set realistic objectives, bearing in mind that although mass media can successfully raise awareness, transmit relatively simple information and produce a positive attitude to the way the message is presented, they cannot create complex understandings nor teach the skills needed to support health-related behaviour, nor can they affect beliefs and influence attitudes where these are not consistent with the existing values and motivation of the target group.
- Ensure that the delivery of the media programme will ensure the target receives sufficient exposure: individuals may need to receive the same message several times before they manage to absorb and remember the message and, of course, it should be delivered through media that are used by and accessible to the target group.
- Repetition of messages may need to continue for a long period of time if the main purpose is not just to ensure that the message is remembered but rather to act in a 'norm-sending' way, i.e. to breed familiarity but not contempt.
- Analyse the nature of the message to be transmitted, focusing on the audience's likely perceptions of the benefits and costs implicit in the message. Remember that costs are not merely financial but also have to do with experiencing inconvenience, discomfort, pain or loss of gratification. Even minimal costs are likely to result in a failure to influence behaviour (though the message may set the agenda for subsequent successful inter-personal influence).
- Adopt an appropriate style for message delivery (i.e. 'branding'); a positive affect is more likely to be effective than a negative affect. Take account of the fact that long-term, 'distal benefits may have zero attraction, especially for young people; short-term gains are more attractive. Beware using fear appeal; it is hardly ever the most effective strategy in the long run and may create defensive avoidance. If fear is to be aroused, there must be some means of reducing any anxiety generated (e.g. by accessible personal support, direct or via phone 'hot lines').
- The message can often be crafted to provide 'inoculation' against anticipated negative messages and products. When handled with care, this can be a useful function for media work.
- Use an appropriate source, even if this is just a 'voice-over'; the source must be credible and, preferably, provide an attractive model for the adoption of recommended attitudes or behaviours. Credible sources can lose their credibility in a remarkably short period of time, for instance, youth audiences are notoriously fickle in their allegiances.
- Do not patronise, demean or otherwise antagonise the audience!
- More effective campaigns use multiple media.
- All mass media should be pre-tested following recommended guidelines for formative research.

6. The mass media are still frequently seen as a panacea. They are also especially attractive to politicians since the appearance on television of dramatic and attractive 'commercials' (e.g. on the evils of drug abuse) may at least convince voters that their government is taking positive action (however ineffective). It is, therefore, essential to submit campaigns having unrealistic goals to critical appraisal and evaluation.

# REFERENCES

Aitken, P. P., Leathar, D. S., O'Hagan, F. J. and Squair, S. I. (1987) *Children's awareness of cigarette advertisements and brand imagery. British Journal of Addiction*, 82, 615–622.

Ajit, T. C. (1982) *A life worth living. Public Relations*, Winter, 3–5.

Amos, A., Currie, C., Gray, D. and Elton, R. (1998) *Perceptions of fashion images from youth magazines: does a cigarette make a difference? Health Education Research*, 13 (4), 491–501.

Atkin, C. K. (1981) *Mass media information campaign effectiveness*. In R. E. Rice and W. J. Paisley (Eds) *Public Communication Campaigns*. Sage, Beverly Hills, CA.

Auger, T. J., Wright, T. J. and Simpson, R. H. (1972) *Posters as smoking deterrents. Journal of Applied Psychology*, 56, 169–171.

Backer, T. E., Rogers, E. M. and Sopory, P. (Eds) (1992) *Designing Health Communication Campaigns: What Works?* Sage, Newbury Park, CA.

Ball-Rokeach, S. J. and de Fleur, M. L. (1976) *A dependency model of mass media effects. Communication Research*, 3, 3–21.

BBC (1982) *'Play It Safe': Child Accident Prevention Campaign*, BBC Broadcasting Research Special Report. BBC, London.

Bell, J. and Billington, D. R. (1985) *Annotated Bibliography of Health Education Research Completed in Britain from 1948–1978 and 1979–1983*. Scottish Health Education Group, Edinburgh.

Berger, A. A. (1991) *Media Analysis Techniques*. Sage: Newbury Park, CA.

Best, G., Dennis, J. and Draper, P. (1977) *Health, the Mass Media and the National Health Service*. Unit for the Study of Health Policy, London.

Best, J. A. (1980) *Mass media, self-management and smoking modification*. In P. O. Davidson and S. M. Davidson (Eds) *Behavioral Medicine: Changing Health Lifestyles*. Brunner/Mazel, New York, NY.

Blane, H. T. and Hewitt, L. E. (1977) *Mass Media, Public Education and Alcohol: a State-of-the-Art Review*. National Institute on Alcohol Abuse and Alcoholism, Rockville, MD.

Blane, H. T. and Hewitt, L. E. (1980) *Alcohol, public education and mass media: an overview. Alcohol, Health and Research World*, 5, 2–16.

Block, M. (1965) *Alcoholism: Its Facets and Phases*. Oxford University Press, Oxford.

Bonaguro, J. A. and Miaoulis, G. (1983) *Marketing a tool for health education planning. Health Education*, January/February, 6–11.

Botvin, G. J., Eng, A. and Williams, C. L. (1980) *Preventing the onset of Cigarette smoking through life skills training. Preventive Medicine*, 9, 135–143.

Bouman, M., Maas, L. and Kok, G. (1998) *Health education in television entertainment – Medisch Centrum West: a Dutch drama serial. Health Education Research*, 13 (4), 503–518.

Bouman, M. (1999) *The Turtle and the Peacock: the Entertainment Education Strategy on Television*. Wageningen Agricultural University, Wageningen, The Netherlands.

Bourgeois, J. C. and Barnes, J. G. (1979) *Does advertising increase alcohol consumption? Journal of Advertising Research*, 19, 19–29.

Breed, W. and Defoe, J. R. (1978) *Bringing alcohol into the open. Columbia Journalism Review*, 18, 18–19.

Breed, W. and Defoe, J. R. (1979a) *Drinking on television: a comparison of alcohol use to the use of coffee, tea, soft drinks, water and cigarettes. The Bottom Line*, 2, 28–29.

Breed, W. and Defoe, J. R. (1979b) *Themes in magazine alcohol advertisements: a critique. Journal of Drug Issues*, 9, 511–522.

Breed, W. and Defoe, J. R. (1980a) *Mass media, alcohol and drugs: a new trend. Journal of Drug Issues*, 9, 511–522.

Breed, W. and Defoe, J. R. (1980b) *The mass media and alcohol education: a new direction. Journal of Alcohol and Drug Education*, 25, 48–58.

Breed, W. and Defoe, J. R. (1981) *The portrayal of the drinking process on prime-time television. Journal of Communication*, 31, 48–58.

Breed, W. and Defoe, J. R. (1982) *Effecting media change: the role of cooperative consultation on alcohol topics. Journal of Communication*, 32, 88–99.

Brown, R. A. (1978) *Educating young people about alcohol use in New Zealand: whose side are we on? British Journal of Alcohol and Alcoholism*, 13, 199–201.

Budd, J. and McCron, R. (1979) *Communication and Health Education, A Preliminary Study*. Health Education Council, London.

Burt, A., Illingworth, D., Shaw, T. R. D., Thornley, P., White, P. and Turner, R. (1974) *Stopping smoking after myocardial infarction. Lancet*, i, 304–306.

Cantril, H. (1958) *The invasion from Mars*. In E. E. Maccoby, T. M. Newcomb and E. L. Hartley (Eds)

*Readings in Social Psychology*. Henry Holt, New York, NY, pp. 291–300.

Caudill, B. D. and Marlatt, C. (1975) *Modelling influences in social drinking: an experimental analogue. Journal of Consulting and Clinical Psychology*, 43, 405–415.

Cernada, G. P. and Lu, L. P. (1982) *The Kaohsiung Study. Studies in Family Planning*, 3, 198–203.

Chaffee, S. (1981) *Mass media in political campaigns: an expanding role*. In R. E. Rice and W. J. Paisley (Eds) *Public Communication Campaigns*. Sage, Beverly Hills, CA.

Chapman, S. (1986) *The Lung Goodbye: A Manual of Tactics for Counteracting the Tobacco Industry in the 1980s*, 2nd Edn. International Organization of Consumers' Unions, The Hague, The Netherlands.

Chapman, S. (1994) *What is public health advocacy?* In S. Chapman and D. Lupton (Eds) *The Fight for Public Health: Principles and Practice of Media Advocacy*. BMJ Publishing, London.

Chapman, S. and Egger, G. (1983) *Myth in cigarette advertising and health promotion*. In H. Davis and P. Walton (Eds) *Language, Image and Media*. Blackwell, Oxford.

Chapman, S. and Fitzgerald, B. (1982) *Brand preference and advertising recall in adolescent smokers: some implications for health promotion. American Journal of Public Health*, 72, 491–494.

Charlton, A. (1986) *Children's advertisement-awareness related to their views on smoking. Health Education Journal*, 45, 75–78.

Chesterfield-Evans, A. and O'Connor, G. (1986) *Billboard utilizing graffitists against unhealthy promotions (BUGAP) – its philosophy and rationale and their application in health promotion*. In D. S. Leathar, G. B. Hastings and J. K. Davies (Eds) *Health Education and the Media*. Pergamon Press, London.

Cole, R. and Holland, S. (1980) *Recall of health education display materials. Health Education Journal*, 39, 74–79.

Colver, A. P., Hutchinson, P. J. and Judson, E. C. (1982) *Promoting children's home safety. British Medical Journal*, 285, 1177–1180.

Cuckle, H. S. and Vunakis, H. V. (1984) *The effectiveness of a postal smoking cessation kit. Community Medicine*, 6, 210–215.

Dale, E. and Chall, J. A. (1948) *A formula for predicting readability: instructions. Education Research Bulletin*, 27 (37), 11–20.

Davison, R. L. (1983) *Questions about cancer: the public's demand for information. Journal of the Institute of Health Education*, 21, 5–16.

de Chernatony, L. (1993) *Categorizing brands: evolutionary processes underpinned by two key dimensions. Journal of Marketing Management*, 9, 109–120.

Defoe, J. R. and Breed, W. R. (1989) *Consulting to change media contents: two cases in alcohol education. International Quarterly of Community Health Education*, 9, 257–272.

Dembo, R., Miran, M., Babst, D. V. and Schmeidler, J. (1977) *The believability of the media as sources of information on drugs. International Journal of Addictions*, 12, 959–969.

Department of Health (1999) *Smoking Kills*. HMSO, London.

Docherty, S. C. (1981) *Sports sponsorship – a first step in marketing health?* In D. S. Leathar, G. B. Hastings and J. K. Davies (Eds) *Health Education and the Media*. Pergamon Press, London.

Dorn, N. (1981) *Communication with the working class requires recognition of a working class: a materialist approach*. In D. S. Leathar, G. B. Hastings and J. K. Davies (Eds) *Health Education and the Media*. Pergamon Press, London.

Dorn, N. and South, N. (1983) *Message in a Bottle*. Gower, Aldershot.

Douglas, T. (1984) *The Complete Guide to Advertising*. Macmillan, London.

Dunnigan, M. G., McIntosh, W. B., Sutherland, G. R., Gardee, R., Glebin, B., Ford, J. A. and Robertson, I. (1981) *Policy for the prevention of Asian rickets in Britain: a preliminary assessment of the Glasgow rickets campaign. British Medical Journal*, 282, 357–360.

Durgee, J. F. (1986) *How consumer sub-cultures code reality: a look at some code types. Advances in Consumer Research*, 13, 332–337.

Eakin, E. G., Lichtenstein, H. H., Severson, V. J., Stevens, V. J., Vogt, T. M. and Hollis, J. F. (1998) *Use of tailored videos in primary care smokint cessation interventions. Health Education Research*, 13 (4), 519–527.

England, P. M. and Oxley, D. E. (1980) *Head infestation in Humberside: a health control exercise. Health Education Journal*, 39, 23–25.

Engleman, S. R. (1983) *The Impact of Anti-smoking Mass Media Publicity*. Health Education Council, London.

Evans, R. I., Rozelle, R. M. and Mittlemark, M. B.

(1978) *Deterring the onset of smoking in children. Journal of Applied Social Psychology*, 8, 126–135.

Fairclough, N. (1995) *Ideology*. Arnold, London.

Farhar-Pilgrim, B. and Shoemaker, F. F. (1981) *Campaigns to affect energy behavior*. In R. E. Rice and W. J. Paisley (Eds) *Public Communication Campaigns*. Sage, Beverly Hills, CA.

Finn, P. (1980) *Attitudes toward drinking conveyed in studio greeting cards. American Journal of Public Health*, 70, 826–829.

Flay, B. R. (1981) *On improving the chances of mass media health promotion programs causing meaningful changes in behavior*. In M. Meyer (Ed.) *Health Education by Television and Radio*. K.G. Saur, München.

Flay, B. R., Pentz, M. S., Johnson, C. A., Sussman, S., Mestell, J. et al. (1986) *Reaching children with mass media health promotion programs: the relative effectiveness of an advertising campaign in a community-based program and a school-based program*. In D. S. Leathar, G. B. Hastings and J. K. Davies (Eds) *Health Education and the Media*. Pergamon Press, London.

Flay, B.R., Hansen, W.B., Anderson Johnson, C. (1987) *Implementation effectiveness trial of a social influences smoking prevention programme using schools and television. Health Education Research*, 2, 385–400.

Flesch, R. (1948) *A new readability yardstick. Journal of Applied Psychology*, 32, 221.

Fuglesang, A. (1981) *Folk media and folk messages*. In M. Meyer (Ed.) *Health Education by Television and Radio*. K.G. Saur, München.

Garlington, W. and Dericco, D. (1979) *The effect of modelling on drinking rate. Journal of Applied Behavior Analysis*, 10, 207–211.

Gatherer, A., Parfit, J., Porter, E. and Vessey, M. (1979) *Is Health Education Effective?* Health Education Council, London.

Gemming, M. G., Runyan, C. W. and Campbell, B. J. (1984) *A community health education approach to occupant protection. Health Education Quarterly*, 11, 147–158.

Gerbner, G., Gross, L., Morgan, M. P. and Signorelli, N. (1981) *Health and medicine on television – special report. New England Journal of Medicine*, 305, 90–94.

Gordon, E. (1967) *Evaluation of communications media in two health projects in Baltimore. Public Health Reports*, 82, 651–655.

Grant, A. S. (1972) *What's the use of posters? Journal of the Institute of Health Education*, 10, 7–11.

Green, L. W. and Kreuter, M. W. (1991) *Health Promotion Planning: An Educational and Environmental Approach*. Mayfield, CA.

Greenberg, B. S. and Gantz, W. (1976) *Public television and taboo topics: the impact of 'VD Blues'. Public Telecommunications Review*, 4, 59–64.

Hansen, A. (1986) *The portrayal of alcohol on television. Health Education Journal*, 45 (3), 127–131.

Harris, J. (1983) *Interpretive Summary of Hypothermia Campaign Evaluations, Winter of 1982/3*. Health Education Council, London.

Harrison, C. (1980) *Readability in Classrooms*. Cambridge University Press, Cambridge.

Hartley, J. (Ed.) (1980) *The Psychology of Written Communication*, Part 3. Kogan Page, London.

Hastings, G. B., Stead, M., Whitehead, M., Lowry, R., MacFadyen, L. et al. (1998) *Using the media to tackle the health divide: future directions. Social Marketing Quarterly*, IV (3), 42–67.

Health Education Council (1982) *Report of a Meeting held on 29th April, 1982: The Tyne-Tees Alcohol Education Campaign*. Health Education Council, London.

Health Education Council (1983) *The Tyne-Tees Alcohol Education Campaign*. Health Education Council, London.

Henry, H. W. and Waterson, M. J. (1981) *The case for advertising alcohol and tobacco products*. In D. S. Leathar, G. B. Hastings and J. K. Davies (Eds) *Health Education and the Media*. Pergamon Press, London.

Holcomb, C. and Ellis, J. (1978) *Measuring the readability of selected patient education materials: the Cloze Procedure. Health Education*, 9, 8.

Hutchinson, A. and Thompson, J. (1982) *Rubella prevention: two methods compared. British Medical Journal*, 284, 1087–1089.

Institute for Alcohol Studies (1985) *The Presentation of Alcohol in the Mass Media, Report of a Seminar, January 1985*. Institute for Alcohol Studies, London.

Jackson, R. H. (1983) *'Play It Safe': a campaign for the prevention of children's accidents. Community Development Journal*, 18, 172–176.

Jenkins, J. (1983) *Mass Media for Health Education*. International Extension College, Cambridge.

Katz, E. and Lazarsfeld, P. (1955) *Personal Influence: the Part Played by People in the Flow of Mass Communication*. Free Press, Glencoe, IL.

Katz, E., Blumler, J. and Gurevitch, M. (1974) *Utilisation of mass communications by the individual.* In J. Blumler and E. Katz. (Eds) *The Uses of Mass Communication.* Sage, Beverly Hills, CA.

Kerr, M. and Charles, N. (1983) *Attitudes to the Feeding and Nutrition of Young Children.* Health Education Council, London.

Kinder, B. N. (1975) *Attitudes toward alcohol and drug abuse: experimental data, mass media research and methodological considerations.* International Journal of Addictions, 10, 1035–1054.

King, R. (1979) *Drinking and drunkenness in 'Crossroads' and 'Coronation Street'.* In J. Cook and M. Lewington (Eds) *Images of Alcoholism,.* British Film Institute, London.

Klapper, J. T. (1960) *The Effects of Mass Communication.* Free Press, Glencoe, IL.

Klapper, J. T. (1997) *The effects of mass communication.* In O. Boyd-Barrett and C. (Eds) *Approaches to Media: A Reader.* Arnold, London.

Kotler, P. (1975) *Marketing for Non-Profit Organizations.* Prentice Hall, New York, NY.

Lavigne, A. S., Albert, W. and Simmons, M. (1986) *The application of market segmentation in alcohol and drug education: the APPLAUSE project.* In D. S. Leathar, G. B. Hastings and J. K. Davies (Eds) *Health Education and the Media.* Pergamon Press, London.

Lazarsfeld, P. F. and Merton, R. K. (1975) *Mass communication, popular taste and organised social action.* In W. Schramm (Ed.) *Mass Communications.* University of Illinois Press, Urbana, IL.

Leathar, D. S. (1980) *Defence inducing advertising.* In *Taking Stock: What Have We Learned and Where Are We Going? Proceedings of the ESOMAR Conference*, Monte Carlo, pp. 153–173.

Leathar, D. S., Hastings, G. B. and Davies, J. K. (Eds) (1981) *Health Education and the Media.* Pergamon Press, London.

Leathar, D. S., Hastings, G. B., O'Reilly, K. M., and Davies, J. K. (Eds) (1986) *Health Education and the Media II.* Pergamon Press, Oxford.

Lefebvre, R. C., Doner, L., Johnston, C., Loughrey, K. et al. (1995) *Use of database marketing and consumer-based health communication in message design.* In E. Maibach and R. L. Parrott (Eds) *Designing Health Messages: Approaches from Communication theory and Public Health Practice.* Sage, Thousand Oaks, CA.

Leslie, J. (1981) *Evaluation of mass media for health and nutrition education.* In M. Meyer (Ed.) *Health Education by Television and Radio.* K.G. Saur, München.

Levens, G. E. and Rodnight, E. (1973) *The Application of Research in the Planning and Evaluation of Road Safety Publicity, Proceedings of the European Society for Opinion in Marketing (Budapest) Conference*, pp. 197–227.

Liu, A. P. (1981) *Mass campaigns in the People's Republic of China.* In R. E. Rice and W. J. Paisley (Eds) *Public Communication Campaigns.* Sage, Beverly Hills, CA.

Lovelock, C. H. (1977) *Concepts and strategies for health marketers. Hospital and Health Services Administration*, Fall, 50–63.

Lupton, D. (1994) *Analysing news coverage.* In S. Chapman and D. Lupton (Eds) *The Fight for Public Health: Principles and Practice of Media Advocacy.* BMJ Publishing, London.

Maloney, S. K. and Hersey, J. C. (1984) *Getting messages on the air: findings from the 1982 alcohol abuse prevention campaign. Health Education Quarterly*, 11, 273–292.

Marsden, G. and Peterfreund, N. (1984) *Marketing public health services. International Quarterly of Community Health Education*, 5, 53–71.

McCombs, M. E. and Shaw, D. L. (1972) *The agenda setting function of the press. Public Opinion Quarterly*, 36, 176–187.

McCron, R. and Budd, J. (1987) *Mass communication and health education.* In I. Sutherland (Ed.) *Health Education: Perspectives and Choices.* National Extension College, Cambridge.

McCron, R. and Dean, E. (1983) *Well Being – An Evaluation.* Channel 4 Television Broadcast Support Services, London.

McGuire, W. J. (1973) *Persuasion, resistance and attitude change.* In I. De Sola Pool et al. (Eds) *Handbook of Communication.* Rand McNally, Skokie, IL.

McGuire, W. J. (1981) *Theoretical foundations of campaigns.* In R. E. Rice and W. J. Paisley (Eds) *Public Communication Campaigns.* Sage, Beverly Hills, CA.

McKinlay, J. B. (1979) *A case for refocusing upstream: the political economy of illness.* In E. G. Jaco (Ed.) *Patients, Physicians and Illness.* Free Press, New York, NY, p. 12.

McLaughlin, G. (1969) *SMOG grading: a new readability formula. Journal of Reading*, 12, 639.

McQuail, D. (1994) *Mass Communication Theory: An Introduction*, 3rd Edn. Sage, London.

Mendelsohn, H. (1968) *Which shall it be: mass education or mass persuasion for health? American Journal of Public Health*, 58, 131–137.

Mendelsohn, H. (1973) *Some reasons why information campaigns can succeed. Public Information Quarterly*, 37, 50–61.

Mendelsohn, H. (1980) *Comments on the Relevance of Empirical Research as a Basis for Public Education Strategies in the Area of Alcohol Consumption*. Department of Mass Communication, University of Denver, Denver, CO.

Mendelsohn, H. (1986) *Lessons from a national media prevention campaign*. In D. S. Leathar, G. B. Hastings and J. K. Davies (Eds) *Health Education and the Media*. Pergamon Press, London.

National Cancer Institute, (1998) *Making Health Communication Programs Work: A Planner's Guide,*. Information Projects Branch Office, Bethesda, MD. (http://rex.nci.nih.gov/NCI_Pub_Interface /HCPW/ACKNOW.HTM)

Nelkin, D. (1987) *Selling Science: How the Press Covers Science and Technology*. Freeman, New York, NY.

O'Byrne, D. J. and Crawley, H. D. (1981) *Conquest smoking cessation campaign 1980 – an evaluation*. In D. S. Leathar, G. B. Hastings and J. K. Davies (Eds) *Health Education and the Media*. Pergamon Press, London.

Ogbourne, A. C. and Smart, R. G. (1980) *Will restrictions on alcohol advertising reduce alcohol consumption? British Journal of Addictions*, 75, 293–296.

Palmer, E. (1981) *Shaping persuasive messages with formative research*. In R. E. Rice and W. J. Paisley (Eds) *Public Communications Campaigns*. Sage, Beverly Hills, CA.

Pichert, J. W. and Elam, P. (1985) *Readability formulas may mislead you. Patient Education and Counselling*, 7, 181–191.

Piepe, A. *et al.* (1986) *Does sponsored sport lead to smoking among children? Health Education Journal*, 45, 145–148.

Player, D. A. (1986) *Health promotion through sponsorship: the state of the art*. In D. S. Leathar, G. B. Hastings and J. K. Davies (Eds) *Health Education and the Media*. Pergamon Press, London.

Player, D. A. and Leathar, D. S. (1981) *Developing socially sensitive advertising*. In D. S. Leathar, G. B. Hastings and J. K. Davies (Eds) *Health Education and the Media*. Pergamon Press, London.

Puska, P., Koskela, K. and McAlister, A. (1979) *A comprehensive television smoking cessation programme in Finland. International Journal of Health Education*, XXII (suppl. 4).

Raw, M. and de Plight, J. V. (1981) *Can television help people stop smoking?* In D. S. Leathar, G. B. Hastings and J. K. Davies (Eds) *Health Education and the Media*. Pergamon Press, London.

Quinn, J. R. (1991) *Letter to the editor, New York Times*, March 31.

Raw, M., White, P. and McNeill, A. (1990) *Clearing the Air: a Guide for Action on Tobacco*. British Medical Association, London.

Redman, B. K. (1984) *The Psychology of Written Communication*, Part 3. Kogan Page, London.

Reid, D. (1985) *National No Smoking Day*. In J. Crofton and M. Wood (Eds) *Smoking Control*. Health Education Council, London.

Rhodes, A. (1976) *Progaganda: the Art of Persuasion, World War II*. Angus and Robertson, London.

Robbins, A. (2000) Unpublished Ph.D. thesis, University of Leicester.

Rogers, E. M. and Singhal, A. (1990) *The academic perspective*. In C. Atkin and L. Wallack (Eds) *Mass Communication and Public Health: Complexities and Conflicts*. Sage, Newbury Park, CA.

Rogers, R. S. (1973) *The effects of televised sex education at the primary school level. Health Education Journal*, 32, 87–93.

Romano, R. (1984a) *Pre-testing in Health Communications*. National Cancer Institute, Bethesda, MD.

Romano, R. (1984b) *Making PSAs Work*. National Cancer Institute, Bethesda, MD.

Romano, R. (1985) *Pre-testing smoking messages*. In J. Crofton and M. Wood (Eds) *Smoking Control*. Health Education Council, London.

Rothschild, M. L. (1979) *Marketing communications in nonbusiness situations or why it's so hard to sell brotherhood like soap. Journal of Marketing*, 43, 11–20.

Rubin, A. M. (1983) *Television uses and gratifications: the interactions of viewing patterns and motivations. Journal of Broadcasting*, 27, 37–51.

Rubin, A. M. (1994) *Media uses and effects: a uses and gratifications perspective*. In J. Bryant and D.

Zillmann (Eds) *Media Effects: Advances in Theory and Research*. Lawrence Erlbaum, Hove.

Russell, M. A. H., Wilson, C., Taylor, C. and Baker, C. D. (1979) *Effect of General Practitioner's advice against smoking. British Medical Journal*, 2, 231–235.

Shaw, M. (1986) *Health promotion and the media: the soap opera. Health Promotion*, 1, 211–212.

Singhal, A. (1990) Entertainment-education communication strategies for development, unpublished doctoral dissertation, University of Southern California.

Singhal, A. and Rogers, E. (1989) *Prosocial television for development in India*. In R. E. Rice and C. K. Atkin (Eds) *Public Communication Campaigns*. Sage, Newbury Park, CA.

Smith, W. (1978) *Campaigning for Choice; Family Planning Association Project Report No. 1*. Family Planning Association, London.

Solomon, D. S. (1989) *A social marketing perspective on campaigns*. In R. E. Rice and W. J. Paisley (Eds) *Public Communication Campaigns*, 2nd Edn. Sage, Beverly Hills, CA.

Spencer, J. (1984) *General Practitioners' Views of the 'Give Up Smoking (GUS) Kit'*. Health Education Council, London.

Stein, J. A. (1986) *The cancer information service: marketing a large-scale national information program through media*. In D. S. Leathar *et al.* (Eds) *Media in Health Education II*. Pergamon Press, London.

Taplin, S. (1981) *Family planning campaigns*. In R. E. Rice and W. J. Paisley (Eds) *Public Communication Campaigns*. Sage, Beverly Hills, CA.

Tapper-Jones, L. and Harvard Davis, R. (1985) *A Project to Develop Publications to Support Health Education Within the General Practice Consultation*. Health Education Council, London.

Tones, B. K. (1981) *The use and abuse of mass media in health promotion*. In D. S. Leathar, G. B. Hastings and J. K. Davies (Eds) *Health Education and the Media*. Pergamon Press, London.

Tones, B. K. (1986) *Preventing drug misuse: the case for breadth, balance and coherence*. Health Education Journal, 45, 223–230.

Tones, B. K. (1994) *Marketing and the mass media:*

*theory and myth. Health Education Research*, 42 (3), 165–169.

Tones, B. K. (1996) *Models of mass media: hypodermic, aerosol or agent provocateurs? Drugs Education Prevention and Policy*, 3 (1), 29–37.

Transport and Road Research Laboratory (1967) *Testing a Children's Poster*, Report SRU 2). TRRL, Crowthorne, Berkshire.

Transport and Road Research Laboratory (1970) *Design of Road Safety Exhibitions*, Leaflet SRU 6. TRRL, Crowthorne, Berkshire.

Transport and Road Research Laboratory (1972) *Improving Driving by the Use of Posters Beside Roads*, Report SRU 28). TRRL, Crowthorne, Berkshire.

Wallach, L. M. (1980) *Mass Media Campaigns: the Odds Against Finding Behavior Change*. University of California Social Research Group, School of Public Health, Berkeley, CA.

Wallach, L. M. (1990) *Media advocacy; promoting health through mass communication*. In K. Glanz, F. M. Lewis and B. K. Rimer (Eds) *Health Behavior and Health Education: Theory, Research and Practice*. Jossey-Bass, San Francisco, CA.

Wallack, L. and Barrows, D. C. (1983) *Evaluating primary prevention: the California 'Winners' alcohol program. International Quarterly of Community Health Education*, 3, 307–336.

Wallack, L., Dorfman, L., Jernigan, D. and Themba, M. (1993) *Media Advocach and Public Health: Power for Prevention*. Sage, Newbury Park, CA.

Wellings, K. (1986) *Help or hype: an analysis of media coverage of the 1983 'pill scare'*. In D. S. Leathar *et al.* (Eds) *Health Education and the Media II*. Pergamon Press, London.

Wells, W. W. (1989) *Planning for R.O.I.: Effective Advertising Strategy*. Prentice Hall, Englewood Cliffs, NJ.

Winnard, K., Rimon, J. and Convisser, J. (1987) *The impact of television on the family planning attitudes of an urban Nigerian audience*, Paper presented at the *American Public Health Association*.

Zaltman, G., Kotler, P. and Kaufman, I. (Eds) (1972) *Creating Social Change*. Holt Rinehart and Winston, New York, NY.

# 9 THE COMMUNITY

This chapter is mainly concerned with a particular approach to working in the community setting based on the conviction that health promoters should work *with* communities and seek to facilitate the achievement of the health goals which the communities have themselves identified. This approach typically has a broader, ecological perspective on health, is concerned with fostering empowerment and is oriented largely towards a bottom-up approach. The origins of this way of working, typically described as community development, will be discussed and some of the difficulties associated with it will be considered. Its relationship to other ways of working with communities will be examined. Mostly we will be focusing on work with either the whole or elements of localised communities and also on work with what are described as communities of interest. In the former we might be concerned with a locality in an urban setting or with specific ethnic minorities in that locality and in the latter, for example, with dispersed homeless young people. To a degree the projects we will discuss will have been undertaken with communities who are in some sense or other disadvantaged. Work with communities which has been designated as community development has differed over time and these differences will be examined. Particular features of community project evaluation will be considered before discussing the achievements of such projects.

Strengthening community action was one of the five action areas identified in the Ottawa Charter (WHO, 1986):

> *health promotion works through concrete and effective community action in setting priorities, making decisions, planning strategies and implementing them to achieve better health. At the heart of this process is the empowerment of communities.*

While there are many health promotion initiatives working with this understanding of community action, there are others where the goal of community involvement differs. Types of community participation have been categorised by Kickbusch and O'Byrne (1995) as:

- marginal – community input is limited and transitory and has little direct action on the outcome of the activity;
- substantive – the community is actively involved in determining priorities and carrying out activities even though the mechanism for these activities may be externally controlled;
- structural – the community is an integral part of a project and its participation becomes the ideological basis for the project itself.

Participation in the structural sense is congruent with the modern idea of community development, although it should be pointed out that many projects designated as community development fit the second category rather better than the third.

## THE MEANING OF COMMUNITY

Before attempting to provide some insight into the distinctions between various approaches to working in communities, we should note that while differentiating the various forms of community work can be difficult, there are also problems in deciding on the meaning of the term 'community' itself! A very large number of definitions have been generated, in part reflecting the diverse uses of the term. A much quoted finding is that of Hillerly (cited in Rose, 1990), who found 90 uses of the term community from a review of the community studies literature and the only thing that they had in common was that they were about people. The word community can be applied to units of very differing size; the local community, the European community, the global community. The term is also frequently evoked as Rose (1990) observes:

> *the seductive promise of community is linked by the frequency of its use within political and policy discourses. Concepts of community care, community development, community action jostle on the lips of every speaker, above all politicians and those close to them who wish to indicate that the longing for social solidarity and greater well being is about to be met.*

For many of the projects to be discussed later in the chapter a community is distinguished from any other social aggregation in respect of its relative size, geographical contiguity and the nature of the social networks and norms prevailing within this circumscribed locality. The report of the Calouste Gulbenkian Foundation (1984) provided an apt description of geographically based communities:

> *'Community' ... refers to a grouping of people who share a common purpose, interest or need, and who can express their relationship through communication face to face, as well as by other means, without difficulty. In other words, in the majority of cases we see a community as being related to some geographic locality where the propinquity of the inhabitants has relevance for those interests or needs which they share.*

Some writers have tried to put size limitations on what should be defined as a community of this kind, although it is questionable how useful this is. Henderson and Thomas (1980), for example, defined community as a relatively small geographical neighbourhood and argued that the appropriate catchment area for community development should be between 6000 and 20,000 people. A large number of community development projects are with communities very much smaller than the lower limit. It is the nature of processes to be achieved in such projects that sets limitations on their size. The potential for face-to-face communication and achieving social networks are of major importance in planning 'typical' community projects. There is obviously no clear-cut distinction between a community and a geographical area of more than Henderson and Thomas' upper limit of 20,000 people. In addition to geographically based communities, what can be termed 'relational' communities or 'communities of interest' are important to our discussion. Heller (1989) observed that since modern communication systems make it possible for people to transcend geographical boundaries, relational communities become possible. It can be argued that these have become, for many people, very much more important than geographically located communities.

A term akin to community which has been used for some time and is increasingly being used in health promotion is that of neighbourhood. It is frequently being used to convey the 'seductive promise' noted above. Wellman and Leighton (1979) provided an interesting critique of the way in which urban sociology has tended to focus on neighbourhoods, arguing that the notions of boundedness and density of relationships associated with this geographical concern may not in fact be as beneficial for the well-being of communities as is commonly supposed. We will revisit this point later when we consider the health benefits claimed for community development.

## The healthy community: the community ideal and the ideal community

Implicit in much discussion of community is an ideal which for many is associated either with some close entity represented by the traditional rural village of the past or a certain type of close knit locality within urban settings: the neighbourhood. There are also assumptions that a traditional community is a good one and moreover that a good community is a healthy one. These are typifications of the concept *'Gemeinschaft'*. The classical opposition proposed in the late 19th century was between *Gemeinschaft* and *Gesellschaft* (Tönnies, 1955). The former 'ideal type' community had social bonds based on close personal ties of friendship and kinship with an emphasis on tradition, consensus and information and was closely approximated by agricultural societies. This was contrasted with a *Gesellschaft* society in which secondary relations predominated; contractual, expedient, impersonal and specialised. This was typically represented by modern urban society with allegedly weaker family organisation, an emphasis on utilitarian goals and the relatively impersonal and competitive nature of social relationships.

The change from traditional to modern society has been described as one where *Gesellschaft* characteristics have increasingly taken over from *Gemeinschaft*. These changes have frequently been defined as necessary ones where modernisation has been sought, but, at the same time, a sense of loss has commonly been associated with such changes. This occurs because the positive attributes of *Gemeinshaft* have typically been emphasised and the negative and often health diminishing ones have been ignored.

For many people, therefore, the idea of 'sense of community' would be seen as part and parcel of *Gemeinschaft* and for some would form an integral dimension of community empowerment. McMillan and Chavis (1986) consider that a clear definition of a sense of community is a necessary prerequisite for the development of policy measures designed to create or preserve the intrinsically beneficial features of 'community'. They argue that a sense of community has four elements:

1 membership – a feeling of belonging;
2 influence – a sense of mattering, ... *of making a difference to a group and of the group mattering to its members*;
3 integration and fulfilment of needs – ... *a feeling that members' needs will be met by the resources received through their membership in the group*;
4 shared emotional connection – ... *the commitment and belief that members have shared and will share history, common places, time together, and similar experiences.*

Raeburn (1986) also endorsed the importance of *Gemeinschaft*, arguing that:

*... when people do enjoyable and worthwhile things together at a local level, positive bonds will form between them. This, in turn, leads to residents' overall awareness of local talents, issues and values, so that there is less tendency to look outside one's place of residence for a satisfactory life experience.*

(pp. 392–393)

These rather cosy views of sense of community and the perceptions of loss of key attributes of *Gemeinschaft* in modern societies have been challenged. Wellman and Leighton (1979) commented on the tendency of many urban sociologists to lament the loss of the traditional community in its transformation into a more modern and alienated form. As they put it:

*Lost scholars have seen modern urbanites as alienated isolates who bear the brunt of the transformed society on their own.*

(p. 369)

And so, if the traditional community is 'healthy' the modern community would appear to be sick. The characteristics of this sick 'community lost' are listed by Wellman and Leighton in terms of *Gesellschaft*: 'urbanites' are no longer full members of 'solidarity communities'; they are limited members of several social networks. Primary contacts with people are fewer and more narrowly defined. These ties ... *tend to be fragmented into isolated two-person relationships rather than being parts of extensive networks.* Relationships are weaker in intensity and those networks which do exist are 'sparsely knit', i.e. interfacing with only a small proportion of potential contacts. Networks are 'loosely bounded' having few separate clusters or primary groups. Little structural support is provided for 'solidarity activities or sentiments'. As a result of these features the 'modern' community is less able to provide support and assistance for network members.

A major goal of many community workers and sociologists has been to use community development and other techniques to 'save' the traditional community (or rather recreate it). The characteristics of 'community saved' are the obverse of 'community lost'. As Wellman and Leighton (1989) put it:

> *Many saved social pathologists have encouraged the nurturance of densely knit, bounded communities as a structural salve for the stresses of poverty, ethnic segregation and physical and mental diseases.*

There is, however, according to the authors, a third category of community: 'community liberated'. They argue that the focus of community analysis should not be so much on geographical neighbourhood but rather on networks. At a theoretical level this makes it easier to identify both 'communities without propinquity' and the existence of 'urban villages'. Moreover, they argue that in terms of the mobilisation of support, being able to move among a number of social networks may be more beneficial than being limited to those existing within the confines of a neighbourhood. Indeed, modern communication systems render this close geographical contact irrelevant. The authors do concede that the 'liberated community' may be particularly suited to more affluent sectors of (American?) society insofar as it places a premium on ... *a base of individual security, entrepreneurial skills in moving between networks, and the ability to function without the security of membership in a solidarity community.*

They do, on the other hand, caution that solidarity does not necessarily mean egalitarianism: *... not all of the community's resources may be gathered or distributed equally.* Moreover, there may actually be disadvantages for working class and ethnic minority communities in the 'community found' situation:

> *Concerns about conserving, controlling and efficiently pooling those resources which the beleaguered community possesses also resonate with its members' inability to acquire additional resources elsewhere. A heavy load consequently is placed on ties within the saved community.*

While a strong strand in efforts to work with communities has been to build the characteristics of *Gemeinschaft* communities, the attributes of such communities have, at other times, been viewed negatively and active processes to change them have been instituted. The sense of tradition and the reluctance to change of traditional communities have been focused on by those seeking to modernise societies in the interests of achieving 'development' and economic progress. Over time, the term community development has been associated with a number of views about community change and the residues of earlier meanings are still present. We will now outline some features of the historical development of community work with specific reference to community development.

## THE COMMUNITY DEVELOPMENT TRADITION

Diverse projects have been informed by a community development approach and we will be concerned to review the effectiveness of examples of these later in the chapter. While contemporary associations of the term community development are generally positive ones, this is not invariably the case and awareness of the origins of community development is important in understanding some of the differing views about this particular way of working with communities.

The selection of any specific starting point and the content of a brief review is somewhat arbitrary and can be contested. The intention is to provide some indication of the complexity of the community work tradition. Beginning from the 19th century there were, very simply, two historical strands: the development of work with communities in the countries subject to colonisation (described as the non-industrialised South[1]) and the work in response to problems of industrialised societies (described as the North[1]). In the North changes from traditional society which were already under way accelerated with the industrial revolutions in Europe and North America. Various collective activities developed within the working class communities of the new cities in the 19th century. Some, such as the mutual aid organisations in the UK in the 19th century, were about creating mutual support and maintaining characteristics of the communities that were 'lost', while others were the forerunners of what would now be labelled social action. For example, in World War I rent strikes were examples of communities coming together to bring change, as were the squatters movements after the war (Craig, 1989).

In the South missionaries and colonial governments sought to change the societies they encountered, initially introducing those activities deemed necessary in order to govern and control and later, in the 20th century, in preparation for independence. A commonly identified point for examining community development as a planned activity is the period from the late 1930s onwards. An approach which was used initially to achieve modernisation in agricultural practice, particularly in the USA, was subsequently applied more widely in countries of the South to achieve modernisation in whole societies. According to the United Nations (1971) the term community development came into international usage:

> *to connote the processes by which the efforts of people themselves are united with those of governmental authorities to improve the economic, social and cultural conditions of communities, to integrate those communities into the life of the nation, and to enable them to contribute fully to national progress.*

Community development was part of a three-way strategy for achieving modernisation:

- political modernisation to create viable nations; community development projects to serve as units for implementing programmes;
- individual modernisation to develop personality types needed to operate in a modern society.

Community development was, therefore, a necessary component in achieving consciously accelerated economic, technological and social change. The village community was typically selected as the development unit and nothing smaller than a village was thought to be adequate. Action would combine outside assistance and organised community activity to achieve material outcomes such as wells and schools and non-material gains such as literacy and improvements in health.

In the North a number of countries had by the 1960s become increasingly aware of problems in their own societies. In the context of rising prosperity overall there were disadvantaged communities and demonstrable levels of poverty. Responses to this situation included nation-wide social programmes and also the application of the community development ideas as used in the colonies. For example, in the USA Kindervatter (1979) commented that 'community organization' (an alternative term for community development) first appeared in US social work textbooks in the 1920s and 1930s, but ... *not until the War on Poverty in the sixties did the concept and its application receive much attention*. In the UK the government initiated Educational Priority Areas, the Urban Programme and what was known as the Community Development Project (Community Development Project, 1977). This Home Office initiative consisted of teams of workers and researchers in 12 localities and the project as a whole was informed by the conception of those communities as having deficiencies which needed redress. There was, however, a challenge to the ideas which informed the project, in particular to the location of the causes of poverty and disadvantage in people themselves and in community pathology, rather than in structural causes. The workers in individual localities in the project adopted alternative ideas of community development, in line with those described below. In the UK the Calouste Gulbenkian Report (1974) led to the establishment of community development workers within social work and community education departments who worked to a definition of community development as:

> *A process of social action in which the people of a community organise themselves for planning and action; define their common needs and problems; make group and individual plans to meet their needs and solve their problems; execute these plans with a maximum of reliance on community resources; and supplement these resources when necessary with services and material from governmental and non-governmental agencies outside the community.*

While the early community development projects had a generalist focus, there was also the gradual emergence of community health projects, also built on the core principles of community development, and these will be discussed later. A further strand in our history is that of social action, associated with Alinsky (1946), which can be contrasted with community development. According to Kindervatter, locality (community) development ... *essentially enables people to co-operatively and self-reliantly solve community problems.* On the other hand:

> *... social action strategies aim to enable people to jointly challenge and change existing community power relationships. In terms of the relationship between community members and outside authorities, locality development assumes collaboration and co-operation, whereas social action assumes either competition or conflict.*

According to Kirklin and Franzen (1974):

> *In social action people are organized to bring into being a new power aggregate ... to force the existing political/economic power structure to change public and private policies. The battle is classically seen to be between the 'power haves' and the 'power have nots'.*

The flavour of social action projects has been described by Miller *et al.* (1995).

> *An issue was chosen which was visible, winnable, would yield concrete results and mobilise people by focusing on a villain. Then, clever, publicity winning tactics were deployed.*

They note that the social action approach, although common, is used in ways that often contrast with Alinsky's methods.

Some brief comment needs to be made about social movements which impinged on some areas of community development and social action work. The term social movement is applied to various forms of oppositional collective action aimed at securing some form of social reorganisation. Social movements are not usually highly institutionalised. They arise from spontaneous social protest directed at specific targets. From the 1960s a number of social movements grew up outside institutional settings, in opposition to various features of society and oriented to bringing about change. They included the women's, peace, self-care, self-reliance and ecology movements. Many of these movements have relied on middle class and educated groups for leadership and support. The women's and self-care movements in particular had an influence on community development health projects.

Returning again to the South there are two further important elements which have informed thinking and practice of health promotion work with communities. These are the non-formal education activities which contributed to understandings of empowerment, closely associated with the work of Freire (1972), and the developments which informed the primary health care proposals in the 1978 Alma Ata document (WHO, 1978). Grass roots primary care developments, with the involvement of communities, had emerged in countries such as China and to some extent in non-socialist countries such as Kenya. The Alma Ata document drew on the understandings derived from these developments. Primary health care was:

> *essential health care based on a practical, scientifically sound and socially acceptable method, made universally accessible to individuals and their families in the community through their full participation and at a cost country and community can afford at each stage of development in the spirit of self reliance and determination.*

Community development projects, although informed by differing interpretations of the term community development and consequently with varying levels and types of community participation, have been a key part of health developments in the global implementation of primary health care. In the UK, throughout the same period, community development health projects have been a consistent strand in health promotion, although for the period from the late 1970s until the change of government at the end of the 1990s they received a low level of support. During this period there was little recognition at the policy level of issues of inequality and the need for corrective social action and relatively little mainstream support for community development. Nonetheless, during this period there were the important *Healthy Cities* initiatives informed by ideas of *Health For All*, including a commitment to the empowerment of communities. *Healthy Cities* projects have included community development activities funded by the statutory sectors of health, social work and education and also by the voluntary sector. Within recent health strategy documents in the UK there has been a firm commitment to redressing inequalities in health by addressing the determinants of inequality. The importance of 'community' as an entity has been strongly reaffirmed in redressing inequality and the strengthening and development of community-based initiatives is a key element of strategy alongside appropriate organisational development (Department of Health, 1998, 1999).

There have been, and continue to be, different orientations to community work. These differences may, at times, be over technique or over the means necessary to achieve commonly agreed goals. Alternatively, and of greater importance, the differences may reflect disagreements about the goals themselves and reflect quite fundamental variations in ideology. For example, there has been a gradual shift in understandings associated with the term community development, away from the essentially top-down activities associated with colonialism which were then translated into disadvantaged communities elsewhere towards the ideas of community development as a 'bottom-up' approach to enabling communities to become empowered and overcome disadvantage. At the same time there continue to be problematical features of community development and these will be considered after discussing the processes of community activity in more detail.

## APPROACHES TO COMMUNITY CHANGE

There are alternative strategies to generating change in communities: those which seek to cre-

ate change through top-down intervention and those which aim to facilitate change through bottom-up initiatives with maximal community involvement. The generic term 'community development' is now widely used to describe the second of these two opposing strategies. In the USA the phrase 'community organiaation', as noted above, is often used synonymously. Both have a long history, as we have outlined. For instance, Bivins (cited in Lazes, 1979) described community organisation as *an old and reliable grassroots approach to health education identified in the 1940s*. Its overall purpose as defined by Kindervatter (1979) is ... *to enable communities to improve and change their socioeconomic milieu and/or their position in that milieu*. Croft and Beresford (1992) describe the emphasis of community development as:

> ... *on collective rather than individual action. Its focus has been both the workplace and the neighbourhood. It has been concerned with the economic infrastructure, for example, housing and employment; with supporting people's personal growth and development, and with work performed by women in the community – often unpaid – for example, in play schemes, nurseries and carers' groups.*

> *Community development is an activity which may be undertaken by unpaid community activists, specialised community workers or other professionals adopting this approach. The objectives of community development range from encouraging self-help and mutual aid to politicisation and pressure group activity; from collaboration to confrontation*

> *(p. 29)*

They go on to cite Twelvetrees' (1982) three overlapping approaches to community work: (i) community development itself; (ii) 'political action', i.e. a class-based approach involving coalitions and campaigns; (iii) 'social planning', i.e. the promotion of ... *joint action between voluntary and community organizations and the local state to change and improve services.*

These various observations illustrate the variety of approaches appearing under the rubric of community work and the different interpretations which are often associated with the same or similar terminology. However, although terms may be used interchangeably, sometimes they suggest a distinctive approach. The most commonly used terms are: community organization, community development, locality development and social action. According to Nix (1970), locality development is the same as community development, community organisation and the 'process approach'. Likewise, Kindervatter considered locality development to be similar to community development insofar as it involved a non-directive approach to community work. The present chapter will focus largely on community development, although there will also be some reference to social/technical planning and to social action approaches. Community development will be understood in accordance with Ross and Lappin's (1967) definition:

> ... a process by which a community identifies its needs or objectives, orders (or ranks) these needs or objectives, develops the confidence and will to work at these needs or objectives, finds the resources (internal and/or external) to deal with these needs and objectives, takes action in respect to them and in so doing extends and develops co-operation and collaborative attitudes and practices in the community.

The fundamental goal, then, is self-empowerment. This involves, in Kindervatter's words, ... *people gaining an understanding of and control over social, economic, and/or political forces in order to improve their standing in society.* The extent to which this is achievable is a key question when addressing community development. Whether the formula is social action or community development, the goal is fundamentally political, as is apparent from the following extract from the Calouste Gulbenkian Working Party Report (Calouste Gulbenkian Foundation, 1984).

> We see community development as a main strategy for the attainment of social policy goals. It is concerned with the worth and dig-

> nity of people and the promotion of equal opportunity. ... Community work is most needed in communities where social skills and resources are at their weakest. Community work involves working with those most affected by poverty, unemployment, disability, inadequate housing and education, and with those who for reasons of class, income, race or sex are less likely than others to be, or to feel, involved and significant in local community life.

By comparison, what Nix (1970) referred to as technical planning and can be seen as equivalent to Rothman's notion of social planning tends towards a top-down approach. Social/technical planning is concerned with task rather than process goals and seeks to implement change in the community (for the good of the community) but without being concerned with empowerment of the people living therein. The assumption, of course, is that planners know what is best for the community. However, the difference between a sophisticated social planning approach and more naïve (top-down) programmes is that in the former case planners are aware of the need to take account of the dynamics of change in the community. They will thus employ outreach strategies, seek to identify opinion leaders and generally apply the accumulated wisdom derived from communication of innovations research. They will often, therefore, look like community development/organisation programmes at first glance. There is an overlap between such programmes and some of the community-wide interventions to be considered in the next chapter.

## COMMUNITY DEVELOPMENT OR SOCIAL PLANNING?

In the light of our discussion of ideological differences between approaches and the associated implications for evaluation, the difference between Rothman's 'social/technical planning' approach and the other approaches described above merit some further explication.

First of all, let us remind ourselves of the 'ideal type' of the social planning model, which we might usefully characterise as a deliberate strategy

401

to intervene in a given community in order to achieve predetermined objectives which, if successfully achieved, will prevent disease. According to this model, either the community may be seen as whatever remains after more manageable settings, such as school or workplace, have been targeted or, alternatively, it may be viewed as an opportunity to work less formally with people in their natural habitat. Since many of the designated group may be difficult to reach in other settings, for instance because they may be unemployed or because they do not respond to invitations to attend clinics or surgeries, the social planning approach may be seen as a last ditch attempt to 'get through to' disadvantaged groups or others who might be 'resistant' to change.

An alternative and often complementary orientation is that of the 'community-wide strategy' to be discussed in the following chapter. In practice, there is often no hard and fast distinction between types of approach, especially where the exercise is patently undertaken for the good of the community and seeks to meet very real problems. The distinction is, however, nicely made by Hilton (1988). The example he provides is from developing countries and thus especially appropriate given the impetus which Alma Ata and primary health care gave to the recognition of the importance of creating active, participating communities. Hilton provides examples of what he calls a 'community-oriented' approach in which ... *plans are made by outsiders and people are asked to participate*. Examples are provided below:

> *Our hospital staff is overworked treating cases of malaria, dehydration and malnutrition that could be prevented or treated locally. Therefore we are going to build a clinic in some villages 30 miles from the hospital. We will give an employment exam to the district secondary school leavers and select the best to train as health workers to be sent to the clinics. They will learn how to treat malaria, respiratory infections, malnutrition and other common diseases.*

> *We have done a survey and find very poor conditions of sanitation, hygiene and nutri-*

*tion in all of the villages. Therefore we will train the health workers to do health education. They will teach the people that they should construct latrines and dig wells in order to prevent disease. They will have classes in nutrition for the women so that they will learn how to properly feed their children.*

(p. 1)

Hilton goes on to offer a case study in 'community-based' health promotion. This centres on the story of a primary school teacher who became a 'community organiser'. His training taught him *how to listen and really hear what people are saying and feeling*. He worked on a farm but spent as much time as possible getting closely involved in the life of the community. He listened for 'generative themes', *topics that people have strong feelings about*. He gained the confidence of the village people and was soon invited to a number of meetings of women's groups, church meetings, etc. He prepared 'codes' on the generative themes and presented these in picture form or through story and drama. He engaged the people in dialogue about the possibilities of change. One theme considered particularly important was the lack of money to buy vegetables from wealthy landowners. As a result the group pooled their savings and rented land on which they grew their own vegetables. *The best product from the garden, however, was the discovery that they could work together to solve a problem.*

The process described is, of course, based on Freire's methods of adult education. The initiative he described expanded and resulted in enhanced empowerment of local women who learned how to improve the health of their children by working as equal partners with health workers. The final stage in the process of transformation involved collaboration with other towns and villages and election of villagers to the governing council. This community development process is substantially different from the approach adopted by change agents who seek, with greater or lesser success, to 'plug into' community networks and utilise their dynamic to achieve predetermined preventive goals. Measures of success are primarily those which demonstrate the attainment of preventive objectives. In the second case described by Hilton success is defined in terms of the extent to which community and individual empowerment have been achieved. It is, however, important to underline the fact that the achievement of empowerment will, in all probability, have been the most effective way of preventing the various life threatening diseases which faced the villagers described in Hilton's case study.

## PARTICIPATION, EMPOWERMENT AND COMMUNITY DEVELOPMENT

At the heart of the WHO manifesto for primary health care is the ultimate goal of a socially and economically productive life which is to be achieved through the creation of the active, fully participating community. This too is the focus of community development.

Before further exploring community development we should clarify a few points. First, empowerment is not synonymous with participation, despite their constant and reiterated association. As we noted in Chapter 1, an empowered person is more likely to engage in active community participation than someone who is helplessly apathetic. On the other hand, participation may contribute to empowerment. Self-empowerment, as we have seen, has to do with beliefs about control and the possession of efficacy-creating competencies which contribute to the acquisition of power, i.e. a degree of control over environmental circumstances and other people. Again, in Chapter 1 we distinguished self-empowerment from community empowerment. Although in an important sense an empowered community may be said to be the sum of the self-empowered individuals it contains, there are those who view empowered communities as rather more than that, though this distinction is probably a matter of definition.

A second assertion should be made at this point: empowerment and community participation may be conceived either as goals in their own right or as having an instrumental function. The WHO philosophy seems to include both of these. The instrumental function is evident in more recent

definitions of health, i.e. empowerment and health are means to the end of achieving a socially and economically productive life. More precisely, an empowered participating community is not only necessary to galvanise individuals into looking after themselves but is also a prerequisite for achieving equity and remedying inequalities which are, in turn, the single most important barrier to achieving health goals. At the same time, WHO retains its fondness for its earlier broad definition of health as some positive state (not merely the absence of disease) having mental and social dimensions as well as physical attributes. Empowerment and its component parts provide as good an example as any (and better than most) of well-being or positive health, especially in the mental and social domains.

In Chapter 1 we noted that it is possible to produce a typology of individual control ranging from a kind of cursory and token consultation through to the possession of real power.

In the same way we can define degrees of community participation. Arnstein (1971) makes this point in the form of an oft-quoted 'ladder of participation' which is reproduced in Figure 9.1.

Maximal participation is located at the top of the ladder – the community has some degree of genuine control; at the bottom we have zero participation – complete manipulation. At the mid point there are various degrees of tokenism. We are reminded of the Paris students' declension of the verb 'to participate' during the period of unrest: *I participate, you participate, they profit!*

Brager and Specht (1973) devised an equally well-known scheme to describe this 'spectrum of participation' (Figure 9.2).

| DEGREES OF ACTUAL POWER | Control |
| | Delegated Power |
| | Partnership |
| | |
| DEGREES OF TOKENISM | Placation |
| | Consultation |
| | Informing |
| | |
| NON-PARTICIPATION | Therapy |
| | Manipulation |

***Figure 9.1*** Arnstein's Ladder of Participation (Arnstein, 1971)

| Degree | Participants' action | Illustrative mode |
|---|---|---|
| Low | None | The community is told nothing. |
| | Receives information | The organisation makes a plan and announces it. The community is convened for information purposes; compliance is expected. |
| | Is consulted | The organisation tries to promote a plan and develop the support to facilitate acceptance of, or give sufficient sanction to, the plan so that administrative compliance can be expected. |
| | Advises | The organisation presents a plan and invites questions. It is prepared to modify the plan only if absolutely necessary. |
| | Plans jointly | The organisation presents a tentative plan subject to change and invites recommendations from those affected. |
| | Has delegated authority | The organisation identifies and presents a problem to the community, defines the limits and asks the community to make a series of decisions which can be embodied in a plan which it will accept. |
| High | Has control | The organisation asks the community to identify the problems and to make all te key decisions regarding goals and means. It is willing to help the community at each step accomplish its own goals, even to the extent of administrative control of the programme. |

**Figure 9.2** A Spectrum of Participation (Brager and Specht, 1973)

We will now return to consider the distinction made earlier between top-down community programmes and the 'pure type' of bottom-up initiative epitomised by contemporary notions of community development. Figure 9.3 suggests that programmes might, in fact, be categorised into one of five types. Type I would be represented by community development and the leadership would be concerned only to raise consciousness about felt needs and provide the community with the wherewithal to bring those felt needs to fruition. The priority of Type 1 programmes

would be to achieve empowerment and an improvement in socio-economic status.

On the other hand, the priority of Type 5 programmes would be the achievement of preventive medical targets and their associated epidemiological outcomes. The major coronary heart disease prevention programmes discussed in the next chapter would be categorised as Type 4 programmes. The 'community health projects' are described as Type 3, although we will note later some of the complexities in labelling these projects as a single type. As indicated earlier, community developers do not infiltrate a community without an ideological agenda: their overt purpose is at the very least to remedy inequalities and gain better and fairer distribution of resources for the community in question. We might therefore suggest, albeit a little mischievously, that if a community refuses to identify with the facilitator's political agenda and the facilitator persists in persevering with that agenda, then the programme becomes a Type 3 intervention. It is not difficult to imagine the circumstances in which Type 2 projects might emerge. The community worker conducts a survey of felt needs and a disease-related issue arises; for example, child accidents or problems with the medical services. The community itself has acknowledged the issue and the worker then acts as a facilitator. Programme objectives would probably be acceptable to the managers of the health service. It is, of course, possible that a disease-related issue may be generated which is not acceptable because it does not fit into current priorities. For instance, it is highly likely that a disadvantaged urban community would identify damp housing as a problem. While this is clearly a mental health issue, it might not be compatible with health authority goals for mental health, either because they had been marginalised in the face of problems such as AIDS or coronary heart disease or because they did not quite fit the prevailing mental illness model. Furthermore, because of a lack of clear epidemiological proof that damp housing caused significant respiratory illness, the issue might again be relegated. The health worker may then have to compile evidence to demonstrate that the felt need was in fact a genuine medical problem. This might well prove to be an unpopular measure since the cost implications of modifying housing

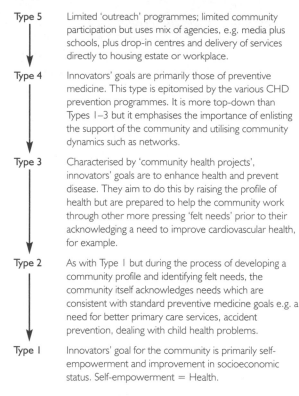

**Type 5** Limited 'outreach' programmes; limited community participation but uses mix of agencies, e.g. media plus schools, plus drop-in centres and delivery of services directly to housing estate or workplace.

**Type 4** Innovators' goals are primarily those of preventive medicine. This type is epitomised by the various CHD prevention programmes. It is more top-down than Types 1–3 but it emphasises the importance of enlisting the support of the community and utilising community dynamics such as networks.

**Type 3** Characterised by 'community health projects', innovators' goals are to enhance health and prevent disease. They aim to do this by raising the profile of health but are prepared to help the community work through other more pressing 'felt needs' prior to their acknowledging a need to improve cardiovascular health, for example.

**Type 2** As with Type 1 but during the process of developing a community profile and identifying felt needs, the community itself acknowledges needs which are consistent with standard preventive medicine goals e.g. a need for better primary care services, accident prevention, dealing with child health problems.

**Type 1** Innovators' goal for the community is primarily self-empowerment and improvement in socioeconomic status. Self-empowerment = Health.

**Figure 9.3** Categories of Community Organisation by Levels of Participation

stock would be politically threatening (see for instance Martin *et al.*, 1987).

The stages of undertaking a community development initiative have been outlined in Chapter 2 and Batten's stages in the process leading to action were presented (Chapter 2, Box 30) The use of a Freirian dialogue approach to identifying felt needs and appropriate actions was also described. Further discussion of the details of undertaking community development projects is beyond the scope of this chapter, but readers are referred to Hope and Timmel (1988).

## NETWORKS, COMMUNITY SOCIAL SUPPORT AND SOCIAL CAPITAL

A considerable number of studies have focused on the beneficial effects of social support in achieving a variety of health outcomes. A review of this area is beyond the scope of the present chapter but we can offer one or two key points.

First, Gottlieb and McLeroy (1992) view social support as one of three features of social health. They noted that early definitions of social health focused on the integration of the individual into the community, participation in community activities, conformity to social norms and appropriate performance of social roles. A more appropriate conceptualisation, in their view, includes 'social integration or involvement' (quantity and quality of relationships); 'social support' (e.g. functional content of relationships such as emotional support); 'social networks' (the structure of relationships with other people within a social system). All three aspects constitute 'social participation', which is, to all intents and purposes, synonymous with community participation.

Gottlieb and McLeroy remind us of the wealth of literature on these various aspects of social participation: they note that *Current Contents* (the journal abstracting service) listed about 100 articles per year from 1989 to 1991 on the effects of social support and social networks. A number of studies have provided quite clear evidence of the direct beneficial effects of participation (as defined above). Gottlieb and McLeroy summarise these for us as follows.

1 The impact of social relationships on physical health is non-specific and is related to all-cause mortality rather than to certain specific causes of death.
2 Risk of dying is increased with very low levels of social relationships (social isolation).
3 The impact of social interaction on health varies with community size and with gender; it is stronger in urban than in rural areas.

The indirect effects on health of social participation must be many and varied. Indeed, the first task is to consider the nature and mechanism whereby social participation exerts its instrumental effect on health promotion and/or the prevention of disease. Various theories have been propounded but we will limit ourselves here to acknowledging the important work of Israel (for instance Israel, 1982, 1987). In 1982, after a review of the literature on the effects of social support and networks on physical and mental well-being, she concluded that five different types of support could be provided through interpersonal relationships. The first of these was affective support, which provided respect and comfort. The second, instrumental support, included material help such as money, food or child care assistance. Cognitive support, on the other hand, was beneficial in providing the information and advice needed to make decisions. A fourth kind of support was referred to as maintenance of social identity and provided 'validation of a shared world view' (cf. Lewis' notion of existential control, which was cited in Chapter 1). Finally 'social outreach' provided access to social contacts (see also House, 1988).

Before moving on, one interesting example of programme success will be provided in this social support context. It refers to a study by Sosa *et al.* (1980) cited by Gottlieb and McLeroy (1992). It concerned 40 pregnant women in Guatemala City who were randomly assigned to treatment and control groups. The former group of women were provided with continuing support from lay women from admission to the birth of the child. The control group, in contrast, underwent the normal delivery process. The length of delivery time for the group which had received social support was 8.7 hours, compared with 19.3 hours for women in the control group.

There has been some mention of social capital in earlier chapters and we can comment further in this section. Although this term has a history of use in general sociology (Putnam, 1993) it has only recently been taken up, somewhat rapidly, in health promotion. Social capital has been described as:

> *the web of cooperative relationships between citizens that facilitate resolution of collective action problems and those features of social structure, such as levels of interpersonal trust, norms of reciprocity and mutual aid, that act as resources for such collective action.*

> (Coleman 1988)

Gillies(1998) has written the following about social capital:

> *Generally social capital is produced by features of the organisation of our societies and communities which facilitate coordination, cooperation and reciprocity. Therefore high levels of trust, positive social norms, and many overlapping and diverse horizontal networks for communication and exchange of information, ideas and practical help will exist where stocks of social capital are high. The relationships and friendships among adults which form the bedrock of social networks provide an informal structure upon which formal citizenship and civic engagement is built.*

Woolcock (in Veenstra, 2000) has identified four main dichotomies that characterise social capital rich communities:

- intra-community ties;
- inter-community ties;
- embeddedness of state society relations at the macro level (synergy);
- institutional coherence and capacity, also at the macro level.

There are studies that have associated social capital with health. In the USA Kawachi *et al.* (1997) found that social capital mediated the relationship between income inequality and health status. Individuals living in states with low social capital were at increased risk of poor self-related health, even when risk factors were controlled for. In the light of such evidence there are initiatives designed to increase social capital in communities. In what way is this different from community development? In some respects it is probably not so different, since community projects build intra-community ties, and to some extent inter-community ones, and also often focus on organisational structures. It is the degree of attention to the macro level elements that distinguishes social capital building from some community development work. However, the two terms are being used together in one, at least, of the *Health Action Zone* intitiatives. The *Wakefield Health Action Zone* plan for action seeks to build social capital and uses the term community development within which social capital will be developed (Wakefield Health Authority, 1999). For community development to be successful their plan states four requirements:

- resourcing of grass roots work;
- networking of grass roots organisations;
- citizen and community participation in strategic organisation and decision making;
- organisational development to open up and facilitate organisations to be responsive to community expressed needs and views.

## COMMUNITY HEALTH PROJECTS

The term 'community health project', mentioned above, is used here to refer to projects which utilise strategies of community development in order to address recognisable health issues, many of which would be congruent with preventive goals. There are many such projects in the UK and they form part of a wider community health movement which has included a number of elements (Blennerhassett et al., 1989):

- community health projects with community workers who apply a community development approach to health issues;
- women's health groups;
- black and ethnic minority health groups;
- self-help groups concerned with health;
- community-based health professionals who are supporting community health groups and voluntary organisations.

Blennerhassett et al. identified two main types of community health project.

1 Neighbourhood based employing one or more community workers. Some of these projects were within the voluntary sector and others related in some way to the NHS.
2 Projects focusing on a community of interest which might cover a wider geographical base than a single neighbourhood. Examples included projects for black and ethnic minority groups and women's health groups.

The work undertaken by the projects included identification of unmet health needs, pioneering new ways of working that might be taken on board by health professionals and providing services which could not be provided by the statutory authorities.

Blennerhasset et al. described the values of the projects as follows:

- they adopted a holistic definition of health;
- a collective approach to health issues was taken through sharing experiences and taking joint action;
- they challenged oppression due to discrimination on the grounds of gender, race, class, age, disability, sexual orientation, etc.;
- they encouraged the empowerment of lay people to express individually and collectively their own health needs;
- a lay, social and democratic view of health issues was adopted rather than a medical model.

Critical appraisals of such projects were produced by the Community Projects Foundation (1988) and Smithies et al. (1990). A well-known example which gives a good impression of the range of activities which can take place within a community development project is described in Box 1.

## PROBLEMATICAL ASPECTS OF COMMUNITY DEVELOPMENT

Various criticisms have been levelled at both community participation and community development. De Kadt (1982), commenting on the success or otherwise of initiatives in developing countries, observed that community development:

> *... hardly ever faced up to the differences in interest that could exist between different members of the 'community' that was to be 'developed', notably in terms of their control over opportunities to make a living. Neither did it have an eye for the unequal (class) relations prevalent within many 'communities'.*
>
> *It thus failed to understand the fundamental social – and political – dynamics of communities in many parts of the world.*
>
> (p. 574)

A similar point was also made by Tumwine (1989) in reflecting on community experience in Zimbabwe:

**Box 1**   Granton Community Health Project

The general aim of the project was to encourage awareness and action on health in the Granton area of Edinburgh.

*Specific Objectives*
- to raise community awareness of health related issues;
- to establish, within the community, a means for initating and maintaining a participatory model of health promotion;
- to monitor and evaluate the process.

*Activities Undertaken by the Project*

*Work with small groups*
women and health
housing and health
courses for elderly
family matters
food and families
tranquillisers group
women and food group
parents and children

*Practical activities*
fruit and veg cooperative
keep fit sessions
relaxation sessions
counselling
pensioners'swim club
pensioners' activities
fitness for big women
outings

*Participatory structures*
Pilton elderly forum
mental health forum
clinic users group

*Campaigns*
feet first chiropody campaign
keep casualty local
tranquillisers

*Audio-visual programmes*
'Who knows best? The range of advice
on feeding babies
'Home Sweet Home': the effects of
'After you leave the surgery';
psychiatric patients speak out

*One-off events*
women's health day
minor tranquillisers
elderly away day

*Training*
sessions with nurses, medical students,
community workers, social workers, etc.

*Granton Stress Centre*
a community mental health
initiative

(Blennerhasset *et al.*, 1989)

*A community is often regarded as a homogeneous entity in which all the members live in the same way, and have the same interests and aspirations. In real life, however, a community is a heterogeneous entity in which the members have different class interests. Even the smallest of communities may reflect the social dynamics prevalent in a region or country. It would be a highly naïve worker who neglects this simple fact.*

On the other hand, De Kadt suggested that Freirean approaches may not have made that mistake, since they started from an assumption of the existence of socio-economic inequalities arising from the nature of capitalist economic systems. Whereas the community developers achieved little because they disregarded inequality, conflict and power relations, the

> ... *conscientisadores ... had over-optimistic, some would say naive, views on the political reaction which their activities were likely to provoke, and on the people's power, or lack of it, to overcome them.*
>
> (p. 574).

As for the process of community participation, he cites a review by David Werner of 40 rural health projects in Latin America:

> ... *when it came to the nitty-gritty of what was going on in the field, many of these ambitious 'king-sized' programmes actually had a minimum of effective community participation and a maximum of handouts, paternalism and superimposed initiative-destroying 'norms'.*
>
> (Werner, 1980, p. 94)

Now it is clear we cannot assume that all community development programmes follow an identical pattern. Indeed, as we have stated, the key feature of recent western, urban community development programmes has been a recognition of the existence of inequalities and a determination to tackle it. However, it may well be the case that even if community development manages to achieve proper community participation, it may be unable to do very much in the face of oppressive environments and socio-economic circumstances. It may, in fact, be true that as Moynihan (cited by Hubley, 1985) said, community work will

> ... *promise a lot; deliver a little. Lead people to believe that they will be better off but let there be no dramatic improvement. Try a variety of programmes, each interesting, but marginal in impact and severely under financed.*

Heller (1989), in defining communities, acknowledged both their geographical and relational elements but insisted that a community should also be defined in terms of 'collective political power'. He distinguished empowerment from collective power. He commented that empowerment means the process of giving power or authority to an individual or group whereas ... *in actuality, meaningful power must be* taken. Ultimately, power is in the community of like-minded individuals who come together to form political coalitions.

A thorough review of this important question of the locus of power cannot be undertaken here and readers are referred to Dixon's (1989) review. We might, however, provide a reminder of our reiteration in this book of the importance of the process of 'reciprocal determinism' of individual action and environmental constraint or facilitation.

There are a number of other problems with community development and it is worth summarising an interesting review by Constantino-David (1982), who provided a detailed and thoughtful critique of community organisation. First she cautions against the members of a community becoming dependent on the workers so that the project collapses once the workers withdraw. Second, she warns of the possibility of creating a new elite of community aides/indigenous workers. Third, she notes the dilemma for workers whose major empowering goal is to facilitate self-empowered choice and promote long-term outcomes such as literacy, autonomy or healthy lifestyles and yet find they must concentrate on specific felt needs; issues which may catch the community's imagination but which may be relatively insignificant in the longer term. She also highlights the 'facilitation versus manipulation' dilemma in which there is a temptation for the worker to manipulate the attitudes and behaviour of the community to conform to the values and political motivation of the worker rather than facilitate empowered choice in the community members. Constantino-David also emphasises the political paradoxes and problems which are usually greater in community organisation than in other health promotion programmes, which are more likely to be congruent with the dominant power structure in society. Loney's (1981) analysis of the British Community Development Projects makes a similar point. The potential for initiating radical action may be limited when funding comes from central government. As Loney says, *It is rather like pacifists sud-*

*denly finding they have army funding*. He does, however, note in his reference to the Community Development Project report *Gilding the Ghetto* (1977)

> *That such a document could emerge from a state sponsored programme and could be printed at government expense must itself encourage a more cautious approach to summary dismissals of the possibilities of working in the state apparatus.*

This is doubtless cheering news for many workers faced with the issue of programme evaluation. They might, however, be excused for a degree of scepticism since community programmes are more likely than most to give rise to a significant gap between the aspirations of funders and those of the workers themselves, to say nothing of the aspirations of the community!

A particular question that has hung over community development, most particularly in the countries of the South, but also frequently relevant in the North, relates to resources. For community development approaches to be used in the context of a commitment to some equal sharing of resources is very different from it being used as a way of extracting work from some communities rather than others. A nice example is provided from South Africa, where rural communities have been encouraged in the context of community development initiatives to develop their own water and sanitation provision while services have been provided in urban communities in the same region (Nene, personal communication).

An extended critique of community development approaches in Latin America which makes reference to resources concerns was provided by Ugalde (1985). He argued that the more stratified a society the less desirable was community participation directed towards extraction of resources from the poor. In contrast, where stratification has been reduced, participation should be encouraged as a means of capital formation and strengthening human dignity. He was also critical of assumptions, informing many community participation programmes, that rural people were disorganised and incapable of collective action:

> *We have the paradoxical situation that governments and international organisations were destroying grassroots organisations and at the same time they were fomenting community organisations under their own control under the rationale that the traditional values of the peasantry were not conducive to effective collective action.*

He also points to evidence of relatively high levels of political community participation in urban Latin American contexts and suggests that international agencies should redirect their efforts towards pressure on governments rather than waste their time organising communities. With reference to case studies from a number of countries he also challenged the emphasis on community participation within primary health care given the widespread lack of success. He also drew attention to the long tradition of blaming the poor for their poverty and disadvantage rather than structural factors. Finally, he reminded us of the history of collective action in many Latin American countries but also emphasised that there was evidence to support the view that democratic community participation will be suppressed if projects raise political awareness.

Many community health initiatives involving community participation have assumed a consensual model and where major inequalities exist this can be challenged. It should also be pointed out that the language of community and community participation is used both by the right and left of the political spectrum and it becomes essential, therefore, to deduce the underlying intentions when empowerment is discussed. Baum (1993) has noted:

> *The new right does use the language of community action. Commentators have noted the tendency for governments to use the rhetoric of community control and empowerment to hide their real agenda of withdrawing support from communities.*

## EVALUATING COMMUNITY PROGRAMMES

Many of the general questions about evaluation do not differ significantly from those in the other settings that we have discussed, although there are some particular issues and challenges. We have noted the small scale localised nature of many projects and the importance attached to adopting an empowerment approach in their work. Particular styles of evaluation will be more appropriate than others to projects of this nature. Participatory research approaches to evaluation have been promoted widely since their philosophy, as typically specified, is coherent with empowerment goals (Tandon, 1981). At the same time, however, projects are often funded from sources which demand a particular type of evidence in order to secure continued funding and the adoption of fully participatory approaches may make such evidence more difficult to obtain. A strategy for evaluation has to be set within a recognition of contextual constraints. Where empowerment and other complex outcomes are project goals we come up against the challenge of developing appropriate indicators to assess achievements. We have also given some mention in this chapter to what have been described as technical/social planning approaches to community organisation. Given that these projects are seeking to achieve goals which have often been set outside a community, they will be less likely to adopt participatory approaches to evaluation and will select evaluation methods that most easily generate evidence of success. At the present time, as noted in Chapter 3, there is some growth in the use of realistic evaluation and theory-based models of change in evaluating community projects.

There are a number of tensions which need to be resolved in the evaluation of community projects. The requirements of the funders of an evaluation may differ from those which a project would itself wish to prioritise. Community health projects have often been asked to justify themselves in terms of health outcomes in addition to, or in place of, the development of empowerment-related attributes. Funding agencies can lack understanding of the principles and practice of community development and this can lead to the setting of unrealistic goals. While expectations should have been explicit from the outset of a project, these may not have been fully acknowledged by all stakeholders and any contradictions in project goals addressed from the early stage. Where an external evaluation is commissioned the questions to be addressed in the evaluation research ought to be appropriate for community development type projects and where this is not the case careful negotiation will be required before work is undertaken.

Debates about appropriate methodology are as prevalent in community project evaluations as in evaluations elsewhere. There is general acceptance of the unsuitability of experimental designs. The people directly involved in a project may hold strong views about their preferred approach to evaluation. Nonetheless, where external funding is provided for evaluation, constraints may be imposed on methodology. At the same time, external funding may also come too late in the life of a project for particular approaches to be adopted. Irrespective of their philosophical commitment to a particular style of evaluation, community projects have also to ensure the continuation of their funding. Evaluators may find it necessary to provide evidence of project success in quantitative terms even where this may not be felt to be the most appropriate evidence to pursue. To refuse to provide such data would not be in the longer term interests of a project. Being able, however, to articulate the limitations of such data and to argue for its combination with qualitative data can be the pragmatic solution. Although we have earlier identified some reservations around methodological triangulation it is clear that there is growing acceptance of its value in evaluating community initiatives.

The power relationships between a funded evaluator and a programme are ones that have to be acknowledged and addressed. Wallerstein (1999), on the basis of a literature review, concluded that despite the growing interest in community-based research and its methodological challenges, little had actually been written about the problematical relationships between communities and evaluators. She provided an interesting discussion of power issues as she experienced them in a four year community project in New

Mexico. While fully committed in general to a participatory research approach and wishing to adopt it in that specific project, she encountered difficulties because, in part, she did not recognise the position of power that she represented to the communities with whom she was working:

> *This lack of recognition of my power served to sabotage genuine community ownership of the evaluation endeavour, which made the interpretation and use of the findings by the communities problematic.*

Her power derived from her University base, membership of the dominant culture and from being a researcher and expert in healthy communities. Where the community was concerned she was also (incorrectly) seen to be part of the state government. In addition, although she explained that the evaluation was separate from funding decisions, this was not accepted by the community. She explains honestly:

> *I introduced the theoretical WHO background, used language that distanced myself and made it difficult for participants to challenge my ideas on the evaluation design. I was not sensitive, in particular, to the power/knowledge I had in constructing the final version of the evaluation plan and interview guide which privileged my own interpretation of the committee's and the communities' ideas.*

She emphasised the need for professionals to recognise the difficulty of engaging community members as partners on an equal power basis. Over time, in her own case, the early difficult relationships evolved towards the participatory model.

Issues in planning and undertaking evaluations of community projects have recently been discussed by Kaduskar *et al.* (1999), with particular reference to the evaluation of community cafes. These are initiatives in the context of efforts to build communities and address inequalities in health. They provide food on a non-profit basis, use volunteer workers and are an initiative in the context of building communities and addressing

inequalities in health. Questions have been raised about the best way to evaluate these innovative developments. In the case reported the researchers opted for a mix of methods which generated quantitative and qualitative data, with an emphasis on triangulation, but acknowledged that this was only one approach that could have been used. As an alternative the possible application of a realist model of evaluation was examined. Instead of asking, as they did, if the café worked they could have asked 'what is it about the café that works for whom in this context? In retrospect they thought this could have been a more appropriate approach, although they do note that the realist approach presupposes some consensus about outcomes which had not initially been in place.

Dixon (1995) has discussed what are often conflicting aspects of community development evaluation. She emphasises the importance of evaluations being undertaken but also proposes the use of a dual track approach which has two complementary elements: a community story approach to the evaluation which communities themselves control and an evaluation led by outside agencies built around the use of community indicators which also reflect community values. The importance of community involvement in evaluation is not simply so that members can become more skilled at such activities but:

> *to enable community members' reflections on their own wins and losses to enhance the never ending struggle to get resources and opportunities for the good life.*

The 'community story' would be produced by groups who would see themselves as co-researchers. An ethnographic approach would be adopted built around participatory action research principles: She lists the community story as an evaluative tool as containing the following elements:

- local control over the research with the focus being the social landscape of organisations, networks, alliances, procedures, practices;
- input from as many sources as possible;

- respect for case study methods and principles;
- a search for meanings and patterns which does not preclude the random, haphazard and contradictory;
- analysis by as many as possible, with some thought to who is not represented by the story;
- the dissemination of insights to influence future community development;
- the establishment of a local archive on which to build.

As an example of dual track evaluations she cites the *Healthy Cities* programme in Australia, which combines community controlled process evaluation and externally controlled programmatic evaluation. The first track involves evaluation consultants teaching process evaluation skills to community participants. The process evaluation is assumed to provide a strong basis upon which the program evaluators can evaluate impacts and outcomes. A dual track evaluation characterises the evaluation of the UK *Health Action Zone* community projects, where there is national and local evaluation with planned integration between the two. Dual track evaluation often takes place in a relatively unplanned manner. Projects frequently undertake their own regular evaluation, often small scale and described in annual reports. At the same time, external funding to support a largely externally managed evaluation can become available at some time in a project history While the case for dual track evaluation can be made for larger projects, in the case of small localised projects it would seem most appropriate to have one evaluation with full community involvement in it whenever possible.

Two reviews of community development projects which provided insights on the nature and processes of evaluation activities have been reported (Beattie, 1995; Smart, 1999). Beattie reviewed reports of 'community development for health' projects covering the period 1979–1990). The review revealed that a variety of evaluation styles were being adopted influenced by accountability arrangements, purposes for which evaluations were undertaken and audiences to which findings were directed. Several of the reports were

bringing together a range of information relevant to the questions posed by the differing stakeholders in community projects and provided good examples of pluralistic evaluation. Beattie suggested that it was the community development for health projects which were most vigorously exploring 'fourth generation evaluation' as discussed earlier. Smart reviewed the strategies adopted in evaluating community development initiatives in Scotland. She conduced documentary analysis and semi-structured interviews within 16 projects, 11 of them in Edinburgh. She was concerned to identify the nature of evaluation activity taking place and to assess the extent of negotiation taking place between funders, managers, project workers and community activists prior to undertaking evaluation research. Little evidence of such negotiation was found. She found a predominance of process evaluation but also some impact evaluation. While there was a bias towards the use of qualitative methods, these were not the only ones used. The rationale for the choice of particular methods was rarely stated explicitly. Three distinct evaluation strategies were identified:

- assessment of whether activities were meeting the needs of service users through process evaluation on a continuing basis;
- monitoring of activities undertaken 'as a matter of course' and used in reports to funders;
- larger evaluation of specific services.

Lack of time and resources imposed constraints on evaluation and comment was made about the expectations around evaluation:

> *We are asked to do an awful lot given the amount of money we have and the impact we can make.*

Even though evaluation activities were routinely undertaken in the majority of the 16 projects a lack of confidence was found in relation to the knowledge and skills required. Training needs were expressed not only from those with little community development experience but also from those with a great deal of experience. Other problems were categorised as ethical and philosophical ones and summarised by:

*Evaluation should be an intrinsic part of everything you do but it is written with certain agendas such as hanging onto jobs. It's not honest. Everyone is too vulnerable to admit failures.*

A number of people interviewed felt that funding bodies did not understand the ethos and principles behind community development and this impacted on the type of information being sought from evaluations, typically the demands for quantitative data.

While there is much support for the practice of community projects undertaking their own evaluations some of the difficulties of doing this have been discussed around the evaluation of community café projects described above (Kaduskar *et al.*, 1999). Although initiatives of this kind are a little different from more general community development projects, the points raised by the researchers may be of wider relevance. They point out that project workers may not always have evaluation skills and may not necessarily want to undertake evaluation. In their case the volunteer workers were busy with running the café and held the view that the methodology of the evaluation should be the concern of researchers. Kaduskar *et al.* propose that if community café staff are to carry out evaluations they will need extensive training and support in techniques.

The challenges in achieving successful partnerships in community-based evaluations adopting action research and participatory approaches in general have also been discussed by Beattie (1995) and Boutilier *et al.* (1997). Boutilier *et al.*, after examining the differing models of action research that exist, have proposed their own model of 'community reflective action research' which attempts to address some of the dilemmas faced by practitioners using participatory research as a health promotion strategy.

We can summarise some features of community project evaluations.

1 Experimental designs are not appropriate although in some limited instances quasi designs might be used using comparison communities where projects have not taken place.

2 Most community projects are implemented at small scale locality levels even if a number of localities form part of a larger project. This lends itself to case study approaches to evaluation informed by interpretivist approaches. Alternatively, there is some use of realist and theory of change approaches in evaluations as exemplified in English *Health Action Zone* projects (Wakefield Health Authority, 1999)

3 Community programmes must take account of the different needs of various stakeholders: community, funders, workers, health professionals, etc., and utilise an evaluation design which can respond to their differing goals. Evaluation also needs to address the individuality of the specific contexts.

4 Community development is above all concerned with action research. While funders of initiatives frequently require particular things from evaluations it is inappropriate for evaluators to maintain an Olympian detachment and merely report on whether or not certain programme objectives have been achieved. Innovative programmes require a continual flow of information from formative and process evaluation in order to be able to change course in pursuit of relevant goals and to react to changing circumstances.

5 The participation of communities in the evaluation process from the beginning through to the writing up and dissemination stages is also a key element in the empowering process, although this does not always occur. Where funders of a project and its evaluation do not understand that the participatory research process can take longer, tensions can arise for both evaluators and project participants. The extent and nature of participation in the research process needs to be agreed and appropriate training and support provided.

## WHAT INDICATORS OF SUCCESS?

Dixon (1995) noted a continuing lack of suitable indicators for assessing community projects. She considers that expert developed indicators are often overly ambitious and unrealistic and says:

*community development indicators must refer to local action strategies and thus address issues amenable to local change, so that there is a chance of success.*

Although it is important, through process evaluation, to accumulate evidence which illuminates the reasons for success or failure of projects and provide guidance for more effective action, it is also necessary, in most cases, to examine whether or not objectives have been achieved. Typically the objectives in question would give rise to indirect or intermediate indicators of performance of process. The literature on community development and many of the examples which describe the community development process provide ready-made indicators of this kind. For instance, we have already noted how Batten's (1967) (Chapter 2, Box 30) seven stages could provide a useful basis for process evaluation as the community moves from passivity to self-empowered action (or not, as the case may be!).

A set of exemplars of certain possible indicators of the success of community development programmes was provided by Fawcett *et al.* (1984). The authors presented seven case studies, each of which illustrated success in at least some of the processes necessary for empowering people. These processes were described as follows.

1 Increasing **knowledge of community problems** from the perspective of those most affected by the problems.
2 Increasing **knowledge of solution alternatives** generated by those most affected by the problems.
3 Increasing **knowledge of the possible consequences** of projects proposed by persons outside the affected community.
4 **Involving consumers** in the redesign of social programmes to fit local needs and resources.
5 **Training new behaviours** for increasing the effectiveness of individual citizens.
6 **Training new behaviours** for increasing the effectiveness of leaders of community groups.
7 **Developing and communicating research information** to increase the likelihood of actions taken regarding problems affecting the poor or disadvantaged.

(pp. 148–149)

(Note that phrases shown in bold represent our emphasis and indicate potential programme objectives within an overall empowerment aim.)

More recently Barr (1995), in reflecting on empowerment of communities in Scottish settings, has proposed a set of indicators to assess empowerment strategies (Box 2).

**Box 2**  Suggested Indicators of Empowerment

1 The existence of strong community controlled institutions on both a geographical and interest group basis.
2 Evidence that such institutions have real influence (though not sovereignty) over the public policy agenda.
3 Evidence of increased direct control of resources and affairs, including community ownership of community assets, such as premises, equipment and information.
4 Evidence that the performance of power structures is genuinely open to influence. This will include political committees and departmental decision making procedures.
5 Evidence that equity is a demonstrably central principle in the policy process at all levels.
6 Evidence that material gains are being achieved for disadvantaged people.
7 Evidence that there is strong but accountable and representative local leadership.
8 Evidence that the performance of professionals reflects values of empowerment and is evaluated by users.
9 Evidence, corroborated by the views of oppressed minority groups, that equal opportunities principles are being upheld.
10 Evidence of increasing democratisation and decentralisation of services and resources allocation within an overall policy framework designed to promote equity.
11 Evidence of personal development of citizens measured not only by increased levels of participation or achievement but also self-esteem.

Contributors to the debate about evaluation in community settings and identifying indicators have not always confined discussion to the small scale community development project. Hayes and Manson-Willms (1991), in seeking to develop healthy community indicators for a Canadian *Healthy Communities Project*, characterised this in their paper as *the perils of the search and the paucity of the find*. The *Healthy Communities Project* was set up in order to encourage communities to participate in a process which allowed them to determine the meaning of health in their communities and to develop inter-sectoral models for achieving a healthy community. As a condition of belonging communities were to identify sensitive, relevant and relatively easy to collect indicators in order to monitor progress towards objectives and to provide a basis for comparison with projects in other communities. This is a situation that can readily arise with respect to many community projects and Hayes and Manson-Willms (1990) make the important point:

> *We argue that such concerns with indicators is misguided. Not only is such a requirement likely to stifle community initiatives by wresting ownership of projects away from local groups but it is also extremely unlikely that any indicators of the type being sought will ever be found.*

One problem identified is the conflict between a search for indicators informed by positivist approaches and the process goals of health promotion. As Dean said earlier (1998):

> *We are searching for indicators of the process of translating health resources into health as distinct from indicators of health itself.*

In taking this task forward we would be looking for appropriate indicators for assessing the process towards valued health promotion goals.

Hayes and Manson-Willms rightly point out that it is unlikely that 'one size fits all' indicators will be found for two main reasons:

- communities are encouraged to develop their own approaches to creating healthy outcomes and indicators will be specific to individual goals;
- conditions of social relations are spatially and temporally specific and contextually dependent – comparisons between communities have to be made in the recognition of differing macro and micro factors.

This position would lead us to argue for project-specific indicators and to a readiness to challenge the imposition of indicators which do not take into account the context in which projects are embedded. At the same time there are processes integral to many projects where knowledge of possible ways of assessing them can be useful even if such measures are customised. The importance of having a clear sense of what is being sought within projects has been stated by Hawe (1994):

> *... vague objectives in program documents, such as 'to empower residents', or 'to bring about structural change' or 'to stimulate health promotion activity networks' should be translated into recognisable and meaningful components appropriate to actual programme activities. In this way precise indicators of what enhanced capacity within a community would look like are pre-set with the dual purpose of providing vision and shape to the intervention as well as providing markers or indicators for the evaluation.*

This statement might sound more prescriptive than some would welcome but Hawe does emphasise that the evaluator works actively with programme workers and the programme design is produced interactively. We have noted the lack of perceived evaluation skills within some projects and there is likely to be a welcome for specific indicators which can be adapted as appropriate within individual projects. While continuing to caution against the too ready use of universal measures and indicators, we can comment on an example of one indicator that has been used and assessed.

Rifkin *et al.* (1988) developed a framework which can be used to assess levels of participation in a programme. They used five dimensions of participation as a basis for measurement connected in a spoke-like configuration (Figure 9.4). The dimensions are:

- needs assessment;
- leadership;
- organisation;
- resource mobilisation;
- management.

The points marked from the hub to the periphery indicate increasing community participation.

Assessments made collectively by those involved in a project can provide a visual representation of where a project is at its outset and at varying times during or at the end of a project. Used formatively it is a way of identifying areas needing attention. Figure 9.4 illustrates, for a hypothetical project, plots from the beginning of a project and after a period of time.

This tool was used in assessing community development in a community-based health programme in the Philippines (Laleman and Annys, 1989) and in a community project in Sweden (Bjärås *et al.*, 1991) The former project had as its aims:

- increasing people's awareness of their situation and of the structures that prevent them from fulfilling their basic needs;
- maximising participation in all aspects of decision making affecting their own lives;
- organising community action to solve problems;
- increasing self-reliance in health and development activities.

The writers concluded that the Rifkin analytical tool appeared to be a practical one for structuring discussion on community participation and they said:

*The tool does not aim to produce an objective and quantitative measurement of a particular situation; this would be illusory given the complexity of the process of community participation, and the necessity for subjective and qualitative indicators. However it does provide a common language for the different observers and makes it possible to pinpoint and describe the dynamics of this complex field.*

In the Swedish project (Bjärås *et al.*, 1991) the writers, while identifying some shortcomings, also concluded that the pentagram framework was a useful one. This simple idea can be used with different dimensions and adjusted according to the specifics of a project. Clearly there is a danger of attaching too much significance to points on the individual dimensions and it might be better to use the 'spokes' without the addition of the marked positions, which can encourage somewhat simplistic and inappropriate quantification.

## Forms of data collection

It is in evaluations of community projects that there have, arguably, been some of the most creative approaches to providing information on achievements. While evaluations have adopted all the standard techniques of questionnaires, interviews, observation, use of documentation and so on, additional methods have also been used. These have included diaries, photos, stories and collage development as ways of documenting project achievements. Such methods may be used alone or in combination with more traditional methods and their products often provide a good element in reports which engages the interest of others when they are disseminated. A number of

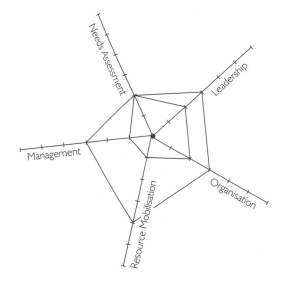

***Figure 9.4*** Sample illustration of Plotting Community Participation

specific techniques have been developed in the context of participatory rural appraisal, used initially in agricultural communities in the countries of the South and, increasingly, in the North. They were developed as methods to find out about people's lives when traditional research methods proved inappropriate. They have been valuable in ensuring that all voices have been heard within community contexts and their use is an acknowledgement that communities are not homogeneous but are structured according to age, gender, ethnicity, disability, poverty and so on. Participatory rural appraisal has been described by Cornwell (1996):

> *It offers ways to open up discussions in a non-threatening way, by focusing on local classifications, local concepts and local explanations. In doing so the objective is not merely to find out. By actively engaging people in a process of exploring and representing what they know, the participatory research process can validate them as knowledgeable, active subjects capable of interpreting and changing their situations themselves.*

A wide variety of participatory rural appraisal methods have been used, some more appropriate to certain situations than others. Very many, however, rely on visualisation, including maps, drawings, dramas, matrix ranking, time lines, chapatti (Venn) diagramming, models and calendars.

When different groups within a community undertake the same activity very different products are generated and these can then form the basis for discussion and planning for future actions. The importance of visualisation has been discussed by Cornwell (1998). As a technique it offers a way of breaking the ice between researchers and communities, especially where previous contacts have not been associated with mutual learning. As techniques they can be contrasted with interviewing. Interviews, if conduced by a researcher, are typically taken away and analysed elsewhere. Using visualisation techniques information is cooperatively produced and in a form that is available for collective reference for cross-checking and analysis. Producing a visual representation is in itself an analytical act and reflections on the products invites further analysis and, maybe, progression to the use of different techniques. For example, use of mapping in a local context may lead to the production of seasonal calendars. Cornwell describes the process of use of seasonal calendars in an Ethiopian project (Box 3). The visual techniques bring out the ideas of people who might remain silent in focus group interviews. The production of the product is a cooperative social act which in itself stimulates discussion and reflection. An important point made by Cornwell is the way that joint products can enable perspectives to be revealed that might not happen through individually focused methods. She says:

> *As images are the products of a group process ownership lies outside identifiable individuals. Attention is focused away from the particular individuals taking part onto an externalised object which acts as a vehicle for views and perceptions.*

Examples are given of ways that such methods have brought out issues that may not have emerged when more traditional methods were used. For example, the use of body mapping in Zimbabwe helped to explain women's use of and reactions to forms of contraception and identified appropriate ways for explanations congruent with women's own representations.

**Box 3**  Use of Seasonal Calendars

Three facilitators worked together with a group of men to construct a seasonal calendar. Using symbols chosen by the participants, an elaborate calendar was produced that showed changes over the year, including disease prevalence, market prices, food availability and labour. One of the participants, a young man, chose to represent malaria with a picture of a mosquito which became progressively larger when the incidence of malaria was high. This provoked a discussion of causes of malaria within a group. From this the team was able to move on to discuss other illnesses. Going back to complete the calendar the facilitators went on to ask questions about connections between various aspects. At first participants did not see any connection. With some probing, connections were made. Participants said with amazement that they had seen for the first time that some of their problems were linked with others and went on to explore ways in which they could address them.

These techniques can be used as part of a slow empowering process or as rapid techniques for obtaining information. In translation to countries such as the UK some of the usage has been rapid but has not necessarily been a component of an empowering process. Such activities, undertaken properly, are time consuming and require particular skills on the part of facilitators. Dockery (1998) reports that in a training exercise to enable health workers to use rapid appraisal techniques the time available was too limited to enable any meaningful community consultation. It was, she said, the 'rapid' in the rapid appraisal approach that appealed to managers.

We mentioned the use of story telling as a method and this has been developed particularly by Labonte *et al.* (1999). Their method was used, as noted earlier, in the evaluation of one of the pilot hospitals in the *Health Promoting Hospitals*.

## COMMUNITY PROJECTS: SOME EXAMPLES OF SUCCESS

While it is probably true to say that many community workers are more concerned with achieving success than with measuring it, there are many examples of project evaluation to draw on. A relatively larger proportion of evaluations than in other settings are found in project reports which do not receive wide dissemination. We will draw mainly on evaluations of community development projects but will also refer to some social action projects and an example of what could be defined as a technical/social planning one. Projects will be drawn from a number of countries. There is no intention to provide a comprehensive review of community project evaluations. We will use the discussion and description of those projects selected to identify the kinds of successes achieved and to refer back to some of the evaluation issues that have been discussed in the earlier part of the chapter. We will begin with a project involving young people in Thailand and then three projects with people who have experienced dispossession of their lands. Many community development activities have taken place with women's groups and we will review several projects which illustrate the range of activities. We will include two projects with women which have incorporated peer teaching approaches and will also describe one systematic review of projects involving women, some of which are described as 'social action' projects. Finally, we will give an example of a project which has characteristics of the social planning model as defined earlier in the chapter.

Kindervatter (1979) has described a series of youth and village development workshops in Thailand. Although at first sight these would not seem to have great relevance for those planning and evaluating community health projects in Western inner city areas the fundamental principles are identical and many parallels can be drawn. For instance, the goals of the organisers of the Thai workshops (which they acknowledged as derived from them rather than from felt needs) was encapsulated in the concept of *khit pen*.[2] This notion is directly comparable with Freire's pedagogical aims as described in Chapter 1. The methods adopted by the 'facilitators' are akin to those recommended for use in UK schools health and life skills teaching, e.g. analysis of felt needs, team building, goal setting, problem solving, etc. The goals of the Thai project, however, proved to be more tangible and immediate and included the acquisition of occupational skills which might be used to help the community by, for example, putting into practice a village project such as building a water drainage system. In other words, we have a scheme which incorporates the two classic goals of community organisation/development: first, the 'ideological' all embracing aim of self-empowering individuals and community; second, the more specific objectives which emerge from the 'felt needs' of the participants.

As for the evaluation planners utilised a number of simple tools to determine:

1 a process effect – participants and facilitators' responses to the programme;
2 intermediate indicators of participants learning – attitudes and behaviours;
3 longer term outcome indicators.

The process evaluation indicated, for instance, that ... *outside resource people tended to present boring lectures!* This fact was taken into account when revising the programme, along with various positive recommendations; that the occupational skills sessions were effective, as were the morning calisthenics. With regard to immediate indicators, various changes in attitudes were recorded, such as greater awareness of village problems and a recognition that the individuals' abilities could be used to improve their lives. At the same time ambivalent results were noted in respect of such items as 'I am confident of my abilities' and 'I think my life will be better five years from now'. Clearly self-empowerment had been tempered by a recognition of the real social and environmental constraints.

As for outcome indicators participants were reported to have become more active in discussion and had acquired increased skills in working in small groups (again it is interesting to note the parallels with school-based life skills evaluation measures). More importantly perhaps, for the good of the community and the experience of success by the participants most of the planned projects had been completed by the end of three months (e.g. raising $300 for village development projects: establishing a day care centre; preparing a village learning centre; construction of three roads; repair of a public hall).

Gordon (1985) described an interesting community development project which was implemented in communities providing labour for a timber-producing company in a rural area of South Africa. Programme goals were to promote community participation by setting up *an infrastructure of decision making bodies in the villages*; to develop a social and recreational programme to foster community solidarity; to increase income levels by *enabling residents to participate in informal income generating activities*. Within a 12 month evaluation period the following indicators of success were reported:

- Community committees were functioning autonomously and further elections organised by the committees were held.
- A number of corporate ventures were organised, such as ploughing fields and hiring cattle herders.
- Equipment for sport and recreation was jointly purchased by the company and the communities.
- By the end of the year, soccer and netball clubs were operating smoothly and two competitions had been supported with great enthusiasm.
- The Community Development Officer organised hearings of two cases in which employees claimed that they had been unfairly dismissed by their supervisors. As a result of the hearings both complainants were rehired. Labour turnover dropped from 80% to 40% over the 12 months of study.

(p. 334)

Despite caveats about expecting too much from a community development mode of working – without the sorts of supplementary help to which reference was made above – it is clear that community development can empower. For instance, O'Sullivan *et al.* (1984) described how a small Native American community was faced with the loss of their homeland as a result of a proposal to build a dam. The results of such a move would have been to damage the physical, psychological, economic and social well-being of that community. Over a number of years a coalition of environmental interest groups (including environmentalists, religious leaders, anti-government advocates, pro-Native American supporters and river recreationists) took up the Native Americans' cause. Apart from various exercises in lobbying and advocacy, a deliberate attempt was made to gain maximal community participation. Subsequently the tribe (the Yavapai)

> *... engaged in an effective, consistent, and intensive media campaign, culminating in a three day march from the reservation to the state capital. They presented a signed petition with an alternative to the proposed dam.*

As the authors put it, *... the tribe publicly demonstrated opposition ... that was forceful, skilful and credible.* To use Bell's (1975) lexicon of political linguistics, the Fort McDowell tribal community entered a power position by communicating to their opponents that *they could and would tie up* (the dam project) *for so long that it could not be built in the foreseeable future.* According to the authors one of the results of this community action (which was more akin to 'social action' in its use of coalitions and conflict than to community development) was that the tribe changed its perception of itself as powerless. One tribal elder stated:

> *... it was the first time the Yavapai had ever won a battle with the government, and we beat the white man at his own game.*

The community had moved towards self-empowerment – and the dam was not built!

In a further project with a community which has experienced dispossession from its lands, disadvantage and poor health is reported from New Zealand (Voyle and Simmons, 1999). The report highlights some of the difficulties in achieving community development when external research requirements have to be prioritised, a pressure that can affect other projects. This project involved the Maori community in a low socio-economic status suburb in Auckland and aimed to promote healthy lifestyles. The writers suggest that the principles of community development and the current cultural renaissance of the Maori may potentially be reinforcing. The project consisted of a community development partnership for health promotion between a health group and the Maori community and took place within a traditional community meeting place, a *marae*. It focused on diabetes awareness, nutrition, exercise, a diabetes support group and other health interventions. In common,

therefore, with many other projects labelled as community development the focus was on specific health topics which have been professionally defined and were not initiated in response to a community's felt and expressed needs. The evaluation included quantitative evaluation of health outcomes and formative and processs evaluation of the development of the health programmes and the factors facilitating success. It was carried out by a community psychologist who participated as an employee of the *South Auckland Diabetes Project* (SADP) and was also a member of the partnership committee. Participant observation and in-depth interviews were the research methods used. Research notes were discussed and corroborated with the appropriate people.

Achievements were reported. In line with the health goals of the project, screening sessions took place together with a variety of other activities: one day health promotion events, diabetes prevention and healthy lifestyles and a diabetes support group. The eventual outcomes were the establishment of a health programme by the *Marae Trust Board* itself. A smoke-free *marae* was declared, successful health promotion days attracting 80–100 people were held, catering to provide low fat and high fibre foods at events was initiated and weekly line dancing took place. In terms of the types of community organisation in Figure 9.3 this project was around Type 4 and moved towards Type 3 over time and possibly had some features of Type 2. The researchers provided an extended reflection on key issues that emerged from the evaluation.

- The *Medical Model* requirements for quantitative pre- and post-programme assessments limited the powers of the partnership committee in planning a programme. Because of the time needed to achieve a specific sample size for baseline measures this again created a loss of momentum for the project as a whole.
- Trust was identified as the most significant issue. Specifically this was distrust among the Maori as a result of their historical and current experiences with Europeans. Within the project itself there was also distrust because the partnership committee did not sufficiently represent all interest groups in the *marae*.

- The health problem of diabetes, although recognised to be a problem, was not one to which the Maori community gave much thought. There was evidence that health protection had low value and the potential benefits of the health programme were seen by the community to be with the SADP partners who might get rewards and kudos from success.

A variety of recommendations were made for future projects which were designed to incorporate more fully the principles of community development. It was also recognised that positivist research models do not fit well with community development strategies.

As noted earlier, a significant number of community development for health projects have involved women. We will begin by reporting on evaluations from a project which is illustrative of those set up in connection with funding for specific aspect of women's health. The evaluations report on a selection of three out of 19 community-based initiatives designed to address smoking among women living on low incomes in Scotland. The *Women, Low Income and Smoking Project* was initiated by *Action on Smoking and Health* (ASH) and funded by the national agency *Health Education Board for Scotland* (HEBS). The project emerged from consultation between community-based projects and health promotion departments. A wide variety of projects were funded (Amos *et al.*, 1999; Barlow *et al.*, 1999; McKie *et al.*, 1999). The three evaluations reported describe a mental health project, a dance and drama group and a project including homelessness and women's aid groups. The dance and drama group project is described in Box 4.

***Box 4*** TAPS Tiree: A Dance and Drama Group for Rural Community Development

Tiree is an island community with 60% on low income and 50% reported as smokers. The project activities encouraged women to think about smoking, although the groups were not primarily about smoking. ASH funding was gained for a pantomine with a health theme with the following objectives:

- to increase self-esteem and a feeling of achievement;
- to enhance community spirit;
- to promote alternative distractions and interests;
- to provide an opportunity for women to develop new skills;
- to provide support for those women trying to change their smoking behaviour.

*Evaluation*
Evaluation included process information: a report of the pantomine and other TAPS initiatives, including newspaper cuttings, telephone interviews with facilitators and in-depth interviews.

*Reported Outcomes*
- Development of confidence and self-esteem.
- Attitudes challenged in an acceptable way and health topics put on the community agenda.
- A more defined community spirit for isolated individuals, particularly women was fostered.
- Some smokers cut down or stopped and perceptions of smoking changed.
- Increased profile for TAPS gave it local credibility and appreciation.

*Two Years Later*
- Work on smoking initiated by the pantomine was being sustained.
- A range of activities which assisted a reduction in smoking had continued: line dancing, keep fit, arts and crafts, etc.

In commenting on the Tiree project Barlow *et al.* (1999) commented that this project out of the 19 showed most clearly how community capacity building needed to be rooted in the community's own experience and there needed to be understanding of community life for supportive professional advice and alliances to become possible. As they said:

*On Tiree difficulties associated with people's location on an island, transport problems, and the lambing season all have an impact on women's abilities to be involved in anything other than caring for the family or working on the crofts.*

A project undertaken in Pakistan also addressed specific aspects of women's health and the associated and highly important issue of women's literacy. The project was undertaken in a group of fishing villages by the *Health Education and Literacy Project* (HEAL). The women in one of the villages had asked for help with basic literacy and learning about health. The women's groups were encouraged to identify actual health issues, how they had been handled and their own feelings and beliefs about the issues. The women then used the information to develop their own stories about appropriate health actions for sharing with others. HEAL provided training in basic literacy to enable women to express their experiences (Knight and Knight, 1995). After 12 months the women had looked at a number of health issues, including diet, child health, hygiene and family planning. Approximately 30 women had learned to read and write and had shared health information with their families. What the women valued most was the way that HEAL staff had looked at problems with them:

*Previous development projects made promises to deliver all sorts of things but never did ... the thing that made this project different was a relationship of trust and care and the fact that we made our own decisions.*

The women in this village made a decision to expand the programme by forming women's groups in three other villages.

Community development approaches have been used in a number of projects addressing the sexual health of young people outside formal schools settings and are seen as the most appropriate ways for working with young people who may be difficult to reach. A number of these projects have used peer education approaches and have revealed some of the differing conceptions of such approaches, as discussed earlier in the schools chapter. One example is a sexual health project for young women in Bradford, UK (Tilford and Alexander, 1998). This project was funded by the Health Authority in response to defined sexual health education needs and specifically to the problem of teenage pregnancy. It was a peer education community-based project in a disadvantaged area on the city outskirts and external evaluation took place during the second year of two years funding. The project was oriented to girls of 14–16 years. The project team included education, health and youth workers and a small group of slightly older girls who fulfilled a peer educator role with the younger ones. The evaluation sought to identify the extent to which the project had been able to develop a group of peer educators who were active in their community and had established a viable support network for them. The indicators agreed with the funders and the project leader were the extent to which:

- peer educators had acquired new information and knowledge about sexual health and related issues;
- levels of understanding about the principles of peer education had been increased;
- personal levels of confidence as peer educators had been enhanced;
- levels of self-esteem had been increased and positive attitudes to sexual health issues achieved;
- peer education skills had been put into practice in all settings.

The methodology adopted was designed to meet the expressed needs of funders for quantitative data on the project together with in-depth information on the processes of the project. The timing of the evaluation in the life of the project and the need to report promptly if further funding for the project was to be secured imposed restrictions on what could be accomplished and the extent to which a participatory style of evaluation could be adopted. All methods of data collection were, however, discussed with project workers, and in some cases with the senior peer educators, and contributions to questionnaire developments were sought. The evaluation used a number of questionnaires, one-to-one interviews with the young women and with project workers and participant and non-participant observations. Data were triangulated. On the basis of the data collected there was good evidence from both the quantitative and qualitative data that the project had responded to the learning needs of its participants and that health knowledge, beliefs and attitudes had been affected. The young women had increased self-confidence and expressed confidence to undertake a range of peer education activities. Although there was some indication that self-esteem had been affected positively, strong conclusions could not be drawn from the information available. The kinds of comments frequently made in interviews with the young women about participation in the project were:

*I feel I have learned a lot since coming to the Group and I also feel I would be able to help others if they need it.*

*I have become more confident.*

*I've looked at myself. I took a step back and looked at my life and it made me change the way I think. It made me grow up more.*

*I think about sexual health more – thinking about safer sex and not just because of getting pregnant, think about it and act on it.*

Full use was made of peer education approaches in the activities within the group. The project was also moving towards activities which would lead to the younger girls also acting as peer educators in their community. The ways that were thought to be most appropriate for doing this were emerging from the young women themselves in tune with the community development ethos of the project. At the end of the two years it could not be concluded that a full team of peer educators who were making a significant impact more widely in their communities had yet emerged. Peer education skills were too strongly associated with a the small number of older girls in the group and were being used largely with the younger girls within the project rather than in the wider local community. The develop-

ment of the skills of younger members had not yet been progressed sufficiently for them to adopt peer educator roles. Ways in which progress to this goal might have been pursued rather more rapidly were identified in the evaluation report. At the same time it could be argued that development had proceeded at the pace that was right for the individuals concerned and the young women had themselves been able to influence the project development. If a project works with an empowerment philosophy it is not easy at the same time to impose a top-down programme designed to achieve goals that have been set, in part, by others. Projects of this kind throw up interesting questions of what should be counted as success. On all the evidence available there were very positive gains for the young women directly involved in the project. Some of the young women had very difficult lives but were gaining significant support from involvement with the project and were coping. For the health authority who funded the project, and who were interested in making some impact on teenage pregnancy levels in the city and also keen to see peer education in action on a wide basis in the project communities, the project hadn't achieved its full goals in the funded time. We do have to ask whether the original goal of training peer educators who could operate effectively was realistic in the time available and within the community development style of the project. That a number of young women gained a great deal from their involvement in the project was an important achievement. Currently the greater readiness to support community development projects is an acknowledgement that such projects are needed if health promotion goals are to be achieved.

A project from a different part of the world but also using peer approaches is *de Madres a Madres* (*From Mothers to Mothers*) (Mcfarland and Fehir, 1994). This project was initiated by project workers and a community health nurse in response to the low use of pre-natal care by Latino pregnant women in the USA. Barriers to use included cultural, linguistic and access barriers, lack of child care and transport. The theoretical basis for the programme was Freire's concept of empowerment education and Wheeler's feminist theory.

The project began with a needs assessment, followed by the identification and training of 14 volunteer mothers as health promoters using 'mother to mother' education, counselling and follow-up for pregnant women and day care services. The project expanded to 30 voluntary mother health promoters. Outcomes reported included: development of a peer network; provision of day care; resisting evictions; obtaining funds to start a community health centre; higher satisfaction and self-esteem.

A somewhat different project that reports on involvement in a community research project as an empowering process is described by Travers (1997). The research took place in the context of a larger research project in Canada oriented to initiating nutrition education for social change among socially disadvantaged women and their families in a community drop-in centre. The research began with participant observation and then progressed to group interviews and meetings with 27 interviews taking place over 16 months. Participant observation also continued over the whole period. Guides were developed for the interviews but topics were also introduced by participants. Triangulation of data was undertaken. A total of 33 women participated, with anything between five and 25 people at sessions and a core group of five or six present throughout. A process of emancipatory education as a result of participation in the groups was reported. This enabled women to initiate collective action for social change to reduce nutritional inequities. The elements of this development were characterised.

- *Consciousness raising as cultural development:* recognition of oppression by gender, race and class and progression to new ways of thinking about and relating to the social world.
- *Developing a social learning community:* the evolution from a collection of individuals to a group with a common sense of purpose. The women described themselves as a learning community.
- *Economic development:* a study of local food pricing; letter writing to stores about inequities in pricing quality and services; direct contact with food sources with data and recommendations for action and positive responses from such actions; the formation of a grassroots cooperative grocery enterprise.
- *Political development:* recognition that difficulties in purchasing adequate food were not rooted in personal adequacy led to letter writing to political leaders, involvement in a grassroots poverty group and saving the drop-in centre from closure.

The gains in the project were analysed in relation to Labonte's (1994) continuum and are illustrated in Box 5. Travers reports that throughout the research process she seldom offered expert advice but enabled the women involved to analyse and reflect on their experiences in ways that explored the social roots of their problems.

***Box 5*** Learning from a Nutritional Inequities Project using Labonte's Continuum

- Personal development: learning to make economical food choices.
- Small group development: through participation in meetings and sharing of experiences small group development took place.
- Community organisation: this occurred in developing the local actions on supermarket pricing inequities.
- Coalition advocacy: coalitions were built with tenants' asssociation and grassroots anti-poverty organisations.
- Political action: moved toward, but did not quite achieve, action at the level of public policy and empowerment at the level of political action.

There is one meta-analysis which it is important to refer to in this chapter. It brings together 40 studies around the theme of empowerment of women for health promotion (Kar *et al.*, 1999) and includes a number of social action projects. Case studies were selected from diverse cultures in which women in negative circumstances had successfully initiated, organised and led effective social action movements which empowered them and improved the quality of life of their communities. The purpose of the review was to identify the conditions, factors and methods which empower women and mothers for social action and health promotion movements. Five criteria were used to select studies for the review:

- availability of reliable written information;
- representativeness – studies from both economically developed and less developed nations;
- the case studies represent what were defined as key domains of quality of life – human rights, equal rights, economic development and health;
- sustainability – the studies should have lasted long enough to achieve goals, wholly or in part;
- uniqueness – studies should have gained national or international recognition and be considered as models for other programmes.

A number of different analyses of the projects were undertaken, including content analysis of the case studies on six dimensions: location; problem; impetus; methods; partners/opponents; context or macro-environment; impact. A meta-analysis of all 40 studies was completed to quantify the factors affecting empowerment. While it could be argued that all studies had a relevance for health promotion 15 of the 40 were specifically defined as having a primary health promotion focus. One of these projects, *de Madres a Madres*, has been described above. The subjects of the other projects are listed in Box 6.

**Box 6**  Health Promotion Studies in Women and Empowerment Review

Mothers Against Drunk Drivers
International Planned Parenthood Federation, Bombay, India
Mother's Clubs in Korea, Colombia, Bangladesh, India
Pueblos Jovenes Community Kitchen Movement, Peru 1980s

Protoype USA Outreach Drug Abuse Program
Women Against Gun Violence, USA
Tri-valley Citizens Against a Radioactive Environment USA
Committee to Rescue Our Health, Puerto Rico
Rape Crisis, Cape Town, Republic of South Africa
South Carolina Aids Education Network
Over 60s Health Center, USA
Traditional Childbearing Group, USA
WORLD (Women Organised to Respond to Life-threatening Diseases), USA
Anti-alcohol Campaign 1993

(Kar *et al.*, 1999)

One key conclusion from the review will be quoted in full:

*Successful case studies from across the globe, from poor and rich nations, diverse sociocultural systems and democratic and oppressive political regimes confirm that under the most adverse conditions, women and mothers can and do lead successful movements that empower them and help promote their Quality of Life. Involvement in social action movements regardless of their specific goals, methods used, or outcomes, has strong empowering effects. These effects are twofold. First, there was an enhancement of the women' subjective well being, their self esteem and self efficacy. The social reputation of women and mothers increased significantly as a result of their involvement in even small scale self help initiatives and local programs. Second, as women acquired important technical and organisational skills, their quality of life and social status were significantly enhanced.*

We described earlier what were defined as social/technical planning projects and identified the key characteristics of such projects. Examples of such programmes can be provided from Latin America, although whether they can always clearly be distinguished as social planning is open to question. Such approaches have been adopted in the context of controlling a number of vector-borne diseases, including dengue fever and Chagas disease (Renshaw and Rivas, 1991; Winch *et al.*, 1992). Winch *et al.*, on the basis of a review, concluded that in those projects which had encouraged participation to improve health few had achieved active participation and many had failed to achieve health benefits. He refers to De Kadt's point, which would also be endorsed by Ugalde, that where material resources are more evenly distributed and governments supportive of, or at least tolerant of, community initiatives, community-based programmes had a better chance of success. He commented:

> *These preconditions for success do not exist in most of Latin America. Sharp inequities in the distribution of power and wealth make government commitment to autonomous community development activity not only uncertain but highly unlikely.*

It is against this context that what the writers actually labelled as a community development approach was used to address Chagas' disease, a major health problem in Bolivia (Renshaw and Rivas, 1991). The programme, undertaken as part of the *Sucre Health Project*, combined four elements: health education, organisational promotion, housing improvement and fumigation. As a result of the health education, mostly based on a dialogue approach with some limited use of mass media, interest was generated in Chagas' disease. Films, which whole villages attended, and drama presentations were used. Although Chagas' disease had a significant impact on health it was not easily recognised by the community because of its slow development, its manifestation through a number of symptoms and deaths from the disease being attributed to other causes. The causal relationship between the *vinchuca* (the assassin bug), which is the transmittor, and Chaga's disease was not understood and the bug was generally tolerated. As a result of discussion the aim was to allow villagers to come to their own conclusions about what to do about the disease. If a community showed interest and met the conditions for participation a local committee was set up and a housing survey undertaken to identify the improvements necessary to eradicate *vinchucas*. All families had to participate since the only effective process was to eradicate the vector from all houses and related buildings. The communities also had to be prepared to undertake the necessary building work as indicated by the project staff. Support to the villagers was available in terms of building materials and food rations, since opportunities to earn outside the community were being lost during the housing improvements. The actual work included demolishing and rebuilding some houses, replastering others and rebuilding animal pens followed by insecticide spraying on completion. In a 1991 report the project was said to have had a significant impact on participating communities. The vector had been virtually eradicated and there appeared to be general improvements in environmental hygiene. Eradication of the disease was not in sight since many people were already infected and were experiencing the disease in a chronic form. The criteria for replication of the achievements reported were seen to be related to the size of communities and the organisation within them. The recommendations were to work with localities of between 20 and 100 families with a similar standard of living where there was a readiness of all to participate. In more heterogeneous communities these conditions would not be met.

This project was directed towards achieving a change in a health problem for which the community had not previously expressed a need. The project did not proceed, however, until, through education, the need was perceived and the community willing to proceed. Direction came essentially from outsiders, as did material support. Very similar strategies have been used in many parts of the world for water and sanitation projects, malaria (Sharma *et al.*, 1991) and other health problems.

We will conclude our selection of evaluation reports with one from Kieffer (1984), which provided valuable insights into the developmental nature of the empowering process from the perspective of the individual member of the community. Quotations from some of these actors describe the changes they were undergoing. In so doing we will also demonstrate the way in which a qualitative research method can provide rich insights into such changes.

Kieffer considered that community members moved through four stages on their journey to empowerment. Following a process of consciousness raising, an initial 'era of entry' is followed by an 'era of advancement'. This stage is in turn succeeded by an era of 'incorporation' and, finally, an 'era of commitment'. The era of entry is characterised by an emergent feeling of *commitment to self-reliance and feelings of attachment and support within a caring community* ... . Kieffer describes the feeling of powerlessness which can exist prior to this first stage in the words of an American living in Harlem.

> *It would never have occurred to me to have expressed an opinion on anything. ... It was inconceivable that my opinion had any value ... that's lower than powerlessness. You don't even know the word 'power' exists. It applies to them. ... I didn't question that that's the way the world was. ... It was their world ... and I was an intruder, you know?*

In the words of Emily

> *People like us ... have a hard enough time copin' with every day livin'. When you have to work every day for your basic food, shelter, clothes, and safety, you're not very much apt to have a lot of energy left to go to meetin's. ... People ... are so busy earnin' a livin' they don't really stop and think about ... what real impact they may have as a citizen.*

The 'era of entry' involves a kind of awakening. Kieffer, however, describes this as happening from a basis of *felt-rootedness in a community* and ... *feelings of attachment and support within a caring community of peers*. Moreover, the initial reaction, he argues, is not fostered by mere consciousness raising but rather by the *immediate and physical violation of the sense of integrity* .... Through a kind of 'trial and error' process they start to develop a *sense of themselves as active political beings*.

Individuals hopefully progress to this second developmental stage. According to Kieffer there are three necessary conditions for satisfactory progress. These are *a mentoring process, ... supportive peer relationships within a collective organizational structure, and the cultivation of a more critical understanding of social and political relations*. This process requires at least a year of ... *intensive engagement and reflection*.

The role of the 'enabler' or mentor is nicely illustrated by Lucinda:

> *When I first got involved ... the (facilitators) all saw beyond me ... they just didn't see me. They saw what I was capable of, what I could be. ... It was so important that somebody cared enough to be there encouraging me, pushing me ... coming back after me ... no matter how afraid I was.*

The third 'era of incorporation' reflects the maturing of 'self-concept', 'critical comprehension' and 'strategic ability'. Emily describes the experience:

> *I've changed. ... I think I'm understanding more of the structure of our society and understanding more of how people operate within our society. But I've still not gotten it straight in my mind where is my little niche. Or do I have one? And what can I really do? One thing's for sure, I won't ever be the same self as I was when this thing first started.*

According to Kieffer,

> *The fundamental empowering transformation ... is in the transition from sense of self as helpless victim to acceptance of self as assertive and efficacious citizen.*

Clearly this goal is eminently desirable in its own right and it is hard to imagine such an empowered individual within an empowered community not responding positively to the narrower preventive objectives of more orthodox health educators and public health specialists.

The words of Lucinda provide us with the kind of performance indicator to which we might well aspire:

*What I've learned in the past four years, I'm applying to all my life. It's changed my whole life – personal, professional, everything. My values have changed. My priorities have changed. Everything has changed.*

## CONCLUSIONS

We have noted a long history of working directly with communities. The outcomes sought from activities have not been and even now are not always consistent, although empowerment has increasingly been seen as a key goal. The attainment of empowerment in communities, as we have seen, is essentially problematical and different tactics and strategies have been proposed to achieve such goals. It is a major assertion in this book that the effort is worthwhile and that it is compatible with the widely endorsed core values and desired goals of health promotion. Community development approaches can be resource intensive and some countries have been reluctant, or unable, to make sufficient resources available to reach all those communities that would benefit. The recent recognition in national policy documents in the UK of the importance of community development has been welcomed. At the same time the critiques of community development approaches need to be borne in mind, in particular concerns about the pursuance of community development unless matched by efforts to address the underlying causes of poverty and disadvantage.

Approaches to evaluation have varied and while strong preferences for interpretivist approaches are often expressed there is plentiful evidence for the pragmatic adoption of methodological pluralism. In those community projects directed fully towards achieving empowerment there is a commitment to participation of community members in evaluation. Resources for projects are often limited and securing sufficient for rigorous evaluation can be difficult. It is more difficult for this setting than others to draw general conclusions about overall effectiveness of community development and related approaches. Projects have demonstrated a range of successes, as we have illustrated, both for communities and for individuals.

## NOTES

1. The terminology for describing parts of the world has been contested. The terms 'developed' 'developing', 'underdeveloped' or First, Second and Third worlds convey particular images that many do not like. The terms North and South have now been fairly widely adopted and will be used here.

2. *Some people translate khit pen as critical thinking, others as rational thinking, still others as problem solving. It is, in fact, the combination of these processes and more. A man (or woman) who has mastered khit pen will be able to approach problems in life systematically. ... If due to outside circumstances or lack of certain necessary knowledge or skills, the solution of his choice can not be implemented right away, a khit pen man will not become frustrated. Instead he will adopt a lesser solution while preparing to make the solution of his choice possible. ... In other words, this philosophy encourages people to change, but not to destroy themselves physically and mentally doing so.* (Dr Kowit Vorapipatana, Thai Adult Education Division, cited in Kindervatter, 1979.)

## REFERENCES

Alinsky, S.D. (1946) *Reveille for Radicals.* Vintage Books, New York, NY.

Allonson, K.R. and Rootman, I. (1996) *Scientific rigor and community participation in health promotion research: are they compatible. Health Promotion International,* 11 (4), 333–340.

Amos, A., Gaunt-Richardson, P., McKie, L. and Barlow, J. (1999) *Addressing smoking and health among women living on low income III. Ayr Barnardo's Homelessness Service and Dundee Women's Aid. Health Education Journal,* 58, 329–340.

Arnstein, S. R. (1971) *Eight rungs on the ladder of citizen participation.* In S. E. Cahn and B. A. Passett (eds) *Citizen Participation: Effecting Community Change.* Praeger Publications, New York, NY.

Barlow, J., Gaunt-Richardson, P., Amos, A. and McKie, L. (1999) *Addressing smoking and health among women living on low income II. TAPS Tiree: a dance and dram group for rural community development.* Health Education Journal, 58, 321–328.

Barr, A. (1995) *Empowering communities – beyond fashionable rhetoric? Some reflections on Scottish experience.* Community Development Journal, 30 (2), 121–132.

Batten, T. R. (1967) *The Non-directive Approach in Group and Community Work.* Oxford University Press, Oxford, UK.

Baum, F. (1993) *Healthy Cities and change: social movements or bureaucratic tool? Health Promotion International*, 8 (1), 31–40.

Beattie, A. (1995) *Evaluation in community development for health.* Health Education Journal, 54, 465–472.

Bell, D. V. (1975) *Power, Influence and Authority: An Essay in Political Linguistics.* Oxford University Press, New York, NY.

Bjäräs, G., Haglund, B. J. A. and Rifkin, S. B. (1991) *A new approach to community participation assessment. Health Promotion International*, 6 (3), 199–206.

Blennerhasset, S., Farrant, W. and Jones, J. (1989) *Support for community health projects in the UK: a role for the National Health Service. Health Promotion International*, 4 (3), 199–206.

Boutilier, M., Mason, R. and Rootman, I. (1997) *Community action and reflective practice in health promotion research. Health Promotion International*, 12 (1), 69–78.

Brager, C. and Specht, H. (1973) *Community Organising.* Columbia University Press. New York, NY.

Calouste Gulbenkian Foundation (1974) *A national centre for community development. Report of a working party.* Gulbenkian Foundation, London.

Calouste Gulbenkian Foundation (1984) *A National Centre for Community Development: Report of a Working Party.* Gulbenkian Foundation, London, UK.

Coleman, J. S. (1988) *Social capital in the creation of human capital.* American Journal of Sociology, 94, S95–S121.

Community Development Project (1977) *Gilding the Ghetto.* Community Development Project, London, UK.

Community Projects Foundation/HEA/SHEG (1988) *Action for Health: Initiatives in Local Communities.* Community Projects Foundation, London, UK.

Constantino-David, K. (1982) *Issues in community organization. Community Development Journal*, 17, 190–201.

Cornwell, A. (1996) *Towards participatory practice: participatory rural appraisal (PRA) and the participatory process.* In K. de Koning and M. Martin (Eds) *Participatory Research in Health.* Zed Books, London, UK.

Craig, G. (1989) *Community work and the state. Community Development Journal.*, 24 (1), 3–18.

Croft, S. and Beresford, P. (1992) *The politics of participation.* Critical Social Policy, 26, 20–44.

Dean, K., (1988) *Issues in the development of health promotion indicators. Health Promotion International*, 3, 13–21.

De Kadt, E. (1982) *Community participation for health: the case of Latin America. World Development*, 10 (7), 573–584.

Department of Health (1998) *Our Healthier Nation: A Contract for Health.* HMSO, London, UK.

Department of Health (1999) *Saving Lives: Our Healthier Nation.* HMSO, London, UK.

Dixon, J. (1989) *The limits and potential of community development for personal and social change. Community Health Studies*, XII (1), 82–92.

Dixon, J. (1995) *Community stories and indicators for evaluating community development. Community Development Journal*, 30 (4) 327–336.

Dockery, G. I. (1996) *Rhetoric or reality? Participatory Research in the National Health Service, UK.* In K. de Koning and M. Martin (Eds) *Participatory Research in Health.* Zed Books, London, UK.

Fawcett, S. B., Seekins, T., Whang, P. L., Muiu, C. and Suarez de Balcazar, Y. (1984) *Creating and using social technologies for community empowerment.* In J. Rappaport, C. Swift and R. Hess (Eds) *Studies in Empowerment: Steps Toward Understanding and Action.* Haworth Press, New York, NY.

Freire, P. (1972) *Pedagogy of the Oppressed.* Penguin, Harmondsworth, UK.

Gillies, P. (1998) *Effectiveness of alliances and partnerships for health promotion. Health Promotion International*, 13 (2), 99–120.

Gordon, A. (1985) *Learned helplessness and community development: a case study. Journal of Community Psychology*, 13, 327–337.

Gottlieb, N. and McLeroy, K. R. (1992) *Social health.* In M. P. O'Donnell (Ed.) *Health Promotion in the Workplace*, 2nd Edn. Delmar Publishing, New York, NY.

Hayes, M. V. and Manson-Willms, S. ( 1990) *Healthy community indicators: the perils of the search and the paucity of the find. Health Promotion International*, 5 (2), 161–166.

Hawe, P. (1994) *Capturing the meaning of 'community' in community intervention evaluation. Health Promotion International*, 9 (3) 199–209.

Heller, K. (1989) *The return to community. American Journal of Community Psychology*, 17 (1), 1–15.

Henderson, P. and Thomas, D. N. (1980) *Skills in Neighbourhood Work*. Allen and Unwin, London, UK.

Hilton, D. (1988) *Community-based or community-oriented: the vital difference. Contact*, 106, 1–4.

Hope, A. and Timmel, S. (1988) *Training for transformation. Contact*, 106, 4–7.

House, J. S. (1988) *Structures and processes of social support. Annual Review of Sociology*, 14, 293–331.

Hubley, J. (1985) *Papers on Community Development*. Mimeograph, Leeds Polytechnic, Leeds, UK.

Israel, B. A. (1982) *Social networks and health status: linking theory, research and practice. Patient Counselling and Health Education*, 4, 65–79.

Israel, B. A. and Rounds, K. A. (1987) *Social networks and social support: a synthesis for health educators. Advances in Health Education and Promotion*, 2, 311–351.

Kaduskar, S., Boaz, A., Dowler, E., Meyrick, J. and Rayner, M. (1999) *Evaluating the work of a community café in a town in the South east of England: reflections on methods, process and results. Health Education Journal*, 58, 341–354.

Kar, S. B., Pascual, C. A. and Chickering, K. L. (1999) *Empowerment of women for health promotion: a meta analysis. Social Science and Medicine*, 49, 1431–1460.

Kawachi, I., Kennedyd, B., Lochner, K. and Prothrow Smith,D. (1997) *Social capital, income inequality and mortality. American Journal of Public Health*, 87, 1491–1499.

Kickbusch, I. and O'Byrne, D. O. (1995) *Community as the focus for health and health changes. Promotion and Education*, II, 17–20.

Kieffer, C. J. (1984) *Citizen empowerment: a developmental perspective*. In J. Rappaport, C.

Swift and R. Hess (Eds) *Studies in Empowerment: Steps Towards Understanding and Action*. Haworth Press, New York, NY.

Kindervatter, S. (1979) *Nonformal Education as an Empowering Process*. Center for International Education, Amherst, MA.

Kirklin, M. J. and Franzen, L. E. (1974) *Community Organization Bibliography*. Institute on the Church in Urban Industrial Society, Chicago, IL.

Knight, A. and Knight, C. (1995) *Learning healthy language. Health Action*, 11, 6–7.

Labonte, R. (1994) *Health promotion and empowerment: reflections on professional practice. Health Education Quarterly*, 21, 253–268.

Labonte, R., Feather, J. and Hills, M. (1999) *A story/dialogue method for health promotion knowledge development and evaluation. Health Education Research*, 14 (1), 39–50.

Laleman, G. and Annys, S. (1989) *Understanding community participation: a health programme in the Philippines. Health Policy and Planning*, 4 (3), 251–256.

Lazes, P. M. (ed.) (1979) *Handbook of Health Education*. Aspem Systems Corp., MD.

Loney, M. (1981) *The British Community Development Projects: questioning the state. Community Development Journal*, 16, 55–67.

Martin, C. J., Platt, F. D. and Hunt, S. M. (1987) *Housing conditions and ill health. British Medical Journal*, 294, 1125–1127.

McFarlane, J. and Mehir, J. (1994) *De Madres a madres: a community primary health care program based on empowerment. Health Education Quarterly*, 21 (3), 381–394.

McKie, L., Gaunt–Richardson, P., Barlow, J. and Amos, A. (1999) *Addressing smoking and health among women living on low income I. Dean's Community Club: a mental health project. Health Education Journal*, 58, 311–320.

McMillan, D. W. and Chavis, D. M. (1986) *Sense of community: a definition and theory. Journal of Community Psychology*, 14, 6–23.

Miller, S. M., Rein, M. and Levitt, P. (1995) *Community action in the United States*. In G. Craig and M. Mayo (Eds) *Community Empowerment: A Reader in Participation and Development*. Zed Books, London, UK.

Nix, H. L. (1970) *The Community and Its Involvement in the Study Planning Action Process*. US Department of Health, Education and Welfare, Atlanta, GA.

O'Sullivan, M. J., Waugh, N. and Espeland, W. (1984) *The Fort McDowell Yavapai: from pawns to powerbrokers*. In J. Rappaport, C. Swift and R. Hess (Eds) *Empowerment: Steps Toward Understanding and Action*. Haworth Press, New York, NY.

Putnam, R. D., Leonardi, R. and Nanetti, R. Y. (1993) *Making Democracy Work: Civic Traditions in Modern Italy*. Princeton University Press, Princeton, NJ.

Raeburn, J. M. (1986) *Toward a sense of community: comprehensive community projects and community houses*. Journal of Community Psychology, 14, 391–398.

Renshaw, J. and Rivas, D. (1991) *A community development approach to Chagas' disease: the Sucre health project, Bolivia*. Health Policy and Planning, 6 (3), 244–254.

Rothman, J. (1979) *Three models of community organisation in practice*. In F. Cox *et al.* (Eds) *Strategies of Community Organisation*. F.E. Peacock, Chicago, IL.

Sharma, R. C., Gautam, A. S., Bhatt, R. M., Gupta, D. K. and Sharma, V. P. (1991) *The Kheda malaria project: the case for environmental control*. Health Policy and Planning, 6 (3), 262–270.

Rifkin, S. B., Muller, F. and Bichmann, W. (1988) *Primary health care: on measuring participation*. Social Science and Medicine, 26 (9), 931–940.

Rose, H. (1990) *Activists, gender and the community health movement*. Health Promotion International, 5 (3), 209–218.

Ross, M. G. and Lappin, B. W. (1967) *Community Organization: Theory, Principles and Practice*. Harper and Row, New York, NY.

Smart, H. (1999) *Evaluating community development for health: a survey of evaluation activity across the Lothians*. Health Education Journal, 58, 355–364.

Smithies, J., Adams, L., Webster, G. and Beattie, A. (1990) *Community Participation in Health Promotion*. Health Education Authority, London, UK.

Sosa, R., Kennel, J. and Klaus, M. (1980) *The effect of a supportive companion on perinatal problems, length of labor, and mother–infant interactions*. New England Journal of Medicine, 305, 597–600.

Tandon, R. (1981) *Participatory research in the empowerment of people*. Convergence, XIV (3), 20–29.

Tilford, S. and Alexander, S. (1997) *Sexual Health Action Group Evaluation*. Centre for Health Promotion Research, Leeds Metropolitan University, Leeds, UK.

Tönnies, F. (1955) *Community and Association*. Routledge and Kegan Paul, London, UK. [Reprint]

Travers, K. D. (1997) *Reducing inequities through participatory research and community empowerment*. Health Education and Behaviour, 24 (3), 344–356.

Tumwini, J. (1989) *Community participation as myth or reality: a personal experience from Zimbabwe*. Health Policy and Planning, 4 (2), 157–161.

Twelvetrees, A. (1982) *Community Work*. Macmillan, London, UK.

Ugalde, A. (1985) *Ideological dimensions of community participation in Latin American programs*. Social Science and Medicine, 21, 41–53.

United Nations (1971) *Popular Participation in Development: Emerging Trends in Community Development*. United Nations, New York, NY.

Veenstra, G. (2000) *Social capital, SES and health: an individual level analysis*. Social Science and Medicine, 50, 619–629.

Voyle, J. A. and Simmons, D. (1999) *Community development through partnerships: promoting health in an urban indigenous community in New Zealand*. Social Science and Medicine, 49, 1035–1050.

Wakefield Health Authority (1999) *Wakefield and District Health Action Zone, Plan and Programme for Action*. Wakefield Health Authority, Wakefield, UK.

Wallerstein, N. (1999) *Power between evaluator and community: research relationships between New Mexico's healthier communities*. Social Science and Medicine, 49, 39–53.

Ward, C. (1990) *Product minded*. New Statesman and Society, 12 October, 31.

Wellman, B. and Leighton, B. (1979) *Networks, neighbourhoods, and communities: approaches to the study of the community question*. Urban Affairs Quarterly, 14 (3), 363–391.

Werner, D. (1980) *Health care and human dignity*. In S. B. Rifkin (ed.) *Health: The Human Factor: Readings in Health, Development and Community Participation*, CONTACT Special Series No. 3. World Council of Churches, Geneva, Switzerland.

Winch, P., Kendall, C. and Gubler, D. (1992)

*Effectiveness of community participation in vector-borne disease control. Health Policy and Planning,* 7 (4), 342–351.

World Health Organization (1983) *New Approaches to Health Education in Primary Health Care,* Technical Report Series 690. WHO, Geneva, Switzerland.

World Health Organization (1978) *Primary Health Care: Report of the Conference on Primary Health Care.* WHO, Geneva, Switzerland.

World Health Organization (1986) *Ottawa Charter for Health Promotion, An International Conference on Health Promotion, November 17–21.* WHO Regional Office for Europe, Copenhagen, Denmark.

# 10 COMMUNITY-WIDE COALITIONS AND INTER-SECTORAL WORKING

## DEFINING COMMUNITY PROGRAMMES

This chapter is predominantly concerned with large-scale programmes involving collaboration between a wide range of organisations, agencies and people in general. Such initiatives are frequently defined as '*community-wide*' programmes. The use of the term 'community' can, however, lead to confusion. For instance, in the last chapter we critically examined the meaning of 'community' and the process of 'community development' and noted the tendency to define community as a relatively small social group, of approximately 'neighbourhood size', having an actual or potential network of inter-personal contacts. The size of the social group targeted in 'community-wide' programmes, on the other hand, is typically much larger and, therefore, it is unlikely that it can have a sense of shared purpose or predicament associated with communities proper. Its size may well be that of a city (e.g. cities researched in the Minnesota project) or a region (e.g. North Karelia) or even a small country (e.g. Wales). Within that aggregate of organisations and people there may well be an intention to stimulate awareness and activity in communities proper and, indeed, community development may be one of a raft of strategies selected to motivate individuals within the broader social structure. It is certainly true that most of the better planned community-wide programmes acknowledge that gaining community participation is essential for project success. However, the projects in question are likely to be more or less driven in a top-down fashion and will frequently not only focus on single issues but be concerned with specific disease prevention goals. They will not, therefore, fit the model of true community development but will be located towards the 'colonisation' end of the spectrum of programme types described in Chapter 9.

The over-riding rationale for community-wide projects relates to a kind of 'economy of scale'. Since a given issue, such as coronary heart disease, is a problem common to a whole region it seems sensible to tackle it a regional level. Moreover, it is assumed that if a coalition of agencies and settings can be established that will work together to provide a common educational programme supported by health policy initiatives, there will be a bigger effect than if a piecemeal approach to health promotion is adopted. Each organisation and setting would play to its strengths and, where relevant, would deploy its power in order to achieve synergistic results.

We can identify two 'community-wide' scenarios, both of which are committed to the principle of collaborative working. The first of these can be characterised (and perhaps somewhat caricatured) as single issue disease prevention programmes. The archetypal example of such an approach is provided by the large number of substantially financed and evaluated international programmes concerned with preventing coronary heart disease. Key examples of these are discussed later in this chapter. The second type of 'community-wide' initiative is less common but increasingly attracting interest and political commitment. Programmes such as this are concerned to achieve broader social goals and will focus on issues such as inequality and community empowerment.

A central feature of such programmes is also collaborative action, though the term used (following *Ottawa Charter* principles) tends to be 'inter-sectoral collaboration' or, perhaps, 'healthy alliances'. Recent exemplars of this approach are provided by current UK health policy, which funded collaborative programmes such as *Healthy Living Centres* and *Health Action Zones*. Reference was made earlier in this book to these initiatives and their origin in concerns with tackling the social determinants of health and illness.

The nature of the political and ideological underpinning of the two types of 'community-wide' programme is typically different in emphasis and, possibly, philosophical commitment. The second type of programme is more likely to centre its activities and strategies on a community development approach whereas the first type may well only seek to involve community representatives in a more tokenistic way but, nonetheless, in the belief that without community involvement the planners' goals will not be achieved. Again, both types of programme acknowledge the importance of macro policy and the provision of supportive environments. Given the complexity of the scenario and the challenge facing programme planners, a theory-driven and systematic intervention design is essential if results of the intervention are not to be random and/or very disappointing. The 'coalition' type of approach has had the greatest levels of funding and experience and has undoubtedly been assiduous in developing systematic programmes. We will, therefore, now provide some examples of programmes, together with their theoretical underpinning and details of the kinds of success they appear to have achieved.

## SYSTEMATIC PROGRAMME PLANNING AND COMMUNITY-WIDE PROGRAMMES

As we have noted elsewhere in this book, there are many respectable models and theories offering guidelines for programme design (for example the PRECEDE–PROCEED Model of Green and Kreuter (1999)). Many programmes, however, adopt theoretical and practical guidelines associated with 'community organisation'. Again, as noted before, this term is itself somewhat ambiguous and is taken by some people to be equivalent to 'community development'. However, it is used here to characterise the approach to relatively top-down, community-wide enterprises. For instance, we might note Farquhar *et al.*'s (1984a) discussion of the field application of 'community organisation' with its three stages of 'development, implementation and maintenance' (Box 1).

**Box I**  Development, Implementation and Maintenance of Community Programmes

*Development*
a) *Goal definition.* A review of the literature and baseline data to determine people's needs for information, motivation, skills, etc. in order to determine target groups and the kind of programme needed to reduce their risks of disease.
b) *Resources definition.* Choice of appropriate resources for each risk factor.
c) *Community recruiting.* Identifying community leaders and enlisting the aid of organisations to achieve programme goals.
d) *Programme definitions.* Gaining feedback *... to fit the community's and the initiators' needs ...*; formative evaluation and design of programme.

*Implementation*
a) *Materials and programme development.* For example, training of leaders; pre-testing materials.
b) *Consulting with community groups.* For example ... *helping advisory boards become functioning community units ....*
c) *Programme field testing.* For example re-designing and refining the programme.

*Maintenance*
This involves *programme monitoring; programme multiplication; programme continuation.* The final goal is institutionalisation and community ownership.

(Farquhar *et al.*, 1984a)

Bracht and Kingsbury (1990) and Bracht *et al.* (1999) have also presented a set of guidelines for community interventions. In so doing they reminded us of Rothman's three 'models' of community work: 'locality development' (i.e. community development), 'social planning' and 'social action'. They also point out that Rothman viewed these models as 'analytical extremes' which would, in practice, often overlap. It would, however, not be unreasonable to suggest that Bracht and Kingsbury's system owes more to 'social planning' than to the other two models. The basis for their approach may be summarised as follows:

- Interventions must be based on a historical understanding of the community;
- multiple interventions are needed;
- health promoters should work through existing structures and take account of existing values and norms;
- active community participation (not tokenism) is required;
- intersectoral collaboration is important to maximise impact;
- long term needs and problems must be addressed to ensure that there will be 'life after the project';
- the community must share responsibility for the problem and its solution.

(Bracht and Kingsbury, 1990, p. 72)

Planning is based on a five stage process:
1  community analysis;
2  design and initiation;
3  implementation;
4  programme maintenance and consolidation;
5  dissemination and reassessment.

Pancer and Nelson (1990) also provide a detailed set of guidelines for 'community mobilisation' in health promotion programmes. This consists of the following 10 point plan:

1  community involvement;
2  planning;
3  needs and resource assessment (health problems and available resources);
4  a comprehensive programme (dealing with multiple risk factors; utilising several different channels; operating at different levels, e.g. families and organisations; designed to change the psychological and social factors which underpin specific disease risk factors);
5  an integrated programme;
6  long-term change (producing stable and lasting change; development of a permanent health promotion infrastructure);
7  altering community norms (requiring partici-

pation of a majority of community members);
8  research and evaluation;
9  sufficient resources;
10  professional and community collaboration (especially between professionals and community leaders).

Clearly, a key issue for those designing such programmes is just how to achieve community mobilisation. Rather than rely on the emergence of community involvement in accordance with pure community development principles, a more proactive process of coalition building is usually recommended.

## CITIZEN PARTNERSHIP AND COALITIONS

One of the central problems facing health promoters is just how people can be converted from a state of passivity into active, empowered community members. Community development suggests a facilitative process which awakens felt needs and helps communities to identify and achieve their own goals. As noted above, the extent to which this is possible has been subjected to challenge and the need to gain the support of already empowered individuals or powerful groups and organisations has been articulated as a more feasible alternative.

The kinds of community-wide programmes we are considering here tend to rely on the latter strategy rather than the former. Indeed, since programme objectives will already have been stated, there is right from the start a limit to the utility of exploring felt needs! As Haglund *et al.* (1990) observe, *A core group of concerned citizens and professionals usually initiates the action process.* Five varieties of 'citizen partnership structure' are offered: 'lead' or official agency; grassroots; citizen panels; networks and consortia. In relation to the first of these, the authors point out that the 'lead agency model' is often used when a single agency has the necessary resources, authority and credibility to take the lead. They cite as an example of this situation the *Pawtucket Project* (to which reference will be made later) in which the local hospital took the major initiative.

The situation which Haglund *et al.* label 'grassroots' is roughly analogous to the community development approach, i.e. it involves people who are not part of more formal structures nor represented by them. 'Citizen panels', on the other hand, work alongside official agencies. Members may be appointed or elected to these panels and, in that capacity, be expected to contribute to policy formulation and implementation. Obviously, there will always be a danger that citizen panels become over-bureaucratised and tokenistic.

'Networks' refer to relatively informal and more transient operations; they tend to be triggered by single issues. The authors distinguish networks from 'consortia', which feature somewhere between the loose aggregate of the network and the more formal and usually hierarchical structure which is described as a 'coalition'. This key phenomenon of North American community organisation merits some consideration, albeit brief.

## Community coalitions

Community coalitions figure quite centrally in US community-wide initiatives [for a more extensive review, see Butterfoss *et al.* (1993) and other papers in the special issue *Community Coalitions, Health Education Research*, 8 (3)]. Essentially they involve inter-organisational collaboration directed at the attainment of common goals.

Bracht *et al.* (1999) define 'coalition' as ... *an organization of individuals representing diverse organizations, factions or constituencies who agree to work together in order to achieve a common goal*. They sum up the key benefits as follows:

> *The major advantage of a coalition is that it involves a breadth and diversity of membership that may make for strange bedfellows but cuts across ideologies and constituencies. The leaders of each organziation are likely to become more committed as the scope of the coalition's membership increases. If existing coalitions can be tapped, much of the work and time of recruitment of community leaders and networking between community factions can be minimized.*
>
> (p. 95)

Green and Kreuter (1999), considering health promotion planning in community settings, suc-cinctly categorise coalitions as 'groups to be reckoned with'. They identify two types of relationship within a community: exchange relationships and coordinative relationships. The former obtain between professionals and clients, the latter between two or more groups with common interests which collaborate to achieve common goals. Coalitions are of the latter type.

Given our discussion in this chapter of the location of power and the feasibility of changing the power and resource structure in the interests of health promotion, we will repeat here a quotation which Green and Kreuter present from Nix (1977).

> *Research findings suggest that reputed community leaders gain influence over others by occupying economic and governmental positions of exchange, which allow them to control, in varying degrees, the lives of other people. In order to distribute effectively this influence over community-wide affairs, community leaders must participate actively in influential organizations of a co-ordinated nature which are composed of representatives of different interest groups and organizations.*

Coalitions seek to counter the substantial influence of governmental, commercial and other powerful interests subsumed in the notion of dominant ideology. We might, incidentally, note at this point that radical social action movements seeking to shift the balance of power as a primary goal would also routinely seek to establish fighting coalitions.

## Citizen boards and task forces

The final type of citizen partnership to be considered here is that of the community or citizen board. The principle is simple and would operate in association with coalitions or other forms of structure discussed earlier. Bracht and Kingsbury list the typical representatives of various community sectors on a community board. They might include: local government officials; local media personnel; schools; commercial and business organisations; unions; health professionals;

**Box 2**  Factors and Skills Important to the Effectiveness of Partnerships and Coalitions

| | |
|---|---|
| *Leadership* | *The extent to which coalitions have one or more members who are well respected and experienced in organizing group activities, garnering resources, facilitating discussion motivating others, negotiating, and recruiting new members.* |
| *Management* | *The extent to which coalitions have the expertise to effectively manage the meeting logistics, resources, and operation for the coalition.* |
| *Communication* | *The degree to which written and verbal communications among coalition members, committee and task force members, staff, and individuals outside the coalition have been clear, timely, and effective.* |
| *Conflict resolution* | *The degree to which friction and tensions arising from turf issues, different personalities, or competing interests of coalition members have been effectively resolved.* |
| *Perception of fairness* | *The extent to which coalition members perceive that they are being treated equitably and the different organizations in the coalition are contributing their fair share in terms of resources and/or work.* |
| *Shared decision making* | *The degree of influence that coalition members have in determining the policies and actions of the statewide coalitions and the amount of authority coalition representatives have to make decisions on behalf of the organizations they represent.* |
| *Perceived benefits versus costs* | *The degree to which individual members and member organizations on state and local coalitions believe the time they have served has been worthwhile.* |

(Bracht *et al.*, 1999, p. 96)

minority and voluntary groups; hospitals; churches; community groups.

The citizen board is commonly supported by a number of task forces, once a given project had been launched. The membership of the task forces might consist of professionals and lay volunteers; they would focus on particular issues such as smoking, diet, exercise or a supportive schools programme. The procedure is well exemplified by the *Minnesota Coronary Heart Disease Prevention Project*, which will be discussed later.

## COMMUNITY-WIDE PROJECTS: EXAMPLES OF SUCCESS?

One of the more obvious conclusions to be drawn from discussions in this book about the effectiveness and efficiency of health promotion programmes is that it is difficult to really know whether or not any given programme has in fact been successful! The nature of the uncertainty may, of course, have to do with apparent weaknesses in the research, both in relation to quantitative/positivist and qualitative/interpretivist designs. It may also derive from a lack of agreement about the nature of a successful result and the appropriateness or stringency of indicators used to assess effectiveness. It would, therefore, be appropriate in the examples of community-wide interventions that are described below to adopt the 'judicial principle'. In other words, in trying to decide whether given programmes justify the time, money and effort spent on them we should ask whether the evidence presented should lead to a conclusion that the balance of probabilities was that the initiative in question had been a success or, more stringently, that the programme had demonstrated effectiveness 'beyond reasonable doubt'.

Most, if not all, of the studies described below cannot be accused of Type 3 error: they have frequently been cited because they do, in fact, adopt systematic, theory-based designs and utilise methods and approaches which should in principle maximise the chance of their achieving their objectives. We have, however, noted in the context of doubts about the degree of effectiveness of the internationally acclaimed heart disease prevention projects that if a very different strategy is required, e.g. the use of horizontal programmes to tackle fundamental sources of ill health, then the omission of radical strategies, for example, to address inequity could technically be categorised as Type 3 error. At any rate, the evaluation strategy employed is also typically robust and the studies are also notable for their extensive use of intermediate and process indicators. Not infrequently though, interim measures rather than final outcome measures are reported, for whatever reason. Insofar as outcome measures are not reported, or are reported but fail to demonstrate a programme effect, we face the dilemma of explaining why apparently well-constructed interventions based on sound theory are apparently ineffective. This dilemma is at its sharpest in reviews of the famous international heart disease prevention projects, particularly because they were usually expensive, based on exemplary principles and used high quality evaluation techniques. The resolution of this dilemma is not easy and possible explanations will be examined later in this chapter.

Before commenting on exemplars of community-wide projects, we should also note that it seems possible to demonstrate evidence of success in programmes which do not meet all, or even most, of the systematic programme requirements discussed earlier. For instance, one of the most impressive and well-evaluated health education programmes was described by Sayegh and Green (1976). This was organised within the American University Medical Center in Beirut. Its purpose was to develop an efficient family planning intervention and although it is perhaps more properly regarded as patient education, its focus was the community. In short, an experimental group of women received education designed to promote the adoption of contraception. The baseline rate of acceptance of family planning was 4.2% but, eventually, contraceptive use settled at a steady rate of some 37%. Bearing in mind that the acceptance rate of a well-known international post-partum programme was 17%, there could be little doubt about the efficiency of this particular intervention. More particularly, the authors demonstrated not only behaviour change but also cost effectiveness: the programme was cheaper per success than alternative methods of family planning education.

Kanaaneh et al. (1976) also demonstrated the effectiveness of a properly organised and realistically targeted outreach programme in Western Galilee. The intervention occurred in a village of 3000 inhabitants and it succeeded in achieving its goal of eradicating scabies which, prior to the campaign, was prevalent in 66% of families.

It would, however, be expected that the prospects of success would be greater where 'community organisation' principles had been fully incorporated into programme design. For instance, Vincent et al. (1987) employed a systematic process of community organisation in a programme designed to reduce adolescent pregnancies. Having raised consciousness about teen pregnancies as a social problem and performed a community assessment, the authors recruited advisory groups, developed 'community linkages', trained adult leaders and produced a joint school and community-based intervention. The evaluation demonstrated that the rate of pregnancy in the South Carolina county where the programme had been in operation had declined significantly compared with rates in comparison counties.

Green and Kreuter (1999) also cite with approval an effective health promotion programme in Kentucky. A significant decline in mortality from cardiovascular disease was recorded in two intervention counties compared with one control county allegedly as a result of a properly structured hypertension control programme. In addition to the impressively hard data on mortality, a reduction in diastolic and systolic blood pressure was recorded together with improved compliance with medication. Green and Kreuter identified 12 features of the programme which met the requirements of systematic community organisation and which were responsible for the impressive results (Box 3).

**Box 3**  Features of an Effective Programme

Appointment of an enthusiastic full-time coordinator; establishment of a task force (*Community High Blood Pressure Control Program Council*) which had membership from schools, health departments, the medical profession, commercial and business interests, the *Cooperative Agricultural Extension Service* and 'interested citizens'; an existing *Nutrition Aide Program* to contact people at high risk identified by their doctors; development of teenage coronary heart disease prevention club using peer teaching; introduction of a school blood pressure screening programme; establishing a volunteer blood pressure screening and monitoring network in churches and small businesses; adding a workplace screening programme to an existing general health programme provided by local health departments; gaining general support from and involvement of local media; providing a continuing education programme for nurses; presenting health education programmes to community clubs, health fairs and large family reunions (a rural Kentucky tradition).

## Programmes promoting mammography in the US and AIDS prevention in Africa

Worden *et al.* (1999) provide an excellent example of theory-based development of a breast screening programme in Lee County. They describe the use of key elements of community-wide programme planning: assessing community characteristics; surveying community leaders; carrying out surveys of population and professional characteristics and attitudes. A major focus is on inter-sectoral working, including the recruitment of volunteers and achieving community participation through fund raising and the development of new community outreach programmes based on focus group work with representatives of African-American women in low income areas. In the first year of the programme a team of eight African-American volunteers recruited women door-to-door and engaged them in small group education combined with clinic visits: 90% of the eligible women had their mammograms. However, a major concern of the programme was not so much the short-term results of the interventions but rather with creating conditions necessary for achieving a sustainable programme, a feature of programme planning that is often ignored and is of particular importance given the number of programmes that collapse when the funding has been exhausted. The indirect indicators of process (Box 4) provide a useful insight into project achievements, especially collaborative working.

**Box 4**  Interim Evaluation of a Community Mammography Programme

*… in one sense the program already has had a positive impact on the Lee County community. During the course of 6 years, the program has encouraged the participation of hundreds of lay volunteers and hundreds of physicians, a group of hospitals that grew from four to six during the period, county and city governments, and a score of public and voluntary health agencies, private foundations, and local businesses. Through "Partners in Health", the program has brought strangers and competitors together to*

> *work on a common problem, providing essential health care to low-income women ... community participation has already benefited at least 660 women receiving help from "Partners in Health" and has also equipped the community with the motivation and skills to address problems thorough cooperative action.*
>
> (p. 81)

Klepp *et al.* (1999) have also provided valuable insights into the complex requirements of programme planning and inter-sectoral working in the peculiar environment of Sub-Saharan Africa. A detailed summary is beyond the scope of this chapter and readers are referred to the original article. However, one item of particular interest is worth noting: the difficulties of reconciling the requirements of international non-governmental organisations with country needs and the problems involved in transferring power to communities and 'institutionalising' programmes within existing structures. It was apparent that the earlier programme had provided evidence of the achievement of important outcomes (Klepp *et al.*, 1997). After 12 months

> *... significant effects favoring the intervention group were observed for exposure to AIDS information and communication, AIDS knowledge, attitudes toward people with AIDS, subjective norms toward having sexual intercourse, and behavioral intention. A consistent, positive, but non-statistically-significant trend was seen for attitudes toward having sexual intercourse and onset of sexual intercourse during the past year (7% vs 17%).*

It was also concluded that it was

> *... feasible and effective to train local teachers and health workers to provide HIV/AIDS education to Tanzanian primary school children.*

Details of the target groups and intervention strategies employed as part of the national AIDS control programme provide further insights, not only into strategies appropriate to community-wide programmes but also into the nature of inter-sectoral working involved. This is reproduced in Appendix 10.1.

Klepp *et al.* remind us of the difficulties of achieving inter-sectoral working. They note that although the activities listed in Appendix 10.1 were implemented within the two study regions, no single community was exposed to all of them and there was no system in place for disseminating programme components or strategies, due substantially to particular geographic, political and cultural features of the study area.

## A quit smoking programme in a minority community

Hunkeler *et al.* (1990) describe a community-wide programme which is of special interest in the context of our current discussion. First, it is based on the kind of systematic community organisation principles exemplified earlier and, second, it seeks to address a significant health problem in a minority community.

The main programme aim was to reduce the prevalence of smoking in the black population of Richmond, CA, by 20%. Black people constituted 47.9% of the population, which would suggest that the term 'minority' is used socially rather than statistically. Forty-six per cent of men and 38% of women were current cigarette smokers. Success was to be decided in two ways: (i) an outcome indicator of smoking prevalence was to be used and smoking rates would be compared with those of a reference group composed of blacks elsewhere in the San Francisco Bay area; (ii) observations in the field would assess community reaction to programme activities and record changes in 'smoking norms, values and practices' as intermediate indicators of assumed ultimate success in outcomes.

The community analysis carried out by the team revealed some interesting features of the community. Of especial interest were strong kinship ties, an influential church presence, a history of community mobilisation, a variety of voluntary organisations including a Black Chamber of Commerce, a strong sense of community pride, a high regard for families and children, *an investment in the city's maintaining a positive public image*.

Clearly these features could be and were taken into account in planning the programme. Certain barriers to implementation were also identified from the community profile: absence of local mass media; the fact that only one-third of the black population actually worked in Richmond; a suspicion of outsiders; greater public concern over crime and drug abuse than with smoking; a high level of billboard and magazine advertising of tobacco targeted at blacks.

In addition to the more general analysis of community characteristics, individual beliefs and attitudes in relation to smoking were assessed.

The programme followed the kinds of recommended procedures discussed earlier. A predominantly black working group of 20 community leaders and medical providers helped formulate activities. A *Community Advisory Board* was established to coordinate the project, consisting of 30 members from the following bodies: schools, local media and the arts, voluntary agencies, *Kaiser Permanente Medical Care Program*, hospitals and clinics, individual health professionals, the *County Health Department*, churches and religious organisations, local government and public institutions, community groups and neighbourhood organisations and representatives from the business community.

Major programme components included: provision of training in counselling and health education techniques for health professionals; an extensive media programme (including, for example, a rap music video entitled *Stop Before You Drop*); a variety of stop smoking materials and services; mobilisation of community organisations; a number of community-wide publicity events; a school-based programme; a volunteer programme.

In the context of earlier discussions about the significance of change agents and 'lay leaders' the function of these volunteers is worth noting (Box 5).

**Box 5** Functions of Volunteers

- Talk to family members, friends and neighbours;
- offer encouragement and support to young people and ex-smokers;
- identify smokers, e.g. in the 'contemplation stage', and provide them with stop smoking self-help materials;
- maintain data on smoking cessation services and make referrals;
- provide a more supportive environment by setting up support groups, stop smoking workshops, etc. and promoting education campaigns.

Reflecting on evaluation of process during the programme the organisers identified a number of necessary strategies for successful community interventions. A summary follows.

1 Meaningful community involvement from the start.
2 Use of methods tailored specifically to the community, taking account of prevailing values and practices.
3 Locking the programme into existing social organisations and networks.
4 As well as appealing to specifically targeted groups, framing the issues so as to unite the whole community (e.g. black community leaders advised that all racial groups should be involved while maintaining a focus on blacks).
5 Designing activities to increase self-esteem and community pride in blacks.
6 Emphasising 'winning strategies' rather than problems.
7 Utilising influence of families, friends and fellow workers.
8 Integrating health issues with other 'felt needs' having higher priority for the black community (e.g. crime and public safety).
9 Employing black staff and spending project funds in the black community.
10 Influencing health agencies to increase resources for black people.

11  Using a variety of exciting and controversial consciousness-raising activities involving large numbers of participants but supporting these with 'solid' cessation services.

12  Enhancing existing community resources by bringing in external funding.

13  Including in initial planning ways of institutionalising the programme so that it survives after the funding runs out.

An interim evaluation was based on a variety of intermediate and indirect/process indicators. For instance, a telephone survey of 400 residents revealed a high level of awareness of the programme (70% in general, 76% in blacks). More significantly, a substantial number of agencies and personnel had agreed to continue the work of the project and incorporate it into their own activities using their own funds. Data were, however, not available on the critical and ultimate goal, rate of smoking cessation.

### The Commit Project

Continuing with the theme of smoking, Mittelmark (1999) singled out the *Community Intervention Trial for Smoking Cessation* (COMMIT) for special comment, largely because it was considered to be particularly well funded and designed (Glasgow *et al.*, 1996). As Mittelmark notes,

> ... the financial backing, planning, study design, intervention, and analysis of COMMIT were very close to as good as a community wide trial could possibly be (Susser, 1995). Yet, the results must be considered disappointing indeed.

In short, the programme had no effect on heavy smoking prevalence; overall smoking prevalence decreased 3.5% in the intervention communities compared with 3.2% in control communities, clearly an insignificant difference.

A follow-up study of COMMIT communities two years after the end of the intervention sought to examine the durability of the project in terms of 'life after the project'. The authors concluded that:

> Although there was evidence that tobacco control activities were continuing in the intervention communities, there was an equal amount of tobacco control effort in the comparison communities. Within the specific tobacco control intervention areas, only the youth area showed more activity in intervention communities than comparison communities ... differential durability was not achieved.

(Thompson *et al.*, 2000, p. 353)

### Project Northland: influencing alcohol misuse

Veblen-Mortenson *et al.* (1999) described lessons learned from a community organisation programme in rural north-eastern Minnesota. It was implemented in 14 randomly assigned intervention school districts. Its purpose was to reduce young people's misuse of alcohol. It utilised the five stage approach to community organisation mentioned earlier in this chapter.

Perry *et al.* (1996) had already demonstrated that after the first phase of the intervention some success had been achieved in influencing 'certain key psychosocial factors', as well as delaying the onset of alcohol use and reducing its prevalence. The current study was mainly concerned to address the social, cultural and physical environmental factors that influenced alcohol use. In other words, its concern was to complement health education with its synergy-inducing companion, 'healthy public policy'. In the authors' words, the aim was to

> shift from a primary focus on ... 'demand factors', reducing teens' desire to drink alcohol through education, development of skills for refusing alcohol, communication with parents and peers, and participation in positive, alcohol-free activities, to more of a focus on 'supply factors', or reducing the availability of alcohol by targeting community-level factors that influence underage drinking.

The acknowledgement of political factors associated with the power structure in rural communities is of particular interest. The success of this venture has yet to be reported but process data imply that the training and support of 11 community action teams has been successful. This training in 'social action' is relevant to later comments about the need to address political issues, especially in relation to inequity. The *Northland* goals are not so radical but involved the use of an action force to influence alcohol-related policy. Box 6 details the 'policy menu' and provides an intrinsically interesting example of alcohol policy measures.

## Accident prevention in Scandinavia

It is fairly apparent (and will become more apparent when we consider the case of preventing cardiovascular disease) that the likely success of community interventions is not only due to sophisticated practice based on sound theory. The characteristics of the health innovation is of paramount importance. This doubtless accounts for the fact that one of the more successful kinds of community intervention concerns accident prevention and injury reduction. Maeland and Haglund (1999) discussed this and other developments in Scandinavian health promotion, during which they cited three examples of reductions in accidental injury as follows:

- a reduction of 29% in all accidental injuries during a two year period (Tellness, 1985; pre-post design);
- reductions of 27% in home accidents, 28% in occupational accidents and 28% in traffic accidents over a three year period (Schelp, 1987; quasi-experimental design);
- a reduction of 53% in burns in children over a seven year period with reductions of 27% in

**Box 6**  Community Policy 'Menu' of Interventions to Reduce Alcohol Access to Teenagers (Northland Project)

*Voluntary Efforts, Community Education*
- Provide alcohol-free recreational events and gathering places.
- Encourage news reporting of alcohol-related problems and crashes.
- Establish an alcohol awareness week with appropriate community activities.
- Educate merchants about alcohol problems, strategies to reduce underage sales.
- Work with youth-oriented adult groups to increase awareness, generate support for policy approaches.
- Publicize server liability laws.
- Call public attention to advertisements that appeal to youth.
- Establish speakers' bureaus.

*Enforcement of Existing Laws*
Encourage enforcement of:
- minimum age-of-sale laws;
- laws against alcohol use in public places;
- laws against adults providing alcohol to youth.

*Local Ordinances, Administrative Policies*
- Require training and certification of alcohol, sellers and servers.
- Restrict alcohol sales at sporting, music and other public events.
- Restrict number, type and location of alcohol outlets, using zoning ordinances.
- Restrict alcohol advertising on billboards at public events, on public property.
- Eliminate alcohol industry and outlet sponsorship of local events.
- Require public hearings for new and renewal liquor licenses.
- Require beer kegs to be tagged with purchaser's name and address.

*Institutional Policies*
- Eliminate alcohol at any school functions.
- Develop sanctions for alcohol users at non-school events.
- Increase enforcement of school-based policies.
- Provide model alcohol policies for recreational settings.

(Veblen-Mortenson *et al.*, 1999)

traffic injuries, 26% in fractures due to falls in elderly (over a five year period) and 15% in skiing injuries over a three year period (Ytterstad, 1995; quasi-experimental design).

## Health promotion in a Mexican-American community

Amezcua *et al.* (1990) described a programme in a Mexican-American community in southwest Texas (the *A Su Salud Project*). This is an oft-cited programme which is of special interest since it was geared to the health needs of low socio-economic status groups. The central feature of this programme was its use of mass media supported by *networks, organization and social reinforcement*. The organisational approach adopted was the *Lead Agency Model*, which, as mentioned earlier, involves a single powerful organisation undertaking responsibility for programme design and implementation together with any necessary coalition building. Programme goals were those of general lifestyle modification designed to achieve a reduction in incidence and prevalence of cigarette smoking, modification of dietary behaviour related to cancer risk, a reduction in alcohol misuse, promotion of car seat belt wearing, an increase in physical activity and fostering appropriate use of preventive services.

The theoretical basis of the programme drew heavily on social learning theory (Bandura, 1986) and, in particular, the notions of modelling and social reinforcement.

After the standard procedure of community analysis a mass media programme was devised which incorporated two sets of television productions. The first consisted of 15 programmes of 5–10 minutes duration utilising role models presenting health 'testimonials' together with the provision of health information in a news format. The second series consisted of four 30 minute documentaries featuring a health education specialist as narrator.

The community organisation aspect of the programme involved two community workers supported by a number of trained volunteers working as community aides. The function of these volunteers was similar to those described in the *Richmond Project* and the *North Karelia Project*, which will be discussed in the next section. It included identification of role models in their own social networks; these models had to be people who had recently made approved changes in lifestyle.

Social reinforcement was to be provided by a coalition of the by now familiar cluster of agencies and organisations: business settings; health care providers; federal, state and local government units; education settings; religious organisations; social clubs; grassroots neighbourhood centres.

The importance of acknowledging the need for a supportive health promoting environment (again based particularly on the North Karelian experience) resulted in attempts to promote voter and consumer demand for healthier products. The process involved: (i) consciousness raising to create demand; (ii) mobilisation of consumers to create public pressure; (iii) consultation with political leaders, administrators and commercial producers and retailers.

The list of barriers identified by the authors is quite illuminating; some of these were also identified in the projects already exemplified here (Box 7).

**Box 7** Barriers to Success in the A Su Salud Project

- The problem of change agents and volunteers competing for the public's attention with other organisations, groups and sales people.
- The problem that many householders migrated to other states to harvest the fields!
- The problem that health professionals were seen as too 'business oriented' rather than being interested in genuine human problems. There was also ... *a great deal of justified fear and distrust of 'official-looking' people who come around asking questions.*
- The problem that strained relations among neighbours due to economic depression made it hard to contact people whose 'felt

needs' were frequently expressed in terms of a desire for jobs and money.

- The problem that community workers seemed to experience stress and feelings of helplessness when faced with the poor social circumstances and economic conditions of community members.
- The problem of ... *small-town dynamics of social control, gossip, and suspicion of one's neighbor's motives.* Husbands do not like to see their wives interacting with other women, attending meetings or participating in social gatherings that they do not control.

The reaction to these perceived problems exemplifies the ways in which process measures can be used formatively during the programme itself. For example, modifications were made to educational aspects of the intervention and community building events were included along with training designed to enhance the image of professional workers and polish their public relations skills.

Again, at the time of writing only interim evaluation results were available centring on process evaluation of volunteer activities. Three hundred and ninety-nine volunteers were interviewed, including 166 of the most active of these in greater depth. Thirty-seven per cent operated within commercial and workplace settings; 30% in neighbourhoods; 21% in religious organisations. A total of 7860 contacts was recorded: these included 6098 adults and 1762 young people. The interviewees had viewed on average 10 TV programmes featuring role models. Seventeen volunteers reported smoking cessation, five reported changes in drinking habits and 196 reported obtaining preventive care. Changes in diet were recorded by 269 volunteers and 226 reported an increase in exercise. The more active volunteers had contacted an average of over 20 people each; their contacts claimed they had seen nine TV programmes featuring role models. Moreover, of these contacts 21 had stopped smoking, 10 had modified alcohol use, 328 received preventive health care, 368 had changed their diet and 353 had increased their levels of exercise.

So again, the question must be asked whether the more difficult goals of lifestyle change would be achieved, a point that will be addressed more specifically in the context of discussing the international heart disease prevention programmes below.

### Fostering healthy ageing: *The Boise Project*

There seem to be relatively few programmes in the community organisation mode that address broader issues of mental and social health. 'Mainstream' preventive medicine programmes such as the heart disease prevention projects find it easier to gain the substantial financial support necessary for integrated community-wide projects.

An exception to this general pattern is, however, provided by a programme reported by Kemper and Mettler (1990), which sought to **build a positive image of aging** and which illustrated *inter alia* the importance of coalition building. Furthermore, it provides evidence of success that might well belong to the 'beyond reasonable doubt' category. The context of the programme was a small American city, Boise in Idaho. A non-profitmaking health promotion research centre acted as lead agency and developed two related programmes for people over 60. These were called *Growing Younger: A Physical Wellness Program* and *Growing Wiser: A Mental Wellness Program*. The programmes were designed to respond to research which had provided a rather bleak consensus view of health professionals.

**Box 8**  A Consensus View about Health Promotion and Older People

- Most older people are not interested in changing health behaviour.
- Older people's habits are too ingrained for change to take place.
- Even if health behaviours are improved, it is usually too late to do much good.

A coalition was duly established including employers, Boise School District, the YMCA and YWCA, the state university, two local hospitals, the District Health Department, the Idaho State Office on Aging and the Idaho Division of Health. A number of committees and task groups were set up and older people themselves were actively involved.

The aims of the first programme were not only to improve fitness and reduce risk but also to influence general community perceptions of and attitudes to ageing. A series of workshops was arranged; these emphasised positive health and included such items as improving quality of home and doctor care and dietary improvements in flexibility, strength and endurance. Successful attempts were made to sustain the impact of the programme in the form of 'neighbourhood groups' which, at the time of writing, had been meeting weekly for seven years.

During the first 30 months 1658 older adults (12% of the target population) had participated in the programme. Subsequently the number grew to more than 3500 senior citizens. Pre- and post-testing indicated significant positive changes in lifestyle and utilisation of services. Participants had lost weight, reduced their body fat, lowered their blood pressure and lipid levels and improved flexibility. Again, in relation to the programme maintenance and diffusion effects a number of spin-off activities occurred, including, for example, 'Happy Hoofers', a walking group which met twice weekly!

The mental wellness programme achieved similarly impressive results. The programme included such items as memory, mental alertness, loss and life change, choices for living and self-image. By the end of the 18 month evaluation, 578 people had participated and a 15 question geriatric depression scale revealed a 24% improvement in risk of depression and memory performance had also improved. Again, a series of spin-offs were noted in the form of a number of 'Meeting of Minds Societies', local discussion groups meeting weekly.

Of particular interest for the broader health promotion perspective was the evidence presented by Kemper and Mettler of the impact of the programme on public policy. Policy changes occurred within the centre for senior citizens, which increased health promotion activities, and in a regional medical centre which ... *greatly expanded its services to older people and created a Senior Life Center to serve their needs better*. At the city and state level increased budgetary support was identified for older people. Moreover, the authors report the diffusion of the initiative to other states: similar programmes had been sponsored in over 100 communities in 30 states at the time of writing.

In fact, this must be one of the most convincing accounts of programme success in that it not only generated lifestyle change (or rather reports of lifestyle change) but it also influenced policy (and did not only achieve sustainability but had a multiplier effect) and appears to have achieved a number of social and mental health goals and generated a good deal of consumer satisfaction.

## INTERNATIONAL HEART HEALTH PROGRAMMES

The reference to the international status of these cardiovascular prevention programmes in the title of this section is somewhat misleading since the programmes which are described in some detail here are, with the one exception of the *North Karelia Project*, from the USA. This is not to say that often quite substantial programmes do not occur elsewhere. It is rather that the programmes discussed below tend to combine in the form of demonstration projects, overt application of theory, community-wide application and, typically, comprehensive and detailed evaluation. They are, however, international in that they have had a major international impact on theory and provided guidelines for the systematic design of community-wide programmes. However, in order to avoid the over-generalisation that such programmes only occur in the USA some reference will be made to certain developments in the UK.

### Coronary heart disease prevention in the UK

In 1988 the National Forum for Coronary Heart Disease Prevention published a review of *Action in the UK, 1984–1987.* It commented on a number of 'special programmes' but, perhaps more importantly, noted a number of efforts both nationally and locally which involved the integration of heart health work into existing activities. One of the strengths of the UK scene compared with the USA is its National Health Service, which incorporates health promotion units at district level and a primary care system which has increasingly over recent years become involved in health education and related preventive and anticipatory care activity. Clearly, if coronary heart disease prevention can be routinely incorporated within general health promotion activities as part of standard service provision, the net effect should be greater than the impact of relatively isolated, albeit high profile, demonstration projects. This is, of course, provided that the delivery of health promotion is efficient; regrettably it is unlikely that any thing as theoretically and organisationally sophisticated as the programmes cited so far will be readily discerned in the UK to date.

One of the best examples of a coherent and integrated approach to the development of health promotion is provided by the *City of Sheffield's Strategic Plan (1990–1993).* This includes a description of the *Heart of Our City,* one of three demonstration projects. This, in turn, relates to an overall strategic programme entitled *Healthy Sheffield 2000* (Sheffield Health Promotion Unit, undated) which, as well as addressing major *Health of the Nation* (Department of Health, 1992) targets, also incorporated a philosophy consistent with the principles of health promotion outlined in Chapter 1. In the light of later discussions we might also note that some features of a community development way of working were built into programmes wherever possible and these moved beyond the tokenism often seen in typical community-wide initiatives. For instance, the *Heart of Our City* project included in its aims: the enhancement of personal skills, self-esteem and general well-being and the stimulation of community participation; the identification and tackling of barriers of a social, economic and environmental nature; the development and refining of evaluative techniques appropriate to community initiatives (p. 116).

The projects mentioned by the National Forum for Coronary Heart Disease Prevention (1988) include seven 'special programmes': *Oxford Prevention of Heart Attack and Stroke Project*; *City and Hackney Heart Disease and Stroke Prevention Project*; *Slough Health Habit*; *South Birmingham Coronary Prevention Project*; *Good Hearted Glasgow*; *Change of Heart* (Northern Ireland); *Heartbeat Wales* (Welsh Heart Programme). Of these, only the last named, *Heartbeat Wales*, could be said to compete in rationale and scope with the international projects, not surprisingly, since it consciously utilised experience from those involved in the US projects. Long-term evaluation results were not available in any detailed or complete form at the time of writing.

## The US approach

Farquhar *et al.* (1983) describe 10 community-based multiple risk factor health education interventions. Four of these will be considered here: the *Stanford Heart Disease Prevention Projects*; the *Minnesota Heart Health Study*; the *Pawtucket Heart Health Study* and the *North Karelia Project* (which is, of course, a Finnish scheme rather than a US project). A detailed review of each is beyond the scope of this chapter which will, therefore, be limited to discussing a number of key features of the projects and their evaluation. First the main characteristics of the programme itself will be described. This will be followed by comments on the nature of the evaluation and, finally, observations will be made on the results of the evaluation where these are available.

As regards evaluation, it should be noted that none of the programmes followed a narrow clinical trials model, with greater or lesser reluctance, and did so for the reasons discussed earlier in this book. Some projects, however, made strenuous efforts to compensate for the lack of a true experimental design by the introduction of various techniques to enhance the internal validity of their quasi-experiments. All projects utilised process evaluation, both to gain illumination and, in its formative mode, to monitor and improve interventions. In some instances a true experimental design might be incorporated within a sub-programme.

Blackburn (1983) described the main strategies which are used to mitigate the effects of what is inevitably an imperfect experiment. These were adopted by the Minnesota project and are listed in Box 9.

**Box 9**  Tactics to Mitigate the Lack of a True Experimental Design (Minnesota Project)

- Creation of a degree of control by matching communities for anticipated important variables such as population structure, service provision, coronary heart disease mortality, etc.
- Staging community entry to the programme thus allowing repetition of the experimental input and the consequent strengthening of inference of cause and effect.
- Sensitive trend measures (allowing time series analysis) by means of cross-sectional surveys of communities and repeated measures of individual change within cohorts.
- Dose–effect measurement which looks for different degrees of response in those subjected to increasing levels of educational exposure and programme involvement.
- Establishing links between responses to specific elements of the educational programme and subsequent changes, e.g. links between participation in a nutrition programme and subsequent change of diet/reduction in risk factors.
- Pooling communities/groups of people exposed to education and comparing them with similar pools in control communities.

(Blackburn, 1983)

## The 'Epidemiological Imperative'

A point we have noted elsewhere and will reiterate later is worth making again at this juncture. Without denigrating the importance of Blackburn's list of tactics, it might be more valuable to challenge the 'scientific gold standard' which leads to apologies for anticipated criticism of the

validity of the research approach. Bearing in mind the political nature of evaluation, mitigating factors will merely serve to confirm the views of 'hard-liners' that a given evaluation falls far short of perfection. And the gold standard is perfection!

It is also worth recalling the preventive rationale of heart disease prevention projects.

Unsurprisingly, their central if not their sole concern is with the prevention of heart disease, a subject that was selected largely because of its prime place in the league table of disease in Western/industrialised nations. Mittelmark (1999) provides a timely reminder of key aspects of this preventive medicine rationale when he cites Rose's (1992) influential statement about the priorities for controlling heart disease (Box 10).

**Box 10**  The Rationale for a Population Approach to Preventing Heart Disease

- Risk factors for heart disease are distributed in populations in a graded manner.
- There is often no obvious and clinically meaningful risk factor threshold that differentiates those at risk and those not at risk for the disease.
- There are many more people in a population at a relatively moderate level of risk than at the highest levels of risk.
- A high risk strategy (focusing effort, after screening, on those located towards the extreme end of the distribution of clinical indicators) is less efficient than improving the risk profile of the entire population (i.e. moving the arithmetic mean level of risk towards the 'healthier' end of the distribution).
- Accordingly, a population-wide approach is the strategy of choice, i.e. to reduce the average level of the population's risk rather than using intensive interventions with relatively small numbers of those at very high risk.

[After Mittelmark (1999) and Rose (1992)]

As with those espousing the intensive high risk approach, the population strategy promoted by Rose and like minded cardiologists and epidemiologists still tends to require that programme effectiveness be evaluated in terms of mortality and morbidity. This requirement, as we will observe below, may be problematical and inappropriate for the effective evaluation of health promotion. In relation to the kinds of evaluation employed, the projects reviewed below will be compared in respect of:

- measures of mortality/morbidity, i.e. disease-related outcomes;
- risk factor reduction;
- intermediate measures of programme outcome ranging from the acquisition of knowledge, attitudes and skills to the various behaviours underpinning risk factor scores;
- indirect measures of programme effectiveness, such as establishing supportive nutrition policies and anti-smoking legislation;
- process/illuminative evaluation.

## The Stanford studies

The *Stanford Three Community Study* began in 1972 and has been extensively documented and described. It sought to examine the impact of two levels of intervention on two Californian towns (Gilroy and Watsonville) by comparison with a control community (Tracy). In addition to their demographic characteristics, towns were selected on the basis of access to Stanford University and their geographic separateness (e.g. by a mountain range!). The populations of the towns ranged from 13,000 to 15,000. The *Stanford Heart Disease Prevention Project* (SHDPP) established the pattern for later schemes by building the interventions on a firm foundation of learning theory. This seems unremarkable but it is worth noting that many preventive interventions prior to that date (and many since!) had been educationally naïve, often making the assumption that providing information was the same as providing education. The theoretical element included an amalgam of social learning theory, attitude and communication theory and social marketing. This produced an almost standard formula which Farquhar *et al.* (1984b) described as a communication–behaviour change framework. Effectively this meant initiating a chain of events that started with agenda setting and moved on to the provision of information and enhanced motivation. Models of good practice were provided together with skills training and 'cues to action' offered. These latter allowed programme participants to acquire self-management competencies. The final step involved ensuring the availability of social and environmental support for newly acquired risk reducing behaviours. There were several points of special theoretical interest in the main interventions used by the SHDPP and these centre on the role of mass media. One community, Gilroy, received only a mass media programme, while Watsonville was subjected to identical media influences but, in addition, was supplied with supplementary intensive instruction. For these reasons the SHDPP found itself a kind of test case in the debate about the capabilities of mass media, a point of some interest in the light of our discussion in Chapter 8. Before examining the impact of these measures, however, we should note the extent of the mass media programming employed by the Stanford team.

**Box 11**  Mass Media Input in the Stanford Three Centre Programme

- Fifty television public service advertisements broadcast by four stations.
- Three hours of television programmes.
- More than 100 radio spots and several hours of radio broadcasting.
- Weekly newspaper columns.
- Advertisements and stories.
- Poster advertising.
- Direct mail, including calendars and cookbooks mailed to each household.
- Kits for schools.
- The programme was continued for nine months (after pre-testing in 1973) and repeated in 1974.

The intensive intervention methodology used in Watsonville was derived from social learning theory and employed a range of behaviour modification techniques. It was delivered to a group of individuals at relatively high risk (two-thirds of a random sample of individuals falling into the top risk quartile) and consisted of home counselling/group sessions for a 10 week period and included spouses who were willing to be involved.

The evaluation strategy involved baseline surveys in the three towns followed by three further surveys of the same samples at one yearly intervals. Participants' knowledge and beliefs about coronary heart disease and its prevention were assessed along with relevant behaviours. The key aspect of the summative evaluation, however, was a measure of reduction in a risk score derived from an equation incorporating cardinal risk factors of age, sex, systolic blood pressure, relative weight, amount of cigarette smoking and plasma cholesterol. Process evaluation was mainly concerned with various mini surveys which monitored the impact of the media, in addition to materials pre-testing and developmental testing of the intensive instruction programme. An additional interesting example of process evaluation was provided by the results of a diffusion survey using network analysis to determine the nature of inter-personal contacts stimulated by the programme. This revealed, for instance, that whereas an individual only receiving a mass media input might have an average number of two inter-personal contacts and a frequency of two conversations with other people about coronary heart disease, someone receiving the media programme together with screening and face-to-face education from a health educator would make contact with eight people and have 13 conversations.

The result of the *Stanford Three Community Study* were convincing. After one year there was evidence of significant shifts on the baseline measures, with Watsonville leading the field, presumably thus justifying the assumption of the superiority of inter-personal education.

For instance, an overall improvement in knowledge about triglycerides and belief in the statement that eating eggs could be harmful had increased. As for behaviour change, there had been a decline in smoking in Watsonville. Bearing in mind the 'borrowing from the future' phenomenon (see Chapter 3), 31% of the Watsonville high risk group had quit smoking during the first year of the programme. In connection with egg consumption, the superiority of Watsonville at the mid-point in the intervention was again in evidence, however, there was also a decline in Tracy, the control community; evidence, perhaps, of the secular trend effect that has bedevilled claims about the effectiveness of community-wide interventions (Maccoby and Farquhar, 1975).

However, what created most interest and debate was the end-of-programme summative evaluation, which demonstrated not only a significant reduction in risk but also revealed that Gilroy, the town exposed only to mass media, had virtually caught up with Watsonville. The relative risk in the control town had increased by some 6% while it had decreased by some 18% in the two experimental towns, yielding a net difference between control and treatment of between 23 and 28%. Among high risk participants the intensive instruction group had a 5% lower risk than the media only group (Farquhar *et al.*, 1977).

**Box 12**  Sample Results from Stanford after One Year

| Indicator | Change |
|---|---|
| Knowledge about triglycerides | Overall Increase from 18 to 45% |
| Belief that egg consumption can be harmful | 65–86% (W); 67–77% (G); no change (T) |
| Decline in smoking | 22% decline (44% in high risk group) (W); 3% (G) |
| Decline in egg consumption | 40% decline (W); 27% (G); 17% (T) |

W, *Watsonville (high intensity intervention)*; G, *Gilroy (media only)*; T, *Tracy (control)*.

(Maccoby and Farquhar, 1975)

What are we to make of these results which suggest that mass media can in fact yield results virtually as good as inter-personal education? The first point to note is that the intensity and extensiveness of the media programme per head of population was very substantial. The second point is, of course, that it is impossible to know the extent to which the media campaign triggered inter-personal education by health professionals and educators. The third point to note is that the media design was based on good learning theory and approximated therefore to inter-personal communication. However, Maccoby and Solomon (1981) themselves state the case very appositely:

*We tentatively attribute much of the success of the community education campaigns to the quality of the media campaign and to the synergistic interaction of multiple educational inputs and to interpersonal communication stimulated by application of these inputs in a community setting (our emphasis).*

Farquahar *et al.* (1977) added:

*Intensive face-to-face instruction and counselling seem important for changing refractory behaviour such as cigarette smoking and for inducing rapid change of dietary behaviour. But we must learn how to use these methods to correct obesity, and to employ them effectively with limited resources (e.g. by training volunteer instructors). Mass media are potentially much more cost-effective than face-to-face education methods.*

The *Stanford Three Community Study*, despite its manifest success, was criticised on several grounds (Levanthal *et al.*, 1980). These objections may be summarised as follows. First, it was argued that the study was wrong to confuse behavioural and medical indicators (a point made in Chapter 3). For instance, health education might well produce a change in behaviour, such as a reduction in dietary cholesterol, without necessarily leading to a reduction in physiological risk and community levels of coronary heart disease. This issue of the wisdom of latching on to epidemiological indica-

tors will be mentioned again later when considering the North Karelia experience. The second objection centres on an accusation that the SHDPP was unduly wedded to a *Medical Model* and missed the opportunity of appraising a genuine community study. As Levanthal *et al.* say, *We believe ... that the Stanford study is better described as a quasi-experimental study of individuals in a community setting and that it retains many of the failings typically ascribed to laboratory investigations*. These critics also regret the lack of sufficient process measures to describe community activities and diffusion of information. The third objection related to problems of internal validity of the kind discussed earlier and which follow failure to employ a true experimental design.

Not surprisingly, the Stanford team reacted somewhat tetchily to these criticisms (Meyer *et al.*, 1980). A detailed discussion of the case is not appropriate here but we might reiterate earlier observations about the impossibility of avoiding criticism on methodological grounds without the talisman of randomisation! We should also note that the follow-up to the *Stanford Three Community Study* sought to meet some of Levanthal *et al.*'s criticisms. This took the form of a five cities study.

The *Five City Project* (FCP), apart from its other goals, attempted to counter criticism of its lack of community focus and Farquhar *et al.* (1984b) have described how it was established. It began in 1978 and was designed to be a genuinely community-based programme which would seek to achieve local community involvement, ownership and control. Community ownership, it was felt, might enhance the mass media components but at a lower cost than the 'individualised instruction' used in the three centre study. It was also hoped that community support might maintain the long-term impact of the intervention. The key features of FCP are listed below.

- Two 'experimental' cities were to receive the health education interventions. These cities are, unlike the original three centres, quite socially complex and larger. The whole city would receive health education and this would consist of a wide range of broadcast media, print media, self-help booklets and the like. The community organisation would involve a number of community groups and organisations and the range of settings described earlier in this chapter. Opinion leaders would be employed to act as health educators alongside more traditional and formal sources. Environmental change would be attempted; for instance, restaurants and shops would be encouraged to provide heart healthy products.

- It was intended that FCP would run for nine years.
- Three moderate sized cities would be used as controls; total population size would be 350,000. A wider age range would be used in surveys (ages 12–74) and repeated samples would be used to monitor programme effects. Annual rates of fatal and non-fatal cardiovascular events would be recorded.

The effects of the programme were discussed by Farquhar *et al.* (1990). The results are summarised in Box 13.

**Box 13** Key Results of the *Five City Study*

- Knowledge of cardiovascular disease risk factors increased steadily during the programme but the improvement in the 'treatment' group was significantly greater at all follow-up points.
- Net reductions (i.e. control minus experimental groups) in cholesterol were recorded (though not substantial); average net decrease was some 2%. Net reductions of some 4% were also recorded for blood pressure.
- A progressive reduction in smoking occurred throughout the study period, *with declines in treatment cities always exceeding those in control cities by about 13%.*
- Weight gain occurred in all surveys but was typically greater in control towns. However, the net decrease in resting pulse rate

was greater in treatment groups in most instances.
- In the words of the authors, *These risk factor changes resulted in important decreases in composite total mortality risk scores (15%) and coronary heart disease risk scores (16%). Thus, such low-cost programs can have an impact on risk factors in broad population groups* (p. 359).

## The *Minnesota Heart Health Program*

The major difference between the *Minnesota Heart Health Program* (MHHP) and the SHDPP is the community organisation aspect and the ways in which a wide variety of agencies and lay people were orchestrated to achieve project goals. Clearly its medical goals were identical to SHDPP and it thus represents a prime example of a community programme that focuses on disease prevention with a top-down orientation but which, nonetheless, makes strenuous efforts to involve the community. The goals of the project were succinctly stated by Jacobs *et al.* (1986). It is interesting to observe how these have taken account of the general downward trend in cardiovascular disease risk in their reference to accelerating the change process.

Major MHHP hypotheses were that a systematic and multiple strategy community-wide health education programme is feasible and will lead to a change in the way people think about heart disease and its prevention, in behaviours related to risk for heart disease, in physiologic risk factors and, ultimately, in disease rates. Some of these changes were occurring naturally. The MHHP aimed to accelerate this change and hypothesised that an intensive education programme of five years duration in a community will initiate risk factor changes leading to decreased disease rates. A further MHHP hypothesis was that the programme would be taken over by the community after the researchers left.

Three pairs of education and reference/control communities were chosen for study and these were enrolled in a phased manner (to enhance evaluation power as indicated earlier). The communities were matched and represent three different types: Mankato paired with Winona represented small free-standing towns; Fargo, ND, paired with Sioux Falls, SD, represented large free-standing cities; Bloomington paired with Roseville, Maplewood and North St Paul represented large suburban areas.

The comprehensive education programme involved three major thrusts: mass media, direct education and community organisation. Education was delivered through health education centres, by means of short courses, lectures, workshops and seminars and, of course, via school programmes. Target groups were community organisations and community leaders, youths, adults and health professionals. An overriding aim was to ensure that there was at least one direct contact with the majority of individuals within the community (Blackburn, 1983).

The intensity of the programme may be judged from an account of the health centre operation (see Box 14).

**Box 14** The Health Centre Operation

Screening was provided together with *exposure to educational and motivational messages*. It involved an audio-visual presentation for the family group to introduce them to the programme. The family then rotated through various screening stations and received further audio-visual inputs about risk factors. Their physical activity level was ascertained at an interactive computer station. Finally, they received a whole family counselling session.

The nature of the schools programme is well illustrated by Perry *et al.* (1985a) who describe a 'needs assessment' of young people's nutrition and exercise status. Perry *et al.* (1985b) also discuss the development of a 20 session heart healthy nutrition education curriculum for third and fourth grade students.

The model of community organisation was described by Carlaw *et al.* (1984). It is defined as a partnership between community and the MHHP development team, and the WHO's (1983) reference to participation is cited by way of philosophical justification:

*Participation – or more correctly involvement – is a process in which individuals and communities identify with a movement and take responsibility jointly with health professionals and others concerned, for making decisions and planning and carrying out activities.*

The procedures described are somewhat different from the classic grassroots bottom-up approach in, for example, disadvantaged inner city communities. The first step involves 'community analysis' by the team, which consists of identifying geographical and interest sector representatives to serve on heart health boards and provision of training. It is followed by the establishment of 'task forces' which identify strategies and seek to influence their communities. Ideally this leads to the third stage, development of 'social system support', which includes skill development sessions in churches, school districts, trade unions, health clubs, etc. This hopefully leads to a 'strengthening of community norms and values'. The final stage should result in *organizational commitment to an improved social environment* and lead to a shift in the balance of power from the initiating researchers to the community itself. However, the impression created is that the main focus is on institutions and community leaders rather than the 'hard-to-reach' targets of traditional locality development initiatives. For instance, as part of the process of 'organisational commitment', i.e. what has been described above as the final stage in the programme, the main target group consists of employers and managers, who are asked to take responsibility for the provision of gentle coercion to lead the population to a healthier lifestyle. Those in authority are asked to encourage and reinforce ... *consistent heart healthy behaviour through financial and other incentive systems* and *insurance companies, banks and related organizations providing favourable rates for heart healthy families and individuals.* These last quotes point up one further way in which the MHHP differs from the SHDPP: it incorporates many of the 'healthy public policy' aspects of health promotion. As Carlaw *et al.* (1984) state:

> *A second aspect of Phase I was the development, in the community, of the opportunities to practice healthful behavior. In practical terms this translated into choices available to the consumer through services such as grocery store labelling, indexing of heart healthy menus in restaurants, improved smoking cessation services and attractive opportunities for physical activity for all age groups. Food packaging and food preparation are directed by marketing factors having little or no relationship to the health of the consumer. Considerable community initiative is needed to modify these services so that heart healthy behavior is encouraged.*

Programme evaluation incorporated a wide range of measures. It is interesting to note that although the possibility existed of random allocation of communities to experimental or reference situations, this tactic was deliberately rejected since the small number of units involved could not guarantee equality: matching was therefore a superior strategy. Intermediate and outcome measures comprised ... *net changes in awareness, participation, cognitions, behaviours, risk factors and disease endpoints* (Jacobs *et al.*, 1985). Process measures included 'linkage' between education components and behaviour change and 'coincidence' of community change with the staged entry of different communities to the programme.

The MHHP provides a nice illustration of three broad categories of measure representing final outcomes, intermediate indicators and indirect indicators. The final outcomes include the disease endpoints: mortality and morbidity data on coronary heart disease and cerebrovascular accident. The intermediate indicators include risk factor measures of blood pressure, smoking, total serum cholesterol and high density lipoprotein (HDL) level together with associated behav-iours relating to blood pressure control, smoking cessation, physical activity in leisure time and diet. More indirect cognitive and attitudinal measures which are related to these variables were also measured.

Jacobs *et al.* (1985) provide an equally useful example of indicators occurring at an early stage on the proximal–distal/input–output chain in their 14 point list of ways in which the community might participate in the programme. These are listed in Box 15. The MHHP also provides a very apposite illustration of the way in which it is possible to utilise true experimental design in community studies. These do of course fall within the broader quasi-experimental framework. As Jacobs *et al.* point out, although ... *it is not possible to randomly withhold from some persons television campaigns, a community walk, or a grocery store labelling program*, it is possible ... *to randomly delay invitation to the MHHP Heart and Health Centre to a random group of persons.*

**Box 15**  Intermediate Indicators of Programme Participation: *Minnesota Heart Health Program*

1  General awareness of the existence of the programme and/or its goals.
2  Coronary heart disease risk factor screening in the MHHP Heart Health Center.
3  Exposure to general MHHP messages in the media.
4  Exposure to specific MHHP messages in the media (such as television programme or a pamphlet or book).
5  Participation in the *Shape-Up Challenge* (a worksite physical activity programme).
6  Recognition/use of the restaurant menu labelling programme.
7  Recognition/use of the grocery store labelling programme.
8  Doing homework with children who participate in an MHHP school programme.
9  Contact with a health professional whose practice has been influenced by MHHP.
10  *Quit and Win* smoking classes and contest.
11  Participation on an MHHP task force.

12 Participation in other MHHP sponsored classes.
13 Social contact with the precepts and ideas of MHHP.
14 Speaking at or hearing a speaker at a club or organisation meeting.

Such sub-experiments serve to test and improve specific methods and interventions.

Process measures/formative evaluation include telephone surveys to check on particular education programmes and the use of focus groups to evaluate media messages. Blake *et al.* (1987) also described in full detail a process evaluation of a physical activity campaign which illustrates the value of such research for programme refinement. They considered community awareness of and participation in five specific kinds of exercise opportunity using telephone surveys and observation of participation. These indicated *inter alia* that participation was highest for activities organised within existing organisations but awareness was highest for heavily publicised general population events.

Several encouraging indications about the likely long-term effectiveness of the project were noted. For instance, Mittelmark *et al.* (1986) reported that initial objectives had been achieved. After two years 190 community leaders were directly involved as programme volunteers, 14,103 residents (60% of adults) had attended a screening education centre and 2094 had attended health education classes and distribution of printed media averaged 12.2 pieces per household.

One of the salient features of the MHHP was the provision of medical education and training for doctors and other health professionals who would act as role models and active educators. After two years 42 of the 65 physicians in Mankato and 728 other health professionals had participated in continuing education programmes offered by the MHHP.

As regards young people's programmes, all third, fifth, sixth and eleventh grade students were involved in the MHHP heart health education teaching and 1665 young people visited the heart health centre with their parents.

Population surveys also revealed higher levels of awareness of the various heart-related risk behaviours in Mankato compared with the reference community. A telephone evaluation revealed that about one-sixth of smokers watched at least one segment of a local television's five day series of cessation hints and 1% stopped smoking. A smoking cessation short course called *Quit and Win* resulted in 5% of all smokers in the community committing themselves to give up smoking. Over 50% of those who signed up stopped for one month and 34% had not relapsed after two months (Schwartz, 1987).

Reference was made above to the inclusion of true experiments within the overall framework. One of these (Murray *et al.*, 1986) compared the level of risk of an experimental group who had received the personalised risk factor screening programme with a control group. After one year the former group had significantly lower risk factor scores in respect of blood cholesterol, diastolic blood pressure, reduced fat and salt consumption and increased regular exercise.

In short, Minnesota's multi-intervention community programme appeared to be having a substantial impact. However, further reflections on its effectiveness will be made later in this chapter.

### The *Pennsylvania County Health Improvement Program* (CHIP)

This community-wide programme laid claim to developing *a new form of social organization: the mobilization of an entire community to improve its health* (Stunkard *et al*, 1985). Its goal was to reduce mortality and morbidity from cardiovascular disease in Lycoming County, PA. It was clearly influenced by the other coronary heart disease projects discussed in this section but allegedly differed from these in the following ways: it had considerably less than 20% of the funding of the other programmes and, as a consequence, had to utilise existing resources and facilities; it involved community participation from the outset and was designed to be owned by the community. Costs were kept as low as possible to facilitate replication.

Details of the history and planning process of CHIP may be consulted in Stunkard *et al.* (1985), as may details of the process of 'coalition building', which is not dissimilar to the strategies described earlier in this chapter. CHIP planners decided to operate via five 'channels'. Two of these were categorised as 'diffuse', namely mass media and voluntary organisations, while three were 'focused', work sites, health organisations and schools.

Rather more detail will be supplied about the planning process involved in developing the workplace programme, given its relevance to Chapter 7. Fourteen steps were involved and these are listed below.

1 Introduction of the programme to management, including a personal presentation.
2 Announcement of the programme to the employees (by company newsletter or a personal letter to employees' homes).
3 Recruitment and organisation of a 'Heart Health Committee' (including a broad cross-section of workers and management).
4 In-house communication planning (by newly created CHIP newsletters).
5 Employee interest and risk factor surveys.
6 Formation of risk factor sub-committees (smoking; hypertension; cholesterol; obesity; physical inactivity).
7 Exploration of communication risk factor reduction programmes (examining existing resources and assessing costs and effectiveness of various programmes).
8 Committee review and programme selection.
9 Development of a programme proposal.
10 Discussion of proposal with the management (e.g. negotiation of release from work and possible financial contributions).
11 Promotion of programmes and recruitment of employees.
12 Scheduling of programmes.
13 Programme implementation.
14 Evaluation and feedback.

Evaluation of the whole CHIP programme was designed as far as possible to be compatible with the other coronary heart disease programmes discussed in this section. Whilst acknowledging the difficulties of conducting 'proper' trials, attempts were made to provide a degree of comparison by selecting Franklin County as a reference area. The major indices of effectiveness would, therefore, consist of comparing changes in these two counties in respect of mortality, morbidity, risk factor reduction, 'community resource inventory' and cost effectiveness.

The nature of the first three measures is self-evident but the community resource inventory may need a little further explanation. Essentially its purpose is to compare changes in activity level of nine different institutions in the study area with those in the control area. It thus provides 'indirect indicators' of effectiveness. Table 10.1 describes the extent of these differences in study and control areas after three years of the programme.

**Table 10.1** Impact of the CHIP programme on resource provision

|  | 1980 | 1983 |
| --- | --- | --- |
| Lycoming County | | |
| Organisations with blood pressure screening | 29 | 52 |
| Organisations with more extensive programmes | 21 | 50 |
| Total organisations with health promotion programmes | 66 | 68 |
| Total organisations in county | 157 | 154 |
| Reference county | | |
| Organisations with blood pressure screening | 29 | 22 |
| Organisations with more extensive programmes | 12 | 13 |
| Total organisations with health promotion programmes | 56 | 32 |
| Total organisations in county | 142 | 126 |

*After Stunkard et al. (1985).*

Taking account of the discussion of economic indicators and cost effectiveness in Chapter 2, it is interesting to note the researcher's calculation of the likely benefit of an effective programme. The costs of CHIP were calculated at $150,000 per year. The direct and indirect costs of cardiovascular disease, on the other hand, were estimated as $33,040,000. A reduction of 10% (half that achieved in Karelia according to Stunkard *et al.*, 1985) would therefore result in savings of $3,300,000.

Additional evidence of programme effectiveness again centred on indirect indicators. For instance, the media output related to hypertension control is shown in Box 16. Again, in relation to the evaluation of effort 58 health promotion programmes were established in 12 different workplaces (employing more than 3800 people). On the other hand, the results of two programmes of weight control in banks and retail stores provided intermediate indicators of effectiveness. Of 172 store workers 34% dropped out of the programme but the remainder lost on average 7.3 lbs. There were virtually no dropouts from the banks and the average weight loss of participants in that setting was 13 lbs.

Moreover, in the context of workplace health promotion the authors reported a decline in the proportion of people with markedly high blood pressure: a fall in workers with a diastolic pressure of over 120 mm from 7.5% in 1981 to 4% in 1982.

**Box 16**  Media Output in One Month: the CHIP Programme

| Media | Messages | Exposure |
| --- | --- | --- |
| Radio | 900 | 113,000 |
| Television | 23 | 45,000 |
| Newspapers | 4.5 | 110,000 |
| Billboards | 5.0 | 470,000 |
| Pamphlet holders | 190 | |
| Pamphlets | 16,500 | 33,000 |

*(Stunkard et al., 1985)*

## The *Pawtucket Heart Health Program*

The special interest of the *Pawtucket Heart Health Program* (PHHP) in the present context is its approach to community organisation and the theoretical rationale which underpins this approach. In short, this project sought to get closer to the grassroots.

The PHHP study community was located in Pawtucket, RI. Its residents were described as predominantly blue collar. The city of Pawtucket had some 72,000 inhabitants and the population was described as very stable. For evaluation purposes it was matched with a control community of some 98,000 people. The project was planned to run from 1980 to 1991; professional guidance was provided for the first four years and thereafter the management would be in the hands of a community volunteer system.

The observations made below are derived from reports by Lefebvre *et al.* (1987) and Elder *et al.* (1986). The authors, in discussing the community-level approach of PHHP, made a distinction between locality development and social planning, as discussed in the previous chapter. Their definition of the former makes reference to the involvement of the people in goal determination and action, democratic procedures, training of indigenous leaders and educational self-help methods. Social planning is seen as an alternative view of community organisation in which social change is planned by designated experts.

> *Citizens are seen as being passive recipients of services ... the practitioner role of 'expert' in social planning strategies contrasts markedly with the 'enabler' posture of locality developers.*

> (Lefebvre *et al.*, 1987)

The PHHP, in practice, aimed to offer a blend of both of these theoretically discrete approaches together with Rothman's (1979) model of social action in which experts *seek to organize coalitions of concerned interests to attack the problem*. Within the framework of PHHP Lefebvre *et al.* see these social action tactics (i.e. advocacy and consciousness raising) as involving:

*... campaign tactics; employment of facts; and persuasion within the context of voluntary association, mass media, and legislative bodies to change institutional and community policies and norms ... citizens can be either recipients or agents of action, while the practitioner role is defined more as that of a coalition builder, fact gatherer, and policy analyst.*

The researchers considered that the PHHP use of churches as heart health delivery systems illustrates this social action approach within Pawtucket.

Elder *et al.* identified four principles operating within the general approach. These are:

* the importance of local ownership;
* the use of inexpensive resources and facilities (to make community ownership more feasible after external funding has ceased);
* the importance of inter-personal education, with media being used as awareness-raising devices;
* the use of multi-level programming, i.e. reciprocal contributions of community, organisational, small group and individual programmes.

Elder *et al.* also recorded the change in emphasis during the first 26 months of PHHP from organisations to community. During the first 11 months the focus was on worksites, churches, schools and other organisations. Progress, however, was slow and this produced a strategic shift after 11 months when an attempt was made to accelerate progress by directing the programme to the community at large in association with media publicity. By the end of this stage perhaps the most singular feature of PHHP had emerged, the 'volunteer delivery system'. Lefebvre *et al.* have argued that there are at least eight reasons for using volunteers in preventive heart health programmes (Box 17).

**Box 17** Eight Reasons for Using Volunteers

* They serve as peer models (cf. the principle of homophily);
* they provide a support network for others who have made changes in lifestyle;

* their own healthy behaviour is reinforced;
* they promote diffusion through social networks;
* effective volunteers can be deliberately 'networked' to help change norms;
* a volunteer system helps promote community ownership;
* it is cost effective;

The goals of PHHP are similar to those of the other major cardiovascular disease prevention programmes and they are similarly 'theory driven'. Lefebvre *et al.* summarised this aspect of the project as an 'intervention cube' where the risk factor and disease endpoints of fitness, weight reduction, fat and cholesterol control, management of blood pressure and reduction of smoking are to be attained via four programme phases. These latter involved motivating the community, providing skills training for risk factor reduction, developing support networks and finally ensuring the maintenance of ensuing change. The programmes are seen as having an impact at four levels: the individual, group, organisation and the community at large.

Evaluation results to date are largely concerned with process but some outcome measures may be discerned! The general situation (Lefebvre *et al.*, 1987) is described in Box 18.

**Box 18** Indirect, Intermediate and Outcome Measures in PHHP

* Children are involved in *Heart Health Clubs*, smoking prevention programmes, and classroom heart health education.
* Parents learn to raise heart healthy children.
* People shop at grocery stores where shelf labels identify foods low in salt, fat and calories and eat in *Four-Heart Restaurants* offering good tasting menu items that are low in fat, sodium and cholesterol.
* Senior citizens are active in *Walk Jog Clubs* and exercise programmes.

- All residents attend community events such as *Octoberfest* or *Meet us in the Park* weekends where the PHHP Heart Check trailer and van are prominently located.
- Fourteen Pawtucket companies sent 23 coordinators to training sessions; 3604 of 5700 eligible employees were screened.
- Twenty-one churches have been involved in social action and devoted some 2105 volunteer hours.
- Trained volunteers have been accepted by both the lay community and the medical professionals. Between 600 and 1000 blood pressure readings are taken monthly at 14 walk-in blood pressure stations. In its first three years more than 30,000 hours have been invested by volunteers in the programme and the PHHP has had over 30,000 contacts with people seeking to improve their heart health.
- People participating in the worksite screening programme succeeded in reducing their blood pressure: prevalence of readings greater than 180/100 dropped from 34 out of 409 screened to zero.
- After a 'community weigh-in' 138 residents recorded a joint loss of 1061 lbs after 10 weeks. Six months later a follow-up interview of 70% of the 211 original participants revealed that 80% had lost weight and 75% were continuing to do so.

In conclusion, we can reasonably say that the PHHP has again demonstrated that a community-wide programme can achieve substantial changes. In the case of PHHP the suggestion has been made that by using a more informal community effort centring on lay workers and volunteers, changes can be produced in a lower socio-economic status community. The methods used, however, still fall short of 'true' community development approaches.

Whether these strategies would be effective within deprived and underprivileged inner city ghettos must remain a matter of conjecture. Two important questions, therefore, still seemed to require answers. First, whether the successful North American experience would generalise to disadvantaged neighbourhoods and to different national populations where health has a lower profile. Second, the question which sceptical clinicians and epidemiologists are constantly posing: will the lifestyle changes recorded by the cardiovascular disease prevention projects result in a demonstrable decline in mortality and morbidity which can unequivocally be attributed to the health promotion? The final example, that of the *North Karelia Project*, demonstrates clear success in fostering lifestyle change in a European setting. It has also claimed to have an impact on mortality and morbidity, but not without challenge!

### The *North Karelia Project*

One of the principal features of the *North Karelia Project* (NKP) is its community focus and the circumstances which led to the establishment of the project are of particular significance. Indeed, one of the most noteworthy features of NKP was the frequently cited popular petition to the Finnish government to deal with the problem of premature death from coronary heart disease, which had apparently forced itself on the consciousness of the population. In fact, following the Seven Countries Study of coronary heart disease mortality (WHO Collaborative Group, 1970) it became apparent that Eastern Finland held the unenviable record of heading the league table of deaths. However, it apparently took three public reports before community leaders, at the end of the 1960s, began to demand action. This coincided with Karvonen, who was leading the Finnish investigation, having a WHO advisory role and being president of the Finnish Medical Association. It is also reported that the awareness-raising effect of epidemiological data was vigorously supplemented by lobbying by the Finnish Heart Association and its volunteer task force; a clear case of advocacy (with or without creative epidemiology!). These somewhat serendipitous circumstances are of importance because it would be wrong to assume that the NKP was the result of some popular upsurge of opinion. Indeed, if the petition to government by community leaders had been a fundamentally grassroots eruption, the generalisability of NKP to other European countries would have been in considerable doubt. On the other hand, it would be wrong to ignore the importance of community awareness: the personal exposure of community members to coronary heart disease deaths in friends and relations doubtless concentrates the mind and creates a level of perceived susceptibility which the *Health Belief Model* requires as an antecedent to preventive action.

At all events, the petition which was signed on 12 January 1971 by the governor, all members of parliament and representatives of official and voluntary bodies signalled the start of a 10 year programme which has continued to have repercussions and has influenced the development of health promotion nationally and internationally. Again, somewhat fortuitously, the start of the project was accompanied by the establishment of a medical school at the University of Kuopio and a new *Public Health Act* which reorganised primary health care. The World Health Organization provided its support and documented the first stages of the project (WHO, 1981) and the thinking underlying the Stanford Project was incorporated.

A full description of the NKP is beyond the scope of this book. Suffice it to say that its theoretical foundation was similar to the projects discussed above and included social learning theory, communication and attitude theory, communication of innovations theory and community organisation principles. It is, however, worth noting one particular point of emphasis which distinguishes the NKP from the North American schemes and which, perhaps, reflects the different political climates of those countries. Unlike the American projects, there was a more overt concern with the socio-economic and physical environment and its effect on the individual's health choices. This is seen in item six (Puska *et al.*, 1985) in the ... *seven key steps to help individuals to modify their behaviour* (Box 19).

**Box 19**  Seven Key Steps to Help Individuals Modify their Behaviour

1 Improved preventive services to help people identify their risk factors and to provide appropriate attention and services.
2 Information to educate people about the relationship between behaviours and their health.
3 Persuasion to motivate people and to promote the intention to adopt the healthy action.
4 Training to increase the skills of self-management, environmental control and necessary action.
5 Social support to help people to maintain the initial action.
6 Environmental change to create the opportunities for healthy actions and improve unfavourable conditions.
7 Community organisation to mobilise the community for broad-ranged changes (through increased social support and environmental modification) to support the adoption of the new lifestyles in the community.

The organisation of the NKP was truly community wide, involving the national health service, and especially the new primary health care centres and the public health nurses, together with the mass media, doctors, social workers, business leaders, voluntary organisations, administrators, trade unions, sports organisations and local political leaders. A special school and youth programme was developed (Vartiainen *et al.*, 1983) and in addition to the kinds of environmental change mentioned in, for example, the MHHP, local industry was prevailed upon to make available low fat dairy products and a new sausage product. This latter move was apparently helped by the fact that two managers had recently experienced heart attacks (McAlister *et al.*, 1982)! Only one aspect of the many interventions described above will receive further comment: the use of voluntary groups and lay leaders.

From the start the NKP sought to gain community involvement. As with the PHHP, it utilised volunteers extensively. Local 'lay leaders' were identified by informally interviewing shopkeepers and other knowledgeable people in the community. These opinion leaders were then trained to act as models and educators. Over a four year period more than 1000 of *the most influential members of the local communities were involved.* The work of these lay opinion leaders was extensively documented (Neittaanmaki *et al.*, 1980; Puska *et al.*, 1986) in the general context of diffusion theory. The picture emerging from this evaluation is one of considerable activity with evidence of genuine influence.

**Box 20** The Work of Lay Leaders in the *North Karelia Heart Disease Prevention Project*: Indirect Indicators of Success

---

- Participation in training.
- Perception of relative ease of discussing the various risk factors with people.
- Attitude to these changes.
- Extent to which leaders had discussed risk factors with three or more people during the preceding week.
- Different modes of action taken (e.g. direct requests to change behaviour, provision of advice, reference to own example, etc.).
- Frequency of discussion with different target groups.
- Frequency of contact with health centre.
- Perception of effectiveness in influencing smoking, dietary behaviours and hypertension problems.
- Involvement in the project's television programmes and involvement in general health education.

(Neittaanmaki *et al.*, 1980; Puska *et al.*, 1986)

---

In addition to the lay leader tactics, the involvement of the MARTTA organisation proved successful. This voluntary local housewives' association introduced *inter alia Parties for a Long Life* in which women were taught how to cook heart healthy meals and as a result of the experience came to believe that healthy cooking could be tasty! Three hundred and forty-four of these sessions were recorded with 15,000 participants. At the 1976 follow up 9% of men and 18% of women in Karelia had been involved at least once (McAlister *et al.*, 1982).

Final observations on the NKP will be concerned with outcome measures. Before considering the customary risk factors it is worth noting an interesting finding on coronary heart disease-related knowledge (Puska *et al.*, 1981). Repeated tests of total coronary heart disease health knowledge during the early phase of the NKP revealed only minimal changes (admittedly from a relatively high starting point). The net change in North Karelia (North Karelia score minus the reference area score) was 4% for men and 2% for women. The researchers comment on interventions which have produced knowledge change but no behaviour change and others which, like the SHDPP, recorded an increase in knowledge and a reduction in risk. They rightfully remark on the dubious relationship between knowledge and behaviour change by comparing the minimal shift in knowledge in North Karelia with the 17 and 12% respective decreases in risk factor levels during the same period.

In relation to behaviour change, changes in self-reported dietary behaviours were recorded which indicated a decline in fat consumption. The influence of the programme on smoking was also extensively analysed (Koskela, 1981). Puska *et al.* (1985) report a net change in North Karelia of 28% in amount of reported daily smoking by men and 14% for women over the period 1972–1982. Elsewhere, in a comparative report of the results of various community projects (Schwartz, 1987), the decline in male smokers in North Karelia is recorded as a shift from 44 to 31% compared with 39 to 35% in the rest of the country. By the fifth year the net percentage decline in prevalence was 2.5% for men and 6.1% for women (bearing in mind that a general decline was also occurring in the reference area and in the country as a whole).

With regard to risk factors generally, a decline was noted in mean serum cholesterol. This decline occurred in both the study and the reference areas but was greater in North Karelia. The net decline was 3% in men and 1% in women for the period 1972–1982. Again, a significant net decline in both systolic and diastolic blood pressure was observed in the experimental area. The net change between 1972 and 1982 was 3% in systolic blood pressure (SBP) and 1% in diastolic blood pressure (DBP) for men and 5 and 2% respectively for women. As with other measures, an overall decline was also occurring in the reference county and the net decline was greater during the first five years of the programme, suggesting a general diffusion effect.

The NKP also evaluated its programme in terms of late primary and secondary prevention. For instance, Salonen *et al.* (undated) state that a higher proportion of men recovering from heart attacks in North Karelia did not resume smoking compared with a similar sample from the reference area. McAlister *et al.* (1982) noted an increase in the proportion of hypertensives receiving medication from a level of 13% in both Karelia and the reference area to 45% in the study area and 33% in the reference county. The proportion of hypertensives was also alleged to be lower in the intervention area.

Before reporting on disease endpoint measures we should consider an outcome measure which did not figure in the North American coronary heart disease prevention projects described above and which serves to illustrate the comprehensiveness and thoroughness of the NKP. The survey questionnaires included questions which attempted to assess the psychosocial consequences of the programme, with a view to checking the possibility that the interventions might have generated hypochondria or other negative side effects. These included: perceptions of health status; perceived levels of stress; psychosomatic symptoms reported. There was in fact no evidence of this and a statistically significant shift for both men and women in the direction of improved subjective health status was reported. The increase was greater in North Karelia than in the reference area while a greater decline in the 20 variable survey of 'complaints' about stress, etc. was

noted in the experimental area. It seems then that subjective well-being was enhanced without creating negative effects, all of which was taken to indicate a greater degree of satisfaction with health enhancement in the intervention county.

## INDICATORS OF SUCCESS: THE PROBLEMATICAL DEMAND FOR EPIDEMIOLOGICAL INDICATORS

The North Karelia Project, along with the other interventions discussed in this chapter, has demonstrated unequivocally that it is possible to mobilise community resources, both professional and lay, and generate changes in knowledge, beliefs and attitudes. Skills can be provided and lifestyle can be influenced such that the risk of premature death and morbidity from contemporary diseases can be reduced. And yet the most important question that is still asked is whether it is possible to demonstrate that the changes wrought in a community like North Karelia would actually reduce the numbers of deaths and the amount of illness caused by the factors which the programme is designed to prevent? The NKP certainly had something to say on the matter and, as the longest running project which has recorded mortality and morbidity events, it would seem to be in a good position to comment. Unfortunately, the issue remains clouded, a situation which is due to the quasi-experimental status of the intervention and the fact that a general decline in cardiovascular disease was occurring in the country as a whole.

It had been quite evident that a decline in mortality from coronary heart disease in Finland as a whole had occurred but, as Salonen *et al.* (1983) have shown, the decline in North Karelia was greater still (Box 21).

***Box 21*** Relative Decline in Cardiovascular Disease Mortality in North Karelia and Finland Generally

- Between 1969 and 1979 there was a reduction in mortality of 24% in men and 51% in women in North Karelia compared with a decline of 12% in men and 24% in other counties in Finland (Salonen *et al.*, 1983)

- The financial implications of this reduction were considered to be substantial, particularly in relation to pension payments. *Estimates from pension disability data already suggest that payment of over $4 million dollars in disability payments may have been avoided by the less than $1 million expended on the project's intervention activities* (McAlister *et al.*, 1982).

- The annual decline in coronary heart disease mortality, from 1969 to 1982, in men was 2.9% in Karelia whereas in the rest of Finland it was 2.0%. For women the respective annual decline was 4.9 and 3.0%. The net decline in North Karelia was 100 deaths per 100 000 men (Tuomilehto *et al.*, 1986).

On the face of it it seems reasonable to ascribe the substantial progress in North Karelia to the NKP. Indeed, Tuomilehto *et al.* (1986) were moved to comment

> *As we cannot think of any reason for the greater decline of mortality from ischaemic heart disease in North Karelia other than the prevention programme it is reasonable to argue that it was a consequence of the project.*

Others, however, could think of alternative explanations and Salonen (1987), one of the principal investigators, felt obliged to produce a disclaimer which acknowledged four potential sources of bias ranging from differential rates of decline in different regions of Finland to the possible effect of general unspecified changes in Finnish society.

Needless to say, this retraction was greeted with barely disguised pleasure by more conservative clinicians (Oliver, 1987), who could not see the logic of changing risk factors unless they had a direct and demonstrable aetological link with disease reduction.

In 1989 Puska *et al.* reflected on the project 15 years after its launch. They noted the level of risk factors in North Karelia, Kuopio (the reference county) and southwest Finland between 1972 and 1987. They argued that the smoking rates in North Karelia were lower than elsewhere, although the serum cholesterol and blood pressure levels were still high (and higher than in southwest Finland). An analysis of mortality trends showed an initial steep decline in North Karelia (in the 1970s) but slowing down in the 1980s. By the mid 1980s the decline in Finland as a whole had reached that of North Karelia. However, a bigger decline seemed to have occurred in North Karelia between 1974 and 1978. Moreover, during the nine years from 1974 to 1983 a significant decline in cancer mortality was observed in North Karelia, considerably more than the reference area and more substantial than the rest of Finland.

Puska *et al.* (1989) also demonstrated a continuing rise in reported levels of subjectively perceived health status. In all areas there was an increase in the percentage of the population rating subjective health as 'very good' or 'good'. The increase varied between men and women (with women reporting higher levels). Between 1972 and 1987 the average increase was from around 33 to 46% for men and from 32 to 51% for women. The authors, rightly, argue that the programme as a whole should be considered a success.

**Box 22**  A Considered View of the Effectiveness of the *North Karelia Heart Disease Prevention Project*

> *Throughout the 15 year period the feasibility of the programme has been good. This has been so despite the fact that – at least in the early years – health service resources were scarce, society's traditional norms militated against change and the diffusion of innovations in lifestyle. Local health services and their staff have cooperated well, thus forming the back bone for the activities. The local population has readily participated in the activities and various community organizations have contributed in various ways to the aims of the project in the area. Because*

*the project aims were integrated with the existing health services and broad community participation was a key feature, the overall costs of the programme have been modest.*

*A major task in North Karelia was how to influence people's health related lifestyles. This is not easy. Even when the hazards of unhealthy habits are well known, many intervention activities meet with limited or no success. The results and experiences presented here indicate major changes and show that, at least in favourable conditions, comprehensive, determined and well planned action can lead to substantial favourable changes.*

(Puska *et al.*, 1989, p. 172)

Similar observations to those made by Puska *et al.* might well be made on other community ventures involving attempts to introduce often problematical changes into individual behaviours and community practices.

## THE INTERNATIONAL HEART DISEASE PROJECTS RE-VISITED: AN APPRAISAL

Reflection on the variety of community-based projects discussed above has revealed a considerable consensus on organisation, methods and evaluation. What is much less clear is the extent of ideological consensus. In particular, many researchers and programme planners endorse community participation, even if this is occasionally somewhat formulaic. We described earlier programmes which are built on the principle of participation, which emphasise the need to work from people's felt needs and which urge community workers first of all to address issues of inequality and imbalance of resources between the 'haves' and 'have nots'. Clearly there will be some sort of divide between programmes of this sort and those which have been rather scathingly defined in terms of 'colonisation'. By definition, of course, the various projects we have just described cannot be considered in any sense as genuine community development initiatives since

they have a 'top-down' disease prevention agenda, even if health workers make not infrequent though occasionally desultory attempts to operate in a 'bottom-up' way. However, the rationale for community involvement is primarily due to the recognition that the preventive goals of the majority of these 'community-wide programmes are more likely to be achieved if maximal community participation can be achieved. After all, given the nature of the programme's preventive medicine orientation and the associated demands from funders, it is not unreasonable to look for measures that will prevent the disease in question and evaluate accordingly. We will, however, argue here that even accepting the preventive philosophy, both the strategies adopted to attain preventive goals and the measures adopted to assess programme effectiveness are, to a greater or lesser extent, fundamentally misplaced. Before developing the argument, though, we will briefly consider current perspectives on the 'showpiece' heart disease prevention projects and will draw on Mittelmark's recent (1999) authoritative analysis.

### Perspective on the projects 25 years on

There are two hypotheses that might be entertained in interpreting the results of the evaluations of the heart disease prevention projects:

- they were actually effective but this effectiveness was masked by the research designs used and the interpretation of the evidence resulting from those designs;
- the projects were ineffective in achieving major and important goals.

If the first hypothesis is justified, then we have cause to be grateful that so much effort and money was not wasted, and we can use the ample process data generated by the projects to develop new programmes.

If the second hypothesis is justified, then we need to ask what more would be needed to achieve success and, given the fact that the major projects seemed to follow best practice, whether a fairly dramatic reorientation of approach, almost amounting to a paradigm shift, would needed in future developments.

465

In any case, we might decide that there are better strategies to be adopted even if the projects are judged to have been effective. Box 23 summarises Mittelmark's succinct assessment of the effectiveness of the 'big four': North Karelia, Stanford, Pawtucket and Minnesota.

**Box 23**   Main Findings of the 'Big Four' Heart Disease Prevention Projects

*North Karelia*
- Beginning with rates that were among the highest in the world, there was a dramatic decline in coronary heart disease death rates of more than 50% over a 20 year period in all of Finland. The decline was even steeper in North Karelia in the 10 years after the project was launched.
- By the early 1980s the rest of Finland had caught up: for instance, the decline in cardiovascular disease mortality in men was 57% in North Karelia and 52% in all Finland (Puska, 1995a,b), a 5% difference.

*Stanford Five City Project*
- Among women there were significant differences between intervention and control communities for knowledge and coronary heart disease risk but not for blood pressure, total cholesterol, smoking, body mass index and all cause mortality risk (Winkleby *et al.*, 1996).
- Among men there were significant differences in knowledge, systolic blood pressure, diastolic blood pressure and body mass index but no significant differences for total cholesterol, smoking, coronary heart disease risk and all-cause mortality risk coronary heart disease risk (Winkleby *et al.*, 1996).
- The greatest differences between intervention and control communities were observed at the end of six years but these differences had begun to fade 4–5 years after the end of the intervention.

*Pawtucket, Rhode Island Programme*
- *The Pawtucket researchers concluded that achieving cardiovascular risk reduction at the community level was feasible, but maintaining statistically significant differences between the treatment and the control communities was not ... the project provided*

*only limited evidence for the feasibility of cardiovascular disease risk reduction by the community-based education approach (Carleton et al., 1995)* (Mittelmark, 1999, p. 9).

*The Minnesota Heart Health Program*
- In many ways the Minnesota project was the most thorough and sophisticated of the four programmes and its use of three intervention and three control communities (as described earlier in this chapter) provided a more rigorous test of observed differences.
- After two to three years, the control communities ... *had greater exposure to cardiovascular disease prevention messages than at the beginning of the study, but the intervention communities had significantly greater exposure that seemed attributable to the special education program ...* (Luepker et al., 1994). *A similar positive pattern was seen for total blood cholesterol, systolic and diastolic blood pressure, body mass index, and physical activity. For cigarette smoking, the trend among women favored the intervention by the midpoint of the education program, but among men no difference between intervention and control communities was observed* (Mittelmark, 1999, p. 10).
- As with the other projects, differences between intervention and control communities were not sustained (with the important exception of cigarette smoking among women (Luepker *et al.*, 1994).
- Coronary heart disease rates decreased to a similar degree in both the intervention and control communities during the course of the study (Luepker *et al.*, 1996). (N.B. The Minnesota project was the only one of the US studies to publish mortality and morbidity results.)

(Derived from Mittelmark, 1999, pp. 8–10)

One of the advantages of the three US studies was the extensive collaboration between the researchers involved in designing and evaluating the projects. Accordingly, it was possible to make direct comparisons between six intervention communities and six control communities and produce an assessment of average gains in respect of risk factors and mortality risk. This joint analysis was obliged to conclude that although there were some differences between intervention and control communities, these never achieved statistical significance (Winkleby *et al.*, 1997).

Mittelmark's (1999) assessment makes rather bleak reading for those who have developed and implemented sophisticated and apparently 'state-of-the-art' interventions,

> *... in the final analysis, the main objectives of these studies were not achieved. Risk factors did not on the whole differ between intervention and control communities, and all communities tended to show improvement. The more limited data on morbidity and mortality are consistent with the overall pattern described here.*

> (p. 11)

However, the situation may not be (quite) as depressing as first appears. We will argue below that, according to at least some criteria, it is possible to claim a degree of success, depending in part on what is being measured. On the other hand, it is probably true that to make impressive gains in communities at serious risk of various kinds of ill health, a new approach is needed, and that approach is one which will seek to focus on the broader social and economic determinants of most diseases. We will also reiterate a point made with some force in Chapter 2: judging the success or failure of health promotion projects (especially in relation to such topics as cardiovascular disease) by using epidemiological indicators of success is fundamentally misplaced.

## Key issues in judging the effectiveness of community-wide projects

Those workers who have invested substantial amounts of time, effort and expertise in the design of major projects, such as the cardiovascular disease prevention group, might be forgiven for being a little depressed at achieving results which were at best disappointing and/or ambiguous. Two broad conclusions might be drawn: first that the projects were, in fact, effective (at least in part) but the wrong measures were used on which to base decisions about effectiveness and/or important changes were ignored or undervalued. Alternatively, it might be concluded that these sophisticated programmes were in fact ineffective. In which case, it is essential to understand why.

The natural tendency after investing considerable effort into a project that reveals disappointing results is to look to improve the research design to demonstrate changes that were there but were masked by insensitive measurement or were actually present but were considered to lack validity because of the failure to adopt a true experimental design. At the same time, since we tend to be reluctant to relinquish strategies that have involved considerable effort, this pursuit of a better research design may be accompanied by the development of a better intervention. If the original intervention seems to have been well designed the tendency is to recommend more of the same rather than consider a substantially different approach. Whereas the second option might well merit serious consideration, the first option can be challenged. Let us first make the assumption that community-wide projects have been effective but the wrong criteria were used to judge success. The remarks which follow are considered to be relevant to the various initiatives discussed in this chapter but of particular relevance to the heart disease prevention projects. The main argument is briefly stated below.

### The projects were effective but the wrong criteria were used to assess effectiveness

*The use of epidemiological indicators was inappropriate.* Although only the North Karelia project and the Minnesota project recorded mortality and morbidity data, the general view was that these epidemiological indicators would furnish the final proof of effectiveness or failure. It is certainly true that some interventions have claimed to demonstrate effectiveness in terms of mortality or morbidity. For instance the *Oslo Study* (Holme *et al.*, 1985), which was a randomised controlled trial, demonstrated a 47% reduction in incidence of the first major coronary heart disease event after health education about diet and smoking in a group of 1232 high risk middle aged men. Again, there seems to have been agreement, even among detractors, that the North Karelia project had produced a sustained decline in cancer mortality that was greater in the intervention area than in the rest of Finland. However, it would be unwise to rely on such epidemiological outcomes, moreover, and more importantly, their use is unnecessary for assessing the effectiveness and efficiency of health promotion. As noted earlier in this book, the basis for this assertion is as follows.

- There will inevitably be a time lag between health promotion inputs and 'medical' outcomes such as a reduction in the incidence and prevalence of a given disease. This delayed impact has been described as a 'sleeper effect' (as noted in Chapter 3). It is not so much that the intervention remains dormant like a virus that is suddenly triggered years in the future but, rather, the intervention generates immediate and deferred changes which themselves have an ultimate effect on the chosen disease measure. Smoking is, of course, a case in point: health promotion influences the psychosocial and environmental determinants of recruitment to and/or cessation of smoking. The disease sequelae that would have resulted for a proportion of the non-smokers and ex-smokers do not therefore follow. The phenomenon is discussed at greater length in Chapter 2 in relation to the notion of a proximal–distal chain of effects.
- A number of risk factors, of greater or lesser importance, exert an influence on a multiply determined condition such as cardiovascular disease. It is accepted, however, that the cardinal risk factors (e.g. for coronary heart disease)

contribute only some 40% to the variance of disease experience. Accordingly, the links between risk factor reduction and the disease in question may be somewhat tenuous in population terms.

- On a purely logical point, the use of epidemiological indicators can be discarded as an irrelevance since the relationship between the risk factors addressed by the community-wide projects discussed above and the disease (however tenuous that might be) has already been demonstrated. If it has not been demonstrated, it is unethical and wasteful to mount a health promotion programme in the first place.
- In other words, it seems that on occasions health promotion programmes are being judged as if they were epidemiological investigations!
- *The Projects have provided useful 'process data'.* This is rather a weak justification for programmes that primarily exist to demonstrate risk factor reduction. It is argued that all of the major projects provide detailed insights into the processes involved in developing and implementing sophisticated and effective interventions. It is undoubtedly true that they do just that: as we have seen, the projects describe and illuminate procedures such as the recruitment and use of lay leaders, the development of supportive health policy, the involvement of citizen groups, etc., etc. However, there would certainly be more illuminating and cheaper ways of achieving those goals. It should, however, be noted that funding agencies would be considerably less willing to support programmes that were not obviously tackling major diseases by seeking to reduce population risk.

### Problems with secular trends, or 'borrowing from the future'

One of the most common and problematical results of evaluations of community-wide projects has been the phenomenon of secular trends. Mittelmark (1999) illustrates this in respect of the Stanford and North Karelia projects (Box 24).

**Box 24**  Borrowing from the Future: the Secular Trend Effect

*The initial progress reports from the European projects and California were electrifyingly positive. The cities and towns that were approached were eager to participate. Community organization models that had been developed for other applications worked well in the new cardiovascular disease prevention programs. Interventions that were grounded in communications and behavior change theories could be implemented at the community-wide level. Early trends in behavior and risk factors favored the hypothesis that the community-based approach to cardiovascular disease reduction was feasible ... beginning with rates that were among the highest in the world (in North Karelia), there was a remarkable decline in coronary heart disease death rates during the decade after the intervention was launched. There were significant declines in some risk factors. ... However, by the early 1980s, the rest of Finland had caught up ....*

The evidence, then, is strong that secular trends within a whole population have commonly invalidated claims about the effectiveness of apparently successful interventions, because 'It would have happened anyway!' What are the implications of the phenomenon? At one level it could be argued that programmes should not be launched where there was evidence of the existence of a (positive) secular trend. Such a conclusion would, however, depend on the reasons why the control community had 'caught up'. There are a number of possibilities.

- The effect was due to 'contamination' of the control area due to 'leakage' from the experimental area, after all, it is now widely recognised that it is virtually impossible to maintain the integrity of the control and, since the use of control communities involves quasi-experimentation without the gold standard of randomisation, the strategy offers few advantages

(see Chapter 3). If the secular effect was due to contamination then, by definition, it was due to the success of the 'experimental' intervention.

- The effect was not due to direct contamination from intervention group to comparison group but rather the comparison group received health promotion from other sources. As Pietinen *et al.* (1989) commented about North Karelia, The original idea to have a reference area for the comparison of trends in risk factor levels and mortality rates has now lost much of its original meaning and importance because the development in all parts of the country quickly became almost identical (pp. 1022–1023) (see also Salonen, 1987). This was certainly the case with the *Heartbeat Wales* cardiovascular disease prevention project where the comparison region (whose identity was kept secret) was exposed to both heart health-related health promotion from the English government and from a variety of local initiatives within the region and its component districts. Perhaps it could have been argued that the patriotic Welsh focus and the more coherent approach of *Heartbeat Wales* should have been superior to the more fragmentary English inputs and there might still have been a difference between intervention and control. However, any difference must, at worst, have been diminished by the competing English programme.

- Some third factor might have been at work influencing not only potential control areas but also the intervention effects. The higher intensity of the experimental intervention might thus have caused a more rapid but temporary superiority to control groups and/or the rest of the nation. This third influence might have been as general and as vague as a change in ethos that favoured lifestyles changes relating to cardiovascular disease risk reduction, directly or indirectly. For instance, the development of policy initiatives that provided active support to, say, smoking cessation or merely served a 'norm-sending' function doubtless developed during the period of the health promotion interventions. The best that can be said,

if this is the general case, is that such developments represent a kind of unattributable health
promotion!

**The projects really were ineffective**
Let us suppose that the failure to achieve anticipated
sustained change in risk factors is not due to Type 2
error (i.e. due to inappropriate or insensitive measurement techniques) and the projects are judged as
ineffective or, more realistically, not as effective as
they were expected to be. If this is true then the
error factor shifts from Type 2 to Type 3. In other
words, there was something wrong with the programmes themselves. It does, however, seem churlish to write off such a variety of sophisticated and
intelligent efforts. If we accept the assertion made
earlier that mortality and morbidity data should not
be used as indicators of success, a more realistic view
is that the projects were indeed successful in many
ways, including the achievement or acceleration of
the achievement of risk factor reduction. Accordingly, we might expect that projects such as those
described above will have a greater impact on
higher socio-economic groups and will not materi-
ally affect those in the alienated and disadvantaged
sectors of the population which harbours the highest rates of disease, disability and malaise. It is,
therefore, more sensible to seek to build health promotion (utilising 'process' evidence from the major
community-wide projects) into institutionalised systems of health and social care.

Whittemore and Buelow (1999) describe an
interesting four-fold categorisation of community-wide health promotion programmes in Latin
America. They compare a 'Reform' approach with
a Radical' approach. The former is concerned
with *permutations of existing social arrangements and culture* whereas a Radical approach is
concerned to make *significant departures from
existing social arrangements*. Two sub-categories
of the Reform approach are identified as 'alternative', i.e. *partial change in individuals' arrangements*. The other is designated 'reformative', i.e.
*changes in the structure of society*. The Radical
approach is viewed as either 'Redemptive', i.e.
*total change in individuals* or 'Transformative',
i.e. *total change in social structures*.

This typology resonates with the models and
discussions in Chapters 1 and 2 of this book.

We argue here that to avoid Type 3 error a
'transformative' category of community programme may be necessary, not only to achieve
social goals but also to better achieve preventive
outcomes.

At any rate, following the observations made in
Chapter 1 of this book it is clear that disease or
specific issue focused programmes will be less
effective than broader based programmes that
seek to address the more fundamental, social
determinants of health, such as working conditions and inequity in general. In other words,
'horizontal programmes' are needed. Models for
such programmes already exist, and initiatives
such as *Healthy Cities* have already been discussed
earlier. Again, in the UK a raft of such initiatives is
being launched at the time of writing under such
names as *Health Action Zones* and *Healthy Living
Centres*. Their major concerns are to address
inequalities and achieve multi-sectoral action.
However, when we discussed evidence of the
effectiveness of *Healthy Cities* we observed that
progress in establishing structures for working, let
alone influencing, policies was typically slow and
complex.

We seem to need the kind of theory-based, systematic programme design that has been (successfully!) employed by the projects discussed above,
in order to generate sophisticated 'social' interventions that are centred on working with the
community, and having the support of broader
coalitions. Quite clearly, inter-sectoral working is
a *sine qua non* for such enterprises. Accordingly,
we will give some final consideration in this chapter to this task.

## INTER-SECTORAL WORKING

Inter-sectoral collaboration is necessary to achieve
effective coalitions and other alliances directed
towards the promotion of health. Drawing a clear
distinction between a coalition and a healthy
alliance is not easy and the terms are frequently
used interchangeably. Coalitions and alliances
involve people from more than one sector work-

ing together. The size and composition of these groupings can vary widely and this will impact on the ways that they are structured and operate. There are factors that apply broadly to inter-sectoral working and it is these on which we will focus. Many of the points may also apply to working across divisions within sectors and across professional groupings. Inter-sectoral/multi-sectoral partnerships have been defined as:

> *Relationships involving the sharing of power, work and/or support with others for the achievement of mutual and/or compatible objectives*
>
> (Ontario Ministry of Natural Resources, in Thompson and Stachenko, 1994)

and as:

> *the pooling of appreciations or tangible resources ... by two or more stakeholders, to solve a set of problems which neither can solve individually.*
>
> (Gray 1985)

There is a clear consensus that inter-sectoral action is necessary if health promotion goals are to be met. It has always been understood that health is the outcome of multiple influences operating at a number of levels but this was overlooked somewhat in the enthusiasm for modern medicine in the earlier part of this century. When the limitations, as well as the strengths, of modern medicine as a determinant of health began to be assessed critically by McKeown (1976) and others there was a return to recognising the multiple determinants of health and to assessing their relative contributions. The corollary of recognising multiple determinants is the necessity to work to secure health through action in all those sectors that have contributions to make. While different sectors make their individual and separate contributions to the promotion of health, advocating inter-sectoral action is built on the assumption that there is a synergistic effect from 'joined up' working. The promotion of inter-sectoral working has been included within key documents from the WHO from Alma Ata onwards and the statements contained are probably familiar to most readers.

The WHO (1996) discussion document is a typical one:

> *health promotion is multisectoral in scope and looks at all sectors of public policy in terms of their potential health creating resources. It builds on intersectoral collaboration in its development and implementation.*
>
> (WHO, 1986)

The idea of inter-sectoral collaboration has been accepted with enthusiasm and the importance of establishing and working through alliances is integral to the settings approach as discussed earlier. Sectors have, for a long time, interacted to varying degrees, although such activity would not typically have been defined as fully collaborative. The nature of these links is exemplified by Rowling and Jeffreys (2000) in discussing the development of health promoting schools:

> *the history of health service/schools links has tended to cast schools in the passive recipient role. The starting point for health workers is usually to see themselves as needing to have something to offer to schools, and neither they nor the school personnel often recognise the capacity of the schools themselves to contribute to the partnership.*

It has also been noted frequently in the literature, and it will also be the experience of many in health promotion, that advocating inter-sectoral action preceded any thorough analysis of how this can most effectively be achieved in the promotion of health.

Very many initiatives incorporating inter-sectoral action have been initiated and many have been less than satisfactory, both with relation to process and to the outcomes achieved, and have been insufficiently underpinned by theory. It was the view of Nutbeam (1994) in an editorial on inter-sectoral action that the evidence for the effectiveness of such partnerships was still rare. Following a literature review O'Neill *et al.* (1997) also concluded that the authors they drew on generally conceded that inter-sectoral work fails more often than it succeeds. They suggested that this was for two main reasons.

- Health-related professionals are used to operating in a very prestigious sector of society. They often approach other sectors, expecting them to 'buy in' to health-related issues without regard for how the health sector can support the legitimate agendas of other sectors.
- Recommendations for inter-sectoral health action are usually based on lessons derived from trial and error rather than on science.

Negative comment on current literature has been made by Light and Pillemer (in Butterfoss *et al.*, 1993), describing it as wisdom literature, largely anecdotal and tending to be based on experiences and impressions. We can, perhaps, take issue with these comments. There have been some careful case studies using qualitative research, undertaken rigorously, and these can often be as valuable, if not more so, for understanding alliances in action as 'scientific' research. We would not challenge the shortcomings of some of the lists of ways to make alliances work where these do not appear to be theory or research based. An editorial in the same issue as O'Neill *et al.*'s paper seemed to take a less pessimistic view:

> *Today health promotion faces a paradox in our understanding of intersectoral collaboration for health. These are the best of times because of the richness and quality of research and theory building that is occurring; but they are also the worst of times in that we are now beginning to grasp the real difficulties of the task.*
>
> (Sindall, 1997)

O'Neill *et al.* drew three main conclusions from their literature review of research on collaboration and organisational relationships:

- it was vital to move beyond the ideological statements and to conceptualise inter-sectoral action in terms of the (often selfish) interests pursued by individual or organisational actors;
- the relative power of actors interacting in inter-sectoral ventures is of paramount importance;
- the nature of the formal and especially the informal ties between the actors is also of central importance in shaping collaborative efforts.

A number of theoretical ideas have been identified as relevant to understanding the theory and practice of inter-sectoral working drawing on organisational theory, coalition theory and areas of social psychology and sociological theory. Theories have been reviewed (Gray 1985; Butterfoss *et al.*, 1993; Delaney, 1994a) and readers are referred to these for a full discussion. We will draw on theoretical ideas raised in reviews as we discuss the phases of inter-sectoral working and identify selected factors which, if applied, may increase effectiveness. We will comment on the composition of alliances, definition of tasks, barriers and drivers of inter-sectoral collaboration, benefits and costs to participants and outcomes. There will be some factors that are particularly relevant to some stages in a history of inter-sectoral action. Butterfoss *et al.*, drawing on innovation literature, say:

1 each stage in the development of a programme may need a different set of strategies;
2 the strategies which apply to one stage may be counterproductive at the next;
3 strategies should be contoured to a programme's stage of development.

(Goodman and Steckler, 1990)

### Initiating inter-sectoral collaboration and establishing direction

Alliances may be newly created but in other cases they are developments built on the basis of some existing interaction. A number of factors can stimulate the formation of an alliance. Policies which recommend closer working together of sectors are an important factor. For example, recent health strategy documents in the UK have promoted the formation of alliances beginning with *Health of the Nation* in 1992. *Saving Lives: Our Healthier Nation* (1999) describes partnerships where organisations and people work together to improve health overall as one of the two main ways through which it will achieve health goals. Moves to inter-sectoral action may also come from recognition of issues at community level, for example in the context of *Healthy Cities* developments or the UK *Health Action Zone* developments. On occasions situations arise which provide the stimulus for people to come together, while at other times what has started as an informal collaboration develops into a more formal one. A large amount of inter-sectoral working occurs because it is required or, alternatively, because it is acknowledged that getting a job done properly is most likely to happen if sectors collaborate. A number of other factors stimulate alliance formation:

- there is a vision about the subject in question;
- positive attitudes towards coordination;
- recognition of a mutual need;
- resource scarcity;
- failure of existing efforts to address a problem;
- compatibility among organisatons and capacity to maintain linkages;
- an effective or motivated catalyst;
- previous history of collaboration.

From a review of the effectiveness of alliances and partnerships for health promotion and the examination of case studies from all over the world Gillies (1998) described the structure of alliances as including the sectors of health, education, social welfare, environment, transport, tourism and employment and they spanned public, private and non-governmental agencies. At the same time some professionals in some sectors are more highly involved in alliances. Scriven (1995), from a survey of specialist health promoters in England and Wales, reported that they were highly active in initiating and managing collaborative initiatives with 98% of health promotion units having alliances in place with the education sector. The education sector played the less active role in alliance maintenance. The composition of alliances in health promotion will differ in part in relation to the specific focus of work. Whether the health sector is or should invariably be involved is a subject for debate. Gillies (1998) concluded from her review of alliances that the stronger the representation of the community and the greater the community involvement in the practical activity of health promotion alliances the greater the impact and the more sustainable the gain.

A critical mass is needed to achieve the goals of a respective alliance together with a group composition that incorporates the necessary skills mix. People bring differing skills and interests to alliances and this pooling of the assets partners bring is a significant factor when resources are limited. An important factor is not to exclude from alliances those people and sectors that have a legitimate contribution to the work of a specific alliance. A case in point, noted in an earlier chapter, is the importance of involving young people in the *National Healthy Award Scheme*, designed to encourage the development of *Healthy Schools* through establishing and consolidating partnerships (Aggleton *et al.*, 2000). They reported that partnerships worked best when they included a wide range of stakeholders while respecting each other's priorities.

Once an alliance is initiated the development of a consensus about the reasons for working inter-sectorally is necessary, plus agreement about the ways that inter-sectoral action will facilitate the work. According to Walker (1992), understanding the defining ideas that inform the organisations of interest is important:

> *A defining idea is widely accepted as carrying meanings and values around which actors can rally, and share a broad consensus despite variations in specifics. It serves as a focus, drawing in areas from other aspects of a culture.*

Some of the rather diffuse goals of health promotion are not always easy to communicate to alliance partners who may not be fully familiar with health promotion concepts and understandings can differ according to sector. Taking the time to identify and explore understandings at the early stage can prevent many subsequent difficulties in alliance working. Butterfoss *et al.* (1993) noted that a common error in efforts to build inter-sectoral partnerships is the definition of the problem only from the health sector perspective and the failure to recognise the legitimate interests of all the partners in joint activity. Not surprisingly, he says, potential partners often react to this health imperialism by withdrawing to find other ways to pursue their interests. Finding the common ground of interest between health and other sectors inevitably involves negotiation, compromise and continuous appraisal of the common ground. Equally as important as developing common purpose in coming together is being clear about what falls outside the purpose of the collaboration.

A number of writers point to the importance of a clear definition of the issues and a guiding purpose at the outset of a project. There is evidence that, in general, the more focused the problem the better the chances of engaging others in solving it (Nutbeam, 1994). It is interesting to note that the pilot health promoting hospitals project had participating hospitals building up work, in collaboration, around general aims and five or more specific sub-projects. Having a shared goal links with the idea of a shared vision. This was a theme which emerged from a study of inter-sectoral working towards *Health For All* in two English towns (Delaney *et al.*, 1993; Delaney, 1994b). A substantial proportion of the 41 people interviewed identified the key role of 'shared vision' in motivating organisations, or groups of health workers, to collaborate. This was articulated by a senior health officer who identified the significance of attempts to create a shared vision of what health is about while recognising that every agency will have its own priorities stated that:

> *they also need to feel that they are part of a broad thrust towards a vision of health which is holistic in nature and which is focusing on the important themes of* Health For All.

## Maintaining the process and achieving tasks

At some point in the early phase of working together the processes of how the alliance will work have to be established. The cultures of working in different sectors can vary significantly and some accommodation may be needed by all parties if the spirit of alliance working is to be honoured. It has been observed that alliances can often be dominated by certain partners and their preferred ways of working become the ones which are adopted. (Hawe and Stickney, 1997). Where coming together is in the interest of pursuing longer term organisational linkages time may more easily be found for exploring such cultural differences at the start of working together more closely. In other situations, and some of the coalitions discussed earlier are cases in point, the alliance is initially set up for a particular period of time and there may be pressures to progress tasks rapidly, thus making it difficult for sufficient attention to be given to matters of process.

Indicating an exit point at the start of activity has been discussed as a significant isssue since people are not usually willing to commit to long-term open ended programmes This is not to overlook the fact that some coalitions and alliances may be set up for long-term action and may become 'institutionalised' McLeroy *et al.* (1994), referring specifically to coalitions, said that relatively little attention had been given to how coalitions terminate and the effects of termination on participating organisations They asked if communities can plan for coalition termination. It would be helpful, they proposed, to study the termination phase of coalitions and develop guidelines on this.

This takes us on to consider the degree of formalisation within coalitions and alliances and the impact this has on their functioning. Some coalitions are highly structured and may operate formally while small community-based alliances are much less so.

Butterfoss *et al.* (1993) concluded that the evidence was mixed on the relationship between the degree of formalisation and successful collaboration. An aspect of formalisation is the issue of leadership. We can ask to what extent alliances should be equal collaborative partnerships with no clearly defined leader and characterised by revolving of responsibilities in relation to the particular tasks in hand. Alternatively, should there be a clear leadership function and a leader who can command respect and can build and maintain partnerships and act as a catalyst for action? The response is to a considerable degree determined by the size and nature of the coalition or alliance. Leadership roles can, of course, change as issues develop and knowing when leadership might usefully rotate is necessary to effective functioning. It has been proposed that alliances dealing with complex ongoing problems require management of interactions between parties, although reallocation of power and responsibilities may change over time (McCann, in Hawe and Stickney, 1995).

Irrespective of the structure of an alliance people will play particular roles, whether or not these are designated formally. The roles that people play in alliances have been examined and the importance of delineating roles and responsibilties and ensuring that each partner is employed in tasks which match skills and interests has been assessed. Role clarity was assessed in Rogers *et al.*'s (1993) study of a coalition to develop a tobacco control plan. Clarity of role was not, it transpired, correlated with any of the intermediary measures of coalition effectiveness. More generally, the relative contributions of members within a collaboration will differ. Contributions can be related to individual style, individual skills, the sector from which a person comes and the centrality of this sector within an alliance. Some members are more attracted to the networking side of a project and others to decision making aspects. The balance between task and process within alliances has been studied (Costongs and Springett, 1997). They emphasised the importance of creating arenas for dialogue so *that people really get to know each other, appreciate each other's roles, exchange values and learn from each other.* Short-term actions can be important in motivating an alliance towards its ultimate goal.

The way that planning takes place in alliances can have implications for satisfaction with the process. Drawing on data from the study mentioned above, Hawe and Stickney pointed out that traditional health promotion planning methods do not have immediate appeal to those outside health promotion. The fact that this model was allowed to dominate in their evaluation of a food policy coalition could have been challenged.

The ongoing processes in the group are important, including the readiness of partners to understand other sectors and to make allowances as and when necessary. Misunderstandings and stereotypes can be held about other sectors. The safe-

guarding of professional territories has also long been recognised. St Leger (1997) noted the mutual stereotypes held by general practitioners and teachers which may explain why partnerships between health and education have been superficial. In addition, stakeholders from one sector may not appreciate the best ways of establishing and sustaining productive inter-sectoral collaboration with other sectors.

Decision making is required in alliances and ways of making decisions need to be established, whether by majority rule or, as often preferred, by seeking consensus. At various points in the life of an alliance conflicts will arise and these require negotiation and resolution. Conflicts can arise for a number of reasons, which include the emergence of differences about task and process or process and perceptions of unequal contributions to an alliance. According to Brown (1984), conflicts generated during the decision making process can be energising, forcing *both sides to develop new options and new ways of working together*. Edelstein (in Butterfoss *et al.*, 1993) suggested several aspects of coalitions that can be useful in understanding the context in which conflicts emerge. These relate to whether the coalitions are voluntary versus required, reactive versus proactive, confrontational versus cooperative or built around consensus versus dissensus. The previous history of participation is also important.

The process of inter-sectoral working can be difficult and making progress does not necessarily happen quickly. The time that *Healthy Cities* developments have taken was noted earlier and similar observations have been made from health promoting schools and hospitals. Aggleton *et al.* (2000), in the study referred to earlier, said that there was evidence that funders and policy makers need to understand and allow for the long lead time that effective partnerships require. Without this there can be inappropriate expectations about what can be achieved within a particular time scale.

The benefits and also the costs of being involved in alliances and coalitions have been explored. There is fairly strong evidence that members will participate in coalitions only if ben-

475

efits (or potential benefits) outweigh the costs (Butterfoss *et al.*, 1993). A wide variety of benefits have been identified from projects and reported in the Butterfoss review.

### Benefits

- Increased networking, information sharing and access to resources;
- involvement in an important case and attaining the desired outcomes from a coalition's efforts;
- enjoyment of the coalition's work;
- receiving personal recognition;
- enhancing personal skills.

### Costs

- Devoting time to the coalition that is taken from other obligations;
- losing autonomy in shared decision making;
- expending scarce resources;
- overcoming an unfavourable image held by others;
- lacking leadership from the leadership or staff of a coalition;
- perceiving a lack or appreciation or recognition;
- becoming burnt out;
- lacking the necessary skills and feeling pressured for additional commitment.

### Outcomes

There are debates about the importance of process versus outcome achievements from alliances. Some literature emphasises the importance of early achievements which can have a number of positive effects: maintaining motivation; attracting attention to the coalition; enhancing its credibility. There is a danger that too much focus on short-term goals might detract from the long-term goal. We have earlier cautioned against developing prescriptive indicators for community programmes and there is a balance to be gained between such prescription and a general lack of direction. Indicators have been suggested and these can be useful guides, if modified as and when appropriate in evaluating a specific alliance. Those suggested by Speller and Funnell (1995) are listed below.

### Process

- Commitment;
- community participation;
- joint working;
- accountability.

### Output

- Policy change;
- service provision and environmental change;
- skills development;
- publicity;
- contact;
- knowledge, attitudes and behaviour change.

## Skills for inter-sectoral working and training

It is necessary to recognise the need for training as well as to identify the nature of such training. People bring many skills to inter-sectoral working but not necessarily all those that may be required. Those needed can include: general group work and communication skills, influencing skills, managing change, decision making; conflict resolution and organisational skills including meeting procedures. Reticulist skills have been identified earlier.

## Conclusion

Means *et al.* (1991) had this to say:

> *Few professionals would challenge the need for working together, collaborative initiatives, building relationships or joint working. And yet public policy is littered with examples of organisational disagreements about how best to concretise such statements of principle.*

There is a growing body of evidence that can be drawn on as well as the 'wisdom literature' referred to above. Some commentators are positive about the effectiveness of alliance working (Gillies, 1998) while others probably continue to share the reservations expressed earlier and call for more research. If, however, training for inter-sectoral working was increased and the competences from such training put into practice the effectiveness of inter-sectoral working could be enhanced.

# REFERENCES

Aggleton, P., Rivers, K., Mulvihill, C., Chase, E., Downie, A., Sinkler, P et al. (2000) Lessons learned: working towards the National Healthy School Standard. Health Education, 100 (3), 102–110.

Amezcua, C., McAlister, A., Ramirez, A. and Espinoza, R. (1990) A Su Salud: health promotion in a Mexican-American border community. In N. Bracht et al. (eds) Health Promotion at the Community Level. Sage, London< Uk.

Bandura, A. (1986) Social Foundations of Thought and Action: A Social Cognitive Theory. Prentice-Hall, Englewood Cliffs, NJ.

Blackburn, H. (1983) Research and demonstration projects in community cardiovascular disease prevention. Journal of Public Health Policy, 4, 398–421.

Blake, S. M., Jeffery, R. W., Finnegan, J. R., Crow, R. S., Pirie, P. L. et al. (1987) Process evaluation in a community-based physical activity campaign: the Minnesota Heart Health Program Experience. Health Education Research, 2 (2), 115–121.

Bracht, N. (Ed.) (1999) Health Promotion at the Community Level: New Advances. Sage, Thousand Oaks, CA.

Bracht, N. and Kingsbury, L. (1990) Community organization principles in health promotion: a five stage model. In N. Bracht et al. (Eds) Health Promotion at the Community Level. Sage, Newbury Park, CA.

Bracht, N. et al. (Eds) (1990) Health Promotion at the Community Level. Sage, Newbury Park, CA.

Bracht, N., Kingsbury, L. and Rissel, C. (1999) A five stage community organization model for health promotion: empowerment and partnership strategies. In N. Bracht (Ed.) Health Promotion at the Community Level: New Advances. Sage, Thousand Oaks, CA.

Brown, C. (1984) The Art of Coalition Building: a Guide for Community Leaders. The American Jewish Committee, New York, NY.

Butterfoss, F. D., Goodman, R. M. and Wandersman, A. (1993) Community coalitions for prevention and health promotion,. Health Education Research, 8 (3), 315–333.

Carlaw, R. W., Mittlemark, M. B., Bracht, N. and Luepker, R. (1984) Organization for a community cardiovascular health program: experiences from the Minnesota Heart Health Program. Health Education Quarterly, 11, 243–252.

Carleton, R. A., Lasater, T. M., Assaf, A. R., Feldman, H. A., McKinlay, S. and the Pawtucket Heart Health Program Writing Group (1995) The Pawtucket Heart Health Program: Community: changes in cardiovascular disease risk factors and projected disease risk. American Journal of Public Health, 85, 777–785.

Costongs, C. and Springett, J. (1997) Joint working and production of a City wide health plan: the Liverpool experience. Health Promotion International, 12 (1), 5–9.

Delaney, F. (1994a) Making connections: research into intersectoral collaboration. Health Education Journal, 53 (4), 474–485.

Delaney, F. (1994b) Muddling through the middle ground: theoretical concerns in intersectoral collaboration,. Health Promotion International, 9, 217–227.

Delaney, F., Cumming, M. and Tilford, S. (1993) Making Connections: Intersectoral Collaboration for Health. Health Education Unit, Leeds Metropolitan University, Leeds, UK.

Department of Health (1992) Health of the Nation. HMSO, London.

Department of Health (1999) Saving Lives: Our Healthier Nation. The Stationery Office, London.

Elder, J. P., McGraw, S. A., Abrams, D. B. et al. (1986) Organizational and community approaches to communitywide prevention of heart disease: the first two years of the Pawtucket Heart Health Program. Preventive Medicine, 15, 107–117.

Farquhar, J. W., Maccoby, N., Wood, P. D., Alexander, J. K., Breitrose, H. et al. (1977) Community education for cardiovascular health. Lancet, i, 1192–1195.

Farquhar, J. W., Fortmann, S. P., Wood, P. D. and Haskell, W. L. (1983) Community studies of cardiovascular disease prevention. In N. M. Kaplan et al. (eds) Prevention of Coronary Heart Disease: Practical Management of Risk Factors. W.B. Saunders, Philadelphia, PA.

Farquhar, J. W., Fortmann, S. P., Maccoby, N., Wood, P. D., Haskell, W. L. et al. (1984a) The Stanford Five City Project: an overview. In J. D. Matarazzo et al. (Eds) Behavioural Health: A Handbook of Health Education and Disease Prevention. John Wiley, New York, NY.

Farquhar, J. W., Maccoby, N. and Solomon, D. S. (1984b) Community applications of behavioural medicine. In W. D. Gentry (Ed.) Handbook of

*Behavioural Medicine*. Guildford Press, New York, NY.

Farquhar, J. W., Fortmann, S. P., Flora, J. A. *et al.* (1990) *Effects of communitywide education on cardiovascular risk factors: The Stanford Five City Project. Journal of the American Medical Association*, 264 (3), 359–365.

Funnell, R., Oldfield, K. and Speller, V. (1995) *Towards Healthier Alliances: A Tool for Planning, Evaluating and Developing Healthy Allliances*. The Wessex Insititue for Public Health Medicine, Health Education Authority, London, UK.

Gillies, P. (1998) *Effectiveness of alliances and partnerships for health promotion. Health Promotion International*, 13 (2), 99–120.

Goodman, R. M. and Steckler, A. (1990) *Mobilising organisations for health enhancement*. In Glanz, K., Lewis, F. M. and Rimer, B. K. (Eds) *Health Behaviour and Health Education: Theory, Research and Practice*. Jossey-Bass, San Francisco, CA.

Green, L. W. and Kreuter, M. (1999) *Health Promotion Planning: An Educational and Ecological Approach*, 3rd Edn. Mayfield, Mountain View, CA.

Haglund, B., Weisbrod, R. R. and Bracht, N. (1990) *Assessing the community, its services, needs, leadership, and readiness*. In N. Bracht *et al.* (Eds) *Health Promotion at the Community Level*. Sage, Newbury Park, CA.

Hawe, P. and Stickney, E. K. (1997) *Developing the effectiveness of an intersectoral policy coalition through formative evaluation. Health Education Research*, 12 (2), 213–225.

Holme, I., Hermann, M. D., Helgeland, A. and Leren, P. (1985) *The Oslo Study: diet and anti-smoking advice. Preventive Medicine*, 14, 279–292.

Hunkeler, E. F., Davis, E. M., McNeil, B., Powell, J. W. and Polen, M. R. (1990) *Richmond quits smoking: a minority community fights for health*. In N. Bracht *et al.* (Eds) *Health Promotion at the Community Level,*. Sage, Newbury Park, CA.

Jacobs, D. R., Luepker, R. V., Mittelmark, M. B., Folsom, M. B., Pirie, A. R. *et al.* (1986) *Community-wide prevention strategies: evaluation design of the Minnesota Heart Health Program. Journal of Chronic Diseases*, 39, 755–788.

Kanaaneh, H. A. K., Rabi, S. A. and Baderneh, S. M. (1976) *The eradication of a large scabies outbreak using community-wide health education. American Journal of Public Health*, 66, 564–567.

Kemper, D. W. and Mettler, M. (1990) *Building a*

*positive image of aging: the experience of a small American city*. In N. Bracht *et al.* (eds) *Health Promotion at the Community Level*. Sage, Newbury Park, CA.

Glasgow, R. E., Sorensen, G., Giffen, C., Shipley, R. H., Corbett, K. and Lynn, W. (1996) *Promoting worksite smoking control policies and actions: the Community Intervention Trial for Smoking Cessation (COMMIT) experience. Preventive Medicine*, 25, 186–194.

Klepp, K.-I., Ndeki, S. S., Thuen, F., Leshabari, M. T. and Seha, A. M. (1965) *Predictors of intention to be sexually active among Tanzanian school children. East African Medical Journal*, 73, 218–224.

Klepp, K.-I., Ndeki, S. S., Leshabari, M. T., Hannan, P. and Lyimo, B. A. (1997) *AIDS education in Tanzania: promoting risk reduction among primary school children. American Journal of Public Health*, 87, 1931–1936.

Klepp, K.-I., Masatu, M. C., Setel, P. W. and Lie, G. T. (1999) *Maintaining preventive health efforts in sub-saharan Africa: AIDS in Tanzania*. In N. Bracht (Ed.) *Health Promotion at the Community Level: New Advances*. Sage, Thousand Oaks, CA.

Koskela, K. (1981) *A Community Based Antismoking Programme as a Part of a Comprehensive Cardiovascular Programme (The North Karelia Project)*. University of Kuopio, Kuopio, Finland.

Lefebvre, R. C., Lasater, R. M., Carleton, R. A. and Peterson, G. (1987) *Theory and delivery of health programming in the community: the Pawtucket Heart Health Program. Preventive Medicine*, 16, 80–95.

Leventhal, H., Cleary, P. D., Safer, M. A. and Gutmann, M. (1980) *Cardiovascular risk modification by community-based programs for lifestyle change: comments on the Stanford study. Journal of Consulting and Clinical Psychology*, 48, 150–158.

Luepker, R. V., Murray, D. M., Jacobs, D. R., Mittelmark, M. B., Bracht, N. *et al.* (1994) *Community education for cardiovascular disease prevention: risk factor changes in the Minnesota Heart Health Program. American Journal of Public Health*, 84, 1383–1393.

Luepker, R. V., Rastam, L., Hannan, P. J., Murray, D. M., Gray, C. *et al.* (1996) *Community education for cardiovascular disease prevention: Morbidity and mortality results from the Minnesota Heart Health Program. American Journal of Epidemiology*, 144, 351–362.

Maccoby, N. and Farquhar, J. W. (1975) *Communication for health – unselling heart disease. Journal of Communications*, 25, 114–126.

Maccoby, N. and Solomon, D. (1981) *Experiments in risk reduction through community health education*. In M. Meyer (ed.) *Health Education by Television and Radio*. K.G. Saur, Munchen, Germany.

McAlister, A., Puska, P., Salonen, J., Tuomilehto, J. and Koskela, K. *et al.* (1982) *Theory and action for health promotion: illustrations from the North Karelia Project. American Journal of Public Health*, 72, 43–55.

McKeown, T. (1976) *The Role of Medicine*. Provincial Hospitals Trust, London, UK.

McLeroy, K. M., Kegler, M., Steckler, A., Burdine, J. M. and Wisotzky, M. (1994) *Community coalitions for health promotion: summary and further reflections. Health Education Research*, 9 (1), 1–12.

Maeland, J. G. and Haglund, B. J. A. (1999) *Health promotion developments in the Nordic and related countries*. In N. Bracht (Ed.) *Health Promotion at the Community Level: New Advances*, 2nd Ed. Sage, Thousand Oaks, CA.

Means, R., Harrison, L., Jeffe, S. S., and Smith, R. (1991) *Co-ordination, collaboration and health promotion: lessons and issues from an alcohol education programme. Health Promotion International*, 6 (1), 31–40.

Meyer, A. J., Maccoby, N. and Farquhar, J. W. (1980) *Reply to Kasl and Leventhal et al. Journal of Consulting and Clinical Psychology*, 48, 159–163.

Mittelmark, M. B., Luepker, R. V., Jacobs, D. R. *et al.* (1986) *Community-wide prevention of cardiovascular disease: education strategies of the Minnesota Heart Health Program. Preventive Medicine*, 15, 1–7.

Mittelmark, M. B. (1999) *Health promotion at the community-wide level: lessons from diverse perspectives*. In N. Bracht (Ed.) *Health Promotion at the Community Level: New Advances*. Sage, Thousand Oaks, CA.

Murray, D. M., Luepker, R. V., Pirie, P. L., Grimm, R. H., Bloom, R. E. *et al.* (1986) *Systematic risk factor screening and education: a community wide approach to prevention of CHD. Preventive Medicine*, 15 (6), 661–672.

National Forum for Coronary Heart Disease Prevention (1988) *Coronary Heart Disease Prevention: Action in the UK 1984–1987*. Health Education Authority, London, UK.

Neittaanmaki, L., Koskela, K., Puska, P. and McAlister, A. L. (1980) *The role of lay workers in community health education: experiences of the North Karelia Project. Scandinavian Journal of Social Medicine*, 8, 1–7.

Nix, H. L. (1970) *The Community and Its Involvement in the Study Planning Action Process*. US Department of Health, Education and Welfare, Atlanta, GA.

Nutbeam, D. (1994) *Intersectoral action for health: making it work. Health Promotion International*, 9 (3), 143–144.

Oliver, M. F. (1987) *Letter to the Editor. Lancet*, ii, 518.

O'Neill, M., Lemieux, V., Groleau, G., Fortin, J. P. and Lamarche, P. A. (1997) *Coalition theory as a framework for understanding and supplementing intersectoral health related intervention. Health Promotion International*, 12 (1), 79–87.

Pancer, S. M. and Nelson, G. (1990) *Community-based approaches to health promotion: guide-lines for community mobilization. International Quarterly of Community Health Education*, 10 (2), 91–111.

Perry, C. L. Griffin, G. and Murray, D. M. (1985a) *Assessing needs for youth health promotion. Preventive Medicine*, 14, 379–393.

Perry, C. L., Mullis, R. M. and Maile, M. C. (1985b) *Modifying the eating behaviour of young children. Journal of School Health*, 55, 399–402.

Perry, C. L., Williams, C. L., Veblen-Mortenson, S., Toomey, T., Komro, K. A. *et al.* (1996) *Outcomes of a community-wide alcohol use prevention program during early adolescence: Project Northland. American Journal of Public Health*, 86 (7), 956–965.

Pietinen, P., Vartiainen, E., Korhonen, H. J. *et al.* (1989) *Nutrition as a component in community control of cardiovascular disease (The North Karelia Project). American Journal of Clinical Nutrition*, 49, 1017–1024.

Puska, P. (1995a) *General discussion, recommendations, and conclusion*. In P. Puska, J. Tuomilehto, A. Nissinen, and E. Vartiainen (Eds) *The North Karelia Project: 20 Year Results and Experiences*, pp. 345–356. National Public Health Institute, Helsinki, Finland.

Puska, P. (1995b) *Main outline of the North Karelia Project*. In P. Puska, J. Tuomilehto, A. Nissinen and

E. Vartiainen (Eds) *The North Karelia Project: 20 Year Results and Experiences*, pp. 23–30. National Public Health Institute, Helsinki, Finland.

Puska, P., Vienda, P., Kottke, T. E. *et al.* (1981) *Health knowledge and community prevention of coronary heart disease. International Journal of Health Education*, XXIV (supplement).

Puska, P., Nissinen, A., Tuomilehto, J., Salonen, J. T., Koskela, K. *et al.* (1985) *The community-based strategy to prevent coronary heart disease: conclusions from the ten years of the North Karelia Project. Annual Review of Public Health*, 6, 147–193.

Puska, P., Koskela, K., McAlister, A. *et al.* (1986) *Use of lay opinion leaders to promote diffusion of health innovations in a community programme: lessons learned from the North Karelia Project. Bulletin of the World Health Organization*, 64, 437–446.

Puska, P., Tuomilehto, J., Nissinen, A. *et al.* (1989) *The North Karelia Project: 15 years of community-based prevention of coronary heart disease. Annals of Medicine*, 21, 169–173.

Rogers, T., Howard-Pitney, B., Feighery, E. C. Altman, D. G. *et al.* (1993) *Charaacteristics and participant perceptions of tobacco control coalitions in California. Health Education Research*, 8 (3), 345–357.

Rose, G. (1992) *The Strategy of Preventive Medicine*. Oxford University Press, Oxford, UK.

Rothman, J. (1979) *Three models of community organization in practice*. In F. Cox *et al.* (Eds) *Strategies of Community Organization*. F.E. Peacock, Chicago, IL.

Rowling, L. and Jeffreys, V. (2000) *Challenges in the development and monitoring of Health Promoting Schools. Health Education*, 100 (3), 117–123.

Salonen, J. T. (1987) *Did the North Karelia Project reduce coronary mortality? Letter to the Editor. Lancet*, ii, 269.

Salonen, J. T., Hamynen, H. and Heinonen, O. P. (Uundated) *Impact of a Health Education Programme and Other Factors on Stopping Smoking after Heart Attack*. Mimeograph, University of Kuopio, Kuopio, Finland.

Salonen, J. T., Puska, P., Kottke, T. E. *et al.* (1983) *Decline in mortality from coronary heart disease in Finland from 1969 to 1979. British Medical Journal*, 286, 1857–1860.

Sayegh, J. and Green, L. W. (1976) *Family planning education: programme design, training component and cost effectiveness. International Journal of Health Education*, 19 (supplement).

Schelp, L. (1987) *Community intervention and changes in accident pattern in a rural Swedish municipality. Health Promotion*, 2, 109–125.

Scriven, A. (1995) *Healthy alliances between health promotion and education: the results of a national audit. Health Education Journal*, 54, 176–185.

Schwartz, J. L. (1987) *Smoking Cessation Methods: The United States and Canada, 1978–1985*, pp. 62–71. US Department of Health and Human Services, Washington, DC.

Sheffield Health Promotion Unit (undated) *Healthy Sheffield 2000: Health Promotion Programme Strategic Plan, 1990–1993*. Programme Steering Group, Sheffield Health Promotion Unit, Sheffield, UK.

Sindall, C. (1997) *Intersectoral collaboration: the best of times, the worst of times. Health Promotion International*, 12 (1), 5–7.

St Leger, L. (1997) *Health promoting settings: from Ottawa to Jakarta. Health Promotion International*, 12 (2), 99–101.

Stunkard, A. J., Felix, R. J. and Cohen, R. Y. (1985) *Mobilizing a community to promote health: the Pennsylvania County Health Improvement Program (CHIP)*. In J. C. Rosen and L. J. Solomon (Eds) *Prevention in Health Psychology*. University Press of New England, Hanover, NH.

Susser, M. (1995) *Editorial: the tribulations of trials: intervention in communities. American Journal of Public Health*, 85, 156–158.

Tellness, G. (1985) *An evaluation of an injury prevention campaign in general practice in Norway. Family Practice*, 2, 9103.

Thompson, B., Lichtenstein, E., Corbett, K., Nettekoven, L. and Feng, A. (2000) *Durability of tobacco control efforts in the 22 Community Intervention Trial for Smoking Cessation (COMMIT) communities 2 years after the end of intervention. Health Education Research*, 15 (3), 353–366.

Thompson, P. R. and Stachenko, S. (1994) *Building and mobilising partnerships for health: a national strategy. Health Promotion International*, 9 (3), 211–215.

Tuomilehto, J., Geboers, J., Salonen, J. T. *et al.* (1986) *Decline in cardiovascular mortality in North Karelia and other parts of Finland. British Medical Journal*, 293, 1068–1071.

Vartiainen, E., Pallonen, V., McAlister, A. *et al.* (1983) *Effect of two years of educational intervention on* adolescent smoking (the North Karelian Youth Project). *Bulletin of the World Health Organization*, 61, 529–532.

Veblen-Mortensen, S., Rissel, C., Perry, C. L., Forster, J., Wolfson, M. and Finnegan, J. R. (1999) *Lessons learned from Project Northland: community organization in rural communities*. In N. Bracht (ed.) *Health Promotion at the Community Level: New Advances*, 2nd Edn. Sage, Thousand Oaks, CA.

Vincent, M. L., Clearie, A. F. and Schluchter, M. D. (1987) *Reducing adolescent pregnancy through school and community-based education. Journal of the American Medical Association*, 257 (24), 3382–3386.

Walker, R. (1992) *Inter-organisational linkages for community health. Health Promotion International*, 7 (4), 257–264.

Whittemore, A. A. and Buelow, J. R. (1999) *Health and health promotion in Latin America: a social change perspective*. In N. Bracht (Ed.) *Health Promotion at the Community Level: New Advances*, 2nd Edn. Sage, Thousand Oaks, CA.

Winkleby, M. A., Taylor, C. B., Jatulis, D. and Fortmann, S. P. (1996) *The long-term effects of a cardio-vascular disease prevention trial: The Stanford Five City Project. American Journal of Public Health*, 86 (12), 1773–1779.

Worden, J. K., Geller, B. M., McVety, J. S., Dorwaldt, A. L. and Lloyd, C. M. (1999) Community capacity for a breast screening program: the Lee County Experience (1991–1998). In N. Bracht (Ed.) *Health Promotion at the Community Level: New Advances*, 2nd Edn. Sage, Thousand Oaks, CA.

World Health Organization Collaborative Group (1970) *Multifactorial trial in the prevention of coronary heart disease. European Heart Journal*, 1, 73–79.

World Health Organization (1981) *Community Control of Cardiovascular Diseases: The North Karelia Project*. WHO European Regional Office, Copenhagen, Denmark.

World Health Organization (1983) *New Approaches to Health Education in Primary Health Care*, Technical Report Series 690. WHO, Geneva, Switzerland.

World Health Organization (1986) *Health Promotion: A Discussion Document*. WHO, Copenhagen, Denmark.

Ytterstadt, B. (1995) *The Harstad Injury Prevention Study: Hospital-based Injury Recording and Community-based Intervention*. Thesis, Institute of Community Medicine, University of Tromso, Tromso, Norway.

# Conclusions

The Introduction signalled the change in this edition towards a focus on health promotion rather than health education and the reasons for this were identified. Developments in health promotion since the last edition were also outlined. It is the purpose of this final chapter to bring together some of the conclusions we have drawn as a result of working on this edition and, as we did in the previous one, offer a few thoughts about future directions in the evaluation of the achievements of health promotion.

There are a few closing remarks that can be offered about the shift to health promotion. It will have been apparent that while health promotion has been the focus, we have continued to work with a model that sees this as including health education as a core component alongside healthy public policy. There is an impeccable logic for policy and environmental actions directed towards the development of health and we would argue, on most occasions, for these to be prioritised in health promotion. There are, however, limits on the extent to which health can be developed through political and environmental action alone. There are situations where policy cannot easily be developed or, where it can be developed, can have little immediate effect on health. The extent to which individual freedoms can and should be curtailed through policy and environmental action in the interests of securing community health is also a matter for continuing debate. The educational component of health promotion continues to be a vital part of the project to develop health. This education is a necessary support to policy and environmental action but traditionally has been heavily oriented towards individual health-related attributes and behaviours.

Although there appears to have been a significant increase in the extent to which the term health promotion is used throughout the world it is also clear that in very many countries health education functions remain the dominant activity and there is, as yet, relatively little attention to the full range of functions associated with holistic health promotion. This is partly because the thinking about health promotion is still being disseminated but it may also reflect the very great barriers to working on policy and related issues in some situations. The current global problem of HIV/AIDS serves to remind us of the continuing importance of health education. Reduction of the problem, as in any other aspect of health promotion, requires action on its underlying determinants but currently, and in the immediate future, health education actions directed towards individual behaviours can make some valuable contributions to the reduction in HIV levels. While such action is not the ultimate answer, failure to offer educational interventions could be seen as unethical and a failure to address the rights of individuals and communities.

In many countries where health promotion is well developed there are large numbers of people whose main focus of activity within it continues to be on the health education component. It would be perverse to marginalise a consideration of the effectiveness of health education actions while these continue to be a significant element of health promotion. For this reason, in reviewing effectiveness in selected settings we have given full consideration to health education alongside examining achievements in relation to health promotion as a whole. Prior to commenting on overall successes to date we will offer a few concluding comments on the processes of evaluation.

Throughout the book we have noted the debates about methodologies for conducting evaluation research. While these are clearly important in the academic development of a discipline and especially where this development is taking place rapidly the debates have equal importance for those concerned with health promotion in practice. The growing emphasis on evidence-based practice throughout health, education and other sectors has been noted in several chapters. There is good evidence from some countries, the UK offering a specific example, that health promoters are alive to the importance of evidence-based practice and committed to achieving it (South and Tilford, 2000). Decisions about the nature of evidence to be sought in health promotion and the methods by which it should be generated have to be made. The last few years have been characterised by active and, at times, polemical debate on these issues, with some resultant confusion. When such confusion exists this may deter practitioners from carrying out evaluation. Establishing areas of consensus about health promotion evaluation as well as acknowledging the areas of disagreement is important and we have noted that this is beginning to happen.

In this edition we have reported the accelerated production of reviews of existing evidence and especially of systematic reviews using procedures widely applied to assessing the effectiveness of health care interventions. A question at the start of this revision concerned the extent to which we should attempt to undertake systematic reviews of the evidence for the topics we were to consider. This would have been both unrealistic and inappropriate. Systematic reviews are extremely time consuming and could not have been undertaken for all areas. We might have confined our use of evidence to that which has already been systematically reviewed. Such evidence, however, would have been limited in that all areas of health promotion have yet to be reviewed and, further, because of the methodological criteria used for deciding on studies to be included in reviews. We would have been left in a situation of being unable to comment on many important areas of health promotion.

As readers will be aware, we have adopted a compromise position, drawing, for convenience, on systematic review evidence when available and in full acknowledgement of the limitations and strengths of reviews but complementing this evidence with that from other types of evaluation study. For those implacably opposed to the use of systematic review evidence we should not have drawn at all on such evidence. It can be argued, however, that the exclusion of systematic review evidence would have been inappropriate in that we are seeking to provide a commentary which would have value for the full range of potential readers. To the extent that recent systematic reviews are incorporating greater attention to the quality of interventions and the processes of their implementation in drawing up inclusion criteria the outcomes of reviews may become more acceptable to some who have hitherto expressed reservations. Those who fully reject the methodology of such reviews will not, of course, be persuaded by what may be seen largely as cosmetic changes.

There are many health promoters, possibly the majority in some contexts and sectors, who want the kind of evidence of success that is more easily generated from evaluations informed by an interpretivist methodology and would argue that this is the only way to approach evaluation of complex health promotion initiatives. Since complex interventions form an increasing proportion of health promotion activity the agreement of criteria for assessing the rigor of qualitative evaluations used in assessing their achievements are important. More compilations of evidence from such qualitative evaluations are also needed. In addition, we have noted the growing advocacy of realist and *Theory of Change* models of evaluation as appropriate ones for evaluating complex health promotion interventions (Pawson and Tilley, 1997; Wimbush and Watson, 2000).

In general, as we have noted throughout the text, there is growing support for pragmatism in selecting approaches to evaluation research. As will be fully apparent to readers, since health promotion includes a diversity of activities carried out in very different contexts the requirements for evidence of effectiveness and the methods for securing it will continue to be diverse. Sometimes quantitative evidence will be needed, sometimes qualitative and at other times a combination will seem best suited to answering research questions.

It will have been evident that the types of evidence of success which have been sought and the methodologies preferred for securing it, the extent of evaluation and the achievements reported differ between settings for reasons which have been discussed within individual chapters. A few observations can be made on the similarities and differences.

- In spite of the popularity of the health promoting settings concept and active developments of programmes to achieve such goals there are, to date, relatively few evaluations of settings which include full attention to all the key components, in contrast to attention to one or more specific elements of settings. Most commonly addressed are health education activities and the development and implementation of specific policies; those directed towards the prevention of smoking or the promotion of healthy eating are frequently reported.

- The sophistication of evaluation-related thinking and practice varies. For example, on the evidence of published literature, evaluation in school settings currently seems to be more developed than that in health promoting hospital settings.

- While there is rapidly growing support for the adoption of participatory styles of evaluation the importance attached to such styles varies between settings. For example, they are commonly, but by no means universally, seen as integral to evaluations of community development projects but are relatively rare in evaluation of interventions in health care settings. It is clear that in the period since the last edition there has been much more attention to facilitating stakeholder involvement in health promotion evaluations.

- Studies appropriate to inclusion in systematic reviews can be found in most settings but are much more likely to be generated in some than others. The systematic reviews evidence which is available also tends to originate from a relatively small number of countries, predominantly from the USA.

- Although certain approaches to evaluation are more likely to be adopted in specific settings

there is evidence of a growing preference, if both published and unpublished literature is considered, for studies which generate both quantitative and qualitative data and which are seen to provide a comprehensive evidence base for use in decision making about activities.

- Although there is nothing new in asserting the importance of building interventions on a sound theoretical basis, it is apparent that this continues to be under-emphasised in many studies, published as well as unpublished. Attention to theory has been rather more evident in some areas of school health education and some patient education interventions.

- If the published literature on evaluations is taken as a whole there appears to be a greater focus on some issues than others. Often these are health topics which are important in specific countries and which may feature in national health planning documents. In countries of the North prevention of smoking and the promotion of sexual health and nutritional health are extensively evaluated. By comparison, the promotion of mental health receives less attention. In the South it appears there is also attention to the evaluation of sexual health interventions and also to those concerned with the prevention of water-related and nutrition-related diseases and to malaria prevention. Overall, the amount of studies published from the South is small in volume.

- Within those topics that have been the subject of activity across most settings there are under-researched aspects. Except in community development, where activities are typically with groups experiencing inequalities, it is still relatively uncommon to find reported evaluations of interventions focused specifically on the reduction of health inequalities, or their intermediate indicators. In the literature as a whole we have also noted the relatively small proportion of reported interventions which have incorporated a gender differentiated approach, even in the prevention of smoking, where the literature on the influences on smoking behaviour indicates the significance of gender. Currently there is evidence, both from published studies and from other literature, that the issues of gender and ethnicity are beginning to be more actively addressed (Gabhainn and Kelleher, 2000; Gadin and Hammarstrom, 2000).

Although we support the adoption of settings approaches and there has been a proliferation of suggestions of places that can be defined as a setting, it is clear that, to date, work has been strongly focused on relatively few of these settings In the light of this it is important to identify those groups who may be excluded from health promotion activities. This point was raised at the end of the last edition and while there have been some welcome initiatives, there is still much to be accomplished. Groups that can be identified include homeless people, out of school children, refugees, especially where such people have been dispersed across geographical areas, minority groups, people with disabilities, nomadic communities and, in general, any people who are isolated from conventional settings. All these groups, and others not listed, typically experience poorer health. Equity considerations demand that these omissions be redressed.

There are two issues which were the subject of Chapter 2 and which merit some concluding comment after completing the reviews of evidence in the succeeding chapters: the nature of theory underpinning interventions and developments in indicators. In the last edition we identified the need for more use of theory derived from disciplines other than psychology, traditionally drawn on heavily in health education. There is evidence that welcome developments have occurred, perforce because health promotion, in contrast to health education, demands this shift. There has been an expanding use of sociological theory as well as that from other disciplines contributing to health promotion. A framework integrating theory from psychology and sociology and designed to inform sexual health interventions provides a good example of an extended theory base (Wight *et al.*, 1998). Nonetheless, in reported evaluations there is still a strong emphasis on the use of psychological theory and it will be a few more years

before the changes that are taking place on the ground and, in academic discussion, filter through fully into published evaluation reports.

The need for appropriate indicators to measure the conceptually complex outcomes of health promotion was discussed earlier in Chapter 2. What has become apparent is that there is growing recognition that careful consideration needs to be given to developing such measurements. For example, the renewed focus on community approaches has seen attention directed towards generating measures for assessing community capacity, community empowerment, community involvement and so on. Other complex outcomes requiring continuing work on measurement indicators, both qualitative and quantitative, include healthy alliances and coalitions, empowerment and the quality of interventions.

In commenting on successes as a whole we can do so with reference to the main elements of health promotion as presented in the *Ottawa Charter*. This categorisation has been disseminated widely and is also being adopted in countries of the South, where health promotion, in contrast to health education, has been slower to emerge. We do not wish to repeat earlier discussion but a few closing reflections may be useful as a preliminary to looking forward.

## BUILDING HEALTHY PUBLIC POLICY

In the documents which attain world wide dissemination, those from the WHO being key examples, the attention to the need for healthy public policy is strongly emphasised. The extent to which concerted international policy making has taken place differs according to the aspect of health. Smoking prevention offers a good example, with the current development of a Framework Convention planned for 2003 revealing many of the challenges to be addressed. Child poverty is a major determinant of health and although the need for global action to reduce such poverty is acknowledged, effective actions are slower to emerge. At the individual country level the significant shift in UK general health policy, which has the potential to lead to the development of health and to a reduction in health inequalities has been noted positively (Ziglio *et al.*, 2000). Within individual countries policies which are single sector ones are likely to be easier to develop and implement. Policies directed towards the development of health promoting schools offer a good example. Where policies directed towards specific health topics are concerned these typically require multi-sectoral action. Those sectors most committed to specific policies are not necessarily those with the greatest power in the policy development process.

## DEVELOPING PERSONAL SKILLS

This is the element of health promotion traditionally addressed through health education activities. It can be suggested that recent developments have mostly been in the amount of reported evaluation rather than the emergence of significant new evidence on effectiveness. Much evidence has also been brought together through systematic and other reviews and disseminated in accessible format. We have welcomed the activities designed to bring together evidence from studies from countries of the South where publication has often been more difficult to achieve and wider dissemination of study evidence has not regularly taken place.

We have commented, particularly with reference to schools' health education, on the extent to which interventions have been theory based and the nature of the theory used. Psychological theory has continued to dominate interventions but has been drawn on much more fully in some health topics than others. In the case of smoking prevention which, for a long time, has seen the use of sophisticated approaches there has been some shift of focus. The recognition of the difficulty of securing wide-scale adoption of these approaches which require careful teacher training and a commitment to fidelity of implementation and, furthermore, the limited impact of health education when not complemented by policy and environmental action has led to some reappraisal of classroom-based work.

A development which has progressed quite rapidly in some countries and some settings has been the increased emphasis on the identification of individual and community needs in making decisions about interventions to implement. Techniques involving rapid appraisal which were developed initially in countries of the South have been adopted widely and have facilitated this process. Where the full principles of health promotion are being adopted there is a commitment to working on felt and expressed needs. There is an obvious tension between this commitment and the growing pressures to implement evidence-based interventions which may not necessarily be in line with expressed needs. There are concerns that in some contexts pressures to implement evidence-based interventions will have a negative impact on health promotion practice.

## CREATING SUPPORTIVE ENVIRONMENTS

The extent to which the health promoting concept has been applied in totality has been referred to frequently in earlier chapters. In particular, we have noted that environmental action can be slower to achieve in some settings than actions which address general policy and health education. Some specific health areas are exceptions to this general observation. Smoking prevention provides an example where environmental actions have been implemented widely, with the result that 'no smoking' has become the norm in many settings and complemented by the removal of advertising in public places and other environmental actions designed to reduce access to tobacco products. Other examples of successes in creating supportive environments have been reported from the *Schools Water Action Programme* (Schreuder, 1997), creation of shady environments in the context of skin cancer prevention (Horsley *et al.*, 2000), healthier environments in workplaces (Price *et al.*, 2000), etc.

## STRENGTHENING COMMUNITY ACTION

In Chapter 9 we discussed the importance given to community involvement in securing the goals of primary health care. While this has often been in the context of achieving health gains in situations where resources from statutory and other sectors have been either unavailable or inadequate there has also been much commitment to the importance of participation as a right. In some countries, particularly some in Europe where there was for periods of time less commitment to community action, the last 5 years have seen what are important developments. The UK, the context in which this book has been written, is one where the national policies have brought back to centre stage the importance of community action, community development, increasing social inclusion, community empowerment and the development of social capital. This change has led to increased resources becoming available for community approaches and a real stimulus to thinking about ways of achieving and measuring successes. Reported evaluations from many of the innovative interventions currently being implemented are awaited with interest.

## REORIENTING HEALTH SERVICES

It has not been a major emphasis of this particular book to fully assess this element of health promotion action although we have examined the developments in attention to health promotion in primary care and health care settings. These developments may provide a proxy indicator for reorientation of services but it should be noted that the introduction of new activities can happen in the absence of any fundamental shift in thinking and in distribution of resources. The health promoting hospitals initiative is still in its early stages and it would be premature to conclude that any significant impact has been made on the nature and orientation of hospital activities. The implementation of primary health care world wide illustrates the problems in achieving reorientation (Mull, 1990). The UK changes in primary care do embody the potential for change in the desired direction and developments will be observed with interest.

Finally, what have we learned about effectiveness, efficiency and equity since the last edition? The extent and nature of achievements as well as the lack of some achievements should have become apparent in reading through earlier chapters. Effective activities have been reported in

each of the settings discussed and for a variety of health-related topic areas where evidence has been available. We have noted many areas where the knowledge base continues to be relatively under-developed. Efficient activities have also been reported but there continues to be less attention to efficiency in reported studies. The growing pressures to undertake evidence-based practice, especially in health care settings, has increasingly directed attention towards effective interventions and to those which are the more efficient ones. Such pressures are likely to continue, so efficiency concerns will need to be addressed even if they sit uncomfortably with some of the principles of health promotion. The achievement of equity and the reduction of health inequalities have become central concerns in health promotion and the new public health. Progress on the development and implementation of interventions and the evaluation of successes in achieving these goals has proceeded rather more slowly and progress differs markedly between and within countries. The UK *Health Action Zones*, mentioned at a number of places in this book, provide one specific example of innovation designed to make an impact on inequity and inequality. Resources have been focused both on geographical areas and on groups of people with greater need. The evaluations which are beginning to emerge will provide evidence on the extent to which interventions have demonstrated successes. While there is a very great deal to be achieved before health promotion can be judged to be highly successful, a recent statement by Raphael (2000) may be one to hold onto:

> *There can be no better argument for health promoters to justify their activities than to state that not only is health promotion an ethical and principled discipline but it is because of its values based approach that it is effective.*

## LOOKING FORWARD

There are a number of things that we expect to happen over the next years if current trends continue.

With reference to health promotion itself we may expect to see wider adoption globally of the activities associated with the term, especially in those countries where the predominant emphasis continues to be on health education. At the same time the links between health promotion and public health and health development will become clearer. With reference to the main activity areas of health promotion a steady expansion of policies at the international and national levels which fully address the promotion of individual and community health should be expected. Policies may be the general ones of education, health and social care as well as policies directed towards specific health issues. We will particularly look for policy actions which have the potential to create greater equity and contribute to a reduction in health inequalities. *The Acheson Report* (Acheson, 1998) in the UK made very many appropriate recommendations. With reference to the critical issue of enhancing health in early childhood, implementation of the *Sure Start* initiative incorporated in the *Saving Lives* document (Department of Health, 1999) is an important initiative. This programme provides support to parents and local communities, is targeted to areas of need and is designed to reduce inequalities in the early stages of life. In some countries advocacy for policy actions is already seen as central to the health promoter and public health roles. In other countries we will look for greater recognition of the need for such actions.

We can also look to the extension of the health promoting settings approach to settings not yet addressed and full attention to all the dimensions of a health promoting setting. Principles of equity need to be considered in settings developments and this has not always been the case to date. Settings developments have made steady progress and with the development of comprehensive indicators for assessing success similar to those being developed for health promoting schools the effectiveness and also the efficiency of these initiatives can be better assessed.

Achieving equity and redressing health inequalities has been registered as an important goal in WHO documentation and accepted as of great importance in many countries. Recognising the need for action is essential but has to be followed through with effective responses. Fuller understanding of the complexities of factors which generate inequities and health inequalities continues to be needed and appropriate interventions implemented. Achieving equity can only occur if this is given priority consideration at all stages of the health promotion planning process and there is a commitment to pursuing it and monitoring and evaluating the actions taken.

In the last chapter we discussed the development of healthy alliances and coalitions and noted the evidence of success in achieving these processes. Given the proportion of interventions designed to promote health which require multi-professional or multi-sectoral action, understanding of the best ways to achieve successes is important. As Ziglio (2000) has pointed out with reference to Europe:

> *current organisational, legislative and institutional mechanisms in the great majority of member states are not yet conducive to intersectoral action for the promotion and maintenance of health.*

Readiness to move towards inter-sectoral action will be a necessary precursor to implementing what is already known about effective actions. Moreover, as the contexts in which alliances are fostered continue to change further research to inform effective alliance building will be needed.

Theory developments and changes were noted in the Introduction. There is some evidence that there has recently been an increase in the emphasis on the importance of developing theory-based interventions. In those sectors of health promotion practice where theory has been less extensively used to date in underpinning practice we can expect to see some changes. Critical reviews of the health promotion theory base, both general and for specific theoretical concepts and models, are ongoing and reviews of areas not recently reviewed will be awaited with interest. Examples of recent reviews have included those of the *Transtheoretical Model of Change* (Whitelaw *et al.*, 2000) and of peer education approaches (Milburn, 1995; Turner and Shepherd, 1999).

Given the wealth of published literature and the need of professionals to be able to access evidence quickly and easily as a basis for determining practice, regular reviews of literature will continue to be needed. Such reviews will need to address the concerns raised by health promoters. The *Cochrane Public Health and Health Promotion Field*, which disseminates evidence of effectiveness of health promotion and public health interventions, is aware of concerns and is motivated to respond, either directly or through identifying other sources of evidence which complement Cochrane evidence.

In each of the previous editions we noted the need for more evidence in total, more evidence in relation to specific outcomes and their intermediate indicators and more evidence in relation to the aspects of health which had been relatively ignored. At the same time we included observations made by various people that we could achieve more if the currently available evidence were to be implemented. While there is a continuing need for evaluations there is no merit in unnecessary replications which could have been avoided if successful dissemination had occurred. This requires that evidence is available in formats and through processes that facilitate access and that people have the necessary skills and other resources to access the evidence and the motivation and resources to implement it. The last few years have seen a very great increase in the importance attached to dissemination processes not only in health promotion but throughout a number of sectors. There is growing evidence on the most effective ways of achieving dissemination and uptake of new ideas and we can look forward to an increase in the use of the existing acknowledge base (Effective Health Care, 1999).

In this edition we have reported on existing evidence and a great deal of this is health issue based, much of it from health education interventions informed by differing approaches. If we accept the definition that activities to be designated as health promotion should be enabling and empowering (MacDonald and Davies, 1998) then quite a number of the interventions included would not meet such a definition. Any future edition of this book would probably confine its attention to health promotion as described in a recent letter to the WHO Director General and leave considerations of health education except where it fitted an *Empowerment Model* to some other text:

> *When ... people are working on matters relevant to health, following a health promotion approach obligates them to encourage openness and participation, strive for the empowerment and autonomy of others, and hold equity and justice as the highest principles.*
>
> (Mittelmark *et al.*, 2001)

We give the last word to Ziglio *et al.* (2000) from their discussion of priorities for future action in health promotion:

> *Health promotion efforts are essential and must be intensified. These require an integrated approach able to link with, and influence social, economic and human development. There is a pressing need for ensuring that health promotion is positioned at the heart of (healthy) social and economic development.*

## REFERENCES

Acheson, D. (1998) *Independent Inquiry into Inequalities in Health*. The Stationery Office, London, UK.

Department of Health (1999) *Saving Lives: Our Healthier Nation,*. The Stationary Office, London, UK.

Effective Health Care (1999) *Getting Evidence into Practice*. NHS Centre for Reviews and Dissemination, York, UK.

Gabhainn, S. N. and Kelleher, C. C. (2000) *School health education and gender: an interactive effect*. *Health Education Research*, 15 (5), 591–602.

Gadin, K. G. and Hammarstrom, A. (2000) 'We won't let them keep us quiet...' gendered strategies in the negotiation of power—implications for pupils' health and school health promotion. *Health Promotion International*, 15 (4), 303–311.

Horsley, L.,Charlton, A. and Wiggett, C. (2000) *Current action for skin cancer reduction in English schools: a report on a survey carried out for the Department of Health. Health Education Research*, 15 (3), 249–259.

Macdonald, G. and Davies, J. (1998) *Reflection and vision: proving and improving the promotion of health*. In J. Davies, and G. Macdonald (Eds) *Quality, Evidence and Effectiveness in Health Promotion: Striving for Certainties*. Routledge, London, UK.

Milburn, K. ( 1995) *A critical review of peer education with young people with special reference to sexual health*. Health Education Research, 10, 407–420.

Mittelmark, M. *et al.* (2001) *Mexico conference on health promotion: open letter to WHO Director General, Dr Gro Harlem Brundtland. Health Promotion International*, 16 (1), 3–4.

Mull, J. D. (1990) *The primary care dialectic: history, rhetoric and reality*. In J. Coreil and J. D. Mull (Eds) *Anthropology and Health Care*. Westview Press, Oxford, UK.

Pawson, R. and Tilley, N. (1997) *Realistic Evaluation*. Sage, London, UK.

Price, G., Mackay, S. and Swinburn, B. (2000) *The Heartbeat Challenge programme: promoting healthy changes in New Zealand workplaces. Health Promotion International*, 15 (1), 49–55.

Raphael, D. (2000) *The question of evidence in health promotion. Health Promotion International*, 15 (4), 355–367.

Schreuder, D. R. (1997) *Issues of inequity , health and water: reflections on the schools water action programmes in post-apartheid South Africa. Health Education Research*, 12 (4), 461–468.

South, J. and Tilford, S. (2000) *Perceptions of research and evaluation in health promotion practice and influences on activity. Health Education Rresearch*, 15 (6), 729–741.

Turner, G. and Shepherd, J. (1999) *A method in search of a theory: peer education and health promotion. Health Education Research*, 14 (2), 235–248.

Wight, D., Abraham, C. and Scott, S. (1998) *Towards a psycho-social theoretical framework for sexual health promotion. Health Education Research*, 13 (3), 317–330.

Whitehead, M. (1991) *The concepts and principles of equity and health. Health Promotion International*, 6 (3), 217–228.

Whitelaw, S., Baldwin, S., Bunton, R. and Flynn, D. (2000) *The status of evidence and outcomes in Stages of Change research. Health Education Research*, 15 (6), 707–728.

Wimbush, E. and Watson, J. (2000) *An evaluation framework for health promotion: theory, quality and effectiveness. Evaluation*, 6 (3), 301–321.

Ziglio, E., Hagard, S. and Griffiths, J. (2000) *Health promotion developments in Europe: achievements and challenges. Health Promotion International*, 15 (2), 143–154.

# APPENDIX 1.1   HEALTH FOR ALL IN THE 21ST CENTURY: PRIMARY HEALTH CARE

## Primary health care (PHC): from Alma-Ata to the 21st century

### Keys to achieving HFA: lessons and progress

- PHC as an approach has provided impetus and energy to progress towards HFA.
- Some progress has been made in ensuring access to the original eight PHC elements.[1]
- PHC remains valid as the point of entry into a comprehensive health care system.
- Inter-sectoral action for health has not been fully achieved.
- Reorientation of health services and personnel to PHC principles remains elusive.
- Community participation takes time and dedication by all.

### HFA in the 21st century: policy objectives to reinforce the PHC approach

- Make health central to development and enhance prospects for inter-sectoral action.
- Combat poverty as a reflection of PHC's concern for social justice.
- Promote equity in access to health care.
- Build partnerships to include families, communities and their organisations.
- Reorient health systems towards promotion of health and prevention of disease.

### Sustainable health systems: some essential components

- Attach greater emphasis to comprehensive quality health care throughout the lifespan.
- Ensure equitable access to the original eight PHC elements.
- Expand PHC elements in response to identification of new threats to health, and opportunities to tackle these threats.

### Essential health system functions that complement and support PHC

- Provide sustainable financing for PHC.
- Invest in human and institutional capacity for health.
- Optimise private and public sector support for PHC through appropriate regulations.
- Strengthen research to support and advance PHC.
- Implement global, national and local surveillance and monitoring systems.

### Note

[1] The original PHC elements included, at least: immunisation against the major infectious diseases; education concerning prevailing health problems and the methods of identifying, preventing and controlling them; promotion of food supply and proper nutrition, an adequate supply of safe water and basic sanitation; maternal and child health care, including family planning; prevention and control of locally endemic diseases; appropriate treatment of common diseases and injuries; promotion of mental health; provision of essential drugs. These should be extended and adapted to include expanding options for immunisation; reproductive health needs; provision of essential technologies for health; health promotion, as defined in the Ottawa Charter and endorsed by resolution WHA42.44; prevention and control of non-communicable disease; food safety and provision of selected food supplements.

# APPENDIX 1.2 RESOLUTION OF THE *FIFTY-FIRST WORLD HEALTH ASSEMBLY* ON HEALTH PROMOTION

**FIFTY-FIRST WORLD HEALTH ASSEMBLY**  **WHA51.12**

Agenda item 20  16 May 1998

## Health promotion

The Fifty-first World Health Assembly,

Recalling resolution WHA42.44 on health promotion, public information and education for health and the outcome of the four international conferences on health promotion (Ottawa, 1986; Adelaide, Australia, 1988; Sundsvall, Sweden, 1991; Jakarta, 1997);

Recognizing that the Ottawa Charter for Health Promotion has been a worldwide source of guidance and inspiration for health promotion development through its five essential strategies to build healthy public policy, create supportive environments, strengthen community action, develop personal skills, and reorient health services;

Mindful of the clear evidence that: (a) comprehensive approaches that use combinations of the five strategies are the most effective; (b) certain settings offer practical opportunities for the implementation of comprehensive strategies, such as cities, islands, local communities, markets, schools, workplaces, and health services; (c) people have to be at the centre of health promotion action and decision-making processes if they are to be effective; (d) access to education and information is vital in achieving effective participation and the "empowerment" of people communities; (e) health promotion is a "key investment" and an essential element of health development;

Mindful of the new challenges and determinants of health and that new forms of action are needed to free the potential for health promotion in many sectors of society, among local communities, and within families, using an approach based on sound evidence;

Appreciating the potential of health promotion activities to act as a resource for societal development and that there is a clear need to break through traditional boundaries within government sectors, between governmental and nongovernmental organizations, and between the public and private sectors;

Noting the efforts made by the 10 countries with a population of over 100 million to promote the establishment of a network of most-populous countries for health promotion;

Confirming the priorities set out in the Jakarta Declaration for Health Promotion in the Twenty-first Century,

1.    URGES all Member States:

(1)   to promote social responsibility for health;

(2)   to increase investments for health development;

(3)  to consolidate and expand "partnerships for health";

(4)  to increase community capacity and "empower" the individual in matters of health;

(5)  to strengthen consideration of health requirements and promotion in all policies;

(6)  to adopt an evidence-based approach to health promotion policy and practice, using the full range of quantitative and qualitative methodologies;

2.  CALLS ON organizations of the United Nations system, intergovernmental and nongovernmental organizations and foundations, donors and the international community as a whole:

(1)  to mobilize Member States and assist them to implement these strategies;

(2)  to form global, regional and local health promotion networks;

3.  CALLS ON the Director-General:

(1)  to enhance the Organization's capacity with that of the Member States to foster the development of health-promoting cities, islands, local communities, markets, schools, workplaces, and health services;

(2)  to implement strategies for health promotion throughout the life span with particular attention to the vulnerable groups in order to decrease inequities in health;

4.  REQUESTS the Director-General:

(1)  to take the lead in establishing an alliance for global health promotion and in enabling Member States to implement the Jakarta Declaration and other local/regional declarations on health promotion;

(2)  to support the development of evidence-based health promotion policy and practice within the Organization;

(3)  to raise health promotion to the top priority list of WHO in order to support the development of health promotion within the Organization;

(4)  to report back to the 105th session of the Executive Board and to the Fifty-third World Health Assembly on the progress achieved.

# Appendix 1.3 Summary of the recommendations of the Independet Inquiry into Inequalities in Health (Acheson) Report

## General recommendations

1. We RECOMMEND that as part of health impact assessment, all policies likely to have a direct or indirect effect on health should be evaluated in terms of their impact on health inequalities, and should be formulated in such a way that by favouring the less well off they will, wherever possible, reduce such inequalities.

    1.1 We recommend establishing mechanisms to monitor inequalities in health and to evaluate the effectiveness of measures taken to reduce them.

    1.2 We recommend a review of data needs to improve the capacity to monitor inequalities in health and their determinants at a national and local level.

2. We RECOMMEND a high priority is given to policies aimed at improving health and reducing health inequalities in women of child-bearing age, expectant mothers and young children.

## Poverty, income, tax and benefits

3. We RECOMMEND policies which will further reduce income inequalities, and improve the living standards of households in receipt of social security benefits. Specifically:

    3.1 We recommend further reductions in poverty in women of child-bearing age, expectant mothers, young children and older people should be made by increasing benefits in cash or in kind to them.

    3.2 We recommend uprating of benefits and pensions according to principles which protect and, where possible, improve the standard of living of those who depend on them and which narrow the gap between their standard of living and average living standards.

    3.3 We recommend measures to increase the uptake of benefits in entitled groups.

We recommend further steps to increase employment opportunities (recommendation 8.1)

## Education

4. We RECOMMEND the provision of additional resources for schools serving children from less well off groups to enhance their educational achievement. The Revenue Support Grant formula and other funding mechanisms should be more strongly weighted to reflect need and socio-economic disadvantage.

5. We RECOMMEND the further development of high quality pre-school education so that it meets, in particular, the needs of disadvantaged families. We also recommend that the benefits of pre-school education to disadvantaged families are evaluated and, if necessary, additional resources are made available to support further development.

6. We RECOMMEND the further development of 'health promoting schools', initially focused on, but not limited to, disadvantaged communities.

7. We RECOMMEND further measures to improve the nutrition provided at school, including: the promotion of school food policies; the development of budgeting and cooking skills; the preservation of free school meals entitlement; the provision of free school fruit; the restriction of less healthy food.

## Employment

8. We RECOMMEND policies which improve the opportunities for work and which ameliorate the health consequences of unemployment. Specifically:

    8.1 We recommend further steps to increase employment opportunities.

    8.2 We recommend further investment in high quality training for young and long-term unemployed people.

We recommend policies which will further reduce income inequalities, and improve the living standards of households in receipt of social security benefits (recommendation 3).

We recommend an integrated policy for the provision of affordable, high quality day care and pre-school education with extra resources for disadvantaged communities (recommendation 21.1).

9. We RECOMMEND policies to improve the quality of jobs and reduce psychosocial work hazards. Specifically:

    9.1 We recommend employers, unions and relevant agencies take further measures to improve health through good management practices which lead to an increased level of control, variety and appropriate use of skills in the workforce.

    9.2 We recommend assessing the impact of employment policies on health and inequalities in health (see also recommendation 1).

## Housing and environment

10. We RECOMMEND policies which improve the availability of social housing for the less well off within a framework of environmental improvement, planning and design which takes into account social networks and access to goods and services.

11. We RECOMMEND policies which improve housing provision and access to health care for both officially and unofficially homeless people.

12. We RECOMMEND policies which aim to improve the quality of housing. Specifically:

    12.1 We recommend policies to improve insulation and heating systems in new and existing buildings in order to reduce further the prevalence of fuel poverty.

    12.2 We recommend amending housing and licensing conditions and housing regulations on space and amenity to reduce accidents in the home, including measures to promote the installation of smoke detectors in existing homes.

13. We RECOMMEND the development of policies to reduce the fear of crime and violence and to create a safe environment for people to live in.

We recommend policies which will further reduce income inequalities, and improve the living standards of households in receipt of social security benefits (recommendation 3).

## Mobility, transport and pollution

14. We RECOMMEND the further development of a high quality public transport system which is integrated with other forms of transport and is affordable to the user.

15. We RECOMMEND further measures to encourage walking and cycling as forms of transport and to ensure the safe separation of pedestrians and cyclists from motor vehicles.

16. We RECOMMEND further steps to reduce the usage of motor cars to cut the mortality and morbidity associated with motor vehicle emissions.

17. We RECOMMEND further measures to reduce traffic speed, by environmental design and modification of roads, lower speed limits in built up areas and stricter enforcement of speed limits.

18. We RECOMMEND concessionary fares should be available to pensioners and disadvantaged groups throughout the country and that local schemes should emulate high quality schemes, such as those of London and the West Midlands.

## Nutrition and the Common Agricultural Policy

19.   We RECOMMEND a comprehensive review of the Common Agricultural Policy (CAP)'s impact on health and inequalities in health.

   19.1   We recommend strengthening the CAP Surplus Food Scheme to improve the nutritional position of the less well off.

20.   We RECOMMEND policies which will increase the availability and accessibility of foodstuffs to supply an adequate and affordable diet. Specifically:

   20.1   We recommend the further development of policies which will ensure adequate retail provision of food to those who are disadvantaged.

We recommend policies which will further reduce income inequalities and improve the living standards of households in receipt of social security benefits (recommendation 3).

We recommend the further development of a high quality public transport system which is integrated with other forms of transport and is affordable to the user (recommendation 14).

   20.2   We recommend policies which reduce the sodium content of processed foods, particularly bread and cereals, and which do not incur additional cost to the consumer.

## Mothers, children and families

21.   We RECOMMEND policies which reduce poverty in families with children by promoting the material support of parents; by removing barriers to work for parents who wish to combine work with parenting; by enabling those who wish to devote full-time to parenting to do so. Specifically:

   21.1   We recommend an integrated policy for the provision of affordable, high quality day care and pre-school education with extra resources for disadvantaged communities (see also: recommendation 5).

We recommend further reductions in poverty in women of child-bearing age, expectant mothers, young children and older people should be made by

increasing benefits in cash or in kind to them (recommendation 3.1).

We recommend measures to increase the uptake of benefits in entitled groups (recommendation 3.3).

22.   We RECOMMEND policies which improve the health and nutrition of women of child-bearing age and their children with priority given to the elimination of food poverty and the prevention and reduction of obesity. Specifically:

We recommend further reductions in poverty in women of child-bearing age, expectant mothers, young children and older people should be made by increasing benefits in cash or in kind to them (recommendation 3.1).

We recommend further measures to improve the nutrition provided at school, including: the promotion of school food policies; the development of budgeting and cooking skills; the preservation of free school meals entitlement; the provision of free school fruit; the restriction of less healthy food (recommendation 7).

We recommend a comprehensive review of the Common Agricultural Policy (CAP)'s impact on health and inequalities in health (recommendation 19).

We recommend policies which will increase the availability and accessibility of foodstuffs to supply an adequate and affordable diet (recommendation 20).

   22.1   We recommend policies which increase the prevalence of breastfeeding.

   22.2   We recommend the fluoridation of the water supply.

   22.3   We recommend the further development of programmes to help women to give up smoking before or during pregnancy and which are focused on the less well off.

23.   We RECOMMEND policies that promote the social and emotional support for parents and children. Specifically:

   23.1   we recommend the further development of the role and capacity of health visitors to provide social and emotional support to expectant parents and parents with young children.

23.2 We recommend local authorities identify and address the physical and psychological health needs of looked-after children.

## Young people and adults of working age

We recommend policies which improve the opportunities for work and which ameliorate the health consequences of unemployment (recommendation 8).

We recommend policies to improve the quality of jobs and reduce psychosocial work hazards (recommendation 9)

24. We RECOMMEND measures to prevent suicide among young people, especially among young men and seriously mentally ill people.

25. We RECOMMEND policies which promote sexual health in young people and reduce unwanted teenage pregnancy, including access to appropriate contraceptive services.

26. We RECOMMEND policies which promote the adoption of healthier lifestyles, particularly in respect of factors which show a strong social gradient in prevalence or consequences. Specifically:

26.1 we recommend policies which promote moderate intensity exercise including: further provision of cycling and walking routes to school and other environmental modifications aimed at the safe separation of pedestrians and cyclists from motor vehicles; safer opportunities for leisure.

26.2 We recommend policies to reduce tobacco smoking including: restricting smoking in public places; abolishing tobacco advertising and promotion; community, mass media and educational initiatives.

26.3 We recommend increases in the real price of tobacco to discourage young people from becoming habitual smokers and to encourage adult smokers to quit. These increases should be introduced in tandem with policies to improve the living standards of low income households and polices to help smokers in these households become and remain ex-smokers.

26.4 We recommend making nicotine replacement therapy available on prescription.

26.5 We recommend policies which reduce alcohol-related ill health, accidents and violence, including measures which at least maintain the real cost of alcohol.

## Older people

27. We RECOMMEND policies which will promote the material well being of older people. Specifically:

We recommend policies which will further reduce income inequalities and improve the living standards of households in receipt of social security benefits (recommendation 3).

We recommend uprating of benefits and pensions according to principles which protect and, where possible, improve the standard of living of those who depend on them and which narrow the gap between their standard of living and average living standards (recommendation 3.2).

We recommend measures to increase the uptake of benefits among entitled groups (recommendation 3.3).

28. We RECOMMEND the quality of homes in which older people live be improved. Specifically:

We recommend policies to improve insulation and heating systems in new and existing buildings in order to reduce further the prevalence of fuel poverty (recommendation 12.1).

We recommend amending housing and licensing conditions and housing regulations on space and amenity to reduce accidents in the home, including measures to promote the installation of smoke detectors in existing homes (recommendation 12.2).

29. We RECOMMEND policies which will promote the maintenance of mobility, independence and social contacts. Specifically:

We recommend the development of policies to reduce the fear of crime and violence and to create a safe environment for people to live in (recommendation 13).

We recommend the further development of a high quality public transport system which is integrated with other forms of transport and is affordable to the user (recommendation 14).

We recommend concessionary fares should be available to pensioners and disadvantaged groups throughout the country and that local schemes should emulate high quality schemes, such as those of London and the West Midlands (recommendation 18).

30. We RECOMMEND the further development of health and social services for older people, so that these services are accessible and distributed according to need.

We recommend a review of data needs to improve the capacity to monitor inequalities in health and their determinants at a national and local level (recommendation 1.2).

## Ethnicity

31. We RECOMMEND that the needs of minority ethnic groups are specifically considered in the development and implementation of policies aimed at reducing socio-economic inequalities. Specifically:

We recommend policies which will further reduce income inequalities and improve the living standards of households in receipt of social security benefits (recommendation 3).

We recommend policies which improve the opportunities for work and which ameliorate the health consequences of unemployment (recommendation 8).

We recommend policies which improve the avail-
~~ social housing for the less well off within a
nvironmental improvement, plan-
which takes into account social net-
works and access to goods and services (recommendation 10).

We recommend policies which aim to improve the quality of housing (recommendation 12).

We recommend the development of policies to reduce the fear of crime and violence and to create a safe environment for people to live in (recommendation 13).

We recommend the further development of a high quality public transport system which is integrated with other forms of transport and is affordable to the user (recommendation 14).

We recommend further measures to encourage walking and cycling as forms of transport and to ensure the safe separation of pedestrians and cyclists from motor vehicles (recommendation 15).

We recommend further steps to reduce the usage of motor cars to cut the mortality and morbidity associated with motor vehicle emissions (recommendation 16).

We recommend further measures to reduce traffic speed, by environmental design and modification of roads, lower speed limits in built up areas and stricter enforcement of speed limits (recommendation 17).

We recommend concessionary fares should be available to pensioners and disadvantaged groups throughout the country and that local schemes should emulate high quality schemes, such as those of London and the West Midlands (recommendation 18).

32. We RECOMMEND the further development of services which are sensitive to the needs of minority ethnic people and which promote greater awareness of their health risks.

33. We RECOMMEND the needs of minority ethnic groups are specifically considered in needs assessment, resource allocation, health care planning and provision. Specifically:

We recommend a review of data needs to improve the capacity to monitor inequalities in health and their determinants at a national and local level (recommendation 1.2).

## Gender

34. We RECOMMEND policies which reduce the excess mortality from accidents and suicide in young men (see also recommendation 24). Specifically:

We recommend policies which improve the opportunities for work and which ameliorate the health consequences of unemployment (recommendation 8).

We recommend policies which improve housing provision and access to health care for both officially and unofficially homeless people (recommendation 11).

We recommend further measures to encourage walking and cycling as forms of transport and to ensure the safe separation of pedestrians and cyclists from motor vehicles (recommendation 15).

We recommend further steps to reduce the usage of motor cars to cut the mortality and morbidity associated with motor vehicle emissions (recommendation 16).

We recommend further measures to reduce traffic speed, by environmental design and modification of roads, lower speed limits in built up areas and stricter enforcement of speed limits (recommendation 17).

We recommend measures to prevent suicide among young people, especially among young men and seriously mentally ill people (recommendation 24).

We recommend policies which reduce alcohol-related ill health, accidents and violence, including measures which at least maintain the real cost of alcohol (recommendation 26.5).

35. We RECOMMEND policies which reduce psychosocial ill health in young women in disadvantaged circumstances, particularly those caring for young children. Specifically:

We recommend further reductions in poverty in women of child-bearing age, expectant mothers, young children and older people should be made by increasing benefits in cash or in kind to them (recommendation 3.1).

We recommend uprating of benefits and pensions according to principles which protect and, where possible, improve the standard of living of those who depend on them and which narrow the gap between their standard of living and average living standards (recommendation 3.2).

We recommend measures to increase the uptake of benefits among entitled groups (recommendation 3.3).

We recommend policies which improve the availability of social housing for the less well off within a framework of environmental improvement, planning and design which takes into account social networks and access to goods and services (recommendation 10).

We recommend the further development of a high quality public transport system which is integrated with other forms of transport and is affordable to the user (recommendation 14).

We recommend policies which will increase the availability and accessibility of foodstuffs to supply an adequate and affordable diet (recommendation 20).

We recommend policies which reduce poverty in families with children by promoting the material support of parents; by removing barriers to work for parents who wish to combine work with parenting; by enabling those who wish to devote full-time to parenting to do so (recommendation 21).

We recommend an integrated policy for the provision of affordable, high quality day care and pre-school education with extra resources for disadvantaged communities (recommendation 21.1).

We recommend policies which improve the health and nutrition of women of child-bearing age and their children with priority given to the elimination of food poverty and the prevention and reduction of obesity (recommendation 22).

We recommend policies which promote the social and emotional support for parents and children (recommendation 23).

We recommend the further development of the role and capacity of health visitors to provide social and emotional support to expectant parents and parents with young children (recommendation 23.1).

We recommend policies which promote sexual health in young people and reduce unwanted teenage pregnancy, including access to appropriate contraceptive services (recommendation 25).

36. We RECOMMEND policies which reduce disability and ameliorate its consequences in older women, particularly those living alone. Specifically:

We recommend further reductions in poverty in women of child-bearing age, expectant mothers, young children and older people should be made by increasing benefits in cash or in kind to them (recommendation 3.1).

We recommend uprating of benefits and pensions according to principles which protect and, where possible, improve the standard of living of those who depend on them and which narrow the gap between their standard of living and average living standards (recommendation 3.2).

We recommend measures to increase the uptake of benefits among entitled groups (recommendation 3.3).

We recommend the development of policies to reduce the fear of crime and violence and to create a safe environment for people to live in (recommendation 13).

We recommend the further development of a high quality public transport system which is integrated with other forms of transport and is affordable to the user (recommendation 14)

We recommend concessionary fares should be available to pensioners and disadvantaged groups throughout the country and that local schemes should emulate high quality schemes, such as those of London and the West Midlands (recommendation 18).

We recommend the quality of homes in which older people live be improved (recommendation 28).

We recommend the further development of health and social sevices for older people, so that these services are accessible and distributed according to need (recommendation 30).

## The National Health Service

37. We RECOMMEND that providing equitable access to effective care in relation to need should be a governing principle of all policies in the NHS. Priority should be given to the achievement of equity in the planning, implementation and delivery of services at every level of the NHS. Specifically:

    37.1 We recommend extending the focus of clinical governance to give equal prominence to equity of access to effective health care.

    37.2 We recommend extending the remit of the National Institute for Clinical Excellence to include equity of access to effective health care.

    37.3 We recommend developing the National Service Frameworks to address inequities in access to effective primary care.

    37.4 We recommend that performance management in relation to the national performance management framework is focused on achieving more equitable access, provision and targeting of effective services in relation to need in both primary and hospital sectors.

    37.5 We recommend that the Department of Health and NHS Executive set out their responsibilities for furthering the principle of equity of access to effective health and social care and that health authorities, working with Primary Care Groups and providers on local clinical governance, agree priorities and objectives for reducing inequities in access to effective care. These should form part of the Health Improvement Programme.

38. We RECOMMEND giving priority to the achievement of a more equitable allocation of NHS resources. This will require adjustments to the ways in which resources are allocated and the

speed with which resource allocation targets are met. Specifically:

38.1 We recommend reviewing the 'pace of change' policy to enable health authorities that are furthest from their capitation targets to move more quickly to their actual target.

38.2 We recommend extending the principle of needs-based weighting to non-cash limited General Medical Services (GMS) resources. The size and effectiveness of deprivation payments in meeting the needs and improving the health outcomes amongst the most disadvantaged populations, including ethnic minorities should be assessed.

38.3 We recommend reviewing the size and effectiveness of the Hospital and Community Health Service (HCHS) formula and deprivation payments in influencing the health care outcomes of the most disadvantaged populations and to consider alternative methods of focusing resources for health promotion and public health care to reduce health inequalities.

38.4 We recommend establishing a review of the relationship of private practice to the NHS with particular reference to access to effective treatments, resource allocation and availability of staff.

39. We RECOMMEND Directors of Public Health, working on behalf of health and local authorities, produce an equity profile for the population they serve and undertake a triennial audit of progress towards achieving objectives to reduce inequalities in health.

39.1 We recommend there should be a duty of partnership between the NHS Executive and regional government to ensure that effective local partnerships are established between health, local authorities and other agencies and that joint programmes to address health inequalities are in place and monitored.

We RECOMMEND that as part of health impact assessment, all policies likely to have a direct or indirect effect on health should be evaluated in terms of their impact on health inequalities and should be formulated in such a way that by favouring the less well off they will, wherever possible, reduce such inequalities (recommendation 1).

(After Department of Health, 1998; http://www.official-documents.co.uk/document/doh/ih/part 2k.htm). Crown copyright material is reproduced with the permission of the Controller of Her Majesty's Stationery Office.

# APPENDIX 1.4   UK GOVERNMENT POLICY INITIATIVES DESIGNED TO IMPACT ON TEENAGE PARENTHOOD

## Programmes which help prevent teenage parenthood

The UK's first government **strategy on sexual health** was launched earlier this year. Over the next year, the Government will work in partnership with health services, voluntary and community groups and pofessionals to develop a framework which will set a programme of action on sexual and reproductive health for all health authorities and local authorities in England. The framework will be published next year. (Lead department: Department of Health.)

The NHS will work with local authorities and other local partners to develop a **Health Improvement Programme** (HImP) to be in place by April 1999. The HImP will identify priorities to improve the health and health care of the local population. It may be appropriate to include teenage pregnancies and teenage parenthood as local priorities for action. (Lead department: Department of Health.)

The first wave of 11 **Health Action Zones** was announced in 1998 and a second wave of 15 HAZs in April 1999, targeting special efforts on areas of deprivation and high health need. They aim to reduce health inequalities and modernise services. Each HAZ has identified priorities within its area, which may include measures to prevent teenage parenthood and services for young parents. (Lead department: Department of Health.)

There are a number of new flexibilities which are being introduced into primary care. **Primary Care Groups** will, from April 1999, introduce increased accountability for primary care provision. There may be a need for targeted incentives to improve access for young people to contraceptive advice in primary care through, for example, appropriate training for GPs and their staff. (Lead department: Department of Health.)

**Sexwise** was established by the Department of Health in March 1995 as part of the Health of the Nation action towards reducing under 16 conception rates. It offers free, confidential telephone advice with the opportunity to talk to a trained adviser about sex and personal relationships and currently receives about 2,500 calls per day. Sexwise has proved very popular which means that a substantial number of callers are unable to get through. (Lead department: Department of Health.)

**NHS Direct** is a telephone advice line, staffed by nurses, which gives patients advice on how to look after themselves as welt as directing them to the right part of the NHS for treatment if they need further medical help. Originally available in three pilot areas, the advice line has now been extended and will be available across the country by the end of 2000. (Lead department: Department of Health.)

**The Quality Protects** programme and other associated initiatives will improve the outcomes far looked-after children in particular and children in need generally and are likely to lead to lower teenage conception rates among this group. The programme will be delivered by local authorities who were asked to submit their action plans to the Department of Health by January 1999. (Lead department: Department of Health.)

The **Healthy Living Centres** initiative was launched at the end of January 1999 by the New Opportunities Fund. This initiative will receive £300 million from Lottery Funds to target the most deprived sections of the population in order to reduce health inequalities and improve the health of the worst-off in society, by 2002. It will be flexible enough to allow for innovative proposals and the different needs of each community, with local key players working in partnership. The type of projects which might be funded could include reproductive health groups and parenting classes. (Lead department: Department of Health.)

**Education Action Zones** are local clusters of schools – usually a mix of not more than 20 primary, secondary and special schools – working in partnership with the local education authority, parents, business, TECs and others. The partnership will encourage innovative approaches to tackling disadvantage and raising standards. (Lead department: Department for Education and Employment.)

## Measures which help teenage parents continue with their education

**New start** aims to motivate and re-engage 14–17 year olds who have dropped out of learning or who are at risk of doing so. At its heart is a multi-agency partnership working at local level. Young people needing extra help in difficult circumstances, including teenage parents, are being targeted by local partnerships in order to bring them back into learning. Funds have been made available to develop New Start activity throughout the country during 1999–2000. (Lead department: Department for Education and Employment.)

As part of the **Excellence in Cities** initiative, to be piloted in six targeted urban areas from September 1999, each secondary school pupil who needs one will have access to a Learning Mentor. The mentors will be based in schools and professionally trained. They will be responsible for making sure that barriers to individuals' learning – in school or outside school are removed by drawing up individual action plans for each child who needs support and having regular contact with pupils and their families. Learning Mentors will have a specific remit in relation to teenage parents. They will liaise with feeder primary schools to identify vulnerable or disaffected pupils who would benefit from targeted help, as well as helping young mothers to return to school and re-engage in education after the birth of their child. They should act as a support mechanism and link

to social services for teenage parents. (Lead department: Department for Education and Employment.)

Pilots for a new **Education Maintenance Allowance** (EMA) will test the effectiveness of a weekly allowance, payable in term time, in increasing participation and achievement in education by 16–19 year olds. The allowance will be available to those who are parents and who live on their own, as well as those who live with low income families. Up to £40 a week will be paid to low income young people in some parts of England to encourage them to stay on in full time education at school or college. The pilots will operate in 15 local education authority areas across the country. If the pilots are successful, then the Government will consider the introduction of EMAs nationally. (Lead department: Department for Education and Employment.)

New national **Student Support** arrangements for post 16s will be introduced from September 1999. Increased access funds will help students with the costs of further education such as transport books and fees. Colleges will also receive more funding for help with child care costs. (Lead department: Department for Education and Employment.) The **Further Education Funding Council** provides funding to allow colleges to provide free child care to students – mostly those in receipt of income-related benefits. (Lead department: Department for Education and Employment.)

## Measures to help teenage parents prepare for work and help with finding work

With resources of £190m, the **New Deal for Lone Parents** (NDLP) offers a personal advisor service delivering a comprehensive package of advice and support on searching for a job, training and child care opportunities tailored to meet the needs of individual lone parents. It is aimed at lone parents whose youngest child is of school age, but parents of younger children are welcome to join. The NDLP can help with child care and travel costs for those who participate in training or attend job interviews, whilst assistance to cover training fees may also be awarded. (Lead departments: Department for Education and Employment, Department of Social Security.)

The **New Deal for Communities** (NDC) designed to tackle multiple deprivation in the very poorest neighbours. It aims to offer people the opportunity of real and lasting change by improving job prospects; bringing together investment in buildings and investment in people; and through better neighbourhood management and delivery of local services. NDC has resources of £800 million over the next three years to support this programme which aims to bring together local people, community and voluntary organisations, public agencies, local authorities and business in an intensive local focus to tackle the problems inherent to these neighbourhoods. Seventeen local authority districts have been selected as eligible Pathfinder Areas, because their problems are very severe, and are now developing their local programmes. More areas will be included in the programme in later years. (Lead department: Department of the Environment, Transport and the Regions.)

The **New Deal for 18–24 year olds** aims to help young people who have been unemployed and claiming Jobseekers' Allowance for six months or more to find work and to improve their prospects of staying in work. Local partnerships will work together to bring down levels of long-term unemployment and to improve the employability of young people in each area. (Lead department: Department for Education and Employment.)

Under **ONE** (formerly Single Work Focused Gateway), people of working age coming into the benefits system will be given support and help in removing barriers to work. The first pilots begin in June 1999. (Lead departments: Department for Education and Employment, Department of Social Security.)

The **Working Families Tax Credit** will be a new tax credit payable to many working families on low or middle incomes and will include a child care tax credit. It will be introduced in October and will replace Family Credit. It will be paid through the wage packet from April 2000. (Lead departments: Department for Education and Employment and Her Majesty's Treasury.)

Under the **National Childcare Strategy**, a Green Paper *Meeting the Child Care Challenge*, published in 1998, set out the Government's plans for good quality child care for all children aged 0–14. The strategy is being taken forward at local level through the **Early Years Development and Child Care Partnerships**. (Lead department: Department for Education and Employment.)

## Measures which support pregnant teenagers and young parents

The Department of Health has provided funding for the National Children's Bureau to develop a self-help guide *Time to Decide*, to support young people in care when making decisions about pregnancy. It includes information about adoption, fostering, abortion, caring for themselves and a new baby, and the further help and support needed to do this. (Lead department: Department of Health.)

A new £540 million programme called **Sure Start** coordinates help for families in greatest need to ensure that their children get the best possible start in life. Help will begin with a visit to every local family from an outreach worker within three months of the baby's birth, in addition to other support currently provided. Sure Start will support parents as much as children and may include training for work and help with parenting problems. The first programmes will be up and running by early summer 1999 and by 2002 there will be over 250 Sure Start programmes across England.

A new **National Family and Parenting Institute** will provide the best possible advice and information on all aspects of family life – particularly the role of parents – to government and to groups working to help families across the country. (Lead department: Home Office.)

The **Child Support** scheme supports the principle that parents should take the main responsibility for maintaining their children. Child support can play an important part in helping young people understand the responsibilities of parenthood by spelling out the costs of raising a child. (Lead Department Department of Social Security.)

The **Housing Investment Programme** is the process by which capital funding is allocated to local authorities to build new housing. Local authorities submit their bids to the Government Offices for the Regions who decide how much funding each local authority receives. (Lead department: Department of the Environment, Transport and the Regions.)

Some teenage parents live in **supported accommodation** which provides a range of special services to meet their needs, such as mother and baby hostels where full time help and support may be given.

The Government is introducing new arrangements for funding supported accommodation from April 2003 and will allocate a budget to local authorities which will encourage local services to work together to meet clients' needs. (Lead departments: Department of the Environment, Transport and the Regions, Department of Health and Department of Social Security.) Crown copyright material is reproduced with the permission of the Controller of Her Majesty's Stationery Office.

# APPENDIX 2.1   AN EXAMPLE OF ILLUMINATIVE EVALUATION: DESCRIBING THE PROCESS IN ESTABLISHING COLLABORATIVE WORKING

The following examples are taken from a 2 day workshop in Melbourne, Australia (August 1996) on the topic 'Creating Partnerships for Health Promotion'.

## Generative theme

Everyone talks about the need to develop new partnerships or inter sectoral collaboration. Our work should lead us beyond ourselves, to partnerships with like-minded groups, organizations, sectors. However, territoriality, competition over resources, different language and concepts, different accounting structures and priorities all seem to get in the way. Power differences/inequalities between partners are often large and are rarely talked about so that they might be resolved. This is particularly true in partnerships involving community people and groups, whose participation is often token, largely because the terms of participation remain largely with institutions. Despite recognition that supports for citizen participation are essential they are often meagre or lacking. There is also a general participation exhaustion with everyone running from one consultation meeting to another in the hopes of not missing something that just might be important, but often is not.

## Case story

I am a medical graduate who has had a lifelong interest in involvement in community-based youth activities. I was recruited 5 years ago to establish an adolescent health program – The Centre for Adolescent Health – which was the first clinical academic program in adolescent health to be established in Australia. Those who came together to stimulate this initiative were three hospitals, a university and VicHealth (the Victoria Health Foundation, an Australian health non governmental organization funded through a special tobacco tax). What quickly became apparent was that these multiple agencies did not share one single vision, had many differing agendas and had chosen me for different reasons. The hospitals' agenda was largely focussed on improving service delivery to young people in problem areas. The academic agenda was more to do with research excellence and education/training. VicHealth had a more politicized agenda informed by the release of a report on youth homelessness emphasizing outreach and development work with youth in the most severe social circumstances. In a similar fashion the agencies valued me in different ways. The hospitals valued my physician status and my knowledge of health service delivery. The university valued my academic achievements. VicHealth looked towards my non-professional commitment to young people as an indication of my understanding of the importance of a social view of health and the promotion of well being as integral components of an adolescent health program.

My initial attempts were to try and please the multiple constituencies by attending management meetings, faculty meetings, staff meetings and key committee meetings at all of these agencies. It quickly became apparent that this was not a good strategy. I was not keeping anyone happy and not achieving core objectives. I came to realize that the true constituency for the Centre for Adolescent Health was young people in the community and that addressing their needs was the key outcome. As I worked towards identifying and addressing these needs, I took a pragmatic decision to focus my partnership building attention on two of the agencies only, one hospital and VicHealth. By slowly building on the particular strengths of these agencies, we were able to begin to develop a common vision that helped us to then take on board other partnerships. The things I learned during this process were, firstly, the need to keep a focus on the big picture and the true constituency for the work of the program; secondly, that there was a need to create a vision around which to rally the partners, rather than to necessarily try and create a hybrid vision from all the different agencies involved; and thirdly, to build on partners' particular strengths and not to try and pursue too many concurrent relationships.

## Theory note

Effective partnerships require the establishment of a clear vision of the role of the organization and a definition of what future role the organization will play. Having agreed on the vision, effective leadership requires working to ensure that the partners have a common goal and a commit-ment~ to share in a true partnership. Effective leadership must focus on the common goal for success, and not try to please all the partners.

Partners may be pre-determined, self-selected or chosen. As development and management of multiple partnerships is difficult, it is essential to identify key partners to ensure any long-term sustainability for the partnership. Key partners may be those who have certain forms of 'power-over' in relation to the issue, often through their control over funding relationships. Changes with partnerships and the external environment require monitoring of power bases – who has power, who has not and how this changes over time. Introduction of new partners, or termination/repositioning of existing partners, may be needed to ensure their ongoing relevance to the issue around which the partnership formed and their effective contribution to achieving partnership goals.

Good partnerships take time to develop. It takes time to develop a shared common goal, a sense of ownership of the project, and an intellectual and emotional commitment to successful outcomes for the project. To accomplish this, the leader needs to be able to unpack the agendas of different partners (which are often hidden) and to understand fully their individual motivations, interests, goals and expectations. The leader may also need to expose the partners to the constituents (those benefiting through the partnership's activities) and the setting at the coalface (where the activities take place). The leader needs to develop and nurture current partnerships while recognizing the need to identify potential new partnerships and train future partnership leaders. The leader also needs to be aware of his or her own personal limitations and be prepared to draw on others' skills to supplement his or her own.

Finally, partners from the constituency (those benefiting from the partnerships activities) need to be provided with opportunities to develop and use skills that empower them to play an active role in the project/organization.

## Benchmarks

The agendas of each partner are clearly stated and a common agenda reached, through agreement on one or more goals

- The partners agree to a process that exposes managers of the partnership to 'coalface' experiences.
- Partnerships establish a process to actively skill the constituency (those benefiting from the partners' activities) so that they are empowered to participate actively in the partnership itself.
- Partners agree on mechanisms to enable skilled constituents to participate in the partnership and methods to monitor that participation.
- Partnerships are strategically managed through establishment of a clear, common vision formally documented and agreed to by all of the partners.

Taken from: Labonte, R.L., Feather, J. and Hills, M. (1999) *A story/dialogue method for health promotion knowledge development and evaluation. Health Education Research,*14(1), pp, 39–50.

# APPENDIX 7.1   CRITERIA FOR SELECTING THE EFFECT STUDIES

1. Changing knowledge/beliefs/awareness, attitudes, values, intentions, skills, health behaviour or lifestyle and the environment *by means of education* should be one of the aims of the intervention in the effect studies. Both health education as well as health promotion interventions are of interest.

2. The interim or final results of interventions should be accessible and obtainable to everyone who has an interest.

3. Studies giving a clear description of the content of the intervention and its objectives are preferred to studies failing to give the reader insight into the intervention studied.

4a The design of the effect evaluation should preferably meet the following conditions:
   - at least one pre-and one post-test measurement;
   - at least one intervention and one comparison group;
   - each group should consist of at last 15 people (preferably randomly assigned).

4b The methods of the evaluation should *preferably* include the presence of triangulation. This refers to the practice of drawing conclusions on a number of different sources of information (which might include different data resources, different respondents or even different researchers).

5. Studies containing extended formative or process evaluation preferred to studies with little or no reflection on the processes involved in programme implementation.

6. Studies discussing the methodology of the intervention and the methodology of evaluation are preferred above studies not discussing these topics.

7. Interventions are *preferably* but not necessarily implemented within the continent of Europe.

8. A maximum of a quarter of the effect studies may originate from your own country.

9. Effect studies evaluating innovative intervention methods are preferred.

10. Recent publications are preferred.

11. For the database (questionnaires/database format), review studies and meta-analysis studies are to be excluded.

12. Good studies which are found to have no effect should also be subject to documentation.

13. Choose a maximum of two publications for each intervention area which deals with another area. This supplementary criterion will minimize duplication of selected publications, since other authors may select some of the same publications you have chosen (because of the overlap of areas in some interventions).

(IUHPE Review Series on Effectiveness of Health Education and Promotion, 1994)

# Appendix 10.1 Target groups and intervention strategies — National AIDS Control Programme implemented by MUTAN

| Target groups | Interventions strategies |
|---|---|
| General public | *Mass media*. Weekly radio programes (15 min) broadcast nationally. Addressed themes related to HIV/AIDS prevention and counseling and treatment of AIDS patients. Responded to questions raised by listeners.<br>*Information centers*. Located in Arusha and Moshi. Provided information, condoms and counseling services to the public.<br>*Public meetings*. Open, outdoor HIV/AIDS education meetings at marketplaces and in conjunction with the Information Centers.<br>*NGOs*. Joint meetings for religious groups and other organizations for information exchange, policy discussions and coordination of efforts. |
| Community leaders | *HIV/AIDS courses*. Five to 10 day intensive courses for party secretaries, village leaders and leaders of youth and women's organisations; the goal was to give them a thorough introduction to HIV/AIDS-related issues. |
| Teachers | *Health education*. Short courses providing information on HIV/AIDS transmission and prevention and effective educational methods. |
| Schoolchildren | *School-based education (Ngao)*. Participatory and behaviour-focused educational programme for students in Standards 6 and 7, taught by teachers with assistance from local health care workers. |
| Health care workers | *STD training*. Training in how to detect, treat and prevent STDs offered at local health care facilities and at the STD clinics in Arusha and Moshi.<br>*Counseling*. Training in how to provide pre- and post-test counseling for AIDS patients and patients taking an HIV test.<br>*Health education*. Short courses providing information on HIV/AIDS transmission and prevention and appropriate care.<br>*Blood screening*. Training in how to secure safe blood transfusions and reporting of data to the NACP. |
| People with HIV or AIDS | *Counseling*. Trained counselors provided in-hospital and home-based follow-up counseling services. |
| Bar workers, truck drivers and miners | *Peer education*. Commercial sex workers in communities regarded as high HIV transmission areas were trained as peer leaders, providing information and condoms to other commercial sex workers, truck drivers and miners.<br>*STD clinics*. The two established STD clinics specifically targetted perceived vulnerable groups such as bar workers and other commercial sex workers. |

(From Klepp, K-I. *et al.* (1999) Maintaining preventive health efforts in Sub-Saharan Africa, in N. Bracht (Ed.) *Health Promotion at the Community level: New Advances*, p. 162.

# AUTHOR INDEX

# Subject Index